THE AMERICAN PUBLIC HEALTH ASSOCIATION

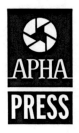

The American Public Health Association (APHA) is the oldest and most diverse organization of public health professionals in the world and has been working to improve public health since 1872. The Association aims to protect all Americans, their families, and their communities from preventable, serious health threats and strives to assure community-based health promotion and disease prevention activities and preventive health services are universally accessible in the United States. APHA represents a broad array of health professionals and others who care about their own health and the health of their communities.

APHA builds a collective voice for public health, working to ensure access to health care, protect funding for core public health services, and eliminate health disparities, among a myriad of other issues. Through its two flagship publications, the peer-reviewed *American Journal of Public Health*, celebrating 100 years of publishing, and the award-winning newspaper *The Nation's Health*, along with its e-newsletter *Inside Public Health*, and a strong books program, the Association communicates the latest public health science and practice to members, opinion leaders, and the public.

APHA is delighted to partner with Jones & Bartlett Learning on important public health issues. More on APHA can be found at www.apha.org.

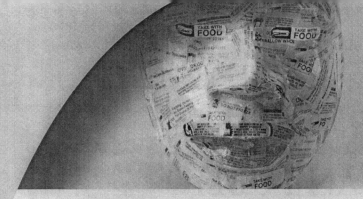

Essentials of
Public Health
Communication

Claudia F. Parvanta, PhD
Professor and Chair, Department of Behavioral & Social Sciences
University of the Sciences
Philadelphia, Pennsylvania
Lead Author and Editor

David E. Nelson, MD, MPH
Director, Cancer Prevention Fellowship Program
National Cancer Institute, National Institutes of Health
Captain, U.S. Public Health Service
Bethesda, Maryland
Editor, Chapter Contributor

Sarah A. Parvanta, MPH
Annenberg School for Communication
University of Pennsylvania
Philadelphia, Pennsylvania
Editor, Chapter Contributor

Richard N. Harner, MD
Adjunct Professor of Neuroscience
University of the Sciences
Philadelphia, Pennsylvania
Editor, Chapter Contributor

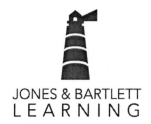

JONES & BARTLETT
LEARNING

World Headquarters
Jones & Bartlett Learning
5 Wall Street
Burlington, MA 01803
978-443-5000
info@jblearning.com
www.jblearning.com

Jones & Bartlett Learning books and products are available through most bookstores and online booksellers. To contact Jones & Bartlett Learning directly, call 800-832-0034, fax 978-443-8000, or visit our website, www.jblearning.com.

Substantial discounts on bulk quantities of Jones & Bartlett Learning publications are available to corporations, professional associations, and other qualified organizations. For details and specific discount information, contact the special sales department at Jones & Bartlett Learning via the above contact information or send an email to specialsales@jblearning.com.

This publication is designed to provide accurate and authoritative information in regard to the Subject Matter covered. It is sold with the understanding that the publisher is not engaged in rendering legal, accounting, or other professional service. If legal advice or other expert assistance is required, the service of a competent professional person should be sought.

Some images in this book feature models. These models do not necessarily endorse, represent, or participate in the activities represented in the images.

Production Credits
Publisher: Michael Brown
Associate Editor: Catie Heverling
Editorial Assistant: Teresa Reilly
Associate Production Editor: Kate Stein
Senior Marketing Manager: Sophie Fleck
Manufacturing and Inventory Control Supervisor: Amy Bacus
Composition: Auburn Associates, Inc.
Art: diacriTech
Cover Design: Kristin E. Parker
Cover Image: Top image: Courtesy of James Gathany/CDC; Bottom images, from left to right:
   Courtesy of Visual Aids/Artist: Fred Weston; Courtesy of James Gathany/CDC
Printing and Binding: Malloy, Inc.
Cover Printing: John Pow Company

Library of Congress Cataloging-in-Publication Data
Essentials of public health communication / Claudia F. Parvanta, lead author and editor-in-chief ... [et al.].
    p. ; cm.
  Includes bibliographical references and index.
  ISBN 978-0-7637-7115-7 (pbk.)
  1. Communication in medicine. 2. Public health. 3. Health education. 4. Medical informatics. I. Parvanta, Claudia F.
  [DNLM: 1. Communication. 2. Health Education—methods. 3. Communications Media. 4. Health Promotion. 5. Public Health Informatics—methods. WA 590 E78 2010]
  R118.E87 2010
  362.101'4—dc22
                                                          2010015270

6048

Printed in the United States of America
16 15 14 13 12   10 9 8 7 6 5 4 3

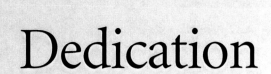

Dedication

To my brother, Michael, for the love and the laughs.
To Abe, who makes life an intergalactic adventure, and
Adam, Sarah, Angela, and Kristina, who provide Ground Control.
To Bibi, an ongoing inspiration. And finally,
to Mom and Dad, who set the course—*Ta shakkor.*

—Claudia F. Parvanta

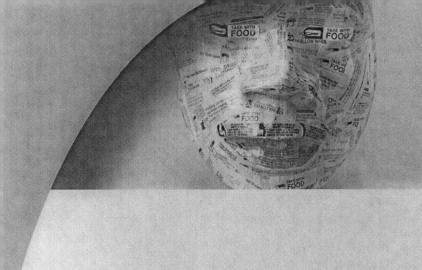

Contents

Chapter 16 Risk and Emergency Risk Communication: A Primer   327
David W. Cragin and Claudia Parvanta

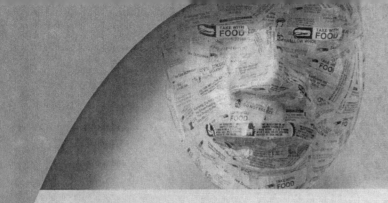

The *Essential Public Health*
Series

Log on to www.essentialpublichealth.com for the most current information on availability.

ABOUT THE EDITOR:

Richard K. Riegelman, MD, MPH, PhD, is Professor of Epidemiology-Biostatistics, Medicine, and Health Policy, and Founding Dean of The George Washington University School of Public Health and Health Services in Washington, DC. He has taken a lead role in developing the Educated Citizen and Public Health initiative which has brought together arts and sciences and public health education associations to implement the Institute of Medicine of the National Academies' recommendation that "...all undergraduates should have access to education in public health." Dr. Riegelman also led the development of George Washington's undergraduate major and minor and currently teaches "Public Health 101" and "Epidemiology 101" to undergraduates.

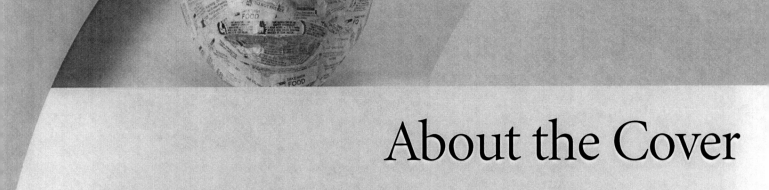

About the Cover

Our cover features Anne Schuchat, MD (RADM, USPHS), Assistant Surgeon General, United States Public Health Service (USPHS) and Director, National Center for Immunization and Respiratory Diseases (NCIRD) at the Centers for Disease Control and Prevention (CDC). Anne Schuchat has worked at the CDC since 1988 on immunization, respiratory, and other infectious diseases. Prior to her current appointment, she served as the director of the CDC's National Immunization Program (NIP). Dr. Schuchat became "Dr. Anne" during the height of the H1N1 crisis. She is a public figure, and we felt that Anne truly represents the best of "Communicating to Inform" a worried public about a potential health risk, as well as what they can do to keep themselves safe.

The cover also features a community library and visiting information specialists. The organization and management of information, long the purview of librarians, is having a new life in our digital world with "health informationalists" appearing as a possible job title, at least at the National Library of Medicine.

Flying off in the left corner is Edward Weston's "Blue in the Face" mask. It is a symbolic reminder of the "do's and don'ts" in health communication. We will speak more about this artwork in the introduction to the book. Photo courtesy of:

Frederick Weston
visualAIDS
526 West 26th Street Suite 510
New York, NY 10001
www.visualAIDS.org

Visual AIDS is an independent arts organization utilizing visual art in the fight against AIDS and supporting HIV+ artists.

Introduction

To me, Frederick Weston's "Blue in the Face" mask speaks to so many of the issues, and challenges, in health communication. Telling someone to do something until you are "blue in the face" is a folksy expression for what "not to do" in health communication. Weston has particularly emphasized the advice to take his medication (presumably for HIV) with food—advice he most likely found difficult, if not impossible, to follow. (One of the complications of HIV is often a lack of appetite, or feeling nauseated.) He has covered the mask, or perhaps even built it up, of the tiny labels affixed to pill bottles dispensed by pharmacies. Prescription drug labels are notoriously confusing, and many of us are working to improve how we share information with patients about their illnesses and their medications.

Moving deeper in the mask, we can ask if Weston modeled it over his own face, or that of a friend. Whether in the making, or in the wearing, there is always a real face behind a mask. And, as health communicators, we must strive to know the real person, and not stop at the level of a "persona." We all use masks; we might call them clothing, hair styles, ways of speaking or posturing, to fit into a culture, or to set ourselves apart as individuals. When we "target" health communication, we often stop at the level of the mask. But when we "tailor," or speak face-to-face, we attempt to take a truer measure of a person to make sure our message fits. Weston is not a "person with HIV," although it is a mask he has to wear at times. He is a person.

As a piece of art, a mask is silent. But, Weston's mask seems to have a "Mona Lisa" smile, with all the mystery that conveys. With its striking color, this mask, and this individual, wants to speak and be heard. Weston speaks not only for himself, but also for Visual AIDS, the organization that represented his work and brought it to a gallery, and the internet, where it could be found. And, Weston speaks for us all, as we all have at least one "imperfection" for which we seek a "cure." And nagging us about it is probably not the way to go.

Finally, throughout human history, we have used masks as part of healing rituals. In some ways, they represent the earliest forms of "health communication," as traditional healers interacted with their deities, or spirits, in an attempt to help the sick. In some ways, the mask represented the humility of the healer, acknowledging that he or she was merely an intermediary between the patient and the source of the cure. Can the same be said of healthcare providers today in how they present themselves to patients?

So, to me, Weston's mask is a powerful symbol of what to do, and what not to do, in health communication. I hope it will serve as an inspiration to those who read this book, and perhaps go on to the career, and calling, of communicating for health.

—Claudia Parvanta

Acknowledgments

Many of the people who helped with ideas or materials for this book are credited where their contributions appear. We thank them for providing cutting edge thinking as well as examples of health communication in action. Their work represents some of the best of the best, and we truly appreciate being able to showcase it in the textbook.

In addition, I (Claudia Parvanta) am indebted to my fabulous teachers, mentors, and employers—who transformed a research anthropologist into a health communications specialist. In chronological order these are: William Novelli (and my immediate boss, Randi Thompson), Mary Debus, Eloise Jenks, William Smith, Margaret Parlato, and most influential of all, Vicki Freimuth. Now at the University of Georgia, Vicki ran the Office of Communication at the CDC. She brought me in to lead a team of health communication specialists, each of whom knew much more than I did in their individual areas of expertise. Vicki served not only as a fount of wisdom, but also as a role model for every form of communication imaginable in a very complex public health agency. Vicki set the managerial tone for letting qualified people do their work with relatively little interference. I tried to copy that style with a fabulous team in the Division of Health Communication (Vicki Beck, Galen Cole, Suzanne Gates, Allen Jannsen, May Kennedy, Susan Kirby, Cheryl Lackey, Clara Olaya, (Huan Linnan before her), William Pollard, Christine Prue, Susan Robinson, and Brandon Varian). The "poodles" (compared to the media relations crew called the "bulldogs") were absolutely unbeatable in terms of their technical capacities, knowledge, and dedication to quality and public service. We all learned from each other, and the synergies (and *CDCynergy*) were worth a score of academic degrees in health communication. Many former "DHCers" contributed examples, insights and resources for this textbook from their current positions within or outside of the CDC.

I remain indebted to the next group of leaders in the CDC Office of Communication (formerly the Health Marketing Center) and the National Center for Health Informatics. These include Jay Bernhardt, Cynthia Baur, Dogan Eroglu, Katherine Lyon Daniels, Cheryl Lackey, and Suzanne Gates who provided access, support, ideas, and encouragement throughout the writing of the book.

On the editorial side, Kristina Parvanta painstakingly prepared the figure logs, as well as several tables. Graduate students in public health, health policy, and marketing at the University of the Sciences contributed to the ancillary materials, chiefly: Patricia Lapera, Rahila Saeed, Raheel Arif, and Erika Hedden. I am indebted to Bill Horton in the U Sciences AT group for overseeing video production and editing. The videos were shot by Sarah Parvanta and edited chiefly by Raheel Arif. The Jones & Bartlett Learning crew of Mike Brown, Sophie Fleck, and particularly Catie Heverling, Tracey Chapman, Kate Stein and Teresa Reilly (ancillaries) all provided great help and support. I thank co-editor, Richard Harner, for having suggested (make that insisted) that I get my "own stuff" out there and providing support to the research, writing, and editing to make that happen. Co-editor David Nelson headed our previous textbook collaboration, providing the voice of experience, while serving as the "Chief Science Officer" on this mission. Co-editor Sarah Parvanta kept us all up to date and writing within the limits of a reasonable graduate workload.

Last but not least, I acknowledge the support of my Dean, Suzanne Murphy, the faculty and staff in the Department of Behavioral and Social Sciences, and my colleagues at the University of the Sciences in allowing me a lot of quality time to write. Lara Schneider provided indispensible and timely help with logistics, and Alison Souley helped with last minute details.

Together with videos and additional materials, there are more acknowledgments on the book website. It really does take a village to write a textbook! Thank you to everyone.

—Claudia F. Parvanta, PhD

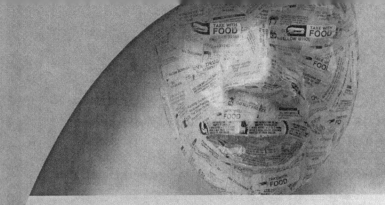

ASPH Competencies for MPH* Featured in the Text

Chapter	BS	E	HPM	SBS	C&I	D&C	L	P	PP
1					1		1	1,6,9	1
2		8	5,6,10	1–5,8,10	2,4,10	5,10	2	1,4,6	1
3	5,8–10	5,8,9	2,9		1-3,5–9	10		3	
4	9,10	4,8–10	9	8	1,4,7–9			3,4	10
5	8-10	1,4,8	4,9,10	6,9	1–3,6–10	3,10	2,7–10	1,3,6, 10	1,9
6	9,10	8,9	4,9,10	3,4,10	2,4,5,7,9,10	9,10	4,6,9	5,7,10	9
7		8		3,6	2–7	3,7,8,10			1
Appendix 7A					1–10	3,8,10			
8			6	1,5,9,10	2,4,6	10			4,5,6
9			6	1–3,5,6,10	4	5,6,9,10			6,7
10	9	9	5,6	1,5,8,10	1, 4–9	10	7	10	2,5
11			6	3–6,9,10	1–4, 6,7,9	9,10	7,9	10	8,9
12			6	1,3–6,9,10	4,6,8,9				7,10
13			6,8,10	5,9	4		7,9		5,8,9
14	9	9	5	5,8	8	10		10	3–7, 9,10
15		8		9	5,7	1,2,8,9	4,9	5	
16	5,9,10	5,9,10	9,10	1,8	2,4,6,7,9	10	1	1,10	2,9

*Abbreviations and numbering per ASPH MPH Core Competency Model, Version 2.3, 2006 (www.asph.org/competency)

DISCIPLINES

BS	Biostatistics
E	Epidemiology
HPM	Health Policy and Management
SBS	Social and Behavioral Sciences
EHS	Environmental Health Science (Chapter 16 provides content for competency EHS 7.)
PHB	Public Health Biology (We do not discuss this.)

CROSS-CUTTING

C&I	Communication & Informatics
D&C	Diversity and Culture
EHS	Environmental Health Sciences
L	Leadership
P	Professionalism
PP	Program Planning
ST	Systems Thinking (This competency is very abstract, but many of the chapters are systematic in their approach.)

Prologue

Essentials of Public Health Communication provides an easy-to-use, comprehensive, and practical approach to understanding and applying principles of communications to a range of public health problems. Health communications and informatics have increasingly been recognized as key cross-cutting and integrative skills for all public health and health-care professionals.

The text is written by a unique group of colleagues who together have laid much of the foundation for today's concept of health communication and informatics. Their joint efforts are reflected in the central role that health communications and informatics play in Healthy People 2020, the national goals for health by the end of the current decade. Their writing, teaching, and practice have given them the extensive and intensive experience that they draw upon in their writing.

Essentials of Public Health Communication provides an ideal text for implementing the health communication and informatics competencies recommended by the Association of Schools of Public Health and incorporated into the Certification in Public Health examination. It can also provide the basis for an undergraduate public health course aimed at integrating public health principles into the education of a wide range of undergraduate as recommended by the Association of American Colleges and Universities. Communications majors and pre-health professional students as well as those pursuing undergraduate public health will find the book engaging and empowering.

The book includes extensive examples drawn from the authors' experience. The materials included in the book have undergone extensive testing in a range of education settings—from classrooms to communities to clinical and public health settings. You will quickly find that you are in the hands of experienced and expert teachers and practitioners. Take a look; I'm confident you will agree.

Essentials of Public Health Communication is a key contribution to the *Essential Public Health* Series. It can be used as a free-standing text or combined with other books in the series such as *Essentials of Health Behavior*. As editor of the *Essential Public Health* Series, I'm delighted that *Essentials of Public Health Communication* is now part of the series.

Richard Riegelman, MD, MPH, PhD
Series Editor

About the Editors

Claudia F. Parvanta, PhD, Professor and Chair, Department of Behavioral & Social Sciences, University of the Sciences, Philadelphia, Pennsylvania
Lead Author and Editor

Dr. Claudia Parvanta, Professor of Anthropology, teaches behavioral science research and culturally competent health communication to public health and health professions students at the University of the Sciences. Before joining the University of the Sciences in 2005, Parvanta headed the Division of Health Communication at the Centers for Disease Control and Prevention (CDC) for six years. She received the U.S. Department of Health and Human Services Secretary's Award for Distinguished Service for her contributions to the CDC's response to the 9/11 and anthrax attacks. Before the CDC, Parvanta was an Assistant Professor at the Rollins School of Public Health, Emory University; the Assistant Director of the U.S. Agency for International Development's Nutrition Communication Project (for Porter/Novelli, a global marketing and public relations agency); and the consulting anthropologist for the Public Health Foundation WIC (Women, Infants and Children) program in Los Angeles, where she provided individualized client counseling to Southeast Asian women. She has designed, managed, or evaluated health and nutrition social marketing programs in more than 20 countries. Together with Nelson, Brownson, and Remington, she is the author of *Communicating Public Health Information Effectively: A Guide for Practitioners* (APHA, 2002).

David E. Nelson, MD, MPH
Director, Cancer Prevention Fellowship Program
National Cancer Institute, National Institutes of Health
Captain, U.S. Public Health Service
Editor, Chapter Contributor

David E. Nelson, MD, MPH, currently heads up the National Cancer Institute's Cancer Prevention Fellowship Program, previously spearheaded efforts to develop the Health Information National Trends Survey (HINTS) for NCI, was the Acting Director of the Bureau of Smoking or Health, and directed the Behavioral Risk Factor Surveillance System (BRFSS) for the CDC. He was the lead author (with Brownson, Parvanta, and Remington) of *Communicating Public Health Information Effectively: A Guide for Practitioners* (APHA, 2002), as well as the author of *Making Data Talk* (Oxford University Press, 2009). He has contributed to, and edited, the chapters in Section II: Informing and Educating People about Health Issues.

Sarah A. Parvanta, MPH
Annenberg School for Communication
University of Pennsylvania
Philadelphia, Pennsylvania
Editor, Chapter Contributor

Sarah A. Parvanta, who received her MPH from the University of North Carolina in 2007, is now enrolled in a PhD program in Health Communication at the Annenberg School for Communication, University of Pennsylvania. As a journalism student, Parvanta interned with the Health Unit of CNN in Atlanta, working for Dr. Sanjay Gupta, among others. She also spent two years supporting the Division of Cancer Prevention and Control at CDC, as a consultant. Despite these years of professional experience, Parvanta brings a youthful perspective to the material, helping to ensure that the text makes sense not only to new learners, but also to her generation of students. She is the co-author for the chapters on theory and new media, and she edited all the chapters in Section III: Being Persuasive: Influencing People to Adopt Healthy Behavior.

Richard N. Harner, MD
Adjunct Professor of Neuroscience
University of the Sciences
Philadelphia, Pennsylvania
Editor, Chapter Contributor

Richard N. Harner, MD, is a clinical neurologist with more than three decades of clinical, teaching, and research experience. He directed the Neurology Department at the Graduate Hospital of the University of Pennsylvania and established the first center for the comprehensive medical and surgical treatment of epilepsy in the eastern United States. After 20 years, he moved to become Professor and Vice Chairman of Neurology at the Medical College of Pennsylvania, where he established a second epilepsy center and directed postgraduate neurology education. He has authored numerous scientific articles, does private consulting for the biotech and pharmaceutical industry, and teaches as an Adjunct Professor in the Department of Behavioral and Social Sciences at the University of the Sciences in Philadelphia. Harner is the lead author for the chapter on patient–healthcare provider communication, and he provided constructive input and expertise to virtually all of the chapters in the book.

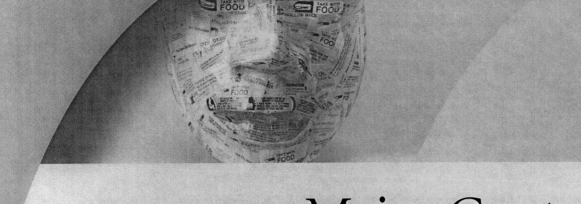

Major Contributors

Bridget C. Booske, PhD, is a Senior Scientist, Population Health Institute, School of Medicine and Public Health, University of Wisconsin, Madison.

Ross Brownson, PhD, directs the Prevention Research Center, George Warren Brown School of Social Work, Washington University in St. Louis, Missouri. He is also affiliated with the Department of Surgery and Alvin J. Siteman Cancer Center, Washington University School of Medicine, Washington University in St. Louis. Brownson is a former member of the Task Force for the Guide to Community Preventive Services and is also the editor or author of the books: *Chronic Disease Epidemiology and Control, Applied Epidemiology, Evidence-Based Public Health, and Community-Based Prevention.*

David W. Cragin, PhD, DABT, is an Adjunct Professor, Department of Health Policy and Public Health, University of the Sciences, Philadelphia, Pennsylvania and Professor of International Pharmaceutical Engineering Management, Peking University, Beijing, China.

Ellen Jones, PhD, is Senior Program Consultant, National Association of Chronic Disease Directors, Atlanta, Georgia, and School of Health Related Professions, University of Mississippi Medical Center, Jackson.

May Grabbe Kennedy, PhD, MPH, is an Associate Professor and Graduate Studies Director in the Social and Behavioral Health Department, Virginia Commonwealth University, School of Medicine, Richmond.

David Kindig, MD, PhD, is Emeritus Professor and Emeritus Vice Chancellor for Health Sciences, School of Medicine and Public Health, University of Wisconsin, Madison.

Patrick L. Remington, MD, MPH, is Associate Dean for Public Health and Professor, School of Medicine and Public Health, University of Wisconsin (UW), Madison. Remington worked as a medical epidemiologist at the CDC and as a State Epidemiologist and Chief Medical Officer for Chronic Disease at the Wisconsin Division of Health prior to joining the UW faculty. He is an author, with Brownson, of *Chronic Disease Epidemiology and Control*, and of numerous articles demonstrating the use of surveillance data to improve population health. He currently is on the advisory committee for Healthy People 2020.

Section Contributors

Box 9.5   Sarah Bauerle Bass, PhD, MPH, and Tom Gordon, PhD
                 Department of Public Health
                 Temple University

Box 11.1   The Advertising Council, New York

Box 11.2   Sandra de Castro Buffington, Director
                 Hollywood, Health & Society, Norman Lear Center
                 Annenberg School of Communication, University of Southern California

Box 11.3   Ann Aikin, MA; Holli Hitt Seitz, MPH; Janice R. Nall, MBA; Jessica Schindelar, MPH; Centers for Disease
                 Control and Prevention

Box 11.4   Wen-ying (Sylvia) Hou, PhD, MPH
                 Cancer Prevention Fellow, HCIRB
                 National Cancer Institute

Box 11.5   Sarah Marchetti, Digital Influence Strategist
                 Ogilvy Public Relations Wordlwide

Box 11.6   Sabira Taher, MPH, Campaign Manager, Health Media and Marketing
                 New York City Department of Health and Mental Hygiene

Box 11.7   Amy Struthers, PhD, Assistant Professor of Advertising
                 College of Journalism and Mass Communications
                 University of Nebraska, Lincoln

Box 11.8   Jane D. Brown, PhD, and James L. Knight, Professor
                 University of North Carolina
                 School of Journalism and Mass Communication

Box 12.2   Patricia McLaughlin, Assistant Vice President of Communications, LEGACY, Washington, DC
                 Joshua Cogan Photography, images

Case Studies Used Throughout the Book

CDCynergy: Folic Acid

Christine Prue, PhD, Centers for Disease Control and Prevention
Katherine Lyon-Daniel, PhD, Centers for Disease Control and Prevention
Lynn Sokler, MS, Centers for Disease Control and Prevention
(Folic Acid work done while at Prospect Associates.)

Bangladesh Nutrition Education Project

Claudia Parvanta, PI, Emory University, Rollins School of Public Health
Amy Cornelli, PhD, University of North Carolina (photographer)
Kate Thomas, MPH, University of Washington
Sabrina Zahman, Trishna Chaabra, Emory University RSPH student researchers

Linda Keiss and Sultana Rahmann (then of Helen Keller, Dhaka)
Indu Alluwalia, Centers for Disease Control and Prevention
People of Dinajpur, Bangladesh

Additional Chapter Acknowledgements and Comments

Cover: Thank you to Frederick Weston for use of his artwork on the cover. Thank you to Amy Sadao, Executive Director, Visual AIDS, for facilitating connection to the artist, as well as providing the image and gallery permission.

Chapter 3: Acknowledgments to Susan Salkowitz, Ruth Gubernick, Anne Turner, Dwayne Jarman, Stephen Marcus, Linda Pederson, Patrick O'Carroll, and Rita Kukafka for their contributions to this chapter.

Chapter 8: Dedicated to Martin Fishbein, PhD (died December 2009).

Chapter 10: Acknowledgments to Matthew Kreuter and Victor Strecher for sharing website resources on tailoring, and to L. Kay Bartholomew and Guy S. Parcel for sharing website resources on information mapping.

Chapter 16: Acknowledgments to Barbara Reynolds, PhD, the CDC, Julia Galdo, Prospect Associates, Peter Sandman, and Vincent Covello.

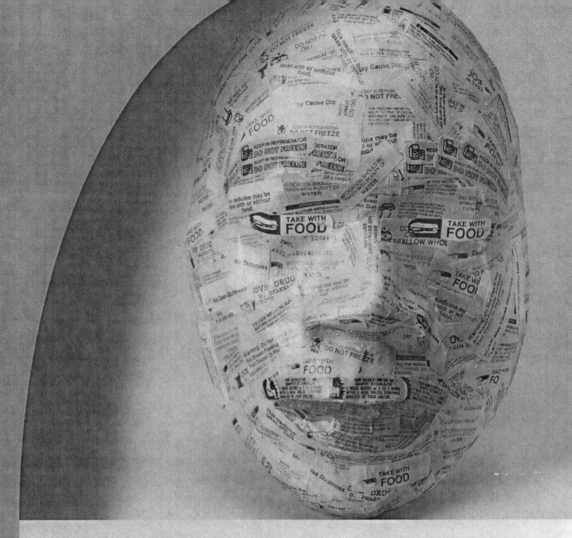

SECTION I

Overview

CHAPTER 1

Introduction to Public Health Communication and Informatics

Claudia Parvanta

INTRODUCTION

Communication and Informatics are broad areas with equally broad definitions. Please see **Box 1–1** for ours.

Box 1–1
Definitions[1,2]

Communication: "How people use messages to generate meanings within and across various contexts, cultures, channels and media" (U.S. Department of Education).

Informatics: "The effective organization, analysis, management, and use of information" (American Medical Informatics Association).

With the January 2009 inauguration of Barack Obama as the nation's 44th president, *Newsweek* columnist Anna Quindlen voiced a widely held opinion that an "era of good speaking" had returned.[3] Obama's successful attainment of the presidency was in no small part due to his ability to articulate complicated ideas in a clear and persuasive manner. The ability to listen, speak, and write well remain among the top skills sought in virtually every field of employment, and are always among the KSAs (knowledge, skills, and abilities) requested of applicants for professional positions at the **Centers for Disease Control and Prevention (CDC).**

But what makes **public health communication** different from the kind of training that most undergraduates receive, or that President Obama, for example, received as a lawyer? It is not so much the processes of developing arguments or being able to write an essay with a "beginning, middle, and an end." The Department of Health and Human Services defined **health communication** as *"the study and use of communication strategies to inform and influence individual and community decisions that enhance health."*[4] Thus, the first difference is the focus on health. The second major difference is the use of *"strategies to inform and influence . . . decisions."*

COMPETENCIES

What do these strategies look like? If you were figuratively flying over this book at 10,000 feet and looking down, you might see the "crop circle pattern" depicted in **Figure 1–1.** Thus, in order to be "outstanding in the field" of public health communication and informatics, there are huge domains of content for you to learn. They are constantly moving, shifting their overlap pattern, and engulfing other domains that seemed

FIGURE 1–1   The View from 10,000 Feet

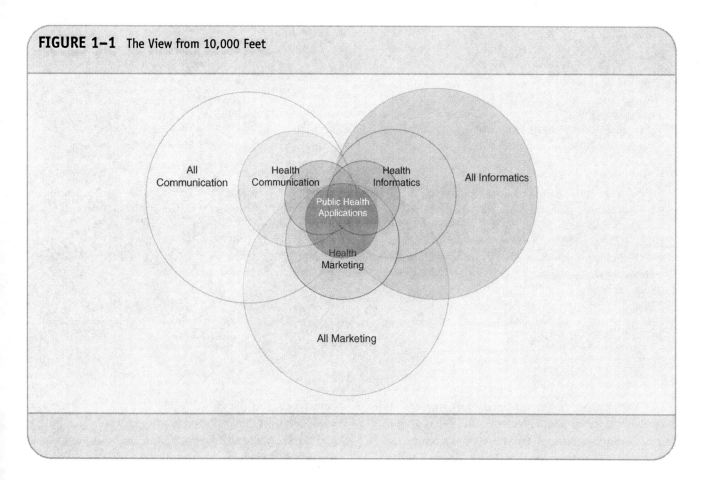

unrelated only a few years ago. The basic foundation for the study of public health communication must be assembled from these shifting domains in order for the novice to begin what we think is a fascinating and rewarding career. This book is designed to help a newcomer aim for and land in the intersection of the nine circles you see in Figure 1–1. Put more directly, we aim to provide the reader with the tools necessary to begin mastering the competencies defined by the **Association of Schools of Public Health (ASPH)**. The **ASPH Core Competencies Development Model** listed the competencies necessary for graduates of master's of public health (MPH) programs in health communication and informatics.

ASPH Core Competencies in Health Communication and Informatics

Like all the ASPH competencies, the ones for health communication and informatics emerged after a two-year modified Delphi process (see **Box 1–2**).

The core competencies shown in **Table 1–1** represent entry-level communication skills, defined as what a graduate from a public health program would be expected to be able to do on the first day of a job. John Finnegan, a noted health communication scholar and Dean of the School of Public Health, University of Minnesota, led the committee that selected and organized these competencies. He noted that, "We thought about separating the communication and informatics competencies, as each can stand alone. But, informatics is the infrastructure for public health in the 21st century the way that water and sanitation were for the 20th . . . the informatics platform will increasingly carry more to the public, but the content will continue to be dominated by communication theory. On this basis, we felt it was best to keep the domains together at this point in public health education."[5]

The Council on Linkages for Academia and Public Health has created more extensive competencies in health communication for practitioners at different administrative levels (see **Box 1–3**).

Box 1–2 Use of the Delphi Method for Health Communication Competencies

Named after the oracle of Delphi in ancient Greece, a "Delphi method" is a small-group research technique that seeks a consensus among experts through sequential rounds of data collection and reduction. The Rand Corporation takes credit for inventing the Delphi method. It is used when there is an insufficient evidence base to make a decision and/or when expert experience and opinion are considered valuable.

The common steps in the process include selecting a set of experts (usually at least 10 people, by tradition), and sending out an initial set of questions. These are usually items that can be ranked or scaled. In the case of the health communication and informatics competencies, the group began with a list of 76 possibilities. In the first round, task group members individually voted to (1) accept, (2) accept with changes, (3) reject, or (4) consider an alternative. They were given the second task of rewording an item if they deemed it acceptable with changes. Working in this manner, the taskforce reduced the list to 10 competencies through 3 Delphi rounds.[*]

Delphi is often used to rank a list of items in terms of priority. For example, Edward Maibach[†] and colleagues conducted a Delphi process on critical elements of social marketing. Published in 1997, it still serves as an important reference tool to define quality in social marketing.

[*]Calhoun, J.G., Ramiah, K., Weist, W.M., & Shortell, S.M. Development of a core competency model for the master of public health degree. *American Journal of Public Health* 98 (2008): 1598–1607.
[†]Maibach E., Shenker A., & Singer, S. Results of the Delphi survey. *Journal of Health Communication* 2, no. 4 (1997): 304–307.

In addition, ASPH is now working on competencies for doctoral-level public health graduates. This focus on competencies is based on the idea that on a human resource level, "quality in" (graduates possessing the health communication competencies) may lead to "quality out" (effective state and local health communication programs). Table 1–1 presents the latest version of the ASPH core competencies for communication and informatics.

Box 1–3 Core Competencies for Public Health Professionals

Adopted May 3, 2010

Communication Skills for Mid-Level Professionals[*]

- Assesses the health literacy of populations served.
- Communicates in writing and orally, in person, and through electronic means, with linguistic and cultural proficiency.
- Solicits input from individuals and organizations.
- Uses a variety of approaches to disseminate public health information.[†]
- Presents demographic, statistical, programmatic, and scientific information for use by professional and lay audiences.
- Applies communication and group dynamic strategies[‡] in interactions with individuals and groups.

[*]Competencies apply to individuals who have earned an MPH or related degree and have at least five years of work experience in public health or a related field (combined pre- and post-master's degree), or individuals who do not have an MPH or related degree but have at least 10 years of experience working in the public health field.
[†]Examples include social networks, media, blogs.
[‡]Examples include principled negotiation, conflict resolution, active listening, risk communication.

Source: Public Health Foundation, the Council on Linkages Between Academia and Public Health Practice. *Core Competencies for Public Health Professionals.* Retrieved August 18, 2010, from http://www.phf.org/link/CCs-example-free-ADOPTED.pdf

> **TABLE 1–1** MPH Core Competency Development Model: Version 2.3 (August 2006)
>
> **COMMUNICATION AND INFORMATICS**
> **The ability to collect, manage, and organize data to produce information and meaning that is exchanged by use of signs and symbols; to gather, process, and present information to different audiences in-person, through information technologies, or through media channels; and to strategically design the information and knowledge exchange process to achieve specific objectives.**
>
> *Competencies:* Upon graduation, it is increasingly important that a student with an MPH be able to . . .
>   1. Describe how the public health information infrastructure is used to collect, process, maintain, and disseminate data.
>   2. Describe how societal, organizational, and individual factors influence and are influenced by public health communications.
>   3. Discuss the influences of social, organizational, and individual factors on the use of information technology by end users.
>   4. Apply theory and strategy-based communication principles across different settings and audiences.
>   5. Apply legal and ethical principles to the use of information technology and resources in public health settings.
>   6. Collaborate with communication and informatics specialists in the process of design, implementation, and evaluation of public health programs.
>   7. Demonstrate effective written and oral skills for communicating with different audiences in the context of professional public health activities.
>   8. Use information technology to access, evaluate, and interpret public health data.
>   9. Use informatics methods and resources as strategic tools to promote public health.
> 10. Use informatics and communication methods to advocate for community public health programs and policies.
>
> *Source:* The Association of Schools of Public Health, ASPH Education Committee. (2006). Master's Degree in Public Health Core Competency Development Model, version 2.3. Retrieved August 18, 2010, from http://asph.org/userfiles/version2.3.pdf

Competency Clusters

We start by reorganizing these competencies into their respective subdomains: primarily, health communication, primarily informatics, and shared competencies.

Competencies That Require More Training in Health Communication

No. 2. Describe how societal, organizational, and individual factors influence and are influenced by public health communications.

No. 4. Apply theory and strategy-based communication principles across different settings and audiences.

No. 6. Collaborate with communication and informatics specialists in the process of design, implementation, and evaluation of public health programs.

No. 7. Demonstrate effective written and oral skills for communicating with different audiences in the context of professional public health activities.

These skills are based on the mastering of theories and approaches to understand the "audiences" for health information and how their information seeking behavior, comprehension, and willingness to act are shaped by multiple factors. The audience may consist of one individual and require the applica-

tion of new "tailoring" technologies. Or, mass communication principles may be applied to reach out to an entire population. Again, the ubiquitous "oral and written communication" skills register here.

Competencies That Require More Training in Informatics

No. 3. Discuss the influences of social, organizational, and individual factors on the use of information technology by end-users.

No. 8. Use information technology to access, evaluate, and interpret public health data.

No. 9. Use informatics methods and resources as strategic tools to promote public health.

These skills look at how health data originate, are stored, transmitted, presented and interpreted. True blue informatics practitioners have strong backgrounds in computer science, statistics, or information science, (e.g., anyone from librarians or database managers to Bill Gates). But public health communicators might be more engaged with the downstream use and interpretation of electronic records and with transforming rates, probabilities, graphs, and other data into useful information for various audiences and purposes.

Competencies That Are Shared

No. 1. Describe how the public health information infrastructure is used to collect, process, maintain, and disseminate data.

No. 5. Apply legal and ethical principles to the use of information technology and resources in public health settings.

No. 10. Use informatics and communication methods to advocate for community public health programs and policies.

These competencies are used chiefly for work in the public arena to ensure that information resources are distributed fairly, ethically, and in support of public health.

How did we arrive at these competencies as the most important? A look at the history of the field of health communication provides some clues.

PUBLIC HEALTH COMMUNICATION: A BRIEF (AND SOMEWHAT PERSONAL) HISTORY

Communication scholars trace their origins to the study of rhetoric (persuasive speaking) by Plato and Aristotle; and journalism has been taught in the United States since the early 1900s. *Health* communication, however, is a relatively young field. Kreps, Bonagura, and Query[6] trace its origins from the "humanistic psychology movement" beginning in 1950s associated with the work of Carl Rogers, Jurgen Ruesch, and Gregory Bateson. The 1960s and 1970s saw a convergence in the fields of psychology, medical sociology, and medicine that produced two distinct tracts in "proto-health communication," healthcare delivery and health promotion. Healthcare delivery included research on the ways:

> interpersonal and group communication influence healthcare delivery, (including) the provider/consumer relationship, therapeutic communication, healthcare teams, healthcare decision-making, and the provision of social support.[7]

In contrast, the health promotion branch grew out of the communication field's long-time focus on media in communication and was concerned with "the development, implementation and evaluation of persuasive health communication campaigns to prevent major health risks and promote public health." The International Communication Association renamed its Therapeutic Communication interest group, which had been formed in 1972, to the Health Communication Division in 1975. The National Communication Association took 10 years to form a health communication group in the United States. The gap in time between the creation of the international and national chapters reflects the earlier use of "social marketing" to achieve international development goals beginning in the late 1970s. Continuing through the 1980s,

the U.S. Agency for International Development (USAID) funded programs to bring this new, strategic approach to what was globally called *information, education, and communication* (IEC). USAID Programs such as "Population Communication Services," "Social Marketing for Change," and "HealthCom" applied lessons learned on Madison Avenue to family planning; child survival, and eventually to all aspects of health, agriculture, and environmental management.

Much of what we have learned about behavior change communication (BCC), which is the term preferred internationally, comes from these early endeavors led by the Academy for Educational Development, the Educational Development Center, Johns Hopkins University, Management Sciences for Health, Manoff International, Porter, Novelli & Associates, the Futures Group, and others, referred to lovingly as "beltway bandits."* Few of the groundbreakers in international health communication published their work in the scientific literature. However, USAID has ensured that its contractors make their program materials and reports available, now on-line, and originally through project clearing-houses.

As a contractor to both USAID and the National Cancer Institute (NCI), William Novelli was one of the early drivers of social marketing in both international and national health communication. Under contract for a range of tasks with NCI, Novelli's agency drafted the 1983 and 1985 publications, *Making P(ublic)S(ervice)A(nnouncement)s Work* and *A Handbook for Health Communication Professionals*. The "blue" and "purple" booklets might have been the first U.S. government publications to put forth a health communication program cycle based on a marketing process. NCI eventually combined these with additional material into what we now refer to as The **NCI Pink Book**, *Making Health Communication Programs Work*,[8] the *de facto* bible for public health communication practice.

So, while scholars of health communication have noted that patient education predominated in the published literature prior to the advent of the journal *Health Communication* in 1989, (see Thomspon[9]); the truth is that a lot was happening in health communication, but not much was being published outside of *gray literature*†. Almost as a footnote, in 1997, the Public Health Education and Health Promotion section within the American Public Health Association formally recognized health communication as part of its group.

---

*Term refers to US 495, the circular highway around Washington, DC. Some of the best beltway bandits were/are actually based in Boston, North Carolina, New York, Seattle, etc.
†Gray literature refers to unpublished, or non-peer-reviewed, reports, usually undertaken for government agencies. Such reports are often highly accurate and authoritative. They are now more commonly available on program websites, or through various agency resources.

Institutionalization of Scientific Health Communication at the CDC[10]

In 1993, the director of the Centers for Disease Control and Prevention, William Roper, formalized the agency's definition of health communication as "the crafting and delivery of messages and strategies, based on consumer research, to promote the health of individuals and communities." The definition characterized the public as consumers whom agency staff needed to understand in order to serve. It also clarified the role of health communication at the CDC as not only providing information, but also working with the public as partners in prevention. Roper also listed three goals for integrating health communication into the internal management functions of the agency:

- Recognize the central role played by health communication in prevention and behavior change programs.
- Integrate marketing and communication considerations into program planning and design.
- Provide staff with sufficient training and technical assistance to manage programs of this nature.

In 1996, Vickie Freimuth was hired to integrate all public relations, media, and prevention communication oversight functions in the Director's Office of Communication (OC). Not long after Freimuth's departure in 2004, the CDC went through a reorganization that resulted in the creation of the National Center for Health Marketing for programmatic communication as distinct from enterprise (i.e., corporate) communication. But, as of this writing, CDC is reorganizing its communication functions once more.

Is Health Education Part of Health Communication, or Vice Versa?

While Freimuth was authorized and supported in creating an integrated office for all communication within the CDC, tensions still existed among programs and personnel who classified themselves as "health educators," "behavioral scientists," or even "scientific writers." In part, this was due to the CDC's kluge-like growth from being the federal focal point for health education in 1974. The National Center for Chronic Disease Prevention and Health Promotion (NCCDPHP), named that in 1988, had previous incarnations as the Bureau for Health Education incorporated within the Office of Smoking and Health. In other centers and division, CDC scientists focused on behavioral science, health promotion, or social marketing. Here are two examples.

> The National Center for HIV, STD, and TB Prevention (NCHSTP) championed the use of behavior change theories in communication strategies to influence high-risk behaviors . . . they legitimized the use of "behavioral epidemiology," allowing ethnographic and other qualitative research methods into the same room as quantitative techniques.

> The chronic disease center (NCCDPHP) . . . innovate(ed) "behavioral surveillance," or counting how many people behave in ways to promote or undermine their health. They established the Behavioral Risk Factor Surveillance System (BRFSS) in 1984 to gave states access to data on the numbers of deaths and magnitude of illness attributable to behavioral risks, such as poor nutrition, tobacco use, unprotected sex, and so on . . . the BRFSS "provides an ongoing mandate to communicate with the public about the state of their health and how it can be improved (through better health behavior)."[11]

To sum up this history, in the late 1970s, USAID launched the use of social marketing to bring (helpful) products to what was then called the "Third World" and convince poor people to plan their families, rehydrate babies stricken with diarrhea, vaccinate against disease, plant green vegetables, etc. The National Institutes of Health (NIH), in particular NCI, adopted social marketing and embraced psychological theory. They were the first to use marketing tactics against the tobacco companies (who were viewed as particularly effective at capturing youth and other vulnerable audiences) as well as apply psychological principles to helping people quit smoking. The CDC made a huge move to apply these principles in HIV/AIDS programs. It integrated the social behavioral focus with a scientific approach to media communication and took the further step of demonstrating how communication fit and flowed with epidemiology.

The CDC Sequence for Health Communication

The CDC's sequence can be simplified as follows:
1. Collect and analyze data (surveillance and field epidemiology) to identify health problems and behavioral/environmental antecedents.
2. Develop communication strategies to modify behavior, modify behavioral antecedents, or lead to improved environmental conditions.
3. Evaluate to see if the communication strategies were effective at changing behavior or conditions.
4. Recollect and analyze health data to measure health outcomes.
5. Repeat step 2–4, if necessary.

It is this *integrated cycle* of health data collection, interpretation, and communication that this textbook will feature as "public health communication." To some extent, the CDC's model of health communication has always embraced informatics as its *alpha* and *omega*. What is different now is that we will also discuss some media strategies that use an informatics platform to create or deliver a health communication intervention.

THE LIMITATIONS OF HEALTH COMMUNICATION

While the CDC and other government agencies have raised health communication to a science, it alone cannot change the face of public health. There are tremendous human and material resources required to keep our water, air, and food clean and healthy, and keep infectious diseases at bay. The U.S. public has come to expect and rely upon a low risk health environment. Rare exceptions make the news—the appearance of a new flu virus (H1N1), the discovery of anthrax in an envelope, or the recall of hamburger meat due to *e coli* infection. But, with healthy conditions, and an active public health workforce, how can we have the highest **infant mortality rate (IMR)** of any developed country? The international ranking in infant mortality for the United States fell from 12th in the world in 1960 to 30th in 2005, where it has remained.[12]

Our infant mortality rate is indicative of the challenges we face in public health communication. In order for the IMR to decrease, environmental conditions, service delivery, and individual behavior would all have to be modified. Similarly, our rates of preventable chronic disease, unintentional injury, sexually transmitted disease, or uninsured children all speak to the limitations of public health communication alone to influence the complex system we portray as the ecological model of public health.[13] Yet, health communication flows in and around every layer of the **ecological model** (see **Figure 1–2**).

THE ECOLOGICAL MODEL

According to the Institute of Medicine (IOM) committee charged with developing recommendations for public health education, understanding the ecological model and using an ecological approach is necessary for all public health practitioners. They write,

> The ecological model assumes that health and well-being are affected by *interaction* among multiple determinants including biology, behavior, and the environment. Interaction unfolds over the life course of individuals, families, and communities ... An ecological *approach* to health is one in which multiple strategies are developed to impact determinants of health relevant to the desired health outcomes. For example, an ecological approach to the reduction of tobacco use would include alteration in physical environment (smoke-free workplaces and public places), alteration in social environment (social marketing of tobacco prevention as a priority), and individual behavior change (smoking cessation classes).[14]

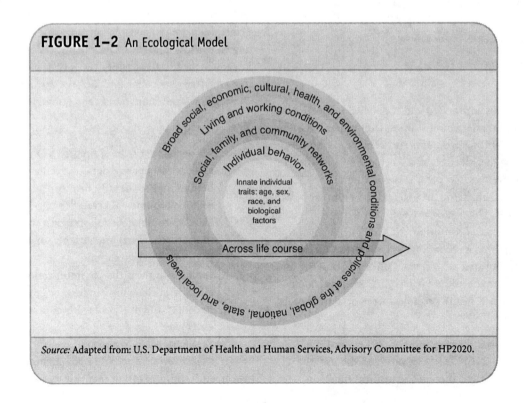

FIGURE 1–2 An Ecological Model

Broad social, economic, cultural, health, and environmental conditions and policies at the global, national, state, and local levels

Living and working conditions

Social, family, and community networks

Individual behavior

Innate individual traits: age, sex, race, and biological factors

Across life course

Source: Adapted from: U.S. Department of Health and Human Services, Advisory Committee for HP2020.

Public health practitioners frequently use a river or stream analogy to refer to the point of entry for an intervention. The source, or "upstream," is considered the broadest or earliest point of entry, while interventions that attempt to modify conditions for individuals are considered the narrowest or latest point of entry, or "downstream." There are parables that go along with this analogy, including whether it makes more sense to rescue drowning people out of a river one by one, or prevent them from falling (or being pushed) in in the first place. **Figure 1–3** features a poster from an international organization attempting to improve water globally, with the clear visual statement that pollution dumped into the water upstream will end up in a child's mouth downstream if we are not careful. The April 20th 2010 explosion of the British Petroleum oil drilling rig in the Gulf of Mexico is a tragic example of a truly "upstream" source of pollution that must now be dealt with through massive clean up efforts. Environmental advocacy efforts to provide more safeguards for off-shore drilling could have prevented it if heard, and acted on, by Congress.

Health communication alone cannot change some upstream (systemic) determinants of poor health, such as an oil spill, or poor social environment, limited healthcare resources, and poverty. But while health communication is not all-powerful, our responsibilities run deeper than we might think. If the individuals who need critical information to protect their health are not seeking or receiving it, understanding it, or being moved to action, we can use health communication to change this. If policymakers who determine national and local services have not received crucial health information, or been moved by it to action, we can use policy advocacy to effect change. An ecological approach to public health communication requires that all factors affecting a particular health condition are explored, and that an effort is made to change the upstream factors while helping individuals achieve the best health outcomes within their control. This is an ethical and professional principle that many practitioners embrace, but for some, their ability to conduct upstream advocacy may be constrained by political forces or regulations.

Health communication strategies can be organized in terms of their relative utility within each level of the ecological model. Some approaches are more effective at influencing the outer (or upstream) layers of the model, including the policymakers who develop regulations or implement programs that provide resources to communities and individuals. Other processes are more effective downstream by influencing community dynamics or facilitating individual behavior change. Several researchers have developed conceptual models for organizing systems-based approaches to health communication. These are discussed in Chapter 2. Now we look at one final model for what health communications is meant to achieve: the **hierarchy of effects**.

HIERARCHY OF EFFECTS MODEL

A final way of looking at our job is through the results we might expect of our efforts. In 1961, Lavidge (a marketer) and Steiner (a psychologist) wrote a pithy article on what advertising was meant to accomplish on the way up to and including actual sales. They outlined six steps moving a potential customer through the cognitive* domains of awareness and knowledge, the affective† domains of liking and preference,

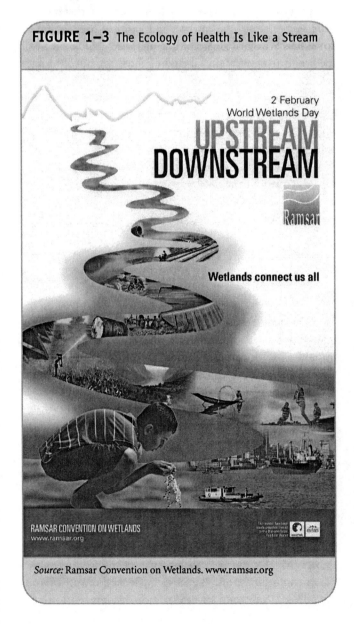

FIGURE 1–3 The Ecology of Health Is Like a Stream

2 February
World Wetlands Day

UPSTREAM
DOWNSTREAM

Ramsar

Wetlands connect us all

RAMSAR CONVENTION ON WETLANDS
www.ramsar.org

Source: Ramsar Convention on Wetlands. www.ramsar.org

---

*Cognitive: how you think.
†Affective: how you feel.

and the decision-to-action domains ("conative," in their parlance) of conviction and purchase. They suggested not only potential advertising vehicles (e.g., sky writing and jingles to create awareness; status and glamour appeals for preference; point-of-purchase for desire to purchase), but market research tools appropriate to each step.[15] The advertising world somehow kept this secret until the 1980s, when McGuire, a social psychologist, first adapted this marketing and advertising model, the Hierarchy of Effects (HOE) Model, to public health communication campaigns.[16]

With a "source" sending information out to a "receiver," the lower-level effects McGuire sought were exposure, attention, interest, and comprehension. A higher order set of effects included acquisition of skills, changes in attitude, short-term retention of information, long-term retention, decision making, one-time performance of a behavior, reinforcement of the behavior, and maintenance of the behavior indefinitely through complex life changes.

Neither the stepwise nature of these effects, nor the relative difficulty of obtaining them, has been the subject of definitive research. However, in practice, many communication programs realized their resources were only sufficient to attain the lower level of effects in the hierarchy. Too many programs did not even achieve adequate exposure to expect any higher order effects—and none were there. It is the post hoc analysis of failed campaigns that has given the HOE considerable credibility. But, failures are rarely reported in the literature. Recently, communications researchers have modified McGuire's steps for program planning and evaluation purposes. McGuire's theory remains a very practical one, and should be credited along with its predecessor for spawning several stage-based and hierarchical models of how people process and act on information they receive.

PUBLIC HEALTH INFORMATICS

The term **informatics,** like communication, can have a very broad definition that encompasses any collection, storage, retrieval, and dissemination of any information anywhere. The Ten Commandments, the Library of Medicine, telemarketing, *EpiX,** Google, and even your cell phone are all based on informatics principles that have contributed to their development.

The CDC published a clear definition of public health informatics in its 2005 call to create centers of excellence for the field. The funding announcement stated, "Public health in-

formatics is defined as the systematic application of information and computer science and technology to public health practice, research, and learning."[17] The CDC has created five centers of excellence in public health informatics with a focus on (1) electronic health record support of public health functions; (2) use of healthcare, population, and other public health data in supporting public health systems and analyses; (3) basic capabilities that support public health practice such as statistical and health surveillance; and (4) public health decision support.[18]

With its origins in public health surveillance systems, "notifiable" diseases, and cancer registries, public health informatics has staked out a population focus in comparison to the healthcare informatics focus on individual medical records. But, the twain meet more often than their pre-Internet progenitors. For example, the creation and multiple uses for a **personal health record** are becoming increasingly popular in all medical care applications, including those provided through publically managed facilities.

The National Center for Public Health Informatics at the CDC manages a number of projects that demonstrate the multiple applications of informatics in public health. The projects and a brief description appear in **Box 1–4.**

Throughout the book we focus on how health communicators access and use databases, survey results, visual representations of data, and digital applications to facilitate health communication tasks.

PUBLIC HEALTH COMMUNICATION AS A JOB: INFORM, EDUCATE, AND EMPOWER

A General Overview

To understand the scope of employment in public health it may help to review the duties for what is arguably the top job in public health communication, the office of the Surgeon General. **Figure 1–4** pictures Vice Admiral Regina M. Benjamin, MD, MBA, Surgeon General, appointed by President Obama. The Surgeon General is appointed by the President of the United States with the advice and consent of the United States Senate for a 4-year term of office.

The **Surgeon General**, in popular mythology, is supposed to be the "Nation's Doctor." More so than administering to the sick, the Surgeon General is meant to keep the public well—and the primary instrument is health communication (see **Box 1–5**).

While the Surgeon General has administrative oversight of the uniformed branch of the U.S. Public Health Service, the position's first five duties describe much of the field of public health communication. The Surgeon General must: "*educate* the public," "*advocate* for effective disease prevention and

---

*EpiX is the Centers for Disease Control and Prevention's Web-based communications system with state and local health departments, poison control centers, and other public health professionals to access and share preliminary health surveillance information.

Box 1–4 Public Health Informatics Projects at CDC

The National Center for Public Health Informatics at CDC sponsors numerous projects that define the state of the art of public health informatics. The overarching program is the Public Health Information Network (PHIN), a national initiative to improve the capacity of public health to use and exchange information electronically by promoting the use of standards and defining functional and technical requirements.

Four projects are featured here from the CDC website, although several others are also described on the site: http://www.cdc.gov/ ncphi/programs-projects.html#cert

- ☑ Assessment Initiative
- ☑ Biosurveillance
  - Communities of Practice
  - Directory, Alerting, and Emergency Operations
- ☑ Electronic Health Records
  - External Workforce Development
  - Knowledge Management
  - Laboratory Systems
  - National Notifiable Disease Surveillance
  - Outbreak Management
  - PHIN Certification
- ☑ Vocabulary/Messaging Standards
  - Global Public Health Informatics

Assessment Initiative
Beginning in 1992 and now in its third 5-year funding cycle, the *Assessment Initiative* is a cooperative program between the CDC and state health departments that supports the development of innovative systems and methods to improve the way data are used to provide information for public health decisions and policy. Through the Assessment Initiative, funded states work together with local health jurisdictions and communities to improve access to data; to improve skills to accurately interpret and understand data; and to improve use of the data so that assessment findings ultimately drive public health program and policy decisions.
The Assessment Initiative supports work in two main focus areas:

- *Community health assessment practice.* Development, implementation, and evaluation of tools, strategies, and approaches to improve the capacity of local public health agencies and communities to conduct effective community health assessments, and demonstrate how the resulting data have been used to affect public health programs and policies.
- *Data dissemination systems.* Implementation of electronic systems for user-friendly analysis and dissemination of public health data (i.e., Internet-based interactive data query systems) and evaluation of the effect of these systems on primary users.

Biosurveillance
The *BioSense* Program goal is to support a national surveillance network through which healthcare organizations, public health, health information exchanges (HIEs), and other national health data sources are able to contribute to the picture of the health of the nation. To achieve its goal, the BioSense program facilitates activity in three areas:

- Local and state public health coordination of data for surveillance.
- Collaboration with partners to develop the workforce.
- Advances in science and technology.

Currently BioSense supports more than 800 registered users; connects with more than 570 hospitals; receives an average of 175,000 near-real-time messages per hour; receives data from more than 1,300 Department of Defense and Veterans Affairs hospitals and healthcare facilities; and receives laboratory data from LabCorp and RelayHealth.

continues

Electronic Health Records
The purpose of the *Electronic Health Records* project is to leverage opportunities created through the increased use in electronic medical records (EMR) systems in healthcare organizations by creating the ability to send actionable public health alerts that can be consumed and distributed by an EMR system. This project explores extending the capability to communicate with EMR systems using a standard messaging format to create actionable alerts that will be delivered to the provider only when applicable to a current patient's situation. By offering a targeted method of delivery, the project aims to avoid alert fatigue. A feedback mechanism will also be included to capture the provider's response to the alert and further improve the effectiveness of the message.

Vocabulary/Messaging Standards
PHIN (Public Health Information Network, CDC) *Vocabulary Standards* is a key component in supporting the development and deployment of standards-based public health information systems. PHIN Vocabulary Services seeks to promote the use of standards-based vocabulary within PHIN systems and foster the use and exchange of consistent information among public health partners. The use of PHIN Vocabulary Standards ensures that vocabularies are aligned with PHIN standards and with appropriate industry and Consolidated Health Informatics Initiative (CHI) vocabulary standards. These standards are supported by the PHIN Vocabulary Access and Distribution System (VADS) for accessing, searching, and distributing standards-based vocabularies used within PHIN to local, state, and national PHIN partners. It promotes the use of standards-based vocabulary within PHIN systems to support the exchange of consistent information among public health partners.

FIGURE 1–4 Vice Admiral Regina M. Benjamin, MD, MBA, Surgeon General

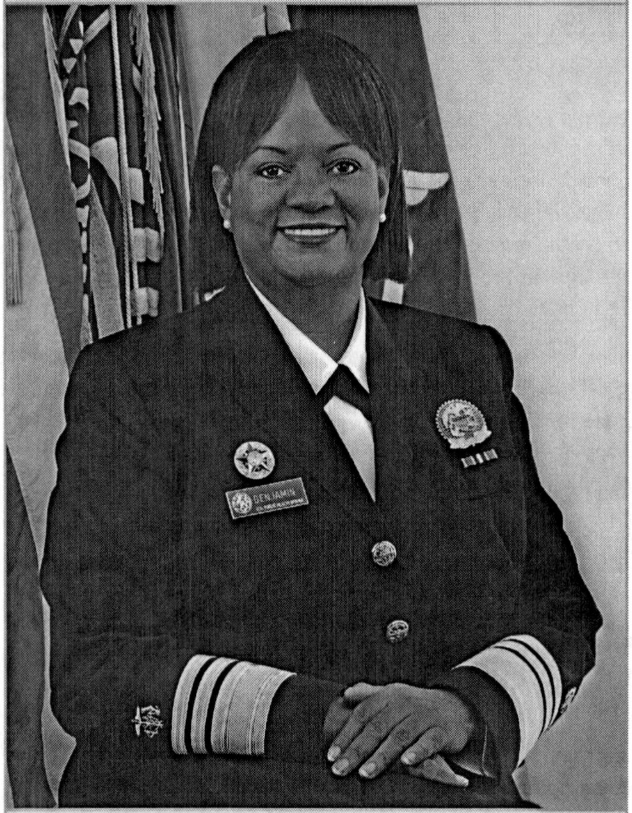

Source: http://www.surgeongeneral.gov/about/biographies/biosg.html

Box 1–5 Duties of the Surgeon General

According to the Department of Health and Human Services, Office of the Surgeon General, the duties of the Surgeon General are to:

- Protect and advance the health of the Nation through educating the public, advocating for effective disease prevention and health promotion programs and activities, and, providing a highly recognized symbol of national commitment to protecting and improving the public's health
- Articulate scientifically based health policy analysis and advice to the President and the Secretary of Health and Human Services (HHS) on the full range of critical public health, medical, and health system issues facing the Nation
- Provide leadership in promoting special Departmental health initiatives, e.g., tobacco and HIV prevention efforts, with other governmental and non-governmental entities, both domestically and internationally
- Administer the U.S. Public Health Service (PHS) Commissioned Corps, which is a uniquely expert, diverse, flexible, and committed career force of public health professionals who can respond to both current and long-term health needs of the Nation,
- Provide leadership and management oversight for PHS Commissioned Corps involvement in Departmental emergency preparedness and response activities
- Elevate the quality of public health practice in the professional disciplines through the advancement of appropriate standards and research priorities and
- Fulfill statutory and customary Departmental representational functions on a wide variety of Federal boards and governing bodies of non-Federal health organizations, including the Board of Regents of the Uniformed Services University of the Health Sciences, the National Library of Medicine, the Armed Forces Institute of Pathology, the Association of Military Surgeons of the United States, and the American Medical Association.

Source: http://www.surgeongeneral.gov/about/duties/index.html. (Accessed November 3, 2009.)

health promotion programs," "provide a highly recognized *symbol* of national commitment" to the nation's health, "*articulate . . . health policy* analysis and advice to the President and the Secretary of HHS," and "provide *leadership in promoting* special . . . health initiatives, e.g., tobacco and HIV prevention . . . both domestically and internationally." The job is an embodiment of public health communication, although not all of its incumbents have been as successful as Dr. C. Everett Koop (Reagan administration) and Dr. Luther L. Terry (Kennedy administration) in focusing the public's attention on critical health issues.

An Essential Public Health Service

Communication is an integral part of virtually every aspect of public health service delivery, and its *outcome* of informing, educating, and empowering people is considered an "essential public health service" in itself, in addition to cross-cutting all the other public health services. **Table 1–2** captures some of the current definitions and functions of health communication,

marketing, and informatics in public health today. This book has been organized to correspond to the tasks of informing, educating, and empowering, as well as persuading the public to act in its best interests.

THE LOGIC OF THIS TEXTBOOK

This book is divided into four major sections:

Section One: Overview. Chapters 1, 2, and 3 provide an overview of public health communications, planning, and informatics.

Section Two: Informing and Educating People about Health Issues. Chapters 4 through 7 describe communication challenges and methods to provide information in a clear and unbiased manner. We focus particularly on translating data into information for different audiences. Section Two concludes with a summary of tips culled from the previous chapters, presented as Chapter 7, Appendix A.

Section Three: Being Persuasive: Influencing People to Adopt Healthy Behavior. Chapters 8 through 12 present theories,

TABLE 1-2 Communication, Marketing, and Informatics in Public Health

Description of the Job of the Surgeon General
The Surgeon General serves as America's chief health educator by providing Americans the best scientific information available on how to improve their health and reduce the risk of illness and injury.

Health Marketing, CDC Definition
Health Marketing involves *creating*, *communicating*, and *delivering* health information and interventions using customer-centered and science-based strategies to protect and promote the health of diverse populations.

The National Center for Public Health Informatics (NCPHI), CDC
NCPHI protects and improves the public's health through discovery, innovation, and service in health information technology and informatics. Informatics can be defined as the collection, classification, storage, retrieval, and dissemination of recorded knowledge. Public health informatics can be defined as the systematic application of information and computer science and technology to public health practice, research, and learning.

National Cancer Institute, Health Communication and Informatics Research Branch
Providing communication leadership across the cancer continuum

Mission Statement: From primary prevention to survivorship and end-of-life care, and all points in between, communication plays a vital role in reducing the burden of cancer. The mission of the Health Communication and Informatics Research Branch is to contribute to the reduction in death and suffering due to cancer by supporting research and development of a seamless health communication and informatics infrastructure. Through internal and extramural programs, the Branch supports basic and translational research across the cancer continuum that will benefit consumers, patients, caregivers and healthcare professionals; from prevention to treatment, through survivorship, and end of life.

National Public Health Practice Standards Program, CDC
Essential Public Health Service #3: Inform, educate, and empower people about health issues. At the local, state, and governance level, this means:

- Health information, health education, and health promotion activities designed to reduce health risk and promote better health.
- Health communication plans and activities such as media advocacy and social marketing.
- Accessible health information and educational resources.

Health education and health promotion program partnerships with schools, faith communities, work sites, personal care providers, and others to implement and reinforce health promotion programs and messages.

Global Public Health Examples
The Communication Initiative (CI) network is an online space for sharing the experiences of, and building bridges between, the people and organisations engaged in or supporting communication as a fundamental strategy for economic and social development and change. It does this through a process of initiating dialogue and debate and giving the network a stronger, more representative and informed voice with which to advance the use and improve the impact of communication for development. This process is supported by web-based resources of summarised information and several electronic publications, as well as online research, review, and discussion platforms providing insight into communication for development experiences.

The Health Communication Partnership (A project of USAID)
Strategic communication for a health competent society.

Communication domains: The Social and Political Environment, Service Delivery Systems, and Health Literate Communities and Individuals.

planning models, and examples of effective strategies for influencing groups of people to adopt healthy behaviors. Everything we said in Section Two applies to Section Three, but persuasive communication adds several layers of complexity to the already challenging task of shaping and disseminating information so that people receive it, understand it, and can act on it. Chapter 13 pulls everything together into an implementation plan, and Chapter 14 describes evaluation of health communication programs.

Section Four: Special Contexts. Chapters 15 and 16 provide snapshots of patient–healthcare provider communication as well as emergency risk communication, respectively. These two circumstances bring unique challenges, as well as tested methods, to public health communication.

Throughout the book you will see boxes featuring examples of exciting research, programs, and resources. These are placed where they make the most sense, but can be read somewhat independently of the chapter material.

CONCLUSION

The fields of health communication and informatics overlap extensively, and public health practitioners have to build skills in both areas to be competent. Through ongoing consultation, the key U.S. public health agencies have developed guidance to help students, and eventually professionals, plan their acquisition of competencies. The goal is a high level of uniform competencies for graduates of public health programs as well as standards of practice for public health agencies at all levels. The competencies are derived from models and theories of how individuals, groups, and societies access, understand, and react to health information. Some of the theories are based on psychological models of individual behavior change; others are based on societal mechanics such as politics and law. Practitioners need to have these tools to contribute to the health promotion and disease prevention objectives we set as a nation. On a global basis, a consensus on objectives and competencies is underway. It is very similar to our national recommendations.

KEY TERMS

ASPH Core Competencies Model

Association of Schools of Public Health (ASPH)

Centers for Disease Control and Prevention (CDC)

Ecological model

Health communication

Hierarchy of effects

Infant mortality rate (IMR)

Informatics

NCI Pink Book

Personal health records

Public health communication

Surgeon General

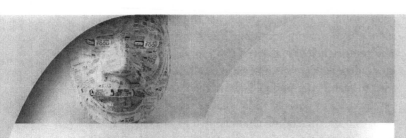

Chapter Questions

1. What distinguishes health communication from everyday communication?

2. Which of the health communication and informatics competencies identified by ASPH do you believe would be needed your first day on the job? Which do you think might be the most difficult to acquire?

3. What is the CDC's approach to health communication?

4. Provide examples of how communication is part of interventions designed to affect different layers of the ecological model.

5. Describe how health communication is used by several government and international organizations.

REFERENCES

1. American Medical Informatics Association [Internet]. Accessed November 4, 2009. Available from https://www.amia.org/inside

2. U.S. Department of Education. Classification of Instructional Programs, 2000; Washington DC. Accessed November 4, 2009. Available from National Communication Association website, http://www.natcom.org/

3. Quindlen, A. The Last Word. *Newsweek,* January 19, 2009. http://www.newsweek.com/id/178844

4. U.S. Department of Health and Human Services, Healthy People 2010, Chapter 11, Health Communication. Accessed November 12, 2009. Available from http://www.healthypeople.gov/Document/HTML/Volume1/11Health Com.htm

5. Dr. John Finnegan, personal communication, June 2009.

6. Kreps, G.L. , Bonaguro, E.W., Query J.L. The history and development of the field of health communication. In: L.D. Jackson & B.K. Duffy, Eds. *Health Communication Research: Guide to Developments and Directions.* Westport, CT: Greenwood Press, 1998, pp. 1–15.

7. Ibid,. pp. 1–2.

8. National Cancer Institute, Making Health Communication Programs Work. Accessed November 19, 2009. Available from http://www.cancer.gov/pinkbook

9. Thompson, T. Chapter 1: Introduction. In: Thompson, T.L., Dorsey, A.M., Miller, K.I., Parrott, R. *Handbook of Health Communication.* Mahwah, NJ: Lawrence Erlbaum Associates, 2003, p. 2.

10. Parvanta, C.F., Freimuth, V. Health Communication at the Centers for Disease Control and Prevention. *Am J Health Behav* 2000;24(1):18–25.

11. Ibid., p. 19.

12. MacDorman, M.F., Mathews, T.J. Behind international rankings of infant mortality: How the United States compares with Europe. NCHS Data Brief, No. 23, November 2009. Accessed December 3, 2009. Available from http://www.cdc.gov/nchs/data/databriefs/db23.pdf

13. Edberg, M. *Essentials of Health Behavior: Social and Behavioral Theory in Public Health (Essential Public Health Series).* See Chapters 1, 2, and 7, for an overview. Sudbury, MA: Jones and Bartlett, 2007, p. 200.

14. Gebbie, K., Rosenstock, L., Hernandez, L.M. (Eds.). Committee on Educating Public Health Professionals for the 21st Century. *Who Will Keep the Public Healthy? Educating Public Health Professionals for the 21st Century.* Washington, DC: National Academies Press, 2003, pp. 32–33.

15. Lavidge, R.L., Steiner, G.A. A model for predictive measurements of advertising effectiveness. *J Marketing* 1961;25:59–62.

16. McGuire, W.J. Public communication as a strategy for inducing health promoting behavioural change. *Prev Med.* 1984;13:299–319.

17. Yasnoff, W.A., O'Carroll, P.W., Koo, D., Linkins, R.W., Kilbourne, E.M. Public health informatics: Improving and transforming public health in the information age. *J Public Health Manage Pract.* 2000:6(6):67–75.

18. Centers of Excellence in Public Health Informatics (P01). Accessed December 10, 2009. Available from http://www.cdc.gov/od/science/PHResearch/grants/fy2005_109.htm

CHAPTER 2

A Public Health Communication Planning Framework

Claudia Parvanta

INTRODUCTION: HEALTH COMMUNICATION IN THE ECOLOGICAL MODEL

Referring back to the ecological model in Chapter 1, our health is affected by our physical environment and limiting or enabling factors created by our society, as well as our own behavior and biology. Reciprocally, our physical condition and behavior affect the health and social welfare of others, and we obviously affect the physical environment. Public health experience has demonstrated that interventions conducted on multiple levels of the model are more effective than those focusing solely on one level. **Table 2–1** shows some of the ways that the CDC used health communication to support interventions directed at the different levels of the ecological model.

A good example of a multilevel intervention is the tobacco policy that addresses taxes on cigarettes, national advertising, worksite activities, and the availability of medical cessation aids (e.g., nicotine gum, patches), presented in Chapter 1.

In this chapter, we introduce the example of the national folic acid[*] campaign managed by the CDC and the National Council on Folic Acid. The CDC and its partners launched advocacy, health provider education, community partnerships, and mass media efforts to increase the availability of foods fortified with folic acid, as well as to increase consumption of folic acid supplements by any woman capable of becoming pregnant. We will come back to the national folic acid program throughout the textbook as an ongoing example that is unusual in scope and longevity.

At the opposite end of the spectrum, many community organizations or public health departments plan and execute small scale interventions on their own. These smaller efforts must work within the limits set by their organizations (chiefly budgetary), and address limited populations defined by specific factors (e.g., geography, health status, age, maternity status, ethnic identity, sexual orientation, church affiliation, school attendance, sports team fans, etc.). **Table 2–2** illustrates the levels of the ecological model and how communication might be used to create or support a public health intervention.

Whether planning for a multilevel, multi-population communication program or a highly focused one, the basic planning process is the same.

---

[*]Folic acid is a B-vitamin that is essential to human health. It is required for the body to make DNA and RNA, the blueprints for development of all cells. It is especially vital to a developing embryo because rapid cell division occurs early in fetal development. Consuming folic acid before conception and through the first months of pregnancy will prevent 50-75% of neural tube defects.

TABLE 2–1 Health Communication at Different Ecological Levels in CDC Folic Acid Program

Ecological Level	Primary Intervention	Communication Intervention
Environmental	Increase number and availability of foods fortified with folic acid. Increase fortification level to 400 µg of folic acid in fortified cereals, bread, pasta, and other prepared foods. Folic acid supplements or multivitamins could be provided at low or no cost to all women.	Advocacy to U.S. Food and Drug Administration (FDA). Education and advocacy to private-sector food and vitamin supplement manufacturers. "Promotional support" for foods and vitamins containing 400 µg of folic acid.
Societal	Policies to promote consumption of folic acid prior to conception. Regulations to define adequate fortification levels in foods. More funding and resources should be committed to neural tube defect (NTD) prevention and education. Health communication normative campaign to promote daily consumption of folic acid supplements—food sources inadequate.	Partner advocacy to federal and state decision makers. Partnership recruitment with national and community organizations. Community, local health department support; media outreach.
Organizational	Educational and technical outreach to obstetricians and gynecologists and pediatricians, concerning reduced risk of NTDs with proper intake of folic acid. Healthcare providers could encourage women to consume folic acid, regardless of their plans for future pregnancies.	Partnership training materials; educational materials for healthcare professionals, managed care, and insurance companies, and health advocacy organizations.
Individual	Health communication: education and persuasion to begin consuming 400 µg of folic acid daily if pregnancy is possible.	Multimedia campaigns using entertainment, public service announcements (PSAs), and print to reach target audiences.

AN OVERALL APPROACH TO PLANNING: BIG WHEEL KEEP ON TURNING

Health communication planning, execution, and evaluation are often depicted together as a circle to emphasize the ongoing nature of program improvement. The National Cancer Institute[1] uses the format shown in **Figure 2–1**.

Another way to look at this is to break down the complex planning process into several sub-plans, each with an inherent research task:

- A **macro plan** that includes analysis of the problem, the ecological setting, the core intervention strategy, and the target population.
  - This stage of planning is normally undertaken after epidemiological data indicate there is a health problem that affects specific groups of people. If there is evidence that a specific intervention has worked to reduce this problem elsewhere, feasibility testing might be conducted to adapt the intervention to the

TABLE 2-2 Communication Interventions in the Ecological Model

Ecological Model Level	Primary Intervention	Communication Support
State, national, global	Policies, laws, treaties, "movements," emergencies. Examples: U.S. seat belt law; EMPOWER tobacco policy (World Health Organization); food fortification or enrichment regulations; small pox or polio vaccination programs; border closing or quarantine to control epidemiological outbreak.	Advocacy to create or maintain policy or law; national and state specific reinforcement advertising; incentive programs; package warnings and labels; government educational campaigns; social mobilization, e.g., national immunization days; multimedia emergency information campaign to advise and calm public.
Living and working conditions	Environmental conditions; hours; policies. Examples: worker safety; time off and vacation policies; creation of walking paths; elimination of lead in gasoline, paint; availability of healthy food choices, healthcare services.	Citizen or worker advocacy (multimedia) to improve conditions; awareness and promotion campaigns for improved facilities, services; state or local lead education campaigns; private-sector advertising for healthy food choices, services.
Social, community, family	Social norms; elimination of social disparities; provision of community health and social services; cultural "rules" for group behavior. Examples: Community Watch, day care, church ministries of health, volunteers.	Grass roots campaigns; radio, TV, Internet, print or locale- (e.g., church, bar) based social marketing or promotional campaigns; opinion leaders and role models; PSAs; health fairs, small media educational materials; reinforcement of norms through group processes.
Individual behavior	Acquisition of beliefs, attitudes, motivation, self-efficacy, products, and services through social marketing, behavior change communications, paid advertising, or psychological counseling.	Multimedia decision aids; educational materials; guidelines; promotional advertising; reinforcement through home, healthcare providers, community.
Individual biology, physiology	Prevention or treatment of illness; healthcare provider visits; screening tests.	Behavior change communication to maintain or establish good health habits; reminders for screening; healthcare provider communication during office visits.

new population. The less we know about the problem, potential solution, or the intended audience, the more formative research must be done before taking the next planning steps.

- A **strategic health communication plan** that focuses on specific change objectives, audiences, messages, and media.
  - Concepts, messages, materials, and media strategies are tested at this stage of planning. This "pretesting" is sometimes referred to as formative research, and at times it is considered "process" research. It should

precede finalization of the implementation plan that comes next.

- An **implementation (or tactical) plan** that says what will be done, when, where, how, with what money, and who is responsible for every piece.
  - Process research is often conducted shortly after the launch of a program to make sure all operations are running smoothly and that messages are getting out and being interpreted as planned. Corrections can be made if this assessment is done early enough.

FIGURE 2–1 Health Communication Planning Cycle

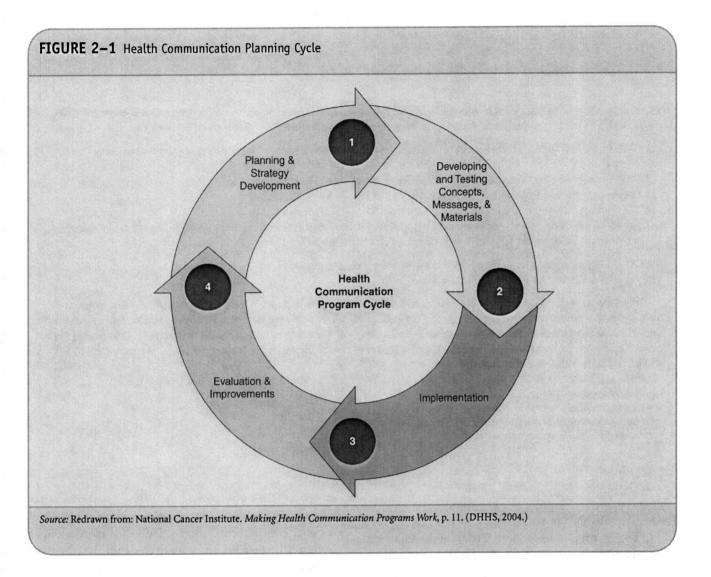

Source: Redrawn from: National Cancer Institute. *Making Health Communication Programs Work*, p. 11. (DHHS, 2004.)

- An **evaluation plan** that says what aspects of the intervention will be monitored or evaluated in order to determine the intervention's worth to key stakeholders. Since most programs want to achieve *measurable* objectives, baseline data often need to be collected before a program is launched. Therefore evaluation planning must begin in the first days of program development.
- A **Partnership, continuation,** and/or **expansion plans** might also be initiated at the outset of a program to ensure a broader reach, diffuse expenses, and provide continuity of leadership and ownership.
- A **Dissemination** and **publication plans**, if desired.

The CDC developed a software tool called *CDCynergy* to help program planners develop and implement health communication programs. CDCynergy refers to each of these plans as "phases." Even though the term "phase" suggests taking one step at a time, in practice several of the phases need to be considered interactively. However, the development of the macro plan is definitely the starting point of the planning process. A health communication program can take more than a year to develop, particularly if a great deal of formative research is necessary. Most interventions run for several months to several years and are followed by evaluations that may also extend from days to years. The involvement of a health communicator in a program from start to finish could turn out to be a five or more year chunk of his or her life.

Several of the best-known approaches and models for planning are discussed in **Box 2–1**.

Box 2–1 Variations in Health Communication Planning

Some of the variation in how health communication planning is approached is based on whether an organization is at the macro stage, developing a communication strategy, or managing the program implementation. Plans that you will commonly encounter include:

- ❑ UNICEF's Triple A Cycle. This consists of "assess–analyze–act," and was developed for any form of planning, not only communication.
- ❑ SCOPE,* created by the Center for Communication Programs at Johns Hopkins University.
- ❑ CDCynergy,† developed by Centers for Disease Control and Prevention (CDC).
- ❑ The six-stage planning model in the National Cancer Institute NCI "Pink Book."
- ❑ The social marketing "wheel" found in multiple social marketing resources, including those supported by the U.S. Agency for International Development (USAID) and the Turning Point Social Marketing National Excellence Collaborative.‡

SCOPE and CDCynergy are among the more complex planning tools and use interactive computer models to build a detailed, multifunctional plan based on individual program data.

International health communication planning models tend to adapt generic planning tools to specific development issues, such as reproductive health, nutrition, and HIV or other infectious diseases. Probably the most comprehensive planning tool ever developed in print is *A Toolbox for Building Health Communication Capacity*.§ The Academy for Educational Development (AED) created this "workbook" using social marketing as well as an "applied behavior change framework" to support child survival programs for USAID. This is available online, free of charge, from AED.

*http://www.jhuccp.org/training/scope/ScopeAbstract.htm
†http://www.cdc.gov/healthmarketing/cdcynergy/
‡http://socialmarketingcollaborative.org/smc/
§http://www.globalhealthcommunication.org/tools/29

DEVELOPING THE MACRO PLAN

The key steps in this plan are:

1. Analyze the problem and the level(s) of the ecological model where you hope to create a change. Based on that analysis, determine what you want to change and where the change must take place.
2. Select the most effective intervention for bringing about this change based on evidence.
3. Choose a core strategy for communication. This identifies target audiences (primary, secondary, and tertiary, discussed later), and the form of interaction with each, for example, education, empowerment, marketing, or political.
4. Identify and recruit partners to accomplish the task.

Let's review each of these steps in detail.

Step 1: Analyze the Problem and Its Place in the Ecological Framework

Diagnosing the Problem: The PRECEDE–PROCEED Model

The **PRECEDE–PROCEED model** has been used to guide countless public health interventions. Developed by Green and Kreuter, and their associates, in the 1970s,[2] the model works backward from a desired state of health and quality of life and asks what environment, behavior, individual motivation, or administrative policy is necessary to create that healthy state. **Figure 2–2** shows the basic PRECEDE–PROCEED model.[3]

PRECEDE–PROCEED divides the process into two phases, assessment and implementation. The needs assessment phase examines the *p*redisposing, *r*einforcing, and *e*nabling *c*onstructs in *e*ducational/*e*nvironmental *d*iagnosis and *e*valuation (*PRECEDE*). The implementation phase addresses *p*olicy, *r*egulatory, and *o*rganizational *c*onstructs in *e*ducational and *e*nvironmental *d*evelopment (*PROCEED*). Predisposing factors include existing beliefs, attitudes, and values (e.g., cultural or ethical norms) that influence whether a person will adopt a behavior. Enabling factors are largely structural, such as the availability of resources, time, or skills to perform a behavior. Reinforcing factors include family and community approval or discouragement.

PRECEDE–PROCEED is discussed extensively in Edberg[4] and will be reviewed in Chapter 9. A comprehensive diagnosis of a problem often reveals that more than one population and more than one level of the ecological model are involved

FIGURE 2–2 PRECEDE–PROCEED Model

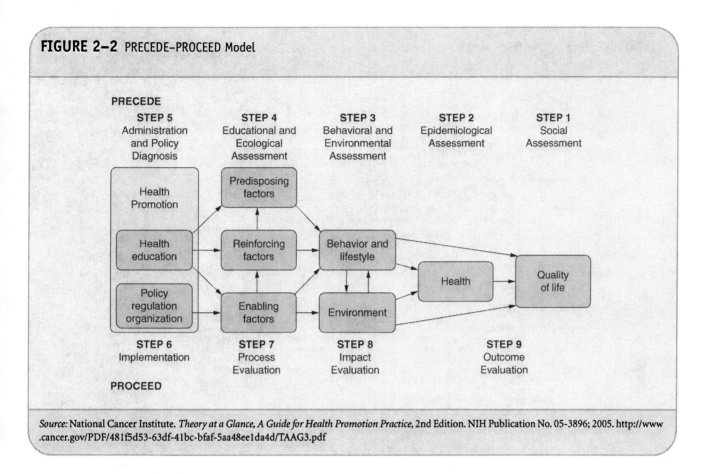

Source: National Cancer Institute. *Theory at a Glance, A Guide for Health Promotion Practice*, 2nd Edition. NIH Publication No. 05-3896; 2005. http://www .cancer.gov/PDF/481f5d53-63df-41bc-bfaf-5aa48ee1da4d/TAAG3.pdf

in creating a problem. All should be addressed in the planning of a successful health communication intervention.

For example, when families share meals, changing the foods served in those meals often requires agreement by several family members (predisposing factors: beliefs about taste and nutrition, food customs and traditions). Food availability can be limited by season of the year, location of markets, as well as food purchasing power (enabling factors). Or if family members criticize the food (e.g., not tasty) the food preparer is unlikely to repeat the performance (reinforcing factors).

As another example, it is well known that many individuals living in the inner city are too afraid of crime to walk around their neighborhood or send their children out to play. All the desire in the world to start an exercise program, and even the offer of free athletic shoes, may not overcome these fears. A "simple" problem in reality is often a complex set of antecedent factors that predispose a belief set, enable or prevent choice, reinforce the status quo, or facilitate change. These factors must be addressed on multiple levels to achieve behavioral change.

The People and Places Framework

Maibach, Abroms, and Marosits[5] have developed a framework to diagram the processes of communication and marketing in terms of their potential for social impact they call the **People and Places Model of Social Change**. Their full model is presented in **Figure 2–3**.

Speaking very plainly, they view the ecological model as people in environments or places, "What about the people, and what about the places, needs to be happening in order for the people (and the places) to be healthy?" Forces that affect people at the individual, social network, or community/population level are referred to as "people fields of influence." Forces that are linked inextricably to a local level or higher administrative level (state, nation, world) are referred to as "place fields of influence." The People and Places Framework (PPF) suggests that organization marketing and business-to-business approaches and policy (legislative, corporate) advocacy are more effective at bringing about change in place fields of influence. Social marketing and health communication, which promote voluntary behavior change based on information,

FIGURE 2–3 People and Places Model

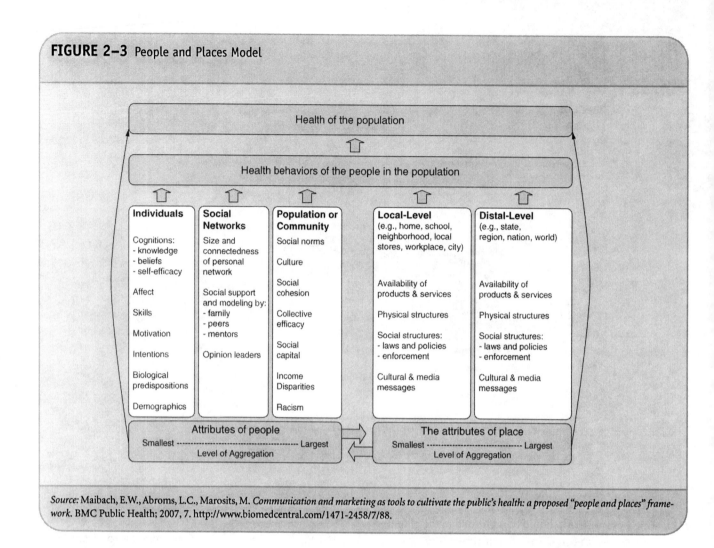

Source: Maibach, E.W., Abroms, L.C., Marosits, M. *Communication and marketing as tools to cultivate the public's health: a proposed "people and places" framework.* BMC Public Health; 2007, 7. http://www.biomedcentral.com/1471-2458/7/88.

motivation, and self-efficacy, among other psychological processes, are more effective at changing people fields of influence. A public health planner can use this information to develop an overarching intervention strategy that will target the desired ecological level(s).

By using the above tools you will develop a fuller understanding of the problem to be addressed, the nature of the required behavioral change, and the levels of the ecological model at which you need to work in order to produce an effective intervention.

Step 2: Select a Primary Intervention Based on Evidence

Unless you are developing an intervention that has never been tried, it is better to adapt an existing **evidence-based intervention** for your community than to develop something from scratch. This way you will be able to estimate your projected

impact and programmatic needs (time, personnel, budget, evaluation needs) more accurately than if planning your approach from a blank sheet of paper. And, it is almost impossible to acquire grant funding without reference to evidence-based interventions (EBIs) in your application.

Chapter 5 will discuss how to consult an evidence base for public health interventions, such as The Community Guide* or Cochrane Reviews.† These are **meta-analyses** of programs and studies that, taken together, provide an estimate of how effective a particular intervention might be in a particular population. Some interventions have not yet generated sufficient evidence to be supported by these resources. It does not mean they do not work, only that there have been

---

*http://www.thecommunityguide.org
†http://www.cochrane.org

an insufficient number of studies with appropriate criteria (sample size, external validity controls, etc.) to be included in a meta-analysis. It is still important to read the primary literature in reputable journals to understand prior approaches and outcomes.

In addition to these research sources, health communication planners need to consult with the target population and its representatives. Interaction with community leaders, either before or after opinion polling, will help you merge what the scientific literature suggests is best with what your community desires. At the conclusion of this stage, you will also determine whether communication will be the primary intervention or will be developed in support of another intervention, such as a new product or service.

Step 3: Identify Relevant Audiences and How You Plan to Interact with Them

Primary, Secondary, and Tertiary Audiences

When planning a communication intervention, you may decide it will be most effective to share information directly with the group of people who are most affected by a problem and whose behavior you hope to change. This group is defined as the **primary audience**. (Sometimes the term "target" is included, as in primary target audience.) For example, if you are trying to get mothers in a developing country to use a more nutritious complementary food for their infants, you might think your best strategy is to speak directly to these mothers (the primary audience) and tell them the benefits of nutrition.

But, after some research in this particular community, you might find that young mothers have very little control over what happens in the household. They live in their husband's home, and their mother-in-law, in fact, makes most of the decisions. So, you decide that before trying to communicate with mothers, you will need to convince the mothers-in-law that their grandchildren can benefit from improved nutrition. In this case, you are reaching out to what is called a **secondary audience**, the group that has a great deal of influences over the behavior of the primary audience.

Finally, you realize that in order to produce change in the behavior of the mothers and mothers-in-law, you will need to reach out to the health workers and other influential people in the community and convince them of the benefits of improved infant nutrition. In this case, you are influencing a **tertiary audience**, or the audience that in some other way affects the behavior of the secondary and primary audiences.

Note that you may sometimes see the term "primary audience" used to refer to the group of people you want to reach first in a sequence. That might be the health workers and community leaders in this example. In fact, if you need to conduct a training program for the health workers to bring them up-to-date with new infant nutrition concepts and empower them to be more effective communicators themselves, then the health workers become the primary audience for this specific intervention. After the health workers are trained, they can then address the mothers and mothers-in-law as *their* primary and secondary audiences, respectively.

In our thinking, and in this book, the primary audience is always the group whose behavior you are trying to change, that is, as a result of this communication intervention this group will think, feel, or act in a certain way. For example, you are planning a teenage anti-smoking campaign in the United States and you hope to enlist the help of musicians and celebrities who appeal to a younger group. While your initial efforts may be directed to these people—the secondary audience—to bring them on-board with your program, you are selecting them to help reach your primary audience—the teenagers.

Choose a Core Communication Strategy for Each Audience

*Decide on whether you plan to "**inform**" or "**persuade**" your intended audience.* According to *Healthy People 2010* health communication "uses communication strategies to inform and influence individual and community decisions that enhance health."[*] Or, put differently, to *inform* and *persuade*. What is the difference?

Informing. As will be explained in Chapter 4, most of the population needs to have raw data and scientific findings decoded into a language they can understand before making an informed decision. The difference between data and information is that *information answers questions*. The same basic fact can be presented in different ways to make it meaningful to whoever is asking the question.

Recent studies of how individuals seek out health information on the internet have provided new ways for health communicators to present information offline as well. Five chapters of this textbook address the various theories and techniques that can be used to transform data into information for different users. The person making a decision might have difficulties reading, using arithmetic functions, or contextualizing information so that it is meaningful to them. Tools to enhance health literacy, numeracy, and cultural competency can be em-

---

*http://www.healthypeople.gov/Document/HTML/Volume1/11HealthCom.htm: 1

ployed to make health information more understandable and meaningful. Advocacy and informatics tools make numbers more eloquent for upstream decision makers. The essential public health service of "inform, educate and empower"* uses the tools from this section of the text.

Persuasion. The more the health communicator is vested in the response to his or her information, the more he or she is venturing into the zone of persuasion. As mentioned later in the chapter, marketing provides an approach to make certain choices seem more favorable to a potential adopter. These approaches can include many of the same factors that make units of information meaningful and understandable, such as cultural cues and references. But persuasive communication takes the next step of employing theories about how individuals or groups make decisions to change behavior. Most of these theories come from the field of social or health psychology, where they have been used extensively to persuade individuals to adopt healthier lifestyles. Their application to group dynamics is relatively new but at least 20 years of practice has provided good results.

There has been a debate in the field about the ethics of using persuasive techniques in health communication. We stick by the stance we put forth in 2002:[6]

> In public health, ethics are largely determined by the extent to which there is scientific consensus about a health issue and the intended and potential unintended outcomes of interventions for all persons. When there is consensus about the beneficial value of a given health behavior for the individual and for society, it is considered ethical to attempt to persuade individuals to adopt a behavior (e.g., not using tobacco, being physically active), or to persuade policy makers to enact policies, support programs, or provide resources to improve health (e.g., mandatory immunization laws for school-age children). Failing to advocate for such individual and social changes when the scientific evidence is strong has ethical dilemmas of its own. When scientific consensus does not exist on a specific topic, when there are potentially serious side-effects involved, or when personal values are critical to a decision, it may be more appropriate to enable individuals to make informed decisions.

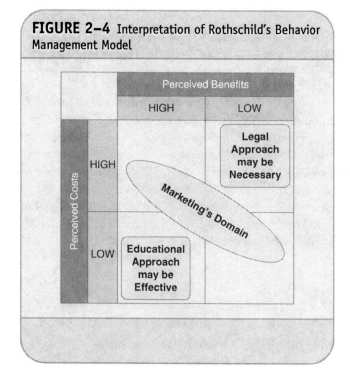

FIGURE 2–4 Interpretation of Rothschild's Behavior Management Model

Health communicators have to decide what is their intention, informing or persuading, before planning their communication strategy. The science, the situation, the community and the principles of the public health practitioner are all included in the ethical calculus of this choice.

Select an overall approach to informing or persuading your audience. According to **Rothschild's Behavior Management Model,**[7] and to economists at large, when a rational individual is asked to adopt a new behavior, he or she evaluates that behavior in terms of its costs and benefits, as well as the individual's motivations and opportunities to act. The motivation behind this change, and the strategy for best facilitation, are depicted in **Figure 2–4.**

Educational approaches. As Figure 2–4 illustrates, if an individual perceives they have much more to gain than to lose (i.e., benefits are obvious and costs are low), then merely providing information or educational approaches might be all that is necessary to prompt a change. A paramount example of this has been the ongoing "Back to Sleep" campaign[†] in which simple informational materials are given to new parents explaining that placing healthy babies on their backs to sleep reduces the risk of sudden infant death syndrome (SIDS). It does not take a lot

---

*http://www.cdc.gov/od/ocphp/nphpsp/EssentialPublicHealthServices.htm#es3

†http://www.nichd.nih.gov/sids/

of persuasion to convince parents to adopt an easily accomplished, no-cost, high-return behavior. **Box 2–2** lists some conditions when educational approaches are most effective.

Legal approaches. At the opposite side of the spectrum, behaviors that appear to offer the individual few personal benefits, are perceived as difficult to maintain, or are costly might require legislative means to enforce. Most public health hygiene laws, smoke-free restaurant regulations, or requirements to strap children into rear safety seats in motor vehicles fall into this category. In order for new laws or regulations to be developed, organizations (government agencies, concerned citizen groups) collect data demonstrating the harm being done, propose solutions to mitigate the problem, and begin an advocacy effort to convince a policymaker at some level (congressional or local legislatures) to take up the issue. Informatics, as well as advocacy communication, is involved in this process. (And it is discussed in Chapter 6.) **Box 2–3** presents some situations where legal or advocacy approaches are more appropriate.

Social marketing. In between compulsion and information is a gray zone where a cost and a benefit is a matter of negotiated exchange. This is the domain of marketing. **Social marketing** can be defined as the "design, implementation, and control of programs aimed at increasing the acceptability of a social idea, practice [or product] in one or more groups of target adopters. The process actively involves the target population, who voluntarily exchange their time and attention for help in meeting their health needs as they perceive them."[8]

Box 2–2
Educational Approaches

Educational approaches work best if:

- The recipient of the information has expressed an interest in, or commitment to, the desired behavior.
- The recipient needs answers to factual questions such as: What? Who? Where? How?
- The information is simple, clear, and unambiguous. And, it is:
  - Written at an appropriate reading level.
  - Communicated in the language of maximum understanding.
  - Age appropriate.
  - Matched to the communication medium.

Box 2–3
Legal Approaches

Advocacy frames issues for public attention, the media, and policymakers. For maximum impact, advocacy should:

- Answer the question: Why should we care?
- Be focused on one or a very limited number of issues.
- Get to the point quickly and end quickly.
- Add emotional content.
- Address local concerns.

In the world of marketing, people are "consumers" who are trying to solve problems. Sometimes the problems are obvious to them, and at others times, their needs are latent. A **latent need** is one of which you are blissfully unaware. Famous examples include body odor, bad breath, and dry, dull skin. If a product can be developed to solve such a latent need and if the price and convenience factors are reasonable, the marketer who develops the product should realize a profit. Hence, we have Dial soap, Listerene, and Jergens with Gold Ribbons, (and scores of other brands). Social marketing has taken this approach and used it to address problems of public health. Unlike commercial marketing, social marketing normally does not focus on a profit margin, although more recent efforts do build a **sustainability*** margin into a product's price. Like marketing, social marketing uses many dimensions to "position" a product, including the product's image, its price, where it is available, and how it is promoted. The four Ps—product, price, place, and promotion—form the basis for a marketing strategy. Social marketing involves more dimensions than health communication alone. Social marketing has also been used to promote intangible "products," that is, behaviors. In this case the dimensions of price, place, and product image are metaphorical. A good example is the well-known "Friends Don't Let Friends Drive Drunk" campaign created by the Advertising Council for the U.S. Department of Transportation, National Highway Traffic Safety Administration (NHTSA). It is explained by social marketing expert Nedra Weinreich in **Box 2–4**.

Thus, depending on whether the change that is proposed is easy or difficult to do or accept, and whether the benefits are obvious or need to be emphasized to overcome resistance,

---

*Sustainability is when the monetary inputs to a program can support its costs. Giving products away for "free," besides being a bad psychological strategy, will not keep a program afloat.

Box 2–4 The 4 Ps in a Drunk Driving Campaign

Friends Don't Let Friends Drive Drunk: How It Satisfied the 4 Ps

By: Nedra Klein Weinreich

This campaign positioned the designed action (product) of friends keeping an eye on each other's level of alcohol impairment, and providing alternative transportation for those too drunk to drive, as a cool and responsible thing for young adults to do. The promotion strategy of television PSAs portraying the potential negative consequences of drunk driving—friends being injured or killed—was designed to lower the perceived social price of "nerdy vigilance." The place where the audience would engage in this action was anywhere young adults gathered to drink. All four marketing Ps worked together to try to persuade the audience to adopt this behavior.

Source: Weinreich NK, personal communication, April 20, 2010.

---

a public health planner might choose education, marketing, or legislative routes as the core strategy.

Step 4: Choose Partners[9]*

No one organization has the time, energy, and resources to make a very large impact on a community, and certainly not on a statewide or national level. Working with partners has been an essential aspect of health communication planning for at least three decades, if not longer. The term *coalition* is often used to refer to a group of different organizations working together for a common cause or campaign. Such coalitions may be formal or informal, with operational rules and governance depending on the group's mission and resources. There are numerous advantages for establishing coalitions to assist you in reaching your programmatic goals. Before you begin to invite organizations to join your coalition, you must decide whether supporting a coalition is a commitment your organization is willing to undertake. Partners selected for a health communication intervention should be able to focus their attention on a target audience and have a high level of credibility within and connection to this group. In order to achieve

objectives and sustain interest in a long-term program, partners must be sought and committed. The following sections describe two effective ways to select partners.

Audience-Oriented Approach

The health communication program identifies groups to receive program messages and services—for example, pregnant women, adolescents, household heads, and isolated geographic groups. You should find out which groups already work most effectively with the intended audience. Partners also may be chosen on the basis of their connection with the intended beneficiaries. Next, the lead agency and the partners develop a plan of action to reach each audience.

Task-Oriented, Problem-Solving Approach

A health communication program may want to accomplish certain tasks—for example, delivering vitamin supplements to all health posts in the country or seeing that all municipalities draft ordinances for bike paths. Which groups can help get the job done? Partners are selected on the basis of what they have to offer: resources, influence, power, logistical support, access.

Box 2–5 lists the numerous benefits as well as the barriers you must consider before involving others in your project.

Later in the book (Chapter 13) we will discuss strategic planning tools such as the SWOT analysis (assessment of strengths, weaknesses, opportunities, and threats). A SWOT analysis, in particular, helps you assess your own, or your organization's strengths, as well as where you need to fill in gaps. You would be well served in selecting partners who have knowledge, skills, resources, or connections to a target audience that you lack. You can choose partners who are in the same field as your organization, but also look beyond to other organizations that may benefit from this coalition. It is important to consider the private sector in this effort, which will be discussed later in this book.

In sum, you should strive to find partners who:

- Share your vision.
- Have experience in the community or with an approach.
- Possess skills that complement your own.

And most critically, the partners should be "stakeholders". They have something "at stake" (their lives, health, reputation, or funding) that depends on the success of the program. Stakeholders might include, among others:

- Representatives of the Primary, or "target" audience for behavioral change

---

*Much of this section is from a draft of the CDC *Physical Activity Guide*. A final version of this guide can be obtained by contacting the CDC. See http://www.cdc.gov/nccdphp/dnpa/pahand.htm.

Box 2–5 Benefits and Barriers of Health Communication Coalitions

There are several possible benefits to forming coalitions. They can:

- Provide the knowledge, expertise, perspective, resources, or credibility needed to bridge gaps in your overall program.
- Conserve resources by avoiding duplication of services, combining resources, and decreasing costs through collective resource-saving opportunities.
- Increase visibility and credibility of your program with decision and policymakers, funders, and the media.
- Use their relationship with the community to mobilize them toward action through collective advocacy.
- Combine the forces of leaders, agencies, gatekeepers, and influential people that may be needed to reach your program's goals.
- Reach specific subgroups within the total population or reach more people within your target audience.
- Broaden community support and strengthen the community's trust in your program.
- Identify gaps in current services and then the members can work together to create programs to eliminate those gaps.
- Make a bigger impact.

Consider these potential problems when deciding if a coalition is the best way to accomplish your goal:

- Coalitions are a time-consuming effort that may take your time away from other projects.
- You must identify potential members of your coalition, convince them to work with you, gain internal approvals, and possibly undergo training—all before you can plan the details of your program.
- The coalition members may require significant alterations in your program ideas.
- Coalitions may also result in a loss of your "ownership" and control for your program.
- The coalition, or individual members, may take credit for the program's results.

You also will need to handle the difficulties that occur when groups work together. Some of these obstacles are:

- Historical or ideological differences.
- Institutional disincentives to collaboration or partnering.
- Competition for resources.
- Lack of leadership and a clear sense of direction.
- Domination by one organization or individual.
- Inadequate participation by important groups.
- Unrealistic expectations about partners' roles, responsibilities, or required time commitments.
- Disagreements among partners regarding values, vision, goals, or actions.
- Inability or unwillingness to negotiate or compromise on important issues.

Source: Centers for Disease Control and Prevention, Division of Nutrition and Physical Activity. *Guide to Working with Coalitions.* Unpublished; 1993.

- Secondary audience, gatekeepers to your target audience— they control access to communicating with your target audience (e.g., religious leaders, block captains, organizational leaders).
- Tertiary audience, influencers, who have earned the respect and admiration of your target audience (e.g., local personalities such as local news anchors, respected politicians, other opinion leaders, national figures such as health authorities or celebrities), if they have a reason to be concerned.

Box 2–6 features the partners who joined the National Council for Folic Acid and some of the resources they brought to the partnership.

CONCLUSION

The first stage of health communication planning involves forgetting about communication details and focusing on the major goals of your project, and the best ways to reach them. This is the macro plan, the big picture, an overall view of the projects and it components. The macro plan is often devel-

Box 2–6 Partners in the National Council for Folic Acid

The Centers for Disease Control and Prevention had resources for beginning the health communication planning process and technical experts to do the process in a systematic manner. Under CDC's leadership, the National Council on Folic Acid (NCFA) was established. Members of the council included:

- American Academy of Pediatrics.
- American College of Obstetricians and Gynecologists.
- Association of Maternal and Child Health Programs.
- Association of State and Territorial Public Health Nutrition Directors.
- March of Dimes Birth Defects Foundation.
- National Coalition of Hispanic Health and Human Service Organizations.
- Shriners' Hospitals for Children.
- Spina Bifida Association of America.
- State health department representative(s).

NCFA served as a steering group, making decisions and broad directives, with ad hoc committees formed to tackle specific projects identified during the planning process. Early in this process, NCFA members delineated their roles based on each of member organization's resources and capabilities. For example, CDC had resources and expertise to conduct the formative and summative research for the campaign, so they took the lead on this activity. March of Dimes and others had the capacity and infrastructure to disseminate materials. The healthcare professional organizations had the capacity to reach their members with information about folic acid. Every member had something to contribute to the overall effort.

Source: From *CDCynergy*, Folic Acid case study. Step 1.3.

---

oped in consultation with organizational partners, each of whom will have a topical focus, a methodological expertise, and a constituency base. Appendix 2A provides an overview of the specific pieces you might include in your own macro plan, as well as an example plan that was developed for the CDC's original Folic Acid program.

KEY TERMS

Continuation plan
Dissemination plan
Evaluation plan
Evidence-based intervention (EBI)
Expansion plan
Implementation (tactical) plan
Inform

Latent need
Macro plan
Meta-analyses
Partnership plan
People and places model of social change
Persuade
PRECEDE–PROCEED Model
Primary audience
Publication plan
Rothschild's behavior management model
Secondary audience
Social marketing
Strategic health communication plan
Sustainability
Tertiary audience

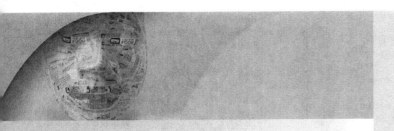

Chapter Questions

1. Name several approaches to health communication planning.

2. What are the key steps to developing a macro plan for a health communication intervention?

3. Sketch out the basics of the PRECEDE–PROCEED model.

4. What are the differences between *informing* and *persuading* your intended audience?

5. Define social marketing. Do you think it is an appropriate approach to use in health communication?

6. What are some criteria for choosing partners for a health communication intervention?

REFERENCES

1. USDHHS, NIH, NCI. *Making Health Communication Programs Work.* NIH Publication No. 04-5145. 2004. Available from: http://www.cancer.gov/pinkbook

2. Green LW, Kreuter MW. *Health Promotion Planning: An Educational and Ecological Approach* (3rd ed.). New York: McGraw-Hill; 1999.

3. NCI. *Theory at a Glance, A Guide for Health Promotion Practice* (2nd ed.). NIH Publication No. 05-3896; 2005. Available from: http://www.cancer.gov/PDF/481f5d53-63df-41bc-bfaf-5aa48ee1da4d/TAAG3.pdf

4. Edberg M. *Essential of Health Behavior. Social and Behavioral Theory in Public Health.* (Sudbury, MA: Jones & Bartlett Publishers 2007).

5. Maibach EW, Abroms LC, Marosits M. Communication and marketing as tools to cultivate the public's health: a proposed "people and places" framework. *BMC Public Health* 2007;7. DOI: 10.1186/1471-2458-7-88. Available at: http://www.biomedcentral.com/1471-2458/7/88

6. Parvanta C, Maibach E, Arkin E, Nelson DE, Woodward J. Chapter 2: Public health communication: A planning framework. In: Nelson DE, Brownson RC, Remington PL, & Parvanta C (Eds). *Communicating Public Health Information Effectively: A Guide for Practitioners.* Washington, DC: American Public Health Association; 2002, pp. 4–15.

7. Rothschild, ML. Carrots, sticks, and promises: A conceptual framework for the management of public health and social issue behaviors. *Journal of Marketing.* 1999;63:24–37.

8. Lefebvre RC, Flora JA. Social marketing and public health intervention. *Health Educ Quarterly.* 1988;15:299–315.

9. USDHHS, Centers for Disease Control and Promotion, Division of Chronic Disease Control and Community Intervention. *Promoting Physical Activity: A Guide for Community Action.* Draft, May 1995; Chapter 5, p. 7.

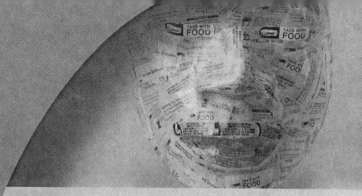

Folic Acid Macro Plan Example

APPENDIX 2A Macro Plan Template

Step	Information	Tools
1	Analyze the problem and its place in the ecological framework.	
1.1	*Health Problem Statement:* What is occurring? What should be occurring? Who is affected, and to what degree? What could happen if problem is not resolved?	Worksheet 2.1 PRECEDE diagnosis
1.2	What needs to change? Individual behavior, policies, environmental conditions?	People and places framework (PPF)
2	*Primary Intervention:* What is it? What is the evidence base? What are its advantages and disadvantages?	
	What needs to happen in order for this intervention to solve the problem? What role will communication play: primary or support?	Review PRECEDE and PPF
3.1	Identify the primary, secondary, and other audiences.	
3.2	For each audience, will you inform, empower, or persuade them?	
3.3	What core strategy will you use (education, marketing, advocacy/law)?	
4	Who needs to be a partner in your coalition? What is their overall partnering role? (Access to people, task specific.)	
5	Logic Model and SWOT analysis*	(See Chapter 13)

*In a "public health reality," you would do these steps now. We will introduce them later in the textbook because you need to learn more before you can accomplish these tasks.

Source: Based on *CDCynergy*, Folic Acid example.

WORKSHEET 2-1   Health Problem Statement

1. What is occurring ?

2. What should be occurring?

3. Who is affected, and to what degree?

4. What could happen if the problem is not addressed?

FOLIC ACID MACRO PLAN EXAMPLE

1.1 Health Problem Statement

What Is Occurring?

The Centers for Disease Control and Prevention (CDC) uses surveillance and epidemiological data to track the prevalence of birth defects in the United States. In 1990, the CDC reviewed data collected since 1983 and reported that the average state level prevalence of neural tube defect (NTD) affected births during this period was 4.6 per 10,000.* NTDs are among the most fatal or debilitating birth defects and include incomplete closure of the spine (spina bifida) and malformation of the brain (anencephaly). Babies born with spina bifida have an opening along their spine, through which the spinal tissue protrudes. These babies often need to have many surgical treatments when they are young, and most grow into adulthood with varying degrees of disability, including paralysis of the feet and legs and lack of control of the bowels and bladder. Mental retardation sometimes occurs, and learning disabilities are com-

mon. Anencephaly is a fatal condition in which most, or all, of a baby's brain and skull are missing. Babies with anencephaly are either stillborn or die within a very short time after birth.

What Should Be Occurring

Folic acid is a B-vitamin that is essential to human health. It is required for the body to make DNA and RNA, the blueprints for development of all cells. It is especially vital to a developing embryo because rapid cell division occurs early in fetal development. In clinical and effectiveness trials, the CDC and multicountry teams were demonstrating that consumption of 400 micrograms (μg) of folic acid prior to conception reduces the risk of NTDs by 50% to 75%.

In 1992, based on strong clinical evidence, the U.S. Public Health Service (PHS) issued the recommendation that women of childbearing age consume 400 μg of folic acid daily to prevent NTDs.

Who Is Affected, and to What Degree?

- Even with this recommendation, there were more babies born between 1992 and 1998 with preventable *spina bifida* and anencephaly than born with defects caused by the thalidomide tragedy of the late 1950s and early 1960s.

*Lary JM, Edmonds LD. Prevalence of spina bifida at birth—United States, 1983–1990: A comparison of two surveillance systems. *MMWR*. CDC Surveillance Summaries. April 19, 1996; 45(2):15–26.

- All women of reproductive age capable of becoming pregnant could be affected by a neural tube defect–affected pregnancy if they consume inadequate amounts of folic acid.
- Specific populations at higher risk for a neural tube defect–affected pregnancy are women with a previously affected pregnancy, women of low socioeconomic status, and women of Hispanic ethnicity.

What Could Happen if the Problem Is not Addressed?

The impact of having a baby with spina bifida or losing a baby born with anencephaly is profound—emotionally, spiritually, and financially. Costs for medical, developmental, and other services for children born with spina bifida are estimated to be about $500 million annually. This does not include any costs associated with counseling or support of parents of children affected by NTDs.

1.2 What Needs to Change?

Policy

While some foods were enriched with folic acid, the level was too low for women to reach the goal of 400 µg/day of folic acid without consuming large volumes. Enrichment or fortification levels needed to be raised to provide 100% of daily need to prevent NTDs.

Environment

- More foods fortified with folic acid needed to be available to women at all income levels.
- Multivitamins containing folic acid or folic acid supplements had to be available for all women at an affordable price, including free.

Organizational Behavior

Physicians—in particular, obstetricians, gynecologists, and pediatricians—had advised women to take folic acid during pregnancy. They needed to understand, and support their patients taking the recommended quantity *prior* to conception.

Individual Behavior

- Knowledge. A 1995 survey by the National March of Dimes Birth Defects Foundation and the Gallup Organization showed awareness of the term "folic acid" at about 52%, but specific knowledge about folic acid to be very low—only 5% of the total sample knew that folic acid helps prevent birth defects, and only 2% knew that a woman should take folic acid before pregnancy in order for it to be effective.

- Vitamin-taking behavior. Studies showed that nonpregnant women under age 25 were least likely to consume a daily multivitamin, with only 19% reporting that they did. This group accounted for approximately 39% of all U.S. births.
- Other dietary behavior. Natural sources of folate, such as orange juice or green leafy vegetables, needed to be consumed in large quantities in order to reach this goal. Women were not generally able, or were often unwilling, to eat the large volumes of food needed to reach the goal.

Biological Level

The neural tube develops very early in pregnancy, about two to four weeks after conception. This is often before a woman knows she is pregnant; therefore, it is often before she can begin taking sufficient amounts of folic acid supplements to prevent NTDs. To provide adequate protection, all women who could become pregnant would need to take in 400 µg/day of folic acid.

2. What Is the Primary Intervention?

The CDC established a goal of increasing the percentage of women consuming the PHS-recommended level of folic acid from 25% to 50%.

Evidence Base

These are examples of key references supporting the primary intervention:

- Centers for Disease Control and Prevention. Use of folic acid for prevention of spina bifida and other neural tube defects—1983–1991. *Morbidity and Mortality Weekly Report* 40 (1991): 513–516.
- MRC Vitamin Study Research Group. Prevention of neural tube defects: Results of the Medical Research Council vitamin study. *Lancet* 338 (1991): 131–137,
- Centers for Disease Control and Prevention. Recommendations for use of folic acid to reduce number of spina bifida cases and other neural tube defects. *Morbidity and Mortality Weekly Report* 41, no. RR-14 (1992): 1–7.
- Berry, R.J., Li, Z., Erickson, J.D., Li, S., Moore, C.A., Want, H., Mulinare, J., Zhao, P., Wong, L.Y., Gindler, J., Hong, S.X., Correa, A., Hao, L., & Gunter, E. Prevention of neural tube defects with folic acid in China. *New England Journal of Medicine* 341 no. 20(1999): 1485–1490.
- Czeizel, A.E. Folic acid and the prevention of neural-tube defects. *New England Journal of Medicine* 350 (May 20, 2004): 2209–2211; author reply, 2011.

What Are its Advantages and Disadvantages?

- The primary advantage to the intervention is that it involves a taking a vitamin supplement or consuming a fortified food product (such as breakfast cereal) on a daily basis. This is a relatively simple behavior change on the part of one individual.
- The primary disadvantage is that women must have the increased level of folic acid in their bloodstream during the first few weeks of gestation. The vast majority of women do not know when this occurs, and therefore, would need to take the vitamin prior to conception. For at least half of the women in the United States, this is an unplanned event. They would, therefore, need to take the vitamin from the time they start having sexual relations.
- The secondary disadvantage is that the additional burden of consuming vitamins or fortified foods falls on young women who are either unaware of the need for or who cannot afford these supplements.

2.1 What Needs to Happen in Order for this Intervention to Solve the Problem?

Changes at the Individual Level

The proportion of women who believe that consuming folic acid daily can help prevent birth defects needs to increase. This requires changes in women's knowledge, attitudes, intentions, and behaviors regarding consumption of folic acid.

Changes at the Healthcare Delivery/Organizational Level

- NTD and folic acid awareness needs to become a routine and standard part of the delivery of preventive healthcare services to women.
- Healthcare providers and healthcare organizations need to be informed about the importance of folic acid and critical timing of its delivery.

Changes at the Health Policy Level

Government organizations and relevant nongovernmental organizations needed to agree on fortification levels, as well as the availability of folic acid as part of routine preventative care for women of procreational age.

Environmental Level

- The level of folic acid in fortified foods needs to be increased to provide an adequate daily dose to prevent NTDs.
- Private-sector food manufacturers needed to be made aware of the importance of adding the appropriate level of folic acid to foods.
- Finding the correct level required additional research, testing, and negotiation with government agencies.

3. Who Are the Various Audiences? How Will You Work with Them?

- Additional research is needed to define the primary audience of "women who can become pregnant" into smaller, more meaningful segments. Following this research, we will use communication to inform and persuade them as a primary intervention.
- Secondary audiences of intermediaries will be empowered to communicate with women about the issue. These include healthcare providers, community organizations, and national organizations concerned with preventing birth defects.
- Tertiary audiences will receive persuasive communications to make taking folic acid a new norm. These audiences include the mass media and college health programs and advisors.
- Information will be provided to agency authorities to facilitate decision making about fortification levels and other regulatory issues.
- Advocacy efforts will be directed to political entities to focus attention on the issue.
- Communication to inform and persuade will be directed to food manufacturers following appropriate legislative action to set levels.
- A combination of information and social marketing will be used to develop the communication interventions.

4. Who Are Your Partners?

See Box 2–6.

Informatics and Public Health

David E. Nelson

INTRODUCTION

What was once considered only possible in the realm of science fiction has become an everyday reality. Public health has embraced Internet and mobile technologies such as smart phones and personal digital assistants (PDAs), as well as advances in digital photography, data visualization, and geographic information systems. Because of these and other technological advances, information is available on a worldwide basis on a scale previously unimaginable, and communication has drastically changed.

Public health is fundamentally based on data. Even as far back as John Snow and the London cholera outbreak in the 1850s, collecting, managing, analyzing, and presenting data efficiently and effectively have been essential to public health practice. Not surprisingly then, the field of public health has been strongly influenced by advances in information technology (IT). The types and uses of technologies are dynamically and fundamentally changing how knowledge and information are obtained, exchanged, interpreted, and disseminated. This

has resulted in the development of a distinct discipline called **public health informatics**, which is related to health communication. Public health informatics arose as a result of the interaction of the sciences and practices related to information, computing, and public health.[1,2]

There is a close relationship between communication and informatics because informatics has substantially improved the availability of information. However in comparison with the field of communication, which heavily stresses messages and audiences, the major emphasis of informatics is on the *information itself and the technological systems through which information is collected, stored, retrieved, analyzed, and displayed.*

Informatics presents important new opportunities for improving communication and influencing public health practice, such as earlier recognition and intervention for disease outbreaks and improved management of chronic diseases.[1,2] It also presents new challenges, such as data security and information overload.[3,4] This chapter presents a broad overview of informatics and its roles in public health, with an emphasis on how these roles are related to communication.

BACKGROUND

Although the term *informatics* is widely used across different health fields, it is helpful to briefly review definitions. Informatics can loosely be considered as **information science**, that is, the science of gathering, managing, storing, classifying, retrieving, and transferring recorded information. Different classification schemes have been used to characterize informatics and its uses in health.

Informatics is applicable to many health areas.[4] These include medical informatics (e.g., use of IT in healthcare settings); bioinformatics, which involves advanced computing techniques and information systems for basic biomedical research (e.g., genetic risk for diseases); and consumer health informatics (e.g., health information seeking or social networking by the public using the Internet). This chapter concerns informatics in public health. *Public health informatics* has been defined as the "systematic application of information and computer science and technology to public health practice, research, and learning."[1] As such, it draws from the expertise of individuals in various disciplines to create and utilize applications to meet the needs of different audiences.[1,5] Some of these disciplines appear in **Table 3–1.**

In contrast to medical care providers, whose major focus is on individual patients (especially treating diseases and injuries), public health practitioners focuses on populations and prevention. There are four key public health principles for public health informatics:[1]

- Promotion of health in the general population (e.g., not simply individuals within a specific medical care clinic).
- Emphasis on prevention of disease and injury by altering the conditions or the environment that place populations at risk.
- Consideration of prevention opportunities wherever they may exist (e.g., public or organizational policy interventions).
- Recognition of the influence of governmental and other contexts on public health information systems and applications (including social, legal, and political considerations).

TABLE 3–1 Disciplines Contributing to Public Health Informatics

Computer science
Information science
Business (e.g., management)
Psychology and other behavioral sciences
Communication
Epidemiology
Statistics
Law
Health promotion and health education
Engineering
Others (e.g., laboratory science, genetics)

Source: Adapted from: O'Carroll PW, Yasnoff WA, Ward ME, Ripp LH, Martin EL (eds). *Public Health Informatics and Information Systems.* New York: Springer-Verlag, 2003.
Kukafka R. Public health informatics: The nature of the field and its relevance to health promotion practice. *Health Promotion Practice,* 2005; 6:23–28.

To date, much of the emphasis of public health informatics has been on the use of IT for the early detection of disease outbreaks, especially those related to infectious diseases.[6] This is not surprising, given that local, state, and federal public health agencies have legally mandated responsibilities to protect populations from certain preventable diseases, such as the contagious diseases of tuberculosis, syphilis, tetanus, and rabies. Therefore, many data collection systems are in place for such reportable diseases. Historically, the collection and entry of data for most reportable diseases involved the use of paper records or phone calls, e.g., between healthcare providers and local health departments or between local and state health departments.

Advances in IT have allowed for much more rapid collection, transmission, availability, and analysis of data, which has led to the earlier recognition of outbreaks and implementation of prevention efforts.[2] Timely global tracking and reporting of information for the 2009 H1N1 influenza epidemic (commonly referred to as "swine flu") in the United States and other countries is one example of how public health informatics systems are used to rapidly identify and monitor an important contagious disease affecting populations.

The level of interest and expansion in public health informatics grew exponentially after the 2001 (9/11) World Trade Center and Pentagon attacks and the subsequent use of weaponized anthrax through mailed letters that same year.[6] Federal funding increased substantially, which supported the creation of several electronic reporting systems designed for early detection of potential biological or chemical threats aimed at populations (e.g., bioterrorism).[7] Increases in funding also lead to enhancements and improvements for existing data collection systems used for the surveillance of health conditions and events. **Box 3–1** provides descriptions of several national and international public health IT systems for the early detection of selected acute diseases or conditions.

The practice of public health is far more comprehensive than preventing or controlling disease outbreaks; thus public health informatics extends far beyond data systems used for infectious disease surveillance. Information technologies that promote healthy behaviors and other forms of preventive health (e.g., disease screening, immunization) are important informatics tools for impacting the health and well-being of populations. IT advances for public health systems related to the environment, chronic disease, and injury prevention and control have greatly increased the speed at which data are obtained, analyzed, and summarized and have made data much more rapidly available to audiences on a broad scale.[1,2,4–7]

Informatics approaches are used for health-related data systems such as population-based registries for persons with cancer, birth defects, certain types of injuries, and other health

Box 3–1 Examples of Data Systems Designed for the Early Detection of Potentially Acute Public Health Diseases or Conditions

GeoSentinel Surveillance Network. GeoSentinel is a worldwide communication and data collection network for the surveillance of travel-related illnesses that may occur among immigrants, refugees, and persons who travel for business or pleasure. Co-sponsored by the International Society of Travel Medicine and the Centers for Disease Control and Prevention (CDC), it consists of 48 medical clinics on six continents that specialize in travel or tropical medicine. Anonymous surveillance data based on information obtained during clinic visits with patients are contributed to a shared database. It has been used to examine and control internationally important infectious diseases such as malaria and rabies, as well as environmental hazards and injuries.

Source: GeoSentinel: The Global Surveillance Network of the ISTM and CDC. http://www.istm.org/geosentinel/main.html.

Global Public Health Intelligence Network (GPHIN). GPHIN is an Internet-based early warning system designed to track and disseminate information about various issues of public health relevance such as infectious disease outbreaks; natural disasters; bioterrorism and exposure to toxic chemicals; and the safety of drugs, medical devices, and other health products. The GPHIN data system was developed and operates under the auspices of the Public Health Agency of Canada. Information is based on monitoring and collecting data from global media sources such as news wires and websites. The system uses an automated process to filter and information prior to analysis by agency staff. Information can be used as an early warning system for outbreaks and other events and to track events nationally or internationally; this system has the capability to send automated e-mail messages about potential adverse events. GPHIN is designed to complement other public health surveillance activities.

Source: Public Health Agency of Canada, Global Public Health Intelligence Network (GPHIN). http://www.phac-aspc.gc.ca/media/nr-rp/2004/2004_gphin-rmispbk-eng.php.

National Electronic Disease Surveillance System (NEDSS). State health departments use a variety of different electronic systems to collect public health data for surveillance purposes. Examples include systems for specific diseases such as HIV, outbreak management, and reporting of certain laboratory values. A major challenge is integrating state electronic surveillance systems such that data can be transferred securely from healthcare providers to state health departments. Electronic information system products exist that were developed by commercial vendors, the CDC or state health departments themselves. NEDSS is a Web-based system that uses standardized health information technology codes to integrate data from these different systems. Interoperability of data systems—that is, the ability to transmit data between computer systems—is essential to improve their efficiency and quality.

Sources: CDC, NEDSS: National Electronic Disease Surveillance System. http://www.cdc.gov/NEDSS/; and Reference 15.

Electronic Surveillance System Early Notification of Community-Based Epidemics (ESSENCE). ESSENCE is a surveillance system designed and run by the U.S. Department of Defense for early recognition of disease outbreaks. It is available for health departments and has been adopted by the District of Columbia, Maryland, and Virginia health departments for the greater Washington, DC, metropolitan area to identify potential bioterrorism or other acute health events (e.g., surveillance related to the spread of West Nile Virus encephalitis). ESSENCE essentially conducts "surveillance" of other data systems, which include a variety of systems such as physician outpatient records, community over-the-counter drug sales, school absentee reporting, nurse advice records, emergency departments, and other data sources. ESSENCE is an example of using a database for syndromic surveillance; that is, it attempts to identify data based on nonspecific symptoms (e.g., fever, headache, bronchitis) that may indicate the start of a more serious health problem.

Source: Reference 2.

conditions.[7] National, state, and local risk behavior survey data on adults and youth (e.g., alcohol use and physical activity) are routinely collected, analyzed, and made available to audiences for program planning, evaluation, and intervention (e.g., health promotion and education; health policies).[7]

Public health informatics continues to influence how data are analyzed and visually presented, such as the use of more sophisticated approaches for analyzing and mapping data. Finally, a growing array of IT options allows public health information to be made directly and rapidly available to members of the public, media, and policymakers; examples include accessing written or numeric information from websites and downloading video or audio materials (e.g., podcasts). Many aspects of public health informatics are increasingly converging with consumer and medical informatics, such as the increased adoption of electronic medical records and use of social media (e.g., Facebook and Twitter) to reach large numbers of people with health messages.

EXAMPLES OF PUBLIC HEALTH INFORMATICS IN ACTION

In this section, we illustrate the contributions of public health informatics in three distinct real-world applications.

A Multistate Infectious Disease Outbreak of Salmonella

As discussed later in this chapter, there is a close relationship between informatics and public health surveillance, that is, the routine collection of tracking of certain diseases, and health conditions in populations on an ongoing basis. One such disease is caused by infections with salmonella bacteria. Salmonella can result in outbreaks of gastroenteritis (e.g., "food poisoning") among large numbers of people, which are characterized by severe nausea, vomiting, abdominal cramps, diarrhea, and fever. Salmonella is estimated to cause more than 1 million cases of gastroenteritis and result in several hundred deaths in the United States each year. Most outbreaks are associated with eating raw or undercooked meat, eggs, or egg-related products. In late 2008 and early 2009, a large multistate outbreak of Salmonella occurred that was found to be related to the consumption of peanut butter.[8]

PulseNet* is a network of public health and food regulatory agency laboratories throughout the United States that is coordinated by the Centers for Disease Control and Prevention (CDC). Using biological samples obtained from persons with suspected disease, participants in PulseNet perform DNA tests, often referred to as **DNA fingerprinting**, to identify clusters of food-borne diseases. These DNA fingerprints are submitted electronically to a database at CDC on a regular basis where they are available for analyses by CDC staff and PulseNet participants.

Using PulseNet data, CDC staff identified a small but highly dispersed cluster of salmonella cases from 12 states in November 2008 with a similar but unusual DNA pattern not previously seen in this data system. In conjunction with state and local partners, the CDC began a more intensive and widespread investigation over subsequent weeks. By late January 2009, a total of 529 persons from 43 states and 1 person from Canada were identified as having been infected; peanut butter consumption was found to be the common thread. Eventually,

one particular peanut butter manufacturing plant in Georgia was identified as the source of the infection. Production at the plant was halted and voluntary recalls of potentially affected products containing peanut butter began. Subsequently, the number of salmonella cases declined.[8] The PulseNet system played a crucial role in assisting scientists to rapidly identify, investigate, and ultimately stop this disease outbreak.

Visualizing State Trends in Adult Obesity

The **Behavioral Risk Factor Surveillance System,** or **BRFSS,** uses monthly telephone surveys of randomly selected adults in states to estimate the prevalence of various health risk factors (e.g., smoking, cancer screening). Data are collected under the auspices of state health departments and sent to the CDC for processing and summarization. Findings from the BRFSS are used by health departments and other organizations to establish and track health objectives, develop and evaluate public health policies and programs, and identify emerging health problems.

State data on the percentage of obese adults date back to the 1980s. Usually, public health surveillance system data from the BRFSS and other surveys are presented in dense tables, which can be hard for persons who are not "data people" to understand.[9] In the late 1990s, CDC scientists presented BRFSS state obesity trend data using a series of color-coded maps. These maps allowed scientific and nonscientific audiences to easily understand the obesity epidemic in a way not possible with data-containing tables and have been well received and widely acclaimed.[9] **Figure 3–1** shows selected state obesity trend maps for selected years from 1990 through 2008. The spread of the obesity epidemic is even more striking when color-coded state maps are viewed sequentially online.†

The wide-scale availability of BRFSS data coupled with improvements in data visualization demonstrate the advancements in data presentation made possible through informatics. These, and similar state trend maps for diabetes and other topics have been widely used in presentations and are available on websites. The obesity maps helped raise awareness about of the obesity problem in the United States, and similar approaches are being used in other countries.

Promoting Health Behavior Change through Internet Interventions

The expansion of access and technologic improvements have spawned the development of advanced Internet applications. Public health interventions designed to promote healthier be-

---

*http://www.cdc.gov/pulsenet/

†http://www.cdc.gov/obesity/data/trends.html

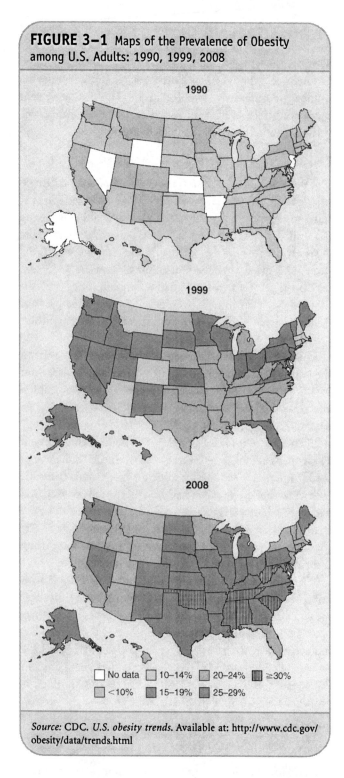

FIGURE 3-1 Maps of the Prevalence of Obesity among U.S. Adults: 1990, 1999, 2008

1990

1999

2008

| | No data | | 10–14% | | 20–24% | | ≥30% |
| | <10% | | 15–19% | | 25–29% | | |

Source: CDC. *U.S. obesity trends.* Available at: http://www.cdc.gov/obesity/data/trends.html

pabilities of the Internet. In addition to being used for health behavior change, such as smoking cessation or weight loss, Internet interventions also can address certain health conditions. These include such as things as decision support for cancer screening or treatment, or for managing chronic diseases such as asthma or diabetes.[11] These applications demonstrate the growing convergence between public health and medical care systems.[5]

A major benefit of Internet interventions, as compared to one-on-one activities in health clinics or similar settings, is that they can reach far more people at lower cost. For example, a smoking cessation online tool was made available to more than 130,000 IBM employees, of whom 8,700 were smokers. Among all smokers, more than 1,700 participated in an Internet smoking cessation intervention.[12]

Internet interventions involve much more than simply putting health information on a website and encouraging people to visit it. Research has shown that more effective Internet interventions are highly structured and personalized; that is, messages are tailored to the characteristics of individual users. Tailoring involves developing different health messages based on factors of individuals such as age, gender, readiness to change, or level of self-efficacy. Providing social support for users, either through readily accessible counselors (e.g., health professionals or coaches via e-mail or telephone) or peers with a similar health issue, are also important intervention components.[10] (Tailoring is discussed in Chapter 10.)

Internet health interventions continue to undergo extensive research and are increasingly becoming more "mainstream." For example, Health Media®, a private company originally developed by Dr. Victor Strecher, a researcher at the University of Michigan, delivers Digital Coaching™ for weight loss, adherence to medication regimens, and other health issues to members of large healthcare organizations or health insurance enrollees. This company was purchased by the Johnson & Johnson Company in 2008.*

INFORMATICS AND PUBLIC HEALTH DATA SYSTEMS

Public Health Surveillance

Public health surveillance involves ongoing systematic data collection, analysis, and interpretation for public health practice.[7] The timely dissemination of data to those responsible for prevention and control is a key public health function. Informatics, because it encompasses data systems, is closely tied to public health surveillance.[1,2,13] Even if you never analyze

haviors are increasingly being delivered through Internet applications and other platforms.[10] Rather than simply including static information in the form of text, interventions can take advantage of the video, audio, and social networking ca-

*http://www.healthmedia.com/index.htm

surveillance data yourself, it is essential to know the basics about surveillance systems to understand the quality of data, the costs, and decisions involved in starting, maintaining, or even discontinuing such systems, and the validity of data underlying public health messages used in communication.[1,2,7,14]

Detailed information about public health surveillance systems, including evaluation of such systems, is covered by others (e.g., Reference 7 and 14) and is beyond the scope of this chapter. Here are some basic principles about surveillance systems relevant for informatics.

Purpose and Uses

Knowing why a data system has been created is an important first step. Developing and maintaining a data system involves the use of resources; thus, there should be a clear and compelling purpose for collecting and using data for public health action. For some health events, there may be a legal requirement for data collection, such as a notifiable (reportable) health condition. Examples of objectives might include considering immediate public health action (e.g., suspected cases of botulism) or program planning and evaluation (e.g., behavioral surveillance).

Intended Audiences

The intended data users and the intended use will influence data collection, analysis, and presentation. An important distinction is between persons who are **data users** and those who are **results users**.[9] Data users, such as epidemiologists or researchers in other fields, tend to be more interested in analysis, hypothesis testing, and so forth. Results users tend to be individuals such as public health program directors, policymakers, advocates, or news media representatives. They are most interested in finding summaries and the implications for action (e.g., issuing warnings about drinking water; increasing educational efforts designed to increase condom use).

Definition of a Health-Related Event

Another basic principle of data systems is how a public health event or condition is defined, i.e., what is actually being counted as data. While this may seem obvious, definition decisions can have profound consequences. If a health event or condition is defined too broadly (e.g., self-reported fever, weakness, and cough), then a lot of time, energy, and money can be wasted collecting and reporting data of little value for public health action. In information science terms, this is referred to as a low **signal-to-noise ratio.** Conversely, a too narrow definition may result in missing potentially important and preventable health problems.

Data Collection and Management

Many of the day-to-day activities of informaticists involve attending to the details of data collection and management for information systems.[1,2] Much of this is technical in nature, but some aspects are relevant for those with general public health training so you can better understand informatics and its contributions. Data sources collected on the "front line" of public health can range from laboratory values submitted electronically to a national database, individual nurses in local public health clinics or doctors' offices making phone calls to state health department employees to report health concerns.[1,7]

The sources of data ultimately collected and included in a public health data system are often decentralized (e.g., performed by different local or state health departments, healthcare facilities, etc.[1,2,9,15]) or derived from individuals at various locations). The quality of information contained in a data system is strongly dependent on the ability and expertise of these individuals and organizations, their training and experience with data collection and their familiarity with the system. Without attending carefully to data quality issues, there is a risk of the GIGO problem—Garbage In, Garbage Out.

Data submitted for entry into a public health information system is usually processed for accuracy. This is typically automated in such a way as to identify ("flag") potential outlying values for further consideration. For example, in an adolescent or adult survey about alcohol use, a data value of consuming an average of "50 alcohol-containing beverages per day" would be flagged for further review because such a value is not physiologically feasible.

An additional challenge posed by decentralized data collection is that data may be in different formats or be entered and stored in systems that use dissimilar software or hardware, even for the same health event under surveillance. Sharing and integrating data from dissimilar systems is a major public health informatics challenge referred to as **interoperability.**[1,2,6,13,15]

Over the years, many public health data systems were created to track just one disease or health condition. Although useful for the specific public health program, such systems cannot exchange data with other information systems. Growing efforts in informatics are under way to improve the interoperability of public health surveillance systems through the development, adoption, and promotion of data standards to facilitate electronic data sharing (receiving and transmitting data) to integrate surveillance systems designed for different data collection purposes.

Legal and Ethical Principles

Ethical and **legal principles** are essential to public health information systems.[3,16] Local, state, and federal government agencies have legal obligations to identify and control threats to public health, and to evaluate and improve public health programs and services.[3,16] Meeting these obligations requires agencies to collect, store, and utilize data from individuals that are often quite personal in nature.

The privacy and confidentiality of public health data and the need to protect human subjects from potential misuse are major concerns in informatics,[3,13,16,17] and careful attention is needed to ensure that the collection and maintenance of data are safeguarded. Information systems can contain data that could potentially be used in ways damaging to individuals. Databases may include full names, dates of birth, phone numbers, and addresses of individuals with certain types of diseases, health treatments, or genetic information. When making data available to others, great care must be taken to prevent identification of individuals, such as not providing extensive demographic information about a few people with a health condition in a sparsely populated rural area where everyone knows everyone else.

Some approaches that are used to ensure proper use of information technology in public health settings are: strong privacy and ethical guidelines and standards security measures such as physical protection and data encryption, and password requirements to limit those with access to potentially compromising data. As has been shown with financial data systems, technologic advances have allowed more data to be readily available in electronic formats to more people. This has resulted in increased privacy and security risks from inadvertent or malevolent release of individual identifying information (such as by computer hackers[3,17]). Imagine, for examine, the implications if credible information from a public health data system was released to a news media representative and revealed that a prominent politician or celebrity was undergoing treatment for a sexually transmitted disease or for substance abuse.

DATA ANALYSIS, INTERPRETATION, DISSEMINATION, AND PRESENTATION

Analysis and interpretation of public health data is based on a good understanding of statistics, epidemiology, evaluation research, and related fields. Historically, researchers obtained or generated an electronic dataset, and then wrote computer programs using statistical software such as SAS® or SPSS® to obtain results. Analysis also necessitated using specialists well versed in quantitative data analysis. This often caused delays in interpreting results, data dissemination, and public health ac-

tion. Advances in informatics have increased the speed and efficiency of data analysis and dissemination around the world. Visitors to public health data system websites, for example, can view preselected summary findings in tables or figures. Many websites allow users to select and analyze data of their own choosing, such as the number of cases or the percentage of a population with a health condition or risk factor by age group, gender, or geographic region. **Figures 3–2** and **3–3** provide examples of user-selected data analyses available from the CDC and National Cancer Institute websites.

With its ability to obtain and integrate data from multiple sources, informatics has advanced the development of the ability to map and analyze public health data using geographic information system (GIS) software and statistical approaches. The most common commercial use of GIS is the global positioning system (GPS) device now frequently used in automobiles and handheld devices. **Figure 3–4** provides an example of using GIS to identify specific New Orleans housing areas by level of flood damage associated with the 2005 hurricanes.[18]

GIS is just one example of how informatics has changed how data can be presented and influence interpretation. Publicly available state **dashboards** (software application control panels) created by the U.S. Agency for Healthcare Quality (**Figure 3–5**) demonstrate how data from more than 100 measures can be summarized into an overall rating of healthcare quality. Extensive amounts of data from different datasets can now be graphed and presented in rapid sequence as video clips using computer software such as Windows Media Player®. The Gapminder Foundation (gapminder.org) allows users to view long-term health and other data trends from many countries. For example, the association between longer average length of life and smaller family size since 1800 can be easily and dramatically visualized by the rapid sequential presentation of annual graphs.

FACTORS INFLUENCING USE OF INFORMATION TECHNOLOGY IN PUBLIC HEALTH

We have considered informatics principles and examples of how informatics is used in public health. The adoption, implementation, integration, and effective use of information systems, however, is complex and influenced by several other broad factors at the individual, social, and organizational level,[19,20] many of which form the basis of well-known theories and models (e.g., Social Cognitive Theory, Theory of Reasoned Action, PRECEDE–PROCEED Model, Diffusion of Innovation, Technology Acceptance model, and Task-Technology Fit Model). Not recognizing and adequately addressing these factors has led to the failure of many IT systems in public health and elsewhere.

Figure 3–2 Results for Miami-Dade County 2007, Youth Risk Behavior Survey, Unintentional Injuries and Violence

Results for Miami-Dade County 2007 compared with United States 2007*						
Unintentional Injuries and Violence						
	2007 Miami-Dade County Results		2007 United States Results			
Question	Percent	95% Confidence Interval	Percent	95% Confidence Interval	p-Value**	Difference***
Among students who rode a bicycle during the 12 months before the survey, the percentage who rarely or never wore a bicycle helmet	89.6	(86.5–92.0)	85.1	(82.3–87.6)	0.02	Different
Percentage of students who rarely or never wore a seat belt when riding in a car driven by someone else	13.3	(11.7–15.2)	11.1	(8.9–13.8)	0.14	Not Different
Percentage of students who rode one or more times during the 30 days before the survey in a car or other vehicle driven by someone who had been drinking alcohol	26.5	(24.3–28.7)	29.1	(27.1–31.2)	0.08	Not Different
Percentage of students who drove a car or other vehicle one or more times during the 30 days before the survey when they had been drinking alcohol	8.6	(7.4–10.0)	10.5	(9.3–11.9)	0.04	Different
Percentage of students who carried a weapon such as a gun, knife, or club on at least 1 day during the 30 days before the survey	14.2	(12.3–16.4)	18.0	(16.3–19.8)	<0.01	Different
Percentage of students who carried a gun on at least 1 day during the 30 days before the survey	5.5	(4.4–6.9)	5.2	(4.4–6.0)	0.60	Not Different

* Only locations that have weighted results in at least one survey year are available for this report.
** p-values were determined using a t-test.
*** Difference is statistically significant for p< 0.05.

Source: Centers for Disease Control and Prevention. "Youth Risk Behavioral Surveillance System. Youth online: comprehensive results." http//apps.nccd.cdc.gov/yrbss/. (Accessed July 8, 2010.)

FIGURE 3–3 Age-Adjusted Death Rates for Lung Cancer, White, Non-Hispanic Females, United States 2006

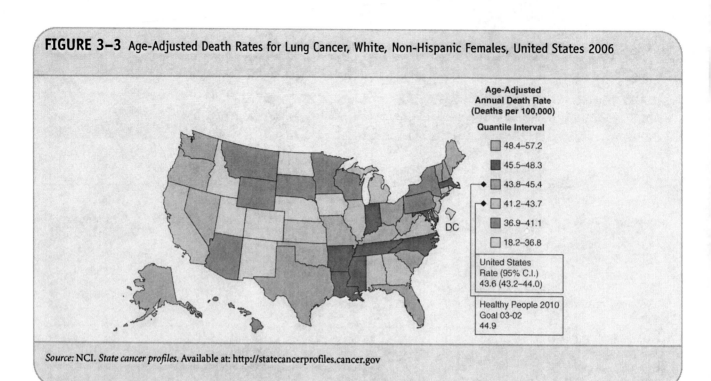

Source: NCI. *State cancer profiles.* Available at: http://statecancerprofiles.cancer.gov

FIGURE 3–4 Geographic Information System (GIS)-Generated Map of Flood-Damaged Housing in New Orleans Associated with Hurricanes Katrina and Rita, 2005

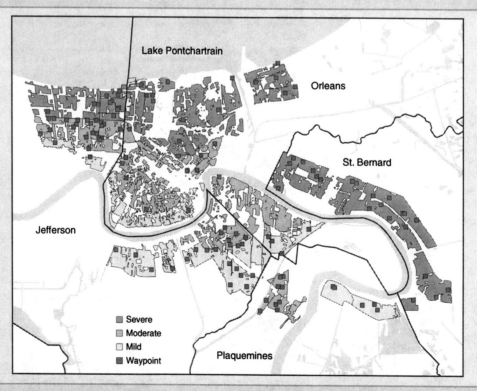

Source: CDC. Health concerns associated with mold in water-damaged homes after Hurricane Katrina and Rita—New Orleans area, Louisiana, October 2005. *MMWR.* 2006; 55:42. Available at: http://www.cdc.gov/mold/pdfs/mmwr55(2)41-44.pdf

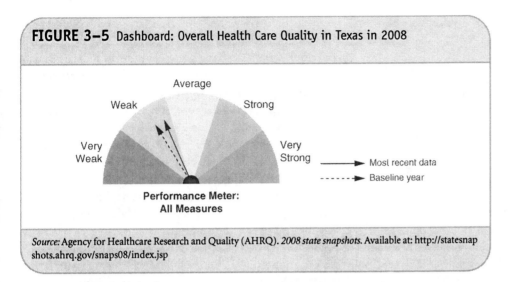

FIGURE 3–5 Dashboard: Overall Health Care Quality in Texas in 2008

Source: Agency for Healthcare Research and Quality (AHRQ). *2008 state snapshots*. Available at: http://statesnap shots.ahrq.gov/snaps08/index.jsp

At the individual level, there are several psychological traits and other characteristics that are highly influential in terms of adopting or rejecting IT.[19,20] Psychological trait examples include personal innovativeness (openness to trying and using new products), self-efficacy (beliefs about one's ability to perform IT-related tasks, skill level), and motivation. IT adoption is also influenced by how individuals assess its attributes, such as perceived ease of use; perceived usefulness; the "fit" of task to the technology; relative advantage over what is currently being used; compatibility with values and past experience; and the power and ability to make modifications.

At the social level, peers have a role in level of acceptance of IT and sometimes are the dominant factor affecting adoption and use.[20] The experiences and recommendations of other people (e.g., professional colleagues within one's organization or elsewhere), social group norms, and pressure to adhere to those norms are examples of social influences. Shared beliefs and the extent to which individuals consider themselves as valued and accepted by management within an organization are additional examples.

Organizational factors relate to the capability of IT to meet the needs and goals of an organization and fit it to the environment in which an organization operates. This can vary greatly from organization to organization.[19] Assessment of organizational needs and goals should be based on a thorough understanding of the way in which existing tasks are being conducted and on identification of tasks that are potentially amenable to IT. Understanding and addressing organizational factors is greatly enhanced if members of an organization, especially those who would use an IT application are empowered to contribute to its development, design, and adoption and participate actively.

CHALLENGES

Public health informatics presents a number of challenges. We have just discussed data collection management, ethical, and legal issues. Other major challenges remain, including overselling, applications and systems that are not user-centered, and funding.

Overselling the Benefits

Public health and medical care have not been spared from excessive hype and lofty expectations of informatics.[4,11] Public health practice is a complex and complicated endeavor. Mere availability of more health-related data and other types of information presented in understandable formats will not address the longstanding root causes of many public health problems, such as population health disparities or lack of health insurance. Complex individual, organizational, and societal problems are not resolvable by quick and easy technological fixes. Because information overload is now such a large challenge, the fundamentals of communication, such as developing messages based on the purpose and audience characteristics, are more applicable than ever to the area of public health informatics.[9]

No Easy Button

Many consider public health information systems and technology too complex and difficult for general use.[4,9,11] This stems from the failure of public health information technology and system developers to thoroughly understand the processes and organizations in which data and other information are collected[19] and from underutilization of user-centered design approaches to IT.[9] Look at Google and Amazon.com to find examples of IT that are user-focused.

Expense

IT systems can be financially expensive to acquire, develop, operate, and maintain. It is necessary to remember that just because data can be digitized and stored electronically in information systems (e.g., automated) does not mean they should be. Much of the funding for public health comes from government, that is, from taxpayers. During economic downturns like the current recession in the United States, public health agencies usually face funding cuts. IT systems may not be obtained or continued, and resources for IT training are likely to be reduced.

CONCLUSIONS

Public health informatics present new opportunities. Two of the most important are:

- Enhanced ability to communicate directly with the public.
- Increased convergence of public health and medical healthcare information systems.

IT advances provide unprecedented opportunities for the general public to receive or obtain health information, whether through information seeking (e.g., on websites) or by active communication efforts on the part of public health agencies, voluntary health organizations, or private companies (e.g., through listservs, social network sites, podcasts). Many consumers now take charge of their own health affairs and are well-versed in health prevention and treatment options.[4,11]

Informatics and IT advances allow segmentation of audiences by demographics, preferences and activities. Detailed segmentation can produce sharply focused target opportunities for tailored communication, e.g., to individuals with insulin-resistant diabetes who are at risk for stroke.

There are expanding possibilities for public health government agencies to partner with nongovernmental organizations, including businesses, to potentially reach a large number of people with credible and up-to-date health information. Such information can increasingly be presented in formats likely to appeal to the general public and other lay audiences.

Finally, there will be increased blurring of the lines between public health and medical informatics.[4,5,11] Continued development and expansion of electronic medical records (EMR) means that medical and other health information from a larger proportion of the population will be available for data analyses, especially among persons enrolled in large health care or health insurance programs. This will increase opportunities to integrate prevention and medical treatment, tailored to the needs of individuals, that may ultimately influence population health. Electronically generated reminders to doctors and nurses for prevention purposes (e.g., about the need for a flu shot or counseling about physical activity) are already in use in many healthcare facilities. The concept of the lifelong "personal health record"[19]—which could contain a large volume of clinical data, health-promoting activities, environmental exposures, and more in electronic format—may become a reality.

KEY TERMS

Behavioral Risk Factor Surveillance System (BRFSS)
Dashboard
Data user
DNA fingerprinting
Ethical principles
Information science
Interoperability
Legal principles
Public health informatics
Public health surveillance
Results user
Signal-to-noise ratio

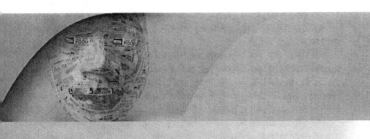

Chapter Questions

1. How is public health informatics related to medical and consumer health informatics? How is it uniquely different?

2. What are three different types of health conditions or events for which data are routinely collected and analyzed by public health agencies using informatics approaches?

3. What is the relationship between informatics and public health surveillance?

4. What are the informatics-related challenges involved in ensuring high-quality data are collected and maintained in public health data systems?

5. Why are the legal and ethical aspects of public health information systems so important?

6. How has informatics led to improvements in data analysis and visualization?

7. How do individual, social, and organizational factors influence decisions to adopt or reject information technology?

ACKNOWLEDGMENTS

We thank Susan Salkowitz, Ruth Gubernick, Anne Turner, Dwayne Jarman, Stephen Marcus, and Linda Pederson. In particular, Patrick O'Carroll and Rita Kukafka, leading national experts on public health informatics, provided in-depth interviews that will be posted on the book's website.

REFERENCES

1. O'Carroll PW, Yasnoff WA, Ward ME, Ripp LH, Martin EL (eds). *Public Health Informatics and Information Systems.* New York: Springer-Verlag; 2003.

2. Lombardo JS, Buckeridge DL (eds). *Disease Surveillance: A Public Health Informatics Approach.* Hoboken, NJ: John Wiley & Sons; 2007.

3. Lee LM, Gostin LO. Ethical collection, storage, and use of public health data. *JAMA.* 2009; 302:82-83.

4. Hesse BW. Harnessing the power of an intelligent health environment in cancer control. In: Bushko RG (ed). *Future of Intelligent and Extelligent Health Environment.* Fairfax, VA: IOS Press; 2005; pp. 159–176.

5. Kukafka R. Public health informatics: the nature of the field and its relevance to health promotion practice. *Health Promot Pract.* 2005; 6:23–28.

6. Kukafka R, Yasnoff W. Public health informatics. *J Biomed Inform.* 2007; 40:365–369.

7. Lee LM, Teutsch SM, St Louis ME, Thacker SB (eds). *Principles and Practice of Public Health Surveillance.* 3rd edition. New York: Oxford University Press. In press.

8. Centers for Disease Control and Prevention. Multistate outbreak of salmonella infections associated with peanut butter and peanut-butter-containing products—United States, 2008–2009. *MMWR Morbid Mortal Wkly Rep.* 2009; 58:85–90.

9. Nelson DE, Hesse BW, Croyle RT. *Making Data Talk: Communicating Public Health Data to the Public, Policy Makers, and the Press.* New York: Oxford University Press; 2009.

10. Bennet GC, Glasgow RE. The delivery of public health interventions via the Internet: Actualizing their potential. *Annu Rev Public Health.* 2009; 30:273–292.

11. Hesse BW. Public health informatics. In Gibbons MC (ed). *eHealth Solutions for Healthcare Disparities.* New York: Springer; 2007; pp. 109–219.

12. Graham AL, Cobb NK, Raymond L, Sill S, Young J. Effectiveness of an Internet-based worksite smoking cessation intervention at 12 months. *J Occup Environ Med.* 2007; 49:821–828.

13. Koo D, O'Carroll P, LaVenture M. Public health 101 for informaticians. *J Am Med Inform Assoc.* 2001; 8:585–597.

14. CDC. Updated guidelines for evaluating public health surveillance systems. *MMWR Morbid Mortal Wkly Rep.* 2001; 50(RR-13):1–29.

15. Dwyer L, Foster KL, Safranek T. Status of state electronic disease surveillance systems—United States, 2007. *MMWR Morbid Mortal Wkly Rep.* 2009; 58:804–807.

16. Goodman RA, Hoffman RE, Lopez W, Matthews GW, Rothstein MA, Foster KL (eds). *Law in Public Health Practice.* 2nd edition. New York: Oxford University Press; 2006.

17. Lurie N, Fremont A. Building bridges between medical care and public health. *JAMA.* 2009; 302:84–86.

18. CDC. Health concerns associated with mold in water-damaged homes after hurricanes Katrina and Rita—New Orleans area, Louisiana, October 2005. *MMWR Morbid Mortal Wkly Rep.* 2006; 55:41–44.

19. Kukafka R, Johnson SB, Linfante A, Allegrante JP. Grounding a new information technology implementation framework in behavioral science: a systematic analysis of the literature on IT use. *J Biomed Inform.* 2003; 36: 218–227.

20. Park S, O'Brien MA, Caine KE, Rogers WA, Fisk AD, Van Ittersum K, et al. Acceptance of computer technology: understanding the user and the organizational characteristics. *Proceeding of the Human Factors and Ergonomics Society, 50th Annual Meeting.* Santa Monica, CA: Human Factors and Ergonomics Society; 2006; pp. 1478–1482.

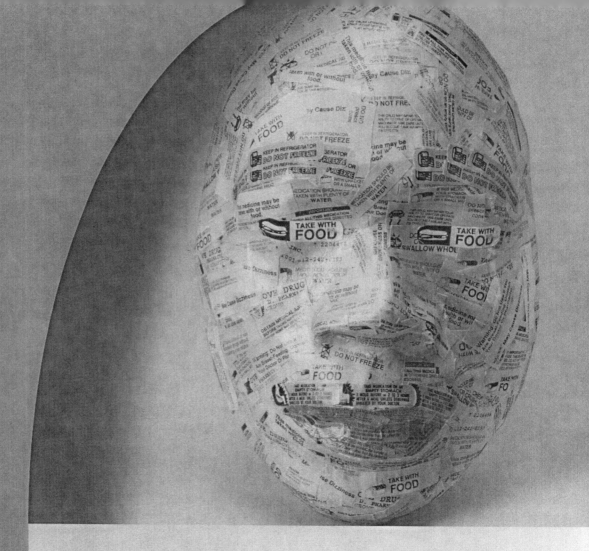

Informing and Educating People about Health Issues

CHAPTER 4

Understanding and Reporting the Science

David E. Nelson

LEARNING OBJECTIVES

By the end of this chapter, the reader will be able to:

- Assess the quality of scientific evidence and level of consensus among scientists on public health issues.
- Identify sources of more credible scientific information.
- Understand factors influencing how "nonscientific audiences" process and understand scientific information.
- Recognize four questions that the general public usually asks concerning a scientific study or report: What did you find (description)? Why did it happen (explanation)? What does it mean (interpretation)? What needs to be done about it (action)?
- Use a single overriding communication objective (SOCO) form to help shape a scientific report for different audiences.

INTRODUCTION

Science is the fundamental basis for public health.[1] The collection, analysis, and interpretation of data using scientific and statistical principles and methods provide the evidence that supports public health actions and recommendations. The effectiveness of public health as a field depends heavily on the synthesis of scientific research and communication of science to those who "need to know it." Two critical but often underappreciated roles for public health practitioners are to:

- Assess the state of scientific knowledge about a specific topic or issue.
- Communicate scientific findings to lay persons, with an eye toward what the findings mean for their audiences.[2,3]

Discussion of scientific principles and methods is beyond the scope of this book and is the subject matter for courses in epidemiology, evaluation, environmental health and behavioral science. Nevertheless, to have a career in public health one must understand and communicate about these areas to persons with little or no training in the public health sciences.

Following are some valuable recommendations for understanding the quality of scientific research and for communicating key scientific findings and conclusions to lay audiences such as the public, policymakers, news media members, and organizational representatives.

EVALUATING QUALITY IN PUBLIC HEALTH SCIENCE

Science is a body of knowledge learned through systemic study using agreed-upon methodologies by others in the same field that attempts to discover generalized truths about phenomena using hypotheses and deductions.[3] Scientific knowledge is primarily gained through analyses of quantitative and qualitative data using mathematical and logical principles. Many types of scientific discipline contribute to public health, ranging from public health policy analysis at one end to molecular studies in laboratories at the other.

Assessing the quality of scientific knowledge means being able to determine characteristics of "better science," that is, being able to separate the wheat from the chaff. It is true that determining scientific quality can be difficult at times, and occasionally experts can be fooled (e.g., when published studies in prominent journals are retracted because of data falsification or failure to report potential conflicts of interest). Nevertheless, there are three broad categories of factors to examine when considering the quality of scientific information relating to the research itself, the level of scientific consensus, and the source of the information (**Table 4–1**).

Research Considerations
Study Designs

There is strong consensus among scientists that some types of research study designs are stronger than others because they

TABLE 4–1 Factors Influencing the Quality of Science in Public Health

- Research considerations
  - Design
  - Representativeness
  - Causality
- Level of scientific consensus
  - Research syntheses
  - Contextual information
- Sources
  - Authors and their institutions
  - Publications and publishers of scientific work

Source: Adapted from:
Turnock BJ. *Public health: What it is and how it works.* Gaithersburg, MD: Aspen; 1997.
U.S. Department of Health, Education, and Welfare, Public Health Service. *Smoking and health: Report of the Advisory Committee to the Surgeon General of the Public Health Service.* Washington, DC: Government Printing Office; 1964. PHS Publication No. 1103.

minimize bias.[4] Without going into detail, the following types of **study designs** are listed from strongest to weakest:

- Experimental or quasi-experimental studies.
- Cohort studies.
- Case-control studies.
- Time-series studies.
- Cross-sectional studies (e.g., surveys).
- Ecologic studies.
- Case studies.

Classic **experimental studies** involve researchers "exposing" group of subjects (e.g., people or animals) to an intervention and comparing the results with those from a group of unexposed subjects who are generally similar to the exposed group. A common example is a drug study in which one group of individuals receives a particular drug and another does not; outcomes are measured in both groups. A quasi-experimental design is one that studies groups in a natural setting (i.e., not controlled by the researcher), e.g., comparing a state with a mandatory immunization law to a state without such a law.

Cohort studies involve a group of individuals for whom data are either collected prospectively (going forward) or for whom historical data exist (retrospective or looking backward). Data are examined for changes over time, such as whether there are changes in one subgroup exposed to some sort of "treatment" or stimulus (e.g., a chemical in an occupational environment) compared with an unexposed subgroup. In **case-control studies** data are collected (often through surveys) about past exposures in a population with a health issue (a disease or condition) and compared with similar data collected from a comparable control group without the disease or condition.

Time-series studies analyze data in one population and typically compare data before and after an intervention occurs, e.g., the percentage of individuals observed wearing a seatbelt before and after a seatbelt law was enacted. A separate comparison population is not used. **Cross-sectional studies** collect data from subjects at one time. The most typical cross-sectional study is a survey. The major drawback of this study design is the collection of data on potential exposures and outcomes at the same time. The lack of sequential data makes it difficult to determine whether or not exposures actually *preceded* potential outcomes of interest.

Ecologic studies typically involve correlating or comparing two types of population-level data. While *such studies of association* can be valuable for generating hypotheses (e.g., smoking prevalence tends to be higher in areas where populations have lower socioeconomic status), they can produce extremely misleading results because association does not mean causation. For example, the association of a higher prevalence of telephone answering machines with lower levels of sexually transmitted diseases (STDs) does not mean answering machines reduce the risk of contracting STDs. Finally, **case studies** report findings from a small number of people or animals having the same disease or symptoms. Case studies are most commonly used in investigations of outbreaks of potentially serious diseases or exposures, such as tuberculosis, pertussis, or to study persons with acute exposures to chemicals (e.g., mercury or hydrogen fluoride).

Population Sample Considerations

In addition to examining study designs, it is important to assess the types of data and whether these data are based on populations that are representative. Although animal models (e.g., studies based on mice) have been extremely useful in science, findings from animal studies may not be applicable to humans. Other important considerations are the number of individuals included in a study and whether or not they are representative of larger populations. Unfortunately, many widely reported studies are based on small numbers of subjects or are obtained from samples of people who are not representative of the general population.

Association and Causality

A longstanding issue in epidemiology and in interpretation of results from scientific studies is the concept of **causality**. For example, if a study demonstrates that risk factor A is strongly associated with health condition B, can we infer that A caused B? Seminal work conducted in the 1960s for the 1964 U.S. Surgeon General's Report on smoking and cancer,[5] and by the noted British statistician Bradford Hill,[6] were identified and remain relevant today as ways to assess the quality of scientific findings and their interpretation.

As is evident from **Table 4–2**, assessing causality involves several considerations. The strength of association means that the greater the size of an observed effect or relationship, the greater is the likelihood that there is a causal relationship (i.e., a study finding that persons using pharmaceutical product Y were 10 times more likely to develop kidney failure than persons not using the product provides much stronger evidence for causality than if exposed persons were only 1.5 times more likely to develop this condition).

Time sequence refers to demonstrating that exposure occurred prior to the development of the observed outcome. *Consistency upon repetition* means that several other research studies have found similar relationships between A and B; *biological gradient* means that persons with greater exposure to A are at higher risk of developing outcome B than those exposed to lower levels of A. *Plausibility* and *coherence of explanation* are closely related to each other. Simply put, an observed association has to be biologically plausible, as well as consistent with other lines of evidence (e.g., with animal studies or time series studies).

Scientific Consensus

Following directly upon the discussion of causation and coherence of explanation, the second major type of factor for assessing the quality of the science is the level of **scientific consensus**. The past two decades have seen an explosion of interest in the compilation and application of "evidence-based" health research findings. Evidence-based findings are obtained by review and classification of available published scientific literature, usually by an expert panel or working group. Such findings now exist for literally hundreds of specific topics, ranging from the relative effectiveness of individual drugs to the selection of community interventions or policies to reduce health risks.[7–10]

While one can debate what constitutes the best research evidence on which to base an **evidence-based intervention**, the key point here is that given the ever-expanding number of health-related studies, there is a great need for syntheses of research such that scientists, practitioners, and lay audiences are provided with consensus information about "the state of the science" and its implications for public health. These types of research syntheses can be invaluable sources of scientific information that are worth communicating to lay audiences. There are four major types of scientific research syntheses:

- Comprehensive organization reports.
- Consensus conference reports.
- Meta-analytic studies of findings from prior research.
- Review articles in professional journals.

Several types of agencies and organizations periodically bring together groups of scientists to conduct systematic reviews of the scientific literature on specific topics. Well-known public health examples include the Surgeon General's Reports on tobacco and other topics, the **Guide to Community Preventive Services**,[7,8] and the **Guide to Clinical Preventive Services**.[9] (**Box 4–1** provides brief descriptions of these resources.)

Other organizations that routinely conduct systematic literature reviews and syntheses include the International Agency for Research on Cancer (IARC) and the Cochrane Collaboration. The completion and publication of these types of reports can be lengthy, sometimes taking several years.

Comprehensive organization reports can be invaluable resources for communication because they are conducted by organizations seen as credible (see the later discussion on sources) and vouch for the results and conclusions. They are usually viewed by other scientists as definitive because of the exhaustive processes used to identify and assess the strength of studies. From a public health practice perspective, they can often be used to develop messages directly relevant for public health practice, e.g., "The United States Preventive Services Task Force recommends screening for colorectal cancer among persons aged 50 to 75 years."

Another resource for ascertaining the level of scientific consensus are consensus conference reports derived from consensus conferences or periodic meetings, whereby leading experts are asked to reach consensus on a topic based on research in their field. The best-known examples of these are the National Institutes of Health (NIH) Consensus Development Statement process[11] and periodic reviews and reports produced by the National Academies of Science (e.g., Institute of Medicine Reports[12]). Both the NIH and National Academies of Science have rigorous processes for selecting scientific experts, conducting extensive literature reviews, and producing summary reports.

Meta-analysis refers to studies where researchers conduct research based on previous research. Using a set of well-defined rules for selecting studies and data sources, statistical approaches have been developed within the past 25 years whereby researchers can pool data from multiple studies on the same topic and calculate a summary measure estimating the level of association between exposure A and outcome B (e.g., motor vehicle safety public health campaigns and their effect on seatbelt use). Meta-analyses have been conducted as part of developing comprehensive reports or for consensus conferences under the auspices of sponsoring organizations, but most are conducted independently and published in scientific journals.

The final type of research syntheses are review articles in scientific journals. For these reviews, researchers usually use keywords and search for available articles on a topic over a period of time from one or more databases (e.g., PubMed or PsychInfo). Authors of review articles then generally provide a list of the articles they reviewed and summarize what they

TABLE 4–2 Important Considerations for Assessing Causality: Hill's Criteria

Label	Meaning	Rules of Evidence
1. Strength of association	What is the magnitude of relative risk?	The probability of a causal association increases as the summary relative risk estimate increases. Hill himself was suspicious of relative risks less than two. Others have set the limits higher. However, a relative risk of less than two does not rule out the possibility of causality.
2. Dose-response	Does a correlation exist between exposure and effect?	A regularly increasing relationship between dose and magnitude is indicative of a causal association. This works for bad things, such as the greater exposure to radiation, the worse your symptoms (usually). And it also works for things we are trying to measure in behavior change, such as if you are exposed to 10 PSA screening tests for prostate cancers as opposed to 1, will your behavior be any different?
3. Consistency of response	How many times has this effect been reported in various populations under similar conditions?	The probability of a causal association increases as the proportion of studies with similar (e.g., positive) results increases.
4. Temporally correct association	Does the exposure precede the effect, or does the occurrence of the disease show the appropriate latency?	Exposure to a causal factor *must* precede the effect. This is an *immutable requirement* that is often ignored.
5. Specificity of the association	How specific is this effect? Do many things influence the effect?	For uncommon health effects (e.g., liver cancer), this evidence can be useful. For diseases with many causes, it is of little use.
6. Biological plausibility	Is the mechanism of action known or reasonably postulated?	See criterion 7.
7. Coherence	Does the cause–effect interpretation seriously conflict with generally known facts of the natural history and biology of the disease?	While a mechanism of action is not a requirement for determining causality, the finding of causality should not be biologically implausible. In contrast, a plausible mechanism of action or other supportive evidence increases the likelihood of a causal association.
8. Experimental evidence	Do laboratory animals show a similar effect?	As in criteria 6 and 7, findings in laboratory animals are supportive of a causal association. However, some chemicals that are notably carcinogenic to humans have tested negative in animal studies.
9. Analogy	Do structurally similar chemicals cause similar effects?	For some classes of compounds, such as nitrosamines, structure-activity predictions can be supportive of a causal association. In contrast, materials such as organotins do not lend themselves to cross-class extrapolations.

Source: Adapted from:
Friis RH, Sellers TA. *Epidemiology for public health practice.* Gaithersburg, MD: Aspen; 1999.
U.S. Department of Health, Education, and Welfare, Public Health Service. *Smoking and health: Report of the Advisory Committee to the Surgeon General of the Public Health Service.* Washington, DC: Government Printing Office; 1964. PHS Publication No. 1103.
Hill AB. The environment and disease: association or causation? *Proc R Acad Med.* 1965; 295–300.

Box 4–1 Guide to Community Preventive Services and Guide to Clinical Preventive Services

The **Guide to Community Preventive Services** is a resource sponsored by the Task Force on Community Preventive Services and hosted on a website at CDC. It is designed to help users select programs and policies to improve health and prevent disease in communities. Rigorous, systematic reviews of scientific research studies, with a particular emphasis on the quality of study designs, are used to determine the effectiveness of programs and policies. When possible, it includes analyses to assess cost effectiveness and other economic-related considerations.

More than 200 interventions have been completed, and the Task Force has issued recommendations covering the following areas:

Adolescent health	Obesity
Alcohol	Oral health
Asthma	Physical activity
Birth defects	Social environment
Cancer	Tobacco
Diabetes	Vaccines
HIV/AIDS, STIs,[a] and pregnancy	Violence
Mental health	Worksite

Here are examples of Task Force recommendations:

- Increasing the unit price of alcohol by raising taxes is recommended based on strong evidence of effectiveness for reducing excessive alcohol consumption and related harms. Public health effects are expected to be proportional to the size of the tax increase.
- Community water fluoridation is recommended based on strong evidence of effectiveness in reducing tooth decay.
- There was *insufficient evidence* to determine the effectiveness of school-based programs to prevent or reduce overweight and obesity among children and adolescents because of a limited number of studies that reported noncomparable outcomes.
- There was *insufficient evidence* to determine the effectiveness of educational and policy approaches in health care or for health-care providers in reducing UV [ultraviolet light] exposure or increasing sun-protective behaviors. Too few articles of sufficient design and execution quality evaluated the effectiveness of these interventions in changing recommendation outcomes.

[a]sexually transmitted infections

The **Guide to Clinical Preventive Services** contains the U.S. Preventive Services Task Force (USPSTF) recommendations on the use of screening, counseling, and other individual-level preventive services that are typically delivered in primary healthcare settings, and it is available on a web site hosted by the Agency for Healthcare Quality Research (AHRQ). Examples include screening for disease, counseling, and preventive medications. USPSTF recommendations have formed the basis of the clinical standards for many professional societies, health organizations, and medical quality review groups. They have been used widely in healthcare settings to teach preventive care.

The USPSTF is an independent panel of experts supported by the federal Agency for Healthcare Research and Quality (AHRQ) and makes recommendations based on systematic reviews of the scientific literature related to the benefits and potential harms of clinical preventive services. The Task Force grades the strength of scientific evidence: A (strongly recommends), B (recommends), C (no recommendation for or against), D (recommends against), or I (insufficient evidence to recommend for or against).

Here are examples of USPSTF recommendations:

Strongly recommends that clinicians screen all adults for tobacco use and provide tobacco cessation interventions for those who use tobacco products. Grade: A recommendation.

Recommends screening for chlamydial infection for all pregnant women aged 24 and younger and for older pregnant women who are at increased risk. Grade: B recommendation.

The *evidence is insufficient* to recommend for or against the routine use of interventions to prevent low back pain in adults in primary care settings. Grade: I statement.

Recommends against screening adults for chronic obstructive pulmonary disease (COPD) using spirometry. Grade: D recommendation.

Sources:

Task Force on Community Preventive Services. *Guide to community preventive services: What works to promote health.* Atlanta, GA: Task Force on Community Preventive Services; 2009. http://www.thecommunityguide.org

U.S. Preventive Services Task Force. *Guide to clinical preventive services, 2008.* Rockville, MD: Agency for Healthcare Research and Quality; 2008. http://www.ahrq.gov/clinic/pocketgd08/

consider as the key conclusions based on the information available in the literature they reviewed.

Keep in mind that although scientific research syntheses are invaluable resources for assessing the quality of the science and consensus among scientists, they have two main drawbacks. First, there is a well-known tendency of scientific journals to preferentially publish articles with positive rather than negative findings—that is, "A is associated with B" rather than "there is no association between A and B." Unless careful attempts are made to uncover studies with negative results, including unpublished studies, research syntheses can be more likely to conclude that potentially spurious associations exist. Second, studies of review articles on tobacco issues and on some pharmaceutical products strongly suggest that conclusions can be biased depending on whether authors have received financial support from tobacco or drug companies.

Another important question to consider that is directly related to the level of scientific consensus and the quality of science is the context in which scientific findings are presented.[3] There is unprecedented, widespread availability of scientific and other types of information now available through the Internet and other sources. Probably every reader of this book has received a widely disseminated e-mail containing some type of startling new finding that was later discovered to be a hoax.

Given the level of hype that can surround certain scientific studies or findings, it is more important than ever to ascertain from a journal article, oral presentation, news story, or other source whether the contextual considerations for a scientific finding are addressed. Unfortunately, over generalization and over interpretation of scientific findings are widespread problems.[2] Table 4–3 includes a list of questions to consider whenever you learn about new scientific information. The individuals and organizations responsible for completing and publishing high-quality scientific studies and research syntheses should be able to readily provide answers to all of these questions without hesitation.

Sources

A common mental shortcut that people use to assess information quality is the perceived *credibility* (trustworthiness and expertise) of the source of that information.[3] For example, you are more likely to believe the information you learn about an automobile radiator from a mechanic than from someone with no experience repairing automobiles. Persons or institutions with potential conflicts of interests, such as alcohol beverage companies, are not likely to be good sources of information about the health risks associated with misuse of alcohol. The same principle holds true when assessing scientific information: some information sources are far more likely than others to have scientific information of higher quality.

TABLE 4–3 Contextual Questions to Consider When Evaluating New Scientific Information

- Have findings been included in a scientifically credible publication?
- Are these findings preliminary?
- Are these new findings, or have they been previously reported?
- How do they compare with previous research? (If findings are different, why should these results be considered more believable than prior research?)
- How certain is it that the results are not due to chance?
- What are potential alternative explanations?
- Can these results be generalized to other populations?
- What are the limitations of these findings?
- What is potentially missing?
- Should judgment be withheld until more evidence is available (e.g., completion of other studies)?
- What do other scientific experts in the same field say about these findings?

Source: Adapted from: Nelson DE, Brownson RC, Remington PL, Parvanta C (eds). *Communicating public health information effectively.* Washington, DC: American Public Health Association; 2002.

Source credibility for scientific information can be considered along two dimensions: (1) the reporting scientists and their respective institutions and (2) the publication or publisher of the reports. The credibility of individual researchers is based on their prior research, reputation within their field among other scientists, and the institution at which they work. With the great availability of searchable databases and Internet search engines such as Google, it is fairly easy to search for prior research publications by individual scientists.

The prominence of the organization a scientist works for is of additional importance. Persons employed at more renowned scientific research organizations (e.g., Johns Hopkins University, NIH) are likely to have higher credibility—although this is certainly not *always* the case—because obtaining and retaining positions in these organizations is highly competitive. Furthermore, for some governmental health agencies such as the CDC, scientific publications go through an extensive review process during which other scientists have the opportunity to review and make suggested improvements prior to publication.

Just as credibility can be based on "whether" scientists' research findings are published, credibility can also be based on "where," or in which publications, the findings are published. Obviously, scientists who have been published extensively in more prominent scientific journals have more proven track records, and thus are likely to be more credible. As mentioned previously, the organizations or institutions responsible for publishing major research syntheses (e.g., the Task Force for Preventive Services and the Institute of Medicine) have high credibility in the scientific community because of the rigorous nature of their research review process. Furthermore, scientists and the news media consider certain prestigious scientific journals, such as *Science, New England Journal of Medicine,* the *Journal of the American Medical Association* (*JAMA*), and *The Lancet,* as being highly credible sources.

Keep in mind that some organizations whose major emphasis is not science publish reports on public health topics related to their area of interest, and these publications can sometimes garner much attention from the media and others. Such reports are not to be confused with comprehensive organization or consensus conference reports. There is great variability among these organizations concerning the level of scientific review, quality of information, and soundness of recommendations. For example, a report on cancer screening from the American Cancer Society, an established voluntary health organization with a long history of scientific involvement, is likely to be highly credible. On the other hand, you should be especially wary of research reviews and recommendations by advocacy-oriented organizations: they may "cherry pick" studies (take findings out of context) to promote particular points of view or recommendations.

In sum, there are many factors that can influence the quality of science and scientific information. You don't have to be a practicing scientist, however, to assess quality. Careful consideration of the factors described here and a healthy dose of skepticism will go a long way toward ensuring that you can locate high-quality scientific information to communicate to others.

HOW LAY AUDIENCES EVALUATE AND PROCESS SCIENCE-BASED PUBLIC HEALTH INFORMATION

There are a number of factors that affect the way non-scientists process and understand scientific information in public health. It is essential to remember that people are not empty vessels—they have different health-related experiences, preexisting beliefs about health, and worldviews.[3,13]

Interest

Readers of this book are especially interested in health issues but health is of only low to moderate interest in the population at large.[3] Research has shown that people who are most interested in health issues tend to be older, female, and have generally better personal health. Others who tend to have strong health interest are those who have experienced health problems themselves or who have close family members with such problems, referred to as *involvement*.[14] The vast majority of people are not thinking about health on a daily basis. Extra ef-

fort is required to gain their attention and let them know why they should care about a particular public health issue.

Culture and Worldview

Many of us in public health do not appreciate the extent to which people have formed their own theories about health. When coupled with broader societal beliefs this complicates communication about scientific findings. Some people have grown up with a completely different tradition of medicine, for example, European homeopathy and botanical cures or southeastern and southern Asian systems that seek equilibrium in bodily humors or energy flow *(chi)*. The NIH is devoting resources to exploring the efficacy of alternative medical therapies. As of this writing, few have attained the level of scientific evidence described by the standards described earlier.

While not a "medical tradition," Americans have several homegrown health beliefs: exposure to cold temperatures causes the common cold, stress gives you high blood pressure, spicy food gives you ulcers, or large doses of vitamins are beneficial to health. These and other deeply held beliefs, some of which stem from a **worldview**, can interfere with scientific health information. Worldview refers to how people perceive their level of control over their own lives and how they think about power and wealth distribution. Examples include fatalism, individualism, egalitarianism, or respect and trust for authority. People with a strong individualistic worldview, for instance, may be opposed to mandatory motorcycle helmet or immunization laws, believing that these laws constitute an unacceptable infringement on individual choice. People with a strong fatalistic worldview often do not believe in screening tests, thinking that if they are meant to die of cancer, they will. People who think the government is untrustworthy might apply this view to all governmental branches and divisions, including the CDC or local health departments. Arguments based on scientific evidence may be ignored by persons with such worldviews.

Trust and Belief

With all that has been discussed about what constitutes strong scientific evidence, sometimes it has nothing to do with the "credibility" people give to a piece of information. People may trust their friends, family members, work colleagues, clergy, the mass media, the Internet, community organization leaders, and others before they trust anything a "pointy headed scientist" has to say. Often anecdotes are viewed as highly credible, for example, "My sister-in-law's friend has been on the pizza diet for 2 weeks and lost 20 pounds. It really works." The anecdotes of others who tried the diet and lost nothing go unconsidered.

The acceptance or disbelief of health information is strongly influenced by two psychological principles: confirmation bias and selective exposure.[15] **Confirmation bias** means that we tend to interpret messages as confirming what we already believe. A classic example of this is a cigarette smoker who, when he or she learns of someone who smoked all of his or her life and died at age 85, sees this as confirmation that the adverse health effects from smoking are exaggerated and that he or she does not need to quit smoking.

Selective exposure means that people like to obtain information from sources with which they agree. We generally like people or mass media sources that espouse opinions similar to our own and that tell us what we want to hear. This is especially challenging now that people have so many communication resources available to them. It has become difficult and expensive to produce a distinctive, scientifically sound public health message that can attract the attention of a nonempathetic or distracted audience.

We discuss Information Processing Theory in Chapter 7. This suggests that our ability to process large quantities of information is limited. Thus, when people are exposed to a lot of information, particularly information that may be complex or unfamiliar, they may "tune it out" or just remember the first or last item. What this means is that we need to be careful how much information we use in our messages, striving to highlight the key points without overwhelming people. Except among persons highly involved in a particular health issue, providing more information will rarely help audiences better comprehend your key messages.

Keep in mind when seeking information, people usually want to get right to the bottom line: what is the key point or gist? This is related to **satisficing**,[15] a term coined (*satisfy* + *suffice*) to describe what happens when people search for information quickly. Since they do not want to expend much time or energy searching, when they find what they need, they search no further. Satisficing is especially common among busy people, such as journalists and policymakers.

People have a strong desire for certainty.[3] When they hear advice from experts, regardless of their field, they want the advice to be definitive. Public health professionals often come up against this challenge. For some types of situation, such as public health outbreaks or potential clusters of disease (e.g., cancer), the cause or solution might take time to discover. In other cases it can take time to realize that no action is warranted because there is no causative agent. When scientists cannot provide definitive answers, or provide an answer that suggests "no action be taken," the public can become fearful and angry. (More on this in Chapter 16.)

A further complication is that many people have difficulty accepting that explanations or recommendations by scientists can change on the basis of further research. For example, healthcare providers for many years recommended that per-

sons with acne avoid consuming high-fat foods because of a presumed causal link. Later, as the result of well-designed research studies, this presumed association was disproved (Of course, this does not mean that consuming diets lower in fat is not a good for health for other reasons).

As should be clear by now, communicating scientific information for public health improvement is complex. Much more is involved than simply explaining findings and making recommendations with the expectation that audiences will believe what we say and do what we want them to do. Even when a public health intervention is supported by strong scientific evidence and consensus, communicating the science will not necessarily lead to a change in behavior.

COMMUNICATING SCIENTIFIC INFORMATION TO LAY AUDIENCES

Content

An important lesson from the fields of communication research and practice is to carefully consider what audiences want from public health and other types of experts.[3,16] From a practical perspective, most people want the answers to these four questions:

1. What did you find (description)?
2. Why did it happen (explanation)?
3. What does it mean (interpretation)?
4. What needs to be done about it (action)?

Description is the journalist's basic "who, what, where, and when?" In a hypothetical example, "*more than 100 people experienced a severe bout of gastrointestinal illness within 24 to 72 hours after attending a church picnic in Anytown, Anystate on June 15, 2009. Further research demonstrated that the affected individuals had a salmonella infection.*"

Explanation and **interpretation** are closely related because they attempt to answer the questions "how" and "why." For example, the explanation for a food-borne outbreak might be, "*Research indicates that those people who ate cheese sauce were more likely to develop the symptoms. The laboratory confirmed that the cheese sauce was heavily contaminated with salmonella.*" Interpretation typically involves trying to determine why findings were what they were, such as hypotheses or theories to explain causal relationships or associations, "*The cheese sauce was inadequately refrigerated, thus providing an opportunity for salmonella to grow.*"

Many scientists focus heavily on description, explanation, and interpretation of scientific information such as research results or public health surveillance findings. However, using messages that raise awareness about a public health problem can create emotional tension, particularly fear. When fear, anger or outrage are raised, people may deny the importance of the problem, become overly optimistic that they are not at risk, or search for someone or something to blame.

The public, policymakers, the press, and others look to public health experts for advice on what should be done to address the problem, that is, what action(s) is needed. Simply put, people want to know how to use information they receive to make decisions.[3] At an individual level, this might mean taking steps to avoid certain adverse health effects (e.g., drink bottled water because of water-borne parasites). For policymakers, this means enacting (or continuing) a remedial recommendation or policy, such as closing a manufacturing plant producing contaminated food products or enacting legislation requiring health insurers to cover contraceptive services. Recommending sources for additional information (government agency, emergency number, TV channel, website, etc.) is another way help to those who want to learn more.

Context

Another key aspect of communicating scientific findings is placement in proper context. Scientific findings always need to be considered in the general context of prior research and recommendations (see Table 4–3). For effective health communication it can be useful to present the same results in the context of the target community. For instance, if a major scientific study demonstrated the value of a screening test, local news could identify where people in a given community may obtain the test. If the news reports about a disease outbreak occurring in another state, it would be a good time to share information on hygiene habits to reduce the risk of contracting a methicillin-resistant *Staphylococcus aureus* (MRSA) skin infection.

Overload

Finally, interpretation of scientific information can be mentally taxing, especially when too much is presented and the information is as complex. It is important to present only the essential information to avoid problems of information overload. Carefully consider, for example, whether numbers should be used in messages at all, let alone which numbers to select (see Chapter 7). For text or visual materials, highlighting key points can be done in several different ways:

- Providing short executive summaries or including key points or conclusions up-front (especially for longer reports).
- Bolding key words.
- Ensuring an adequate amount of open (white) space to avoid crowding.
- Using arrows in figures to demonstrate key points or relationships.
- Including short and descriptive labels or legends in figures.

SOCO

There are communication tools to help you learn to be succinct in writing or speaking about health and science information. The CDC Media Relations office developed a template called the **single overriding communication objective (SOCO)** form. The idea of a message that "socks you in the mouth" (or wherever) was intentional.

Box 4–2 shows a SOCO template in use at the CDC today.

CASE STUDIES

We think a good way to learn how to prepare a news report or other reports of scientific findings is to first deconstruct two scientific publications used extensively in public health. The first example comes from a short research study about a 2003 outbreak investigation reported in the *Morbidity and Mortality Weekly Report* (MMWR),[17] published by the CDC. The second example is based on a lengthy report published by the U.S. Surgeon General in 2006 on the adverse health effects of exposure to secondhand smoke from tobacco products.[18,19] These examples were selected because they represent opposite ends of the spectrum of scientific documents that public health professionals may be asked to assess scientifically, summarize, and communicate about to different audiences.

MMWR Article

Box 4–3 contains an MMWR article about a measles outbreak at a Pennsylvania boarding school in 2003.[17] As of 2003, this outbreak of 11 confirmed cases was the largest of its kind in the United States since 1998. Nearly all cases identified could be linked to a student who had been exposed to measles while traveling in Lebanon and became ill after returning to the Pennsylvania school. The outbreak was controlled through vaccination and through exclusion, or isolation, of students and staff who had interacted with the infected child.

Assessing the science supporting health communication involves considering the research itself, the level of scientific consensus, and the sources (see Table 4–1). As discussed previously, even though a case study is generally considered the weakest study design, it is appropriate for a measles outbreak. Measles is now a rare, but highly contagious disease. Therefore, even a single laboratory-confirmed case is a cause for concern. Noteworthy in the example was the extensive effort of the researchers to ascertain the vaccination status of students and staff so that appropriate control efforts were implemented in the proper groups. Issues of representativeness and causality did not warrant consideration in this study. Instead, the workers had an urgent need to define the diagnostic criteria for measles clearly (symptoms, such as rash, fever, runny nose, and laboratory tests), identify cases, and treat

Box 4–2 CDC SOCO Template

Office of Communication/Media Relations

2   MMWR FACT SHEET

Single Overriding Health Communication Objective (SOHCO)

In one paragraph, please state the key point or objective of your MMWR submission. This statement should reflect what you, the writer, would like to see as the lead paragraph in a newspaper story or in a broadcast news report about your submission.

List three facts or statistics you would like the public to remember as a result of reading or hearing about your article?

What is the main audience or population segment you would like this article to reach?

Primary	Secondary

What is the one message the audience needs to take from this article?

Who in your office will serve as the point-of-contact for media questions?

Name: Degree(s):   Phone:

Title: Division/Center:

Date and time available:

Box 4–3 MMWR Article about Measles

Measles Outbreak in a Boarding School—Pennsylvania, 2003

Measles has not been endemic in the United States since 1997, although limited outbreaks continue to be caused by imported cases (*1,2*). In 2003, CDC assisted in investigating the largest school outbreak of measles in the United States since 1998 (*3*). The outbreak consisted of 11 laboratory-confirmed cases: nine cases in a boarding school in eastern Pennsylvania and two epidemiologically linked cases in New York City (NYC). This report summarizes the results of the outbreak investigation, which indicated that measles continues to be imported into the United States and that high coverage with 2 doses of measles-containing vaccine (MCV) among students was effective in limiting the size of the outbreak. Health-care providers should maintain a high index of suspicion for measles, especially in those who have traveled abroad recently, and recommendations for 2 doses of MCV in all school-aged children should be followed.

In April 2003, the Pennsylvania Department of Health reported to CDC two cases of measles in unvaccinated twins aged 13 years in a boarding school with 663 students. Active surveillance for measles[a] was conducted in the school, hospitals, and doctors' offices through May 2003. Patients were interviewed, acute- and convalescent-phase sera were collected for measles IgM enzyme-linked immunosorbent assay testing, and throat swabs and urine samples were collected for viral genotyping. Efforts to control the outbreak included vaccinating or excluding from campus and isolating all students and staff members with no evidence of immunity to measles.[b] School and personal vaccination records were reviewed to identify susceptible students and staff members, respectively.

For evaluation of vaccine effectiveness, only students enrolled in the school at the beginning of the outbreak were included. All staff members and those students who received measles vaccination during the outbreak were excluded. Vaccine effectiveness (VE) was calculated as VE (%) = [(ARU − ARV) / ARU] × 100, where ARU is the attack rate in unvaccinated persons and ARV is the attack rate in students who had received 2 doses of MCV previously (*4*).

A total of 11 laboratory-confirmed cases of measles were identified. The source patient was a student aged 17 years who had received 2 doses of MCV. On March 15, 2003, the student had returned to the United States from Beirut, Lebanon, where measles was known to be circulating. He had cough and fever the following day and rash on March 21, when he visited an emergency department and was diagnosed with a viral exanthem. Upon returning to school, the patient stayed at the school health center before returning to his dormitory.

Five persons with laboratory-confirmed measles were linked epidemiologically to the source patient. These five included the unvaccinated twins who lived in the same dormitory, the dormitory houseparent, and two other students in different dormitories. One of these latter students infected two additional students in his dormitory and an unvaccinated child aged 13 months in NYC, who was linked epidemiologically to an unvaccinated immigrant aged 33 years, who was diagnosed with measles and who lived in the same apartment building. The ninth school patient was linked epidemiologically to, and might have been infected by, any one of five infected persons from different dormitories.

All nine measles cases in the school were confirmed serologically. Measles genotype D4 was identified in two school patients and the child in NYC. The last date of rash onset in a boarding school patient was April 15. No deaths or major complications were reported; two students with measles, who were unvaccinated because of religious exemptions, required hospitalization for dehydration.

The median age of the nine patients in the school was 17 years (range: 13–26 years). Of the nine, two had not received any doses of MCV, one had received 1 dose, and six had received 2 doses. Patients with 1 or 2 doses of MCV had milder illness than unvaccinated patients, including a shorter duration of rash (median: 5 days versus 10 days; p <0.05) and fewer days of school or work missed (median: 5 days versus 8 days; p <0.05).

Of the 663 students in the boarding school, eight (1.2%) students had never received any doses of MCV, 26 (3.9%) students had received 1 dose, and 629 (94.9%) students had received 2 doses before the outbreak. Thus, vaccine coverage for 2 doses was 94.9% and for >1 dose was 98.8%. Vaccination with measles, mumps, and rubella vaccine was begun on April 3. Of the eight unvaccinated students, four had claimed religious or philosophical exemptions. Of these four students, two contracted measles, one was excluded from the school, and one was vaccinated during the outbreak. All of the remaining four unvaccinated students who did not claim any exemptions were vaccinated during the outbreak as well as other susceptible students and staff members.

continues

Excluding five previously unvaccinated students who were vaccinated during the outbreak and two students who had 2 doses of MCV previously but were inadvertently revaccinated during the outbreak, the measles attack rate was 66.7% (two of three) among unvaccinated students and 1.0% (six of 627) among students who had received 2 doses of MCV. All vaccinees with 1 dose of MCV received a second dose during the outbreak; no measles cases were diagnosed among these students. VE was 98.6% among students who had received 2 doses of MCV.

Reported by: *P Lurie, MD, P Britz, J Bowen, P Tran, MEd, H Stafford, Pennsylvania Dept of Health. YA Gillan, DrPH, New York City Dept of Health and Mental Hygiene. W Bellini, PhD, P Rota, PhD, J Rota, MPH, Div of Viral and Rickettsial Diseases, National Center for Infectious Diseases. E Eduardo, MPH, National Center for HIV, STD, and TB Prevention. G Dayan, MD, S Redd, M Papania, MD, J Seward, MBBS, Epidemiology and Surveillance Div, National Immunization Program. RJ Berry, MD, Birth Defects and Developmental Disabilities Div, National Center on Birth Defects and Developmental Disabilities. L Yeung, MD, EIS Officer, CDC.*

Editorial Note: Measles is rare in the United States, with only 42 confirmed cases in 2003, according to provisional data (2). The limited outbreak described in this report highlights both the success of the U.S. vaccination program and the continuing risk for imported measles despite a high immunity among the U.S. population. The last reported U.S. school outbreak occurred in 2000 and involved nine persons, including six high school students (1). Five of those six student patients had received only 1 dose of MCV, which was in compliance with state requirements at that time (1).

Before 1989, when the Advisory Committee on Immunization Practices recommended a routine 2-dose MCV schedule for school-aged children, larger measles outbreaks with >100 cases occurred in schools (5,6). All states but one now require 2 doses of MCV for children attending school (7). However, exemptions for religious or philosophical reasons are permitted in the majority of states, resulting in exemption for 0.6% of the nation's children (8). These children have a higher likelihood of acquiring and spreading measles than those who have been vaccinated (9).

In the outbreak described in this report, consistent with previous evaluations (10), 2 doses of MCV were highly effective in preventing the spread of measles, although a substantial number of exposed students, combined with a 1% failure rate among recipients with 2 doses, resulted in two generations of transmission in the school. Recipients of 2 doses of MCV had milder symptoms and shorter duration of illness than unvaccinated patients. Two unvaccinated students were hospitalized for dehydration, but none of the vaccinated students required hospitalization.

If an outbreak occurs, all persons whose illness is consistent with the definition for suspected measles[c] should be tested for both measles IgM and measles virus by culture or reverse transcriptase polymerase chain reaction. A convalescent serum should be obtained if the acute IgM is negative. This investigation highlighted the importance of viral specimens to document importation from overseas, confirm spread of the same genotype to NYC, and provide continued evidence for the absence of endemic transmission in the United States (1).

This outbreak of measles was caused by importation; the source patient was infected in Lebanon. Although the patient had classic signs for the disease (e.g., fever, rash, cough, and coryza), measles was not diagnosed initially, and the outbreak was not recognized until two unvaccinated students were hospitalized. A history of recent travel outside the United States should raise suspicion for a diagnosis of measles in a patient with appropriate clinical signs, regardless of vaccination status.

Footnotes
[a]Surveillance was conducted by using the 1997 case definition for measles issued by CDC and the Council of State and Territorial Epidemiologists: illness characterized by a generalized maculopapular rash lasting >3 days; a temperature of >101.0° F (>38.3° C); and cough, coryza, or conjunctivitis.
[b]Students and staff members were classified as having no evidence of measles immunity if they were born after 1957 and could not document history of physician-diagnosed measles illness, positive serology of measles IgG, history of 2 doses of MCV at least 28 days apart (students), or 1 dose (adults) with the first dose at or after age 1 year.
[c]Suspected measles is a febrile illness with a generalized maculopapular rash.

References
1. CDC. Measles—United States, 2000. *MMWR* 2002;51:120–3.
2. CDC. Progress toward measles elimination—Region of the Americas, 2002–2003. *MMWR* 2004;53:304–6.
3. CDC. Epidemiology of measles—United States, 1998. *MMWR* 1999;48:749–53.

continues

4. Orenstein WA, Bernier RH, Dondero TJ, et al. Field evaluation of vaccine efficacy. *Bull World Health Organ* 1985;63:1055–68.

5. CDC. Measles prevention: recommendations of the Immunization Practices Advisory Committee (ACIP). *MMWR* 1989;38(No. S-9):1–18.

6. Hutchins S, Markowitz L, Atkinson W, Swint E, Hadler S. Measles outbreaks in the United States, 1987 through 1990. *Pediatr Infect Dis J* 1996;15:31–8.

7. CDC. 2001–2002 State Immunization Requirements. Atlanta, Georgia: U.S. Department of Health and Human Services, CDC, 2002.

8. CDC. National Vaccine Advisory Committee. Report of the NVAC Working Group on Philosophical Exemptions, Minutes of the National Vaccine Advisory Committee, January 13, 1998. Atlanta, Georgia: National Vaccine Program Office, 1998:1–5.

9. Feikin DR, Lezotte DC, Hamman RF, Salmon DA, Chen RT, Hoffman RE. Individual and community risks of measles and pertussis associated with personal exemptions to immunization. *JAMA* 2000;284:3145–50.

10. CDC. Epidemiology and Prevention of Vaccine-Preventable Diseases, 6th ed. Atlanta, Georgia: U.S. Department of Health and Human Services, CDC, 2000.

Source: Centers for Disease Control and Prevention. Measles outbreak in a boarding school—Pennsylvania, 2003. MMWR 2004;53:306–309.
Note: The table and figure from this article were omitted.

potentially affected persons to prevent further transmission of the disease.

As for level of scientific consensus, this short MMWR article is obviously not a research synthesis. However, it does contain important contextual information to allow readers to understand where the findings "fit" based on prior research. Here are several examples of useful contextual information in the article:

1. Measles is rare in the United States; the last U.S. outbreak occurred in 2000 and it was the largest outbreak (i.e., most number of cases) since 1998.

2. Imported cases (i.e., infected persons traveling from one country to another) are an important source for outbreaks.

3. Two doses of the measles-containing vaccine are highly effective.

4. Findings were consistent with other studies, e.g., unvaccinated persons and persons receiving one vaccine dose are at greater risk.

Assessing the quality of scientific information depends heavily on the credibility of the source, and this article on the measles outbreak is no different. Source factors (e.g., authors and their institutions; the publication itself and its publisher) for an MMWR are essentially one and the same: the CDC.* The MMWR is an official publication of this federal agency and has been published on a weekly basis by the CDC since 1961.[20]

The CDC stands behind the content of this and all other MMWR articles. Articles submitted for publication undergo an extensive review process at multiple levels of the agency and by higher-level officials at the U.S. Department of Health and Human Services. Given CDC's long history of credibility as the federal government's leading public health agency, particularly with regard to infectious disease outbreak investigations (for many years, it was called the Communicable Disease Center), it is reasonable to assume that the scientific findings, conclusions, and recommendations reported in CDC publications are valid and trustworthy.

After assessing the quality of the science, the process of deconstructing the MMWR data and text into messages for communication begins.

Before getting into the specifics of the measles outbreak, the first consideration should be to determine the SOCO. There is no simple formula or one "right way" to decide on the SOCO; however, here's a suggested SOCO for the measles study based on text from the first paragraph of this article:

> Despite high levels of immunization, some people are still at risk for contracting measles from people who recently traveled to countries where measles is common. To minimize the risk, all school-aged children should receive 2 doses of a measles vaccine, and healthcare providers need to consider measles as a diagnosis among people who return from traveling abroad.

Prior to developing main messages based on this scientific article, it is essential to consider if lay audiences such as the public, the press, or policymakers know what measles is and

*Several of the authors of the MMWR article worked for the Pennsylvania Department of Health and the New York City Department of Health and Mental Hygiene, but the final responsibility for all the content in an MMWR article rests with staff members at CDC.

understand the health consequences of measles infection (Why is it important?). Providing basic background information about measles familiarizes audiences with these kinds of information. Audiences learn about the actual disease: it presents with a certain set of symptoms including widespread rash, fever, cough, runny nose, conjunctivitis. They learn about the negative health outcomes: severe cases can cause severe dehydration, pneumonia, or even death. Finally, they learn why public health and healthcare providers are concerned about the spread of the disease. Measles is highly infectious and can last for up to two weeks, allowing plenty of time for transmission to others.

When communicating information from scientific publications to lay audiences, use the four key message elements: description, explanation, interpretation, and recommended actions.

Here are some examples of descriptive messages:

- An outbreak of 11 cases of measles occurred in May 2003: 9 cases at a boarding school in Pennsylvania and 2 cases in New York City linked to a person from Pennsylvania with measles. This was the largest measles outbreak in the United States in five years.
- Although no deaths or serious complications occurred, two persons were hospitalized because of dehydration.
- Persons who had not been vaccinated against measles, or who received only one vaccination rather than two vaccinations as currently recommended, were at greater risk for developing measles or for having more severe symptoms.
- The outbreak was controlled by vaccinating individuals and by excluding or isolating students or staff potentially at risk from the school campus.

Here are some examples of explanatory and interpretive messages:

- The outbreak occurred after an individual contracted measles while he was on a trip to Lebanon. After he returned to Pennsylvania, he developed measles symptoms, but there was a delay in the recognition and diagnosis of the disease.
- The infection spread because of contact between persons with measles and others in school dormitories or with individuals in New York City.
- Measles infection remains a risk in the United States because of people who return to the United States from traveling in certain foreign countries.

As mentioned earlier, the emotional reaction of most people who hear messages about a potentially serious and contagious disease is fear. This means action messages, or recommendations, are extremely important.

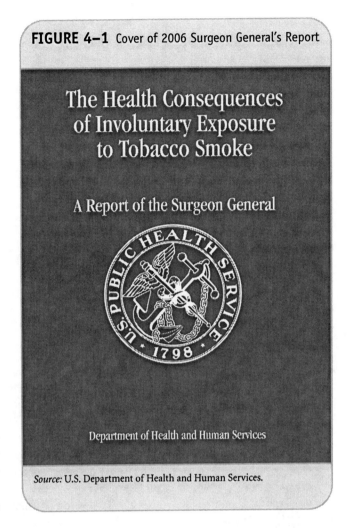

FIGURE 4-1 Cover of 2006 Surgeon General's Report

The Health Consequences of Involuntary Exposure to Tobacco Smoke

A Report of the Surgeon General

U.S. PUBLIC HEALTH SERVICE · 1798 ·

Department of Health and Human Services

Source: U.S. Department of Health and Human Services.

Here are two examples of action messages, both of which are quite similar to the SOCO (note that healthcare providers are the intended audience for the second message):

- To reduce the risk of infection, all school-aged children need to receive two doses of a measles-containing vaccine.
- Healthcare providers need to be vigilant and consider the diagnosis of measles among persons with compatible symptoms, particularly those returning from foreign travel.

Surgeon General's Report

The 2006 **Surgeon General's Report** (SGR) on secondhand smoke (SHS)* is an example of a comprehensive organization report. This landmark 709-page document, which took sev-

---

*The report title refers to involuntary exposure to tobacco smoke, which was the term used in a publication from the Surgeon General's office in 1986. *Secondhand smoke* is now the generally agreed-upon term in the field of tobacco control and prevention and is synonymous with involuntary exposure and environmental tobacco smoke exposure.

eral years to complete, contains a comprehensive review and synthesis of the scientific research literature about the health impacts of SHS exposure. As evidenced by the Table of Contents in **Box 4–4**, it covers a broad range of studies examining the potential adverse health effects of secondhand smoke on many systems within the human body.

While we still need to assess the science and deconstruct this publication for communication purposes, the process is somewhat different than for the previously described MMWR article. In particular, much of the assessment of the science is already done because the authors reviewed hundreds of studies and reached consensus about the quality of the science and strength of association (causality) between SHS exposure and health outcomes.

The document contains an executive summary that highlights the findings, which makes identifying key scientific points for messages much easier. It must be noted that Surgeon General's Reports do not make policy recommendations. Communications about the report, however, could target policymakers—there is strong evidence that SHS laws or regulations are successful at eliminating or severely limiting exposure to SHS. Indeed, several communities and at least one state have used the findings from this report in successful initiatives to enact effective SHS laws.

Assessing the science, again, begins with evaluating the study design and representativeness. Neither of these factors is problematic in the SGR because such factors were evaluated by the authors themselves and because of the sheer volume of the

Box 4–4 The 2006 Surgeon General's Report on Secondhand Smoke*

Table of Contents
Chapter 1. Introduction, Summary, and Conclusions
Chapter 2. Toxicology of Secondhand Smoke
Chapter 3. Assessment of Exposure to Secondhand Smoke
Chapter 4. Prevalence of Exposure to Secondhand Smoke
Chapter 5. Reproductive and Developmental Effects from Exposure to Secondhand Smoke
Chapter 6. Respiratory Effects in Children from Exposure to Secondhand Smoke
Chapter 7. Cancer Among Adults from Exposure to Secondhand Smoke
Chapter 8. Cardiovascular Diseases from Exposure to Secondhand Smoke
Chapter 9. Respiratory Effects in Adults from Exposure to Secondhand Smoke
Chapter 10. Control of Secondhand Smoke Exposure
A Vision for the Future

Six Major Conclusions
1. Secondhand smoke causes premature death and disease in children and in adults who do not smoke.
2. Children exposed to secondhand smoke are at an increased risk for sudden infant death syndrome (SIDS), acute respiratory infections, ear problems, and more severe asthma. Smoking by parents causes respiratory symptoms and slows lung growth in their children.
3. Exposure of adults to secondhand smoke has immediate adverse effects on the cardiovascular system and causes coronary heart disease and lung cancer.
4. The scientific evidence indicates that there is no risk-free level of exposure to secondhand smoke.
5. Many millions of Americans, both children and adults, are still exposed to secondhand smoke in their homes and workplaces, despite substantial progress in tobacco control.
6. Eliminating smoking in indoor spaces fully protects nonsmokers from exposure to secondhand smoke. Separating smokers from nonsmokers, cleaning the air, and ventilating buildings cannot eliminate exposures of nonsmokers to secondhand smoke.

Sources:
U.S. Department of Health and Human Services. *The health consequences of involuntary exposure to tobacco smoke: A report of the Surgeon General.* Atlanta, GA: Centers for Disease Control and Prevention, National Center for Chronic Disease Prevention and Health Promotion, Office on Smoking and Health; 2006. http://www.surgeongeneral.gov/library/secondhandsmoke/report/
Centers for Disease Control and Prevention. *Surgeon General's Reports: 2006 Surgeon General's Report.* http://www.cdc.gov/tobacco/data_statistics/sgr/sgr_2006/index.htm
*The terms *involuntary exposure to tobacco smoke* and *environmental tobacco smoke exposure* are synonymous with *secondhand smoke exposure.*

report. (If you were interested in a particular topic, such as SHS and asthma in children, then it would make sense for you to carefully examine the scientific quality of the studies reviewed in that section of the report.) Determining causality was a major goal of the research in this report. The report provides ratings of evidence for causality between exposure to SHS and each particular health outcome. These ratings were strong evidence, suggestive evidence, inconclusive evidence, or no evidence.

Level of scientific consensus was not an issue (the report itself represents a consensus). Contextual information, or prior research, was taken into account when assigning a causality rating. It is evident from the list of contributing authors that a large array of well-known experts from highly credible institutions contributed to the report.

The U.S. Surgeon General and the SGRs on tobacco have long been considered highly credible sources of health information. The process for obtaining and reviewing the scientific information, as well as the extensive review of report drafts by representatives from federal health agencies and outside scientists not affiliated with its writing, help to ensure the integrity of the findings. It is noteworthy that 29 SGRs on tobacco have been published and no conclusion in these reports has ever been retracted.

Communication planning involves first considering the SOCO. Given the comprehensiveness of the Surgeon General's Report, many different SOCOs are possible depending on the target audience (the public, healthcare providers, policymakers, the press) and communication objectives. There are definitive conclusions for each separate chapter in the report. An excellent place to begin thinking about good SOCO information would be the six major conclusions from the report (see Box 4–4). Probably the simplest SOCO would be:

> There is no safe level of secondhand smoke, according to the Surgeon General.

One of the great values of relying on research synthesis reports such as the Surgeon General's Report is that communications materials may have already been developed and made available, which can save you a lot of time and work. For this report, a wealth of supplementary written and visual materials are available at the CDC's Office on Smoking and Health website (www.cdc.gov/tobacco) and the Surgeon General's website (www.surgeongeneral.gov). These materials were designed to communicate different aspects of the report and are readily adaptable for use by others (e.g., fact sheets on secondhand smoke and children and on how to protect yourself and your loved ones from secondhand smoke, consumer summaries, posters).

As with the MMWR article on measles, it is necessary to ensure that intended audiences understand SHS beyond a general definition, such as "smoke inhaled indirectly from cigarettes." One of the Surgeon General's fact sheets provides more detailed information on "What is Secondhand Smoke?"[21] It defines what SHS means, states that cigarette smoke contains more than 4,000 chemical compounds, and states that at least 250 of these chemicals are known to be toxic or carcinogenic (cancer-causing).

Messages based on this report should describe, explain, and interpret the findings and then provide recommendations for action. Here are examples of descriptive messages:

- The U.S. Surgeon General, after a thorough and comprehensive review of the science, has definitively concluded that secondhand smoke is a major cause of disease [general message].
- Millions of children and adults continue to be exposed to secondhand smoke in their homes and at work [specific message].
- Secondhand smoke causes lung cancer among nonsmokers [specific message].
- Secondhand smoke is a cause of sudden infant death syndrome (SIDS) [specific message].

Here are some examples of explanatory messages (e.g., why the Surgeon General made the reported conclusions):

- Multiple biological mechanisms exist by which secondhand smoke exposure damages different parts of the body [general message].
- Secondhand smoke contains more than 50 cancer-causing chemicals [specific message].
- Secondhand smoke exposure reduces cardiovascular functioning [specific message].

Here are examples of potential interpretive messages from the report:

- There is no safe level of exposure to secondhand smoke [general message].
- Only eliminating smoking in indoor locations fully protects nonsmokers from the health consequences of secondhand smoke [specific message].

Given the implications of the findings in the report, here are examples of action messages:

- Strong and comprehensive smoke-free laws need to be enacted in the state of Y to protect people from secondhand smoke [general message and targeted toward policymakers].
- Persons with existing heart disease, because they are particularly vulnerable, should avoid secondhand smoke

exposure at all costs [specific message targeted toward individuals].

- Physicians should counsel parents not to permit smoking inside their homes [specific message targeted toward healthcare providers].

CONCLUSION

Credible scientific evidence takes on several basic characteristics, including where and by whom such evidence is obtained and published. There are straightforward ways to communicate reports of credible scientific findings to the public. Practicing the recommendations in this chapter can greatly increase the chance that good science, communicated well, can result in good public health. Later, in Chapter Summary II, we discuss the added efforts necessary to make health information accessible to persons with limited literacy or quantitative abilities.

KEY TERMS

Case studies
Case-control studies
Causality
Cohort studies

Confirmation bias
Cross-sectional studies
Description
Ecologic studies
Evidence-based intervention
Experimental studies
Explanation
Guide to Clinical Preventive Studies
Guide to Community Preventive Services
Interpretation
Meta-analysis
Morbidity and Mortality Weekly Report (MMWR)
Satisficing
Science
Scientific consensus
Selective exposure
Single overriding communications objective (SOCO)
Source credibility
Study design
Surgeon General's Report
Time-series studies
Worldview

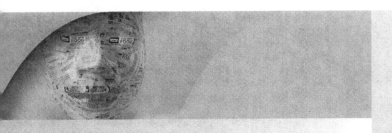

Chapter Questions

1. Why is it important to consider the quality of scientific studies and research syntheses?

2. What are the three broad categories of factors to consider when assessing scientific quality?

3. What are the pros and cons of each type of research synthesis?

4. Why is it important to present findings from a scientific study or report in context?

5. What is source credibility, and why does it matter so much?

6. What are at least five broad factors that influence how people process and evaluate scientific information?

7. How does the concept of acceptable evidence differ between scientists and lay audiences?

8. What are the four basic questions about scientific studies or reports that lay audiences want public health scientists, practitioners, or their representatives to answer?

9. Why do you need to develop a SOCO?

REFERENCES

1. Turnock BJ. *Public health: What it is and how it works.* Gaithersburg, MD: Aspen; 1997.

2. Nelson DE, Brownson RC, Remington PL, Parvanta C (eds). *Communicating public health information effectively.* Washington, DC: American Public Health Association; 2002.

3. Nelson DE, Hesse BW, Croyle RT. *Making data talk.* New York: Oxford University Press; 2009.

4. Friis RH, Sellers TA. *Epidemiology for public health practice.* Gaithersburg, MD: Aspen; 1999.

5. U.S. Department of Health, Education, and Welfare, Public Health Service. *Smoking and health: Report of the Advisory Committee to the Surgeon General of the Public Health Service.* Washington, DC: Government Printing Office; 1964. PHS Publication No. 1103.

6. Hill AB. The environment and disease: association or causation? *Proc R Acad Med.* 1965; 295–300.

7. Zaza S, Briss Pa, Harris KW, et al. *The guide to community preventive services: What works to promote health?* New York: Oxford University Press; 2005.

8. Task Force on Community Preventive Services. *Guide to community preventive services: What works to promote health.* Atlanta, GA: Task Force on Community Preventive Services; 2009. http://www.thecommunityguide.org

9. U.S. Preventive Services Task Force. *Guide to clinical preventive services, 2008.* Rockville, MD: Agency for Healthcare Research and Quality; 2008. http://www.ahrq.gov/clinic/pocketgd08/

10. Strauss SE, Richardson WS, Glasziou P, Haynes RB. *Evidence-based medicine: How to teach and practice EBM.* 3rd edition. Philadelphia, PA: Churchill Livingstone; 2005.

11 National Institutes of Health. *NIH consensus development program.* Bethesda, MD: National Institutes of Health; 2009. http://consensus.nih.gov/

12 The National Academies, Washington DC. http://www.nationalacademies.org/

13. Lum M, Parvanta C, Maibach E, Arkin E, Nelson DE. General public: communicating to inform. In: Nelson DE, Brownson RC, Remington PL, Parvanta C (eds). *Communicating public health information effectively* (pp. 47–57.) Washington, DC: American Public Health Association; 2002.

14. Slater MD. Persuasion processes across receiver goals and message genres. *Commun Theory.* 1997;7:125–148.

15. Plous S. *The psychology of judgment and decision-making.* New York: McGraw-Hill; 1993.

16. Remington PL, Nelson D. Communicating epidemiologic information. In: Brownson RC, Petiti D (eds). *Applied epidemiology.* 2nd edition (pp. 327–351). New York: Oxford University Press; 2006.

17. Centers for Disease Control and Prevention. Measles outbreak in a boarding school—Pennsylvania, 2003. MMWR 2004;53:306–309.

18. U.S. Department of Health and Human Services. *The health consequences of involuntary exposure to tobacco smoke: A report of the Surgeon General.* Atlanta, GA: Centers for Disease Control and Prevention, National Center for Chronic Disease Prevention and Health Promotion, Office on Smoking and Health; 2006. http://www.surgeongeneral.gov/library/secondhandsmoke/report/

19. Centers for Disease Control and Prevention. *Surgeon General's Reports: 2006 Surgeon General's Report.* http://www.cdc.gov/tobacco/data_statistics/sgr/sgr_2006/index.htm

20. Remington PL, Nelson DE. Communicating public health surveillance information for action. In: Lee LM, Teutsch SM, St Louis ME, Thacker SB (eds). *Principles and practice of public health surveillance.* 3rd edition. New York: Oxford University Press. In press.

21. Centers for Disease Control and Prevention. Smoking and Tobacco Use Fact Sheets. "Secondhand Smoke." Available at: http://www.cdc.gov/tobacco/data_statistics/fact_sheets/secondhand_smoke/general_facts/index.htm

CHAPTER 5

"What" to Communicate? Understanding Population Health

Patrick L. Remington, Bridget C. Booske, and David Kindig

LEARNING OBJECTIVES

By the end of this chapter, the reader will be able to:

- Describe how the leading causes of death in the United States have changed over the past 100 years and how health leaders have responded to these causes in terms of assessing and resolving the problems.

- Illustrate how social determinants are related to health among different population groups.

- Understand the four major determinants of health and how we can communicate about these determinants to the public.

- Name major modes of data collection for assessing health determinants and measuring health behaviors.

- List multiple sources of comprehensive information about evidence-based solutions to health problems.

- Consider the challenges involved in communicating about population health.

INTRODUCTION

The goal of this book is to provide the reader with the knowledge and skills needed to become an effective public health communicator. Regardless of the strategy (e.g., to persuade or to inform) or the intended target audience (e.g., individuals or policymakers), the ultimate goal of health communication is to improve the health of individuals. Learning "how" to communicate is necessary—but not sufficient—to achieve this aim. One must also understand "what" needs to be communicated in order to improve population health.

The purpose of this chapter is to help readers develop communication strategies that address the leading health *problems* in a community—not just the leading health *concerns*—to help understand the burden and their causes, and lead to improvements in public health. To better understand "*what*"

needs to be communicated, this chapter focuses on three questions regarding population health in the United States:

- What are the leading health problems in the United States?
- What are the major causes (i.e., determinants) of these health problems?
- What are the most effective programs and policies to address these health problems?

The chapter begins by describing trends in the leading health problems, as well as their causes, over the past 100 years. The next section describes a model of population health that we use to answer the questions shown previously. The sections that follow attempt to answer these questions, with a focus on implications for health communication, using examples from the United States and from our work in Wisconsin. The final section discusses challenges confronting communication efforts today and in the future.

EVOLUTION OF THE LEADING CAUSES OF DEATH IN THE UNITED STATES

Over the past century in the United States, advances in public health and health care have led to dramatic changes in the leading **causes of death** and have increased life expectancy by more than 30 years. Infant mortality has fallen from 150 deaths per 1,000 live births in 1900 to 6.9 per 1,000 in 2005. Some authors have attributed most of this gain to advances in public health.[1,2]

With improvements in sanitation and control of infectious diseases earlier in the 20th century, chronic diseases became the leading causes of death during the middle part of the century. Concomitantly, public health researchers began to shift their focus from the detection of the causes of outbreaks to identifying the complex and interrelated causes of chronic diseases and injuries. To better understand today's leading health problems, we describe the evolution of our understanding of the leading *causes* of death over the past century in four eras: environmental factors, health care, health behaviors, and social and economic factors.

The Era of Environmental Disease (circa 1900)

In the early 1900s in the United States, the leading causes of disease and death were associated with the unhealthy environments in which people lived. In 1900, pneumonia, influenza, tuberculosis, diarrhea, enteritis, and ulceration of the intestines were the leading causes of death, accounting for nearly one-third of all deaths (**Table 5–1**).[3,4] These health problems resulted from poor sanitation (e.g., typhoid), unhealthy food supply (e.g., pellagra and goiter), poor prenatal and infant care, and unsafe workplaces or hazardous occupations.[5]

In response to these health problems, the federal government, state governments, and local departments of public health focused their efforts on laws and regulations intended to improve the health of the environment, such as motor-vehicle safety regulations, occupational safety laws, control of infectious diseases, safer and healthier foods, and fluoridation of drinking water.[2] These policies led to dramatic reductions in communicable diseases and maternal and infant mortality. As mortality rates declined and life expectancy increased, chronic diseases became more important causes of death and disability.

The Era of Expanding Health Care (circa 1950)

By the middle of the 20th century, heart disease and cancer had become the leading causes of death in the United States. Some research began to examine the causes of these chronic diseases. Therefore, the focus of interventions began to shift to healthcare services, including the delivery of **clinical preventive services** such as vaccines for childhood disease, improved maternal and prenatal care, and the detection and treatment of high blood pressure.

Despite some attention to preventive services, most of the attention of the healthcare system focused on the treatment of diseases. Evans[6] commented that "by midcentury the providers of health care had gained an extraordinary institutional and even more intellectual dominance, defining both what counted as health and how it was to be pursued." By the early 1970s, the United States had developed extensive and expensive systems of health care, underpinned by health insurance systems that covered most—but not all—children and adults.[6]

TABLE 5–1 Ten Leading Causes of Death in the United States, 1900 and 2006

Rank	Cause of Death, 1900	Number	Percent	Cause of Death, 2006	Number	Percent
1.	Pneumonia and influenza	40,362	12	Diseases of the heart	631,636	26
2.	Tuberculosis	38,820	11	Malignant neoplasms	559,888	23
3.	Diarrhea, enteritis, and intestinal ulceration	28,491	8	Cerebrovascular disease (stroke)	137,119	6
4.	Diseases of the heart	27,427	8	Chronic lower respiratory diseases	124,583	5
5.	Cerebrovascular disease (stroke)	21,353	6	Accidents	121,599	5
6.	Nephritis (all forms)	17,699	5	Diabetes mellitus	72,449	3
7.	Accidents	14,429	4	Alzheimer's disease	72,432	3
8.	Malignant neoplasms	12,769	4	Pneumonia and influenza	56,326	2
9.	Senility	10,015	3	Nephritis (all forms)	45,344	2
10.	Diphtheria	8,056	2	Septicemia	34,234	1
	All causes	343,217	100		2,426,264	100

Source: CDC. Leading Causes of Death, 1900–1998. http://www.cdc.gov/nchs/data/dvs/lead1990_98.pdf. Accessed September 25, 2009.
CDC. Deaths: Final Data for 2006. *National Vital Statistics Reports.* 2009;57(14).

The Era of Lifestyle and Health Risk Behaviors (circa 1970)

As heart disease, cancer, stroke, and lung disease became the leading causes of death during the mid-1900s, public health researchers began to focus on identifying their causes. Large-scale studies such as the Framingham Heart study, the Seven Countries study, and the British Doctors study began to identify the leading causes of chronic diseases. These studies began to elucidate the important contributions of cigarette smoking, diet, physical inactivity, and high blood pressure to the leading causes of death.

The Lalonde report was published in 1974 in Canada and has been recognized as the first modern government report to state that the emphasis on health care was not sufficient in efforts to improve the health of the population.[7] The report noted that the generally accepted view at that time was that the level of health in a population was equated with the level of *health care*. Instead, it proposed a new framework suggesting that health be considered along four broad dimensions: human biology, environment, lifestyle, and healthcare organization. The report emphasized individuals' roles in changing their behaviors to improve their health.[8]

The publication of the now famous paper entitled "Actual Causes of Death" by McGinnis and Foege[9] in 1993 drew attention to the fact that many deaths were due to preventable causes. Later updated by Mokdad and colleagues,[10] these studies concluded that approximately half of all deaths that occurred in 1990 and 2000 could be attributed to a limited number of preventable factors (**Table 5–2**). Although no attempt was made to further quantify the impact of these factors on morbidity and quality of life, the public health burden they impose is considerable and offers guidance for shaping health policy priorities. These findings, along with escalating healthcare costs and an aging population, argued persuasively for the urgent need to establish a more preventive orientation in the U.S. healthcare and public health systems.

Expert opinion at the time suggested that lifestyle factors had the largest and most unambiguously measurable effect on health.[6–12] Behaviors such as diet, exercise, and substance abuse were also factors most readily portrayed as under the control of individuals. The response by public health was to provide health education to individuals and society, positing that this information alone would be sufficient to change behaviors. The observed model for behavior change at that time was

Knowledge → Attitudes → Practices

or KAP, suggesting that providing knowledge will lead to changes in behaviors. This suggests, for example, that simply providing information about the health risks of smoking should be sufficient to cause people to quit.

About the same time as personal health behaviors received wider recognition as a major contributor to morbidity and mortality, telephone surveys emerged as a feasible method for assessing the prevalence of many health risk behaviors among populations. In 1984, the Centers for Disease Control and Prevention (CDC) implemented the first state-based surveillance system for health behaviors,[13] eventually becoming the largest survey of health behaviors in the world. This system, called the Behavioral Risk Factor Surveillance System (BRFSS),* collects information on health risk behaviors, preventive health practices, and healthcare access primarily related to chronic disease and injury. More than 430,000 adult interviews were completed in 2009, making the BRFSS the largest telephone health survey in the world.

The BRFSS provides valuable information about health behaviors at the state and local level that is of great interest, not only to public health professionals but also to news media

*http://www.cdc.gov/brfss/index.htm

TABLE 5–2 Actual Causes of Death in the United States, 1990 and 2000

Actual Cause	Number of Deaths (%*) in 1990	Number of Deaths (%*) in 2000
Tobacco	400,000 (19)	435,000 (18.1)
Poor diet and physical inactivity	300,000 (14)	400,000 (16.6)
Alcohol consumption	100,000 (5)	85,000 (3.5)
Microbial agents	90,000 (4)	75,000 (3.1)
Toxic agents	60,000 (3)	55,000 (2.3)
Motor vehicle	25,000 (1)	43,000 (1.8)
Firearms	35,000 (2)	29,000 (1.2)
Sexual behavior	30,000 (1)	20,000 (0.8)
Illicit drug use	20,000 (<1)	17,000 (0.7)
Total	1,060,000 (50)	1,158,000 (48.2)

*The percentages are for all deaths. Not all deaths shown.
Source: Mokdad AH, Marks JS, Stroup DF, Gerberding JL. Actual Causes of Death in the United States, 2000. *JAMA.* 2004;291(10):1238–1245.

representatives. The use of a standard questionnaire in all states and over time provides a unique ability to compare and contrast the health of communities. The best-known example of using data to communicate information about the obesity epidemic was presented in a landmark paper in 1999[1,4] followed by the posting of PowerPoint slides on the CDC website.* These slides graphically show the spread of high rates of obesity across the entire United States over time (see also Chapter 3).[10,14]

The Era of Social and Economic Causes (circa 2000)

By the beginning of the 21st century, research had begun to focus farther "upstream" on those factors that increase not only the risk of diseases, but also their predisposing behavioral and other factors. In general, the contribution of physical environment, medical care, and health behaviors to health has been easy for the public and policymakers to understand. One of the reasons for such general appreciation and understanding of these determinants is that the mechanisms by which they biologically affect health and disease (antibiotics, cigarette smoke, air pollution) are relatively easy to understand.

According to the Institute of Medicine's report on the Future of the Public's Health in the 21st Century, "the greatest advances in understanding the factors that shape population health over the past two decades has been the identification of social and behavioral conditions that influence morbidity, mortality, and functioning."[15] Research has increasingly demonstrated the important contributions to health of underlying factors—for example, socioeconomic position, race and ethnicity, social networks and social support, and work conditions, as well as economic inequality and social capital.[15]

In the past 25 years we have built a strong case for the "social determinants" of health such as income, education, occupation, and social cohesion as highly important contributors to health outcomes. The academic field of **social epidemiology** has expanded during this period.[16] Social epidemiology is perhaps best known for the identification of social gradients in health, in which it is not only the extremes of high and low levels of education and income that have health outcome effects, but gradations between them. One of the most important investigators in this field is Sir Michael Marmot, a British social epidemiologist, whose studies of British civil servants clearly illustrates these concepts (**Figure 5–1**).[17]

The four job categories in Figure 5-1 reflect different education and income profiles among British civil servants. It can be seen that there is increased mortality from heart disease at each occupational level (the social gradient). In addition, contributions to this mortality from common risk factors such as blood pressure, smoking, and cholesterol increase with lower

occupational grade can also be seen. But the amount of mortality not explained by these risk factors, in a British system where all have access to medical care, is quite remarkable.

While this example features occupational category as one marker of social class and socioeconomic status, such relationships have also been shown for income, education, and other components of the social determinants of health. While teasing apart the effects of these separate social factors is challenging for researchers, the evidence is convincing; level of education, for example, is probably as important as medical care and other factors in improving health. A large body of evidence supports this claim, including the fact that people in nations, states, and counties with higher levels of education have better health outcomes in many categories.

For example, in 2005 the age-adjusted mortality rate for adults with some education beyond high school was 206 per 100,000 in the United States. However, it was twice as great for those with only a high school education and three times as great for those with less than high school education.[18] People with more education also have fewer disabilities and better physical functioning. One study estimates that eight times more lives would be saved by correcting educational disparities than those saved by medical advances in the same period.[19] One of the most precise studies, which controlled for many

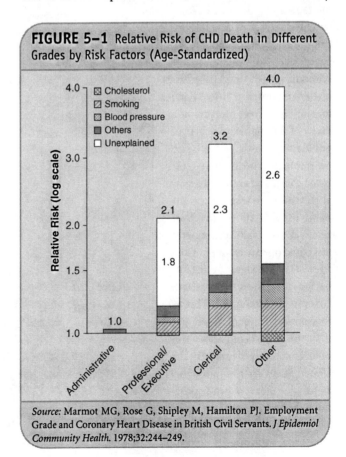

FIGURE 5–1 Relative Risk of CHD Death in Different Grades by Risk Factors (Age-Standardized)

Source: Marmot MG, Rose G, Shipley M, Hamilton PJ. Employment Grade and Coronary Heart Disease in British Civil Servants. *J Epidemiol Community Health.* 1978;32:244–249.

*http://www.cdc.gov/obesity/data/trends.html

other possible explanations, showed a 1% to 3% reduction in mortality rates for each year of additional schooling.[20]

A MODEL FOR POPULATION HEALTH

To communicate effectively and improve the health of the population, it is important to understand how the health of the population is defined and determined. Models of population health are schematic representations of factors that affect the health of populations, measured primarily as the average level of health in the population, but increasingly also considering the distribution of health within populations.[21–23]

Beginning in 2003, we developed a model for population health to measure and rank the health of counties in Wisconsin.[24–26] This model includes two broad categories: **health outcomes** and **health determinants**. The health outcomes included in the model represent both length and quality of life. The summary rank of health determinants in the *Rankings* is determined by a weighted average of data for four components: health care (10%), health behaviors (40%), socioeconomics (40%), and the physical environment (10%). Each measure is a direct measure or a proxy of an important aspect of population health, and is based on publicly available data collected consistently across the state at the county level. The assignment of weights to the four health determinant components was based on expert opinion and a review of the literature regarding how these measures combine. For example, McGinnis, Williams-Russo, and Knickman suggest that "the impacts of various domains on early deaths in the United States distribute roughly as follows: genetic predispositions, about 30 percent; social circumstances, 15 percent; environmental exposures, 5 percent;

behavioral patterns, 40 percent; and shortfalls in medical care, 10 percent."[27] The widely recognized *America's Health Rankings* has four determinant categories with weights currently assigned as follows by an expert panel: personal behaviors, 20%; community and environment, 27.5%; public and health policies, 12.5%; and clinical care, 15%.[28]

This model of population (**Figure 5–2**) has several characteristics that make it relevant to health communicators. First, it demonstrates that the health of the population is determined

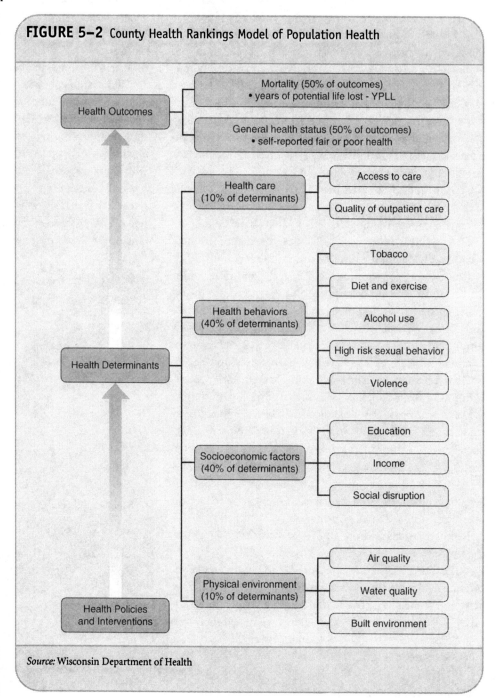

FIGURE 5–2 County Health Rankings Model of Population Health

Source: Wisconsin Department of Health

by multiple factors, ranging from individual health behaviors to the quality of the healthcare and educational systems to the influences of the built environment. This broad definition of health serves as a call to action to the many individuals and organizations in communities to work together toward population health improvement.

This model also demonstrates how interventions (i.e., policies, programs, and information) may affect determinants of health at multiple levels (e.g., individual; social, family, and community; living and working conditions; and broad social, economic, cultural, health, and environmental conditions) to improve outcomes. The results of such interventions can be demonstrated through assessment, monitoring, and evaluation. Through dissemination of evidence-based practices and best practices, these findings would feed back to intervention planning to enable the identification of effective prevention strategies in the future.

To be effective, public health communicators should have a solid understanding of what the important health problems are in their community, the causes of these health problems, and ways to prevent or control them. The previous sections provided an historical perspective on the leading causes of death, as well a model that can be used when considering health communication planning. In the next three sections, we focus on the three major components of population health, including health outcomes, health determinants, and programs and policies.

COMMUNICATING ABOUT THE LEADING HEALTH PROBLEMS

The leading health problems in a community are defined as the *health outcomes* in the models of population health described earlier. They are measured in populations as the rates of mortality (death), morbidity (disease), and health-related quality of life. These health outcomes are considered as the "downstream" effects of those factors that influence health.

Sources of Data on Health Problems

Information about causes of death is reported on death certificates. These certificates are completed by a physician or medical examiner and reported to the county and state health departments, and ultimately to CDC's National Center for Health Statistics, where they are made available to public health practitioners and researchers throughout the United States. The CDC provides easy access to mortality data through its website.*

Disease incidence and prevalence data can be obtained from a number of sources. Cancer incidence data have been available since 1974 for a sample of residents of the United States through the Surveillance, Epidemiology and End Results (SEER) Program at the National Cancer Institute (NCI) and more recently from most state health departments. In addition, administrative data from hospitals and other healthcare providers may provide information about the rates of care for diseases. In addition, data on birth outcomes (e.g., birth weights, prematurity rates) are reported by hospitals to state health departments.

Some information on overall health-related quality of life (HRQoL) is collected at the state level and reported to CDC as part of the BRFSS. Other local initiatives to assess health-related quality of life tend to be disease specific and are driven by healthcare providers and health services researchers interested in studying the health outcomes that result from particular healthcare treatments. These QoL initiatives generally employ quite detailed self-reported assessments of patient conditions but have developed relatively independently. The National Health Measurement Study recently concluded a major effort to examine the performance of a number of HRQoL preference-based summary indices.†

Examples

NCHS Leading Causes of Death by Age Group

Data in **Table 5–3** were obtained from the CDC website and show the leading causes of death overall and for each age group. For persons of all ages, four chronic diseases account for 60% of all deaths (heart disease, cancer, stroke, and lung diseases; see Table 5–1). Cancer is the leading cause of death among persons ages 45 to 74, and Alzheimer's disease is now one of the leading causes of death among persons over the age of 75. Although unintentional injuries are the fourth-leading cause of death overall, they are the leading cause of death for persons under the age of 45 (Table 5–3).[28]

While some disease rates are increasing, heart disease rates are declining. These rates vary considerably by race, gender, and geographic area.

Health Disparities in Wisconsin

America's Health Rankings have ranked states' health annually since 1990. Recently, these rankings have highlighted disparities but until 2008, did not explicitly include them in their overall rankings.[29] The states of Washington[30] and North Carolina[31] also include health disparities in report cards. Interest in assessing Wisconsin's overall health and level of

---

*http://wonder.cdc.gov/

†http://www.disc.wisc.edu/NHMS/index.html

TABLE 5–3 Leading Causes of Death, by Age Group, US, 2006

ALL AGES	< 1 YEAR	1-14 YEARS	15-24 YEARS	25-44 YEARS	45-64 YEARS	65-74 YEARS	75-84 YEARS	85+ YEARS
Heart Disease (26%)	Congenital Anomalies (20%)	Injury (36%)	Injury (47%)	Injury (26%)	Cancer (33%)	Cancer (35%)	Heart Disease (27%)	Heart Disease (34%)
Cancer (23%)	Short Gestation (17%)	Cancer (12%)	Homicide (16%)	Cancer (14%)	Heart Disease (22%)	Heart Disease (24%)	Cancer (25%)	Cancer (12%)
Stroke (6%)	SIDS (8%)	Congenital Anomalies (8%)	Suicide (12%)	Heart Disease (12%)	Injury (7%)	Lung Disease (7%)	Lung Disease (7%)	Stroke (8%)
Lung Disease (5%)	Complications of Pregnancy (6%)	Homicide (7%)	Cancer (5%)	Suicide (9%)	Diabetes (4%)	Stroke (5%)	Stroke (7%)	Alzheimer's Disease (6%)
Injury (5%)	Injury (4%)	Heart Disease (4%)	Heart Disease (3%)	Homicide (6%)	Stroke (4%)	Diabetes (4%)	Alzheimer's Disease (3%)	Lung Disease (4%)

Notes: Injury includes all unintentional injuries (also called accidents)
Statistics were generated using the Web-based Injury Statistics Query and Reporting System (WISQARS) on the CDC National Center of Injury Prevention and Control web site.[28]

health disparity was stimulated by a group trying to assess progress toward meeting two 2010 Wisconsin state health plan goals of promoting and protecting health for all and eliminating health disparities, and through a project advising a foundation on how to "Make Wisconsin the Healthiest State,"* with fewer health disparities.

There are multiple population subgroups across which **health disparities** may occur, but most health disparity measurements focus on a single domain, such as CDC's racial-ethnic Disparity Index.[32] We developed an approach assigning separate grades for both "health" and "health disparity," assessing disparities across multiple domains, and published them in the *Health of Wisconsin Report Card.*[33,34]

Grading curves were established based on data for all 50 states for two outcomes (mortality and unhealthy days) and four life stages (infants, children and young adults, working-age adults, and older adults). Using Wisconsin as an example, grades were assigned for health within each life stage for population subgroups based on sex, race/ethnicity, socioeconomics, and geography. A health disparity grade was also assigned to each life stage. Wisconsin received a B− for health and a D for health disparity. When the same method was applied to all 50 states, no state received an A for either health or health dis-

parity. New Hampshire received the best grades: B+ for health and B for health disparity, followed by Hawaii and Iowa with a B for health and a B for health disparity. Louisiana and West Virginia received grades of F for health and health disparity.

COMMUNICATING ABOUT THE DETERMINANTS OF HEALTH

Public health communication about the leading health problems is an important way to call attention to health problems and serve as a call to action. However, these communication efforts must move upstream to consider those modifiable factors that influence health in the population. Communicators can point out that health in the population is determined by four general areas:

- The way we act: smoking and substance abuse, nutrition and physical activity, unintentional injuries, including driving habits, violence, and risky sexual behavior. These, in turn, are influenced by policies, environment, and culture in our communities, state and nation.
- Our healthcare and public health system: accessibility, affordability, and quality of services.
- Our social and economic situation: child development, education, employment, income and poverty, and social connectedness.
- Our physical environment: housing, the built environment and environmental quality.

*http://www.pophealth.wisc.edu/uwphi/research/healthy.htm

Sources of Data on Health Determinants

Health Behaviors

The primary source of data on adult health behaviors at the national, state, and local levels is the CDC's BRFSS. As noted earlier, BRFSS data are collected monthly in all 50 states, the District of Columbia, Puerto Rico, the Virgin Islands, and Guam. The BRFSS questionnaire consists of a fixed core (asked every year), rotating core (asked every other year), optional modules (standardized sets of questions on specific topics), emerging core (questions for newly arising topics), and state-added modules (questions relevant to the individual state). Items in the BRFSS address smoking, alcohol use, diet, exercise, and other health-related behaviors, such as use of clinical preventive services.

Health Care

Ideally, data on healthcare access, utilization, quality, and costs would be available at the national, state, and local levels. However, there is no single repository of such information. Data on the extent of public and private healthcare coverage is readily available at the national and state levels, for example, from the Current Population Survey. Data on healthcare utilization and costs are collected at nearly every individual healthcare encounter between birth and death in administrative and clinical databases. Similarly, numerous administrative and regulatory requirements lead to the accumulation of data about the providers of these healthcare services. However, the extent to which all of these data are aggregated and accessible for evaluating utilization, quality, and costs widely across the United States, depend on both mandated and voluntary initiatives. Data on health care provided through government-run or -administered programs, such as Medicare, Medicaid, and the Veterans Administration, tend to be more accessible but recent private-sectors efforts, such as those by the National Committee for Quality Assurance (NCQA), HealthGrades, and the Leapfrog group, are increasing the amount of publicly available data on healthcare quality. Other key data sources include the Dartmouth Atlas on Health Care (based on Medicare data), the Commonwealth Fund, the Kaiser Family Foundation, and numerous national- and state-level databases compiled by the Agency for Healthcare Research and Quality.

Social and Economic Factors

Data on social and economic factors are available from a number of sources such as the decennial Census and the more frequent American Community Survey that now provides inter-Census estimates for counties with a population greater than 20,000. Other sources include education data that states are required to collect as part of the federal No Child Left Behind initiative. District- and school-level statistics regarding graduation rates and student performance in reading and math can be accessed online.* As well as being available on a national level from the Bureau of Labor Statistics, unemployment data are generally available at the local and state levels from state government. Information on both violent and property crime are available through the Federal Bureau of Investigation, which collects data on crime reports and arrests from local law enforcement agencies annually, and from the Bureau of Justice. However, data on social cohesion and connectedness are more difficult to access, relying primarily on sporadic population-based surveys and individual research projects, although data on community engagement (e.g., see Civic Life Index from the Corporation for National and Community Service) and civic participation, e.g., voting records, are available.

Physical Environment

Data on environmental factors are available from a variety of sources with differential availability across the different potential units of analysis—for example, national, state, county, city, neighborhood, and so forth. In addition, the quality of these data are also highly variable. For example, data on public water system violations are available in the U.S. EPA Safe Drinking Water Information System, but the quality of the data vary by state. Alternatively, data may be obtained directly from municipal water departments that publish annual reports of water quality. Data on air quality and toxic releases are available from the Environmental Protection Agency (EPA), and food contamination data are collected on a national scale by the Food and Drug Administration (FDA) and the U.S. Department of Agriculture (USDA). Selected measures on the built environment are also available for some geographic units of analysis (e.g., neighborhood "walkability," access to healthy foods in a Zip code, and so forth).

Examples

Action Model to Achieve Healthy People 2020 Goals

Each decade since 1980, the U.S. Department of Health and Human Services (DHHS) has released a comprehensive set of national public health objectives. Known as **Healthy People**, the initiative has been grounded in the notion that setting objectives and providing benchmarks to track and monitor progress can motivate, guide, and focus action.[35] In 2008, DHHS began developing the next decade's objectives, Healthy People 2020,[36] and presented these objectives in 2009. This

---

*www.schooldatadirect.org

plan is best described as a *national health agenda that communicates a vision and a strategy for the Nation.* Healthy People 2020 will provide overarching, national-level goals and serve as a road map showing where the nation should go and how to get there—both collectively and individually.

To communicate the critical role of the multiple determinants of population health—including social and economic factors—Healthy People 2020 is guided by an action model for population health (**Figure 5–3**).[37] This framework was adapted from an Institute of Medicine model that illustrates the determinants and ecological nature of health across the life course.[15] Interventions (i.e., policies, programs, and information) affect the determinants of health at multiple levels (e.g., individual; social, family, and community; living and working conditions; and broad social, economic, cultural, health, and environmental conditions) to improve outcomes.

The Wisconsin County Health Rankings

Since 2003, the University of Wisconsin Population Health Institute has been collecting data and reporting on the multiple determinants of health via the *Wisconsin Health Rankings.* There are three primary goals for the *County Health Rankings:*

1. To increase media attention in local health outcomes and determinants.

2. To highlight the broad range of factors that influence health.

3. To catalyze community health improvement efforts.

An analysis of media coverage from 2004 to 2008 clearly shows that the *Wisconsin County Health Rankings* have succeeded in the first of these three primary goals as the number of *Rankings*-related stories increased from 23 in 2006 to 47 in 2008. Additionally, media outlets appear to be increasingly turning to local sources rather than relying on university-based researchers to put the *Rankings* into context for their readers/viewers/listeners. All but four Wisconsin counties (Barron, Grant, Green Lake, and Richland) have been the focus of a story or mentioned in *Rankings* media during the 2004–2008 period.

News stories largely focus on the rankings/numbers, only sometimes exploring in depth the determinants of health beyond mentioning that the *Rankings* are based on broad determinants. A few more recent articles have made use of accompanying photographs to highlight the determinants of health (e.g., people running and bicycling on paths or exercising in a school's exercise facility). Four in ten stories mentioned real people or programs, although none featured a "real person" or offered narratives illustrating health successes or issues facing the community. Narratives can be especially valuable because they can facilitate attitude and behavior changes

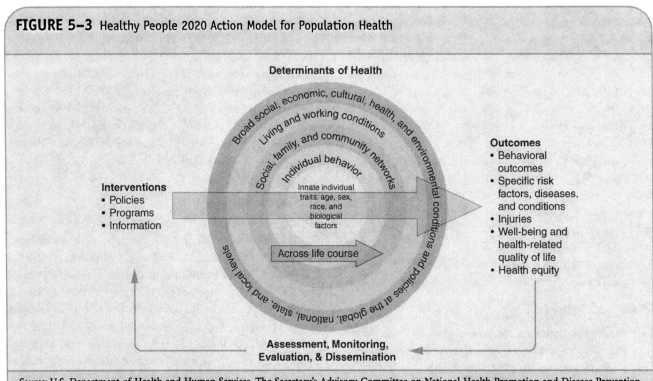

FIGURE 5–3 Healthy People 2020 Action Model for Population Health

Source: U.S. Department of Health and Human Services. The Secretary's Advisory Committee on National Health Promotion and Disease Prevention Objectives for 2020. Section IV. Advisory Committee Findings and Recommendations. http://www.healthypeople.gov/HP2020/advisory/PhaseI/sec4 .htm#_Toc211942918. Accessed January 11, 2010.

among readers, allowing to "connect with broader social groups and populations represented by story characters."[38]

Media coverage of health rankings is not a given. A brief review of media coverage of county health rankings in Kansas, New Mexico, and Tennessee showed mixed results. Kansas saw a similar amount of media interest as Wisconsin in its inaugural county health rankings in 2009, with 29 media stories identified. New Mexico and Tennessee media appeared to be much less engaged in the story. Although, the Tennessee Institute of Public Health has ranked the health of the state's 95 counties since 2006, relatively little media coverage was found. Even less evidence of media coverage was found for the 2008 *New Mexico County Health Rankings*, according to The Institute for Public Health at the University of New Mexico School of Medicine.[39]

COMMUNICATION ABOUT EVIDENCE-BASED SOLUTIONS

The final goal for health communications is to support the translation of science into practice. It is not sufficient to simply communicate about the leading health problems and their determinants. To be effective, health communication strategies must connect information about the problems with potential solutions. Foege applied this concept to epidemiology, when he developed the term "consequential epidemiology" to emphasize that to be effective, the results of epidemiology research must improve public health.[40] Health communications is one important strategy to this end.

Sources of Information on Health Solutions

The volume of information published about the effectiveness of individual programs and policies far exceeds the ability of any person to remain current, summarize, and synthesize. To address this problem, researchers conduct evidence-based **systematic reviews** to consolidate all the information from studies addressing a single clinical or public health question (see also Chapter 4). Systematic reviews use explicit and comprehensive (systematic) methods to identify, select, and critically assess all relevant research on the issue under consideration. To avoid bias, the reviews use standard protocols for searching for data and appraising and combining study data. Over the past two decades, systematic reviews have been increasingly using meta-analysis to provide a more quantitative approach for integrating the findings of individual studies.

Finding information about effective programs and policies is easier today than ever before with the advent of online resources. The Cochrane Collaboration is the most respected source of systematic reviews of healthcare interventions. The PubMed Systematic Review filter is available through the National Library of Medicine. This resource specializes in PubMed searches to retrieve citations identified as systematic reviews, meta-analyses, reviews of clinical trials, evidence-based medicine, consensus development conferences, and guidelines. Additional resources for evidence-based reviews of programs and policies are shown in **Table 5–4**.[41–44]

TABLE 5–4 Sources of Information about Evidence-Based Programs and Policies in the United States

The Guide to Community Preventive Services	The Guide to Community Preventive Services is a free resource to help you choose programs and policies to improve health and prevent disease in your community.[41]
The Guide to Clinical Preventive Services	The U.S. Preventive Services Task Force (USPSTF) was convened by the Public Health Service to rigorously evaluate clinical research in order to assess the merits of preventive measures, including screening tests, counseling, immunizations, and preventive medications.[42]
MMWR Recommendations and Reports	The MMWR Recommendations and Reports contain in-depth articles that relay policy statements for prevention and treatment on all areas in CDC's scope of responsibility (e.g., recommendations from the Advisory Committee on Immunization Practices).[43]
The National Guideline Clearinghouse™	The National Guideline Clearinghouse™ is a public resource for evidence-based clinical practice guidelines. It is an initiative of the Agency for Healthcare Research and Quality, U.S. Department of Health and Human Services, originally created by in partnership with the American Medical Association and the American Association of Health Plans (now America's Health Insurance Plans).[44]

Source: Reprinted from U.S. Census Bureau, International Population

Systematic reviews of the evidence use a pre-defined process for reviewing scientific research to try and answer these questions:

- What interventions have and have not worked?
- In which populations and settings has the intervention worked or not?
- What might the intervention cost? What should I expect for my investment?
- Does the intervention lead to any other benefits or harms?
- What interventions need more research before we know if they work or not?

The Task Force on Community Preventive Services, which oversees the Guide to Community Preventive Services, hopes those who read Community Guide reviews will use more interventions shown to work, use fewer interventions shown not to work, and evaluate research interventions for which there is inadequate evidence to determine whether or not they work.

Examples

Cancer Control PLANET

The **Cancer Control PLANET** (Plan, Link, Act, Network, with Evidence-based Tools) from the National Cancer Institute is a Web-based portal* that helps communicate information about evidence-based cancer control programs and policies. The portal includes five steps for developing a comprehensive cancer control program:

- Step 1: Assess program priorities.
- Step 2: Identify potential partners.
- Step 3: Research reviews of different intervention approaches.
- Step 4: Find research-tested intervention programs and products.
- Step 5: Plan and evaluate the program.

Cancer Control PLANET provides cancer control planners, program staff, and researchers with easy access to resources that can facilitate the transfer of evidence-based research findings into practice.[45] The website provides research reviews of different intervention approaches, showing which approaches have been shown to be effective or ineffective. In addition, the website provides information about recently tested intervention programs and products,

and many of these programs can be downloaded or ordered free of cost.

What Works for Health (Wisconsin)

A report, *What Works: Policies and Programs to Improve Wisconsin's Health,* was developed to move policymakers and other leaders in Wisconsin from information to action, focusing on identifying effective policies and programs that can affect the multiple drivers of health, which in turn affect our health outcomes. The What Works for Health report (and its accompanying database†) provide a menu of policies and programs for possible implementation in Wisconsin. The policies and programs are divided into three categories, based on the overarching goals of improving (1) health behaviors, (2) the social and physical environment, and (3) healthcare and public health systems. It was based on a summary of a wide scan of research to find evidence of effectiveness for policies and programs addressing the multiple drivers of health. The database contains information for each program and policy on:

- Description and intended beneficial outcomes.
- Level of implementation in Wisconsin and other states.
- Evidence rating of policy/program effectiveness.
- Potential population reach, that is, the number of Wisconsin residents potentially affected.
- Potential impact of the policy or program on health disparities.
- Category of decision maker(s) who could enact the policy or program.
- Setting, life stage, and targeted groups.

Effectiveness means whether a policy or program works in real life, while *evidence* is the information on which a judgment can be based or a proof established." However, there can be a range of different types of evidence, from "data resulting from scientific controlled trials and research" through "expert or user consensus, evaluation, or anecdotal information" or personal observation. Our review focused on **scientific evidence** (the accumulation of data through evaluation and research that carefully examines how an intervention is delivered and what improvements result). We searched for the best available research results and for data-driven reviews, rather than intuitive judgment, expertise, or experience. Our gold standard for evidence of effectiveness was based on comprehensive systematic reviews (such as those published in the Community Guide) that found strong

---

*http://cancercontrolplanet.cancer.gov/

†www.whatworksforhealth.wisc.edu

evidence of effectiveness of a particular program or policy. (Systematic reviews involve using a set of specific criteria to perform critical assessment and evaluation of all research studies that address a particular issue.)

In the absence of availability of systematic reviews in particular areas, we conducted direct searches for research evaluating the effectiveness of particular policies or programs. The best direct evidence comes from the gold standard of research designs: **randomized control trials** (RCTs). However, in many areas, it is not feasible, practical, or ethical to evaluate programs and policies using RCTs. In these cases, we looked for good evidence based on other attributes such as relevance, objectivity, and credibility that are considered "effective" but have not been the subject of rigorous scientific study.

COMMUNICATION CHALLENGES

Although the goal of using public health communication to improve the health of the public sounds simple, in practice many obstacles and challenges exist. Despite the overwhelming evidence about the leading causes of disease in society today, the public may be more interested in issues they perceive as being of higher risk but which are likely to have little effect on population health (e.g., an outbreak of a rare or unusual infectious disease that receives extensive news media coverage). Furthermore, messages about health determinants are complex, and there are many competing messages from multiple sources (e.g., political figures, news media spokespeople) offering opinions and anecdotes about "causes" and "solutions."

Confronting Public Perceptions about Risk (Perception versus Realities)

When communicating risk information to the public or policymakers, scientists have discovered that the "actual" risk may have little or no relationship to **risk perception**. Scientists define *risk* precisely as the rate of disease in the population. However, the risks from many environmental exposures, such as chemical toxins, pesticides, or electromagnetic fields, are often difficult to precisely determine in scientific studies. In some cases, the public greatly overestimates the risk and demands costly and difficult interventions. In other cases, the public may greatly underestimate the risk and ignore recommendations that might have a substantial impact on their health.

Risk communication is probably the most challenging problem faced by epidemiologists attempting to translate scientific information because there is often a strong emotional component (especially fear and anger) and distrust of institutions, organizations, or scientists among the affected public. **Risk communication** involves an interactive exchange of information among affected parties (e.g., individuals and organiza-

tions) about the nature, magnitude, significance, and control of risk. It may involve multiple messages about the nature of risk and other messages not strictly about risk, which express concerns, opinions, or reactions to risk messages or to legal and institutional arrangements for risk management.

Complexity of Health Determinants

Messages about the leading causes of death in a community can be newsworthy. People fear these diseases and can relate to information for example, about cancer or heart disease because many have a friend or family member who has been affected. In contrast, stories about the determinants of health may be harder to promote or gain the attention of audiences. This is particularly true regarding the effects of lifestyle, cultural practices, and other social and economic factors. Describing multiple factors in causation with a simple message is challenging. Unlike infectious diseases, where a single cause of the illness is predominant, chronic diseases are caused by many factors over one's lifetime.

Confronting Other "Evidence"

Although the availability of information about evidence-based public health programs and policies has increased, it has not kept pace with the explosion of other sources of information on the World Wide Web. For example, a recent Google search of "weight loss" produces more than 100 million hits, with sponsored links prominently displayed for "Slim Xtreme on Sale," "Lose 21 in 7 Days," and "Jenny Craig Official Site." The leading nonsponsored links include claims such as "The Flat Belly Diet," "Lose Weight Fast," and "9 Best Diet Tips Ever."

CONCLUSION

Advances in public health research and practice over the past century have led to changes in the leading health problems— as well as to changes in our understanding of the contributions of various factors that influence health. Communicators can use population health models when designing communication strategies and focus along the three major areas along the continuum: health outcomes and the leading causes of death and disability; the multiple determinants (behaviors, health care, social and economic factors, and the physical environment); and, effective programs and policies. Communication can be an effective strategy to inform the public about this myriad of health issues. It can even be used to persuade individuals to adopt healthy behaviors or policymakers to promote evidence-based programs and policies. If done effectively, public health communication can be an effective tool to improve the health of the public.

KEY TERMS

Cancer Control PLANET
Causes of death
Clinical preventive services
Health determinants
Health disparities
Health outcomes

Healthy People
Randomized control trials
Risk communication
Risk perception
Scientific evidence
Social epidemiology
Systematic reviews

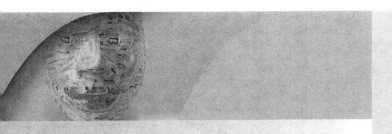

Chapter Questions

1. Why is it important to have a national health behavior surveillance system, like the BRFSS?

2. Describe one of the most important determinants of population health according to the Institute of Medicine. Provide examples of some of the first studies showing evidence for this determinant.

3. What are the four criteria making up health determinant rankings within and among populations? How are these criteria distributed for the entire U.S. population as of 2010 (Hint: *America's Health Rankings*)? How can we communicate these four criteria to the public?

4. Name several of the key data sources of health factors, including for health behaviors, social and economic health determinants, and so forth.

5. List the major sources of evidence-based public health initiatives. Which critical questions do these sources answer (5 total)?

6. Choose one of the following databases of evidence-based health research: *What Works: Policies and Programs to Improve Wisconsin's Health* or Cancer Control PLANET. Describe what information the database includes and what health problem (or problems) it was designed to address.

7. What is the overarching goal of Healthy People 2020?

8. Summarize what is involved in health risk communication.

REFERENCES

1. Bunker JP, Frazier HS, Mosteller F. Improving health: measuring effects of medical care. *Milbank Quarterly.* 1994;72:225–258.

2. CDC. Achievements in public health, 1900–1999: Changes in the public health system. *MMWR.* 1999;48(50):1141–1147.

3. CDC. Leading causes of death, 1900–1998. http://www.cdc.gov/nchs/data/dvs/lead1900_98.pdf. Accessed September 25, 2009.

4. CDC. *National vital statistics reports.* 2009;57(14).

5. CDC. Ten great public health achievements—United States, 1900–1999. *MMWR.* 1999;48(12):241–243.

6. Evans RG, Stoddart GL. Producing health, consuming health care. *Soc Sci Med.* 1990;31:1347–1363.

7. Lalonde M. A new perspective on the health of Canadians. A working document. Ottawa: Government of Canada, 1974.

8. Minkler M. Health education, health promotion and the open society: an historical perspective. *Health Educ Q.* 1989 Spring;16(1):17–30.

9. McGinnis JM, Foege WH. Actual causes of death in the United States. *JAMA.* 1993; 270:2207–2212.

10. Mokdad AH, Bowman BA, Ford ES, Vinicor F, Marks JS, Koplan JP. The continuing epidemics of obesity and diabetes in the US. *JAMA.* 2001;286:1195–1200.

11. Mokdad AH, Marks JS, Stroup DF, Gerberding JL. Actual causes of death in the United States, 2000. *JAMA.* 2004;291(10):1238–1245.

12. Evans RG, Stoddart GL. Models for population health: Consuming research, producing policy? *Am J Public Health.* 2003;93(3):371–379.

13. Remington PL, Smith MY, Williamson DF, Anda RF, Gentry EM, Hogelin GC. Design, characteristics, and usefulness of state-based risk factor surveillance 1981–1986. *Public Health Rep.* 1988 Jul–Aug;103(4):366–375.

14. Mokdad AH, Serdula MK, Dietz WH, Bowman BA, Marks JS, Koplan JP. The spread of the obesity epidemic in the US. *JAMA.* 1999;282:1519–1522.

15. Institute of Medicine. *The future of the public's health in the 21st century.* Washington, DC: National Academies Press; 2002.

16. Berkman L, Kawachi I. *Social epidemiology.* New York: Oxford University Press; 2000.

17. Marmot MG, Rose G, Shipley M, Hamilton PJ. Employment grade and coronary heart disease in British civil servants. *J Epidemiol Community Health.* 1978;32:244–249.

18. Department of Health and Human Services. *Health United States 2007.* CDC/National Center for Health Statistics, March 2008.

19. Woolf SH, Johnson RE, et al. Giving everyone the health of the educated: an examination of whether social change would save more lives than medical advances. *Am J Public Health.* 2007;97:679–683.

20. Elo I, Preson S. Educational differences in Mortality. *Soc. Sci. Med.* 1996;42:47–57.

21. Evans R, Barer M, Marmor T. *Why are some people healthy and others not? The determinants of health of populations.* New York: Aldine de Gruyter; 1994.

22. Friedman DJ, Starfield B. Models of population health: Their value for U.S. public health practice, policy, and research. *Am J Public Health.* 2003 March;93(3):366–369.

23. Kindig D, Stoddart G. Models for population health: What is population health? *Am J Public Health.* 2003;93(3):380–383.

24. Peppard PE, Kindig D, Jovaag A, Dranger E, Remington PL. An initial attempt at ranking population health outcomes and determinant. *WMJ.* 2004;103:52–56.

25. Peppard PE, Kindig D, Dranger E, Jovaag A, Remington PL. Ranking community health status to stimulate discussion of local public health issues: The Wisconsin County Health Rankings. *Am J Public Health.* 2008;98:209–212.

26. Rohan AMK, Booske BC, Remington PL. Using the *Wisconsin County Health Rankings* to catalyze community health improvement. *J Public Health Manage. Pract.* 200915(1):24–32.

27. McGinnis JM, Williams-Russo P, Knickman JA. The case for more active policy attention to health promotion. *Health Affairs.* 2002;21(2):83.

28. CDC National Center for Injury Prevention and Control. WISQARS leading causes of death reports, 1999–2006. http://webappa.cdc.gov/sasweb/ncipc/leadcaus10.html. Accessed January 11, 2010.

29. United Health Foundation. America's health: Weighting of measures. http://www.americashealthrankings.org/2009/component/Weight.aspx. Accessed January 11, 2010.

30. Washington State Department of Health. Report card on health in Washington 2005. http://www.doh.wa.gov/PHIP/reportcard/documents/report_card2005.pdf. Accessed January 11, 2010.

31. North Carolina Department of Health and Human Services. Racial and ethnic health disparities in North Carolina: Report card 2006. http://www.schs.state.nc.us/SCHS/pdf/ReportCard2006.pdf. Accessed January 11, 2010.

32. CDC. Trends in racial and ethnic-specific rates for the health status indicators: United States, 1990-1998—Healthy People 2010. *Statistical Notes.* 23; 2002.

33. Booske BC, Kempf AM, Athens JK, Kindig DA, Remington PL. *Health of Wisconsin Report Card.* University of Wisconsin Population Health Institute; 2007.

34. Booske BC, Rohan AM, Kindig DA, Remington PL. Grading the 50 states on health and health disparities. *Preventing Chronic Disease* (in press).

35. U.S. Department of Health and Human Services. Healthy People 2020: The road ahead. http://www.healthypeople.gov/HP2020/default.asp. Accessed January 11, 2010.

36. U.S. Department of Health and Human Services. The Secretary's Advisory Committee on National Health Promotion and Disease Prevention Objectives for 2020. http://www.healthypeople.gov/HP2020/advisory/PhaseI/default.htm. Accessed January 11, 2010.

37. U.S. Department of Health and Human Services. The Secretary's Advisory Committee on National Health Promotion and Disease Prevention Objectives for 2020. Section IV. Advisory Committee Findings and Recommendations. http://www.healthypeople.gov/HP2020/advisory/PhaseI/sec4.htm#_Toc211942918. Accessed January 11, 2010.

38. Niederdeppe J, Bu QL, Borah P, Kindig DA, Robert SA. Message Design strategies to raise public awareness of social determinants of health and population health disparities. *Milbank Quarterly.* 2008;86(3):481–513.

39. The Institute for Public Health at the University of New Mexico School of Medicine. 2009 (unpublished data).

40. Marks JS. Epidemiology, public health, and public policy. *Prev Chronic Dis.* 2009;6(4). Available at: http://www.cdc.gov/pcd/issues/2009/oct/09_0110.htm. Accessed 10/15/2009.

41. CDC. *Guide to community preventive services.* http://www.thecommunityguide.org/index.html. Accessed November 1, 2009.

42. U.S. Department of Health and Human Services Agency for Healthcare Research and Quality. *Guide to clinical preventive services.* http://www.ahrq.gov/clinic/cps3dix.htm. Accessed November 1, 2009.

43. CDC. *Morbidity and Mortality Weekly Reports.* http://www.cdc.gov/mmwr/mmwr_rr.html. Accessed November 1, 2009.

44. Agency for Healthcare Research and Quality. National Guideline Clearinghouse. http://www.guideline.gov/. Accessed November 1, 2009.

45. Kerner JF. Guirguis-Blake J, Hennessy KD, et al. Translating research into improved outcomes in comprehensive cancer control. *Cancer Causes and Control* 2005;16(Supplement 1):27–40.

CHAPTER 6

Communicating for Policy and Advocacy

Ross C. Brownson, Ellen Jones, and Claudia Parvanta

LEARNING OBJECTIVES

By the end of this chapter, the reader will be able to:

- Understand the importance of policy in influencing health and well-being.
- Describe the characteristics of policymakers and how these help shape communication strategies.
- Identify the role of the message, messenger, and modes of delivery.
- Conduct an environmental scan.
- Understand the barriers and challenges when communicating with policymakers.
- Describe key advocacy strategies.
- Develop several policy and advocacy materials.

INTRODUCTION

In the ecological model, federal and state laws and regulations, as well as local or organizational policies, shape many of the **environmental factors** that affect our health. These include how health-related resources are allocated, managed, and protected. According to the California-based Center for Health Improvement,

> The health of a community is the shared responsibility of many organizations and interests in that community. This includes schools, employers, healthcare providers, local health departments, park and recreation departments, city planners, traffic controllers and the people of the community, to name a few. Negotiating the interests of such a diverse group of concerned citizens and stakeholders is essentially a political

process. In short, politics is the negotiating process by which a civil society decides who gets what, when and how. Politics produces policy. This holds true at any level, from within families, no matter how they are defined, all the way to the White House.[1]

Health policies can be broad in scope[2–4] (e.g., a federal regulation requiring folic acid fortification of bread and other enriched cereal or grain products; state clean indoor air laws) or may involve organizational practices (e.g., a private work-site ban on smoking, school district nutrition and physical activity policies). The healthcare insurance debate of 2009–2010 has given everyone a taste of how passions and politics can shape policy. But sometimes we also manage to influence policy with data. This chapter describes how to communicate about public health data to governmental level policymakers, as well as how to work with partners to bring an issue informed by these data up to a decision-making level, be it for a school, community, or elected official. This is called **advocacy**.

There are a couple of quotations that seem particularly apt in the politics/policy arena. One is the political Golden Rule, that is to say, "He who has the gold, makes the rules." Another is, "For every complex problem, there is a solution that is simple, neat, and wrong." These quotes represent two horns that many policymakers face in the bullring of American politics. There are always powerful groups with large economic interests at stake that have the resources to push a policy agenda. They often pay for surveys and studies that support their positions, trying to ensure they get into the media. And because politicians are elected, and because voters may replace them every two (U.S. representatives, many state legislators), four (the president, state governors), or six years (U.S. senators), it seems that every decision requires a fast solution. How does the acquisition of public health data factor into this process? Sometimes not so well.

Public health practitioners have this annoying need to value accuracy over speed in data acquisition. Most scientific discoveries are achieved through incremental advances in knowledge over years or decades. Data from long-term research studies and surveillance systems provide the best picture of what is happening in public health. And small changes from one year to the next in disease prevalence or behavior change may not be that punchy. Policy makers often want quick, absolute answers to complex questions. Two decades ago, the Institute of Medicine determined that decision-making in public health is often driven by "…crises, hot issues, and concerns of organized interest groups."[5] Indeed, existing public health data from long-term reliable research are often underutilized and sometimes ignored because policymakers regularly make decisions based on short-term demands—like crisis situations—and policies and programs are frequently developed around anecdotal evidence.[6] Changing these patterns is a concern and priority among public health communicators.

We have learned from the corporate world how to make presenting public health data more effective and "business-like," which includes:

- Getting to know our audience.
- Anticipating and answering their questions.
- Presenting our data in a compelling fashion that is easy to grasp.
- Behaving in a professional manner.

STRATEGIC POLICY COMMUNICATION
Get to Know the Audience

The term **policymaker** in this chapter primarily refers to elected officials (e.g., city council members, state legislators, U.S. representatives and senators). There is considerable overlap between the roles and impacts of health policymakers and administrators (e.g., program and agency leaders in the executive branch of government). For example, the director of a state health department makes decisions about how resources are allocated and where an agency's emphasis should be placed when carrying out various health policies. Legislative staff members also play key roles in policy development. Differences among various policy-making audiences are shown in **Table 6–1**.

One example is that executive branch officials can spend more time on a fewer number of issues than legislative staff or elected officials. The opportunities and challenges to effective communication of data have been accentuated by the explosion in information technologies that allow ready access to

TABLE 6–1 Differences in Decision Making among Policy Audiences

Characteristic	Executive Branch, Public Health Administrator	Legislative Branch, Elected Official	Legislative Branch, Staff Member
Time in position	Longer	Shorter	Shorter
Accountability	Governor, board of health, agency head	Constituents by whom they are elected, political party	Elected legislator, committee chair
Personal connection to constituents	Moderate	High	High to moderate
Knowledge span	Deeper knowledge on health issues	Less depth, wider breadth	Less depth, wider breadth
Decision making based on external factors* (aside from research)	Low to moderate	High	High
Time spent on a particular issue	Longer	Shortest	Shorter
Type of data relied upon	Science, empirical studies, experience from the field	Science, media, "real-world" stories, constituents, lobbyists, party priorities	Science, the media, "real-world" stories, constituents, lobbyists, party priorities

*External factors commonly include habits, stereotypes, and cultural norms.

many types of public health data. Although this chapter focuses largely on communicating to policymakers in the public sector, many of the principles and approaches apply equally to private organizations (e.g., health maintenance organizations), voluntary health agencies, and businesses.

There are considerable differences between members of Congress and state or local elected officials. Members of Congress serve full-time. The average age in the 110th Congress was 56 years for the House of Representatives and 62 years for the Senate. Nearly all have a college education, and the most predominant occupation for senators was law, followed by public service/politics. Members of the House were more likely to list public service/politics followed by business and then law. Most members of Congress have little background in public health issues. Among the 538 members, there were 13 medical doctors, 2 dentists, 3 nurses, 2 veterinarians, 1 psychologist, 1 optometrist, and 1 pharmacist. The average length of service was 12.8 years in the Senate and 10 years in the House. There were a record number of women (91) elected to the 110th Congress as well as a record number of Hispanic/Latino individuals (30).[7]

Since the late 1900s, state legislatures have become bodies of increasing diversity. In 1970, most legislatures were composed of white, middle-class males. In 2008, 8% of legislators were African American and 3% were Latino. When legislators classify their profession, 16% indicate they are full-time legislators, 15% are lawyers, and 12% are retired. Professions differed by region: In 2007 the most common profession was attorney (21%) in the Southeast, compared with 13% in the Midwest.[7]

State legislative bodies and procedures differ widely across the United States. The smallest legislature has 49 members and the largest has 424. The National Conference of State Legislatures uses a formula combining the amount of time spent in session, the average monetary compensation, and the number of legislative staff to assess the capacity of state legislatures (see **Table 6–2**).[8]

The formula designates some states as red,* (80% time on the job [in session], higher pay, and larger staff). These states operate most like Congress. White states are in session for about 66% time, or longer, usually need to have outside sources of income to supplement pay, and have intermediate-sized staff. Blue states are in session half-time or less, must earn an income outside of the legislature, and have little or no staff. Average compensation (in 2008) by category varies widely, with the highest salaries for red states ($68,599), followed by white states ($35,326), and blue states ($15,984).[8]

What else do you need to know about your proposed "target" audience? Just about everything. Elected officials usually have websites where they post their voting records, issues of concern to their constituency, and possibly blogs. It is also a good idea to know something about their spouses—many public health initiatives have been instigated through the interests of governors' wives (for the most part), or congressional

---

*This is different than the Republican = Red and Democrat = Blue designation used in election discussions.

TABLE 6–2 Red, White, and Blue Legislatures

Red	Red Light	White		Blue Light	Blue
California	Florida	Alabama	Missouri	Georgia	Montana
Michigan	Illinois	Alaska	Nebraska	Idaho	New Hampshire
New York	Massachusetts	Arizona	North Carolina	Indiana	North Dakota
Pennsylvania	New Jersey	Arkansas	Oklahoma	Kansas	South Dakota
	Ohio	Colorado	Oregon	Maine	Utah
	Wisconsin	Connecticut	South Carolina	Mississippi	Wyoming
		Delaware	Tennessee	Nevada	
		Hawaii	Texas	New Mexico	
		Iowa	Virginia	Rhode Island	
		Kentucky	Washington	Vermont	
		Louisiana		West Virginia	
		Maryland			
		Minnesota			

Source: http://www.ncsl.org/programs/press/2004/backgrounder_fullandpart.htm

spouses, as many have a special interest in an issue. For example, Christopher Shays, a Republican who represented Connecticut's 4th District in the House of Representatives from 1987 to 2009, married his Peace Corps sweetheart, Betsi Shays, who held a high-ranking position in Peace Corps through 1997. If you were not familiar with Shays's conscientious objector status and Peace Corps connection, you might have had the wrong impression of the scope of his interests based purely on his political party and state affiliation. Recognizing the importance of the political spouse, the Centers for Disease Control and Prevention (CDC) chose to work with the Governors' Spouses Association to make October National Breast Cancer Awareness Month, beginning in 1994.

If you are acting in a non-official capacity (you do not represent a government agency) the first rule for interacting with elected officials is that you need to be part of their jurisdiction. If you live in Alabama, and are trying to influence a bill being prepared in Pennsylvania, you need to find someone who lives in Pennsylvania to intercede with the elected official on this issue. Similarly, if you live in a small suburb near Philadelphia, **Figure 6–1** shows who will care about what you have to say, as well as their congressional voting record. Before approaching these elected officials, you need to do at least this level of research to know their predisposition toward your issue.

If you are working in an official capacity (i.e., you work for a state or county health department or for a federal agency), then your voter affiliation and address are not pertinent, although legislative staff will look into it as standard operating procedure. Here is an important lesson from the late Tip O'Neill that should be committed to memory:*

> According to Tip O'Neill, his father, Thomas O'Neill, Sr., shared this wisdom on the occasion of the only election loss of Tip's lifetime—a run for the Cambridge City Council. "(My father) pointed out that I had taken my own neighborhood for granted. He was right: I had received a tremendous vote in the other sections of the city, but I hadn't worked hard enough in my own backyard. 'Let me tell you something I learned years ago,' he said, 'all politics is local.' "[9]

This means that even though constituency shouldn't matter, it will. So again, if possible, find someone from a legislator's voting district to be a spokesperson.

Your first interactions with elected officials will most likely be through their staff. Some of these individuals have in-depth knowledge of health issues or interest in specific health issues, but many do not. Their job is to keep policymakers and administrators informed of the issues and potential pitfalls of proposed legislation. Legislative staff members have a fair amount of influence over the decision about which proposals are put forth as alternatives.[10] When interacting and working with these staff, the communicators' role is to present a compelling argument that leads to a desired action. Also, you should look at *your* job as making *their* job as easy as possible in terms of presenting your thoughts to their boss. When possible, the message should be concise and tied to a policy action. Using sound bites that a policymaker or staffer can later repeat is often helpful. Many public health messages are complicated: policymaking staff members will want to be able to explain their position in simple terms and then call upon experts, such as you or others, to add the details.

Anticipating Their Questions

Regardless of how much information seems to be available, preparing a strategy on an issue requires grasping what members of the relevant public are saying about it. And, the elected official's questions to you are likely to be driven by their reading of the media as well as what the pollsters are saying. So, you need to be prepared with this information as part of your strategy and have the numbers handy. **Figure 6–2** shows a strategy for analyzing issues that can be applied to media coverage, blogs, or polling data.

Media Scanning

In the "good old days" (until about 1995), **media scanning** was still done chiefly by clipping news articles about an issue of interest. The media relations staff of the CDC used to sit in a conference room early in the morning and cut and paste up a photocopy packet from the major papers (*New York Times, Washington Post, USA Today, Atlanta Journal Constitution,* and any local papers where a story was hot). This was distributed across the agency. The CDC switched to a service at the turn of the century that continues to provide print, television, and online reporting of anything of interest to CDC scientists and program managers. The media division posts this on a CDC intranet. You may anticipate that every elected official will make use of media scanning on some level concerning his or her own work, and the constituency's reactions to it.

The amount of information available on the Internet about any issue has made media scanning both easier and more complicated. It is easier because you can see who is talking about an issue, and what they are saying, fairly quickly. And

---

*Among other elected positions, Thomas (Tip) O'Neill was the 55th Speaker of the U.S. House of Representatives from 1977 to 1987, serving under Presidents Gerald Ford, Jimmy Carter, and Ronald Reagan.

FIGURE 6-1 Elected Officials for Wynnewood, Pennsylvania*

Elected Officials-Pennsylvania (19096–2414)

Write Your Elected Officials

Write to your Federal or State elected officials with one click, or just go to the individual pages linked below.

President & Congress	Governor & State Legislators
President	**Governor**
• Barack Obama (D)	• Edward Rendell (D)
Senators	**Senate**
• Arlen Specter (D)	• Daylin Leach (D-17)
• Robert Casey (D)	**House of Representatives**
Representatives	• Tim Briggs (D-149)
• Jim Gerlach (R-6)	

Voting Records for June–November 2009

Key Votes Spotlight   Mega Vote

Senate Votes		Casey (D) Voted	Specter (D) Voted
Confirmed	Confirmation Andre M. Davis, of Maryland, to be U.S. Circuit Judge for the Fourth Circuit 11/09/2009	Y	Y
Passed	H.R. 2847 As Amended; Commerce, Justice, Science, and Related Agencies Appropriations Act, 2010 11/05/2009	Y	Y
Passed	H.R. 3548 as amended; Unemployment Compensation Extension Act of 2009 11/04/2009	Y	Y
Agreed To	Conference Report to Accompany H.R. 2647; National Defense Authorization Act for Fiscal Year 2010 10/22/2009	Y	Y
Rejected	Motion to Invoke Cloture on the Motion to Proceed to S. 1776; A kill to amend title XVIII of the Social Security Act to provide for the update under the Medicare physician fee schedule 10/21/2009	Y	Y
Agreed To	Conference Report to Accompany H.R. 2892; Department of Homeland Security Appropriations Act, 2010 10/20/2009	Y	Y
Agreed To	Conference Report to Accompany H.R. 3183; Energy and Water Development and Related Agencies Appropriations Act, 2010 10/15/2009	Y	Y
Passed	H.R. 3435; A bill making supplemental appropriations for fiscal year 2009 for the Consumer Assistance to Recycle and Save Program 08/06/2009	Y	Y
Confirmed	Confirmation of Sonia Sotomayor, of New York, to be an Associate Justice of the Supreme Court 08/06/2009	Y	Y
Rejected	Thune Amendment on Concealed Firearms 07/22/2009	Y	N
Passed	H.R. 1256. As Amended; Family Smoking Prevention and Tobacco Control Act 06/11/2009	Y	Y

House Votes		Gerlach (R) Voted
Passed	Affordable Health Care for America Act 11/07/2009	N
Passed	Chemical Facility Anti-Terrorism Act of 2009 11/06/2009	N
Passed	Worker, Homeownership, and Business Assistance Act 11/05/2009	Y
Passed	Expedited CARD Reform for Consumers Act of 2009 11/04/2009	NY
Passed	Solar Technology Roadmap Act 10/22/2009	Y
Passed	Bay Area Regional Water Recycling Program Expansion Act 10/15/2009	N
Passed	Making appropriations for Homeland Security FY 2010 10/15/2009	Y
Passed	Cash for Clunkers, Round Two 07/31/2009	Y
Passed	American Clean Energy and Security Act 06/26/2009	N

*Note: This search was run based on zip code.

Source: http://www.votesmart.org/index.htm

FIGURE 6–2 Media Scanning Strategies

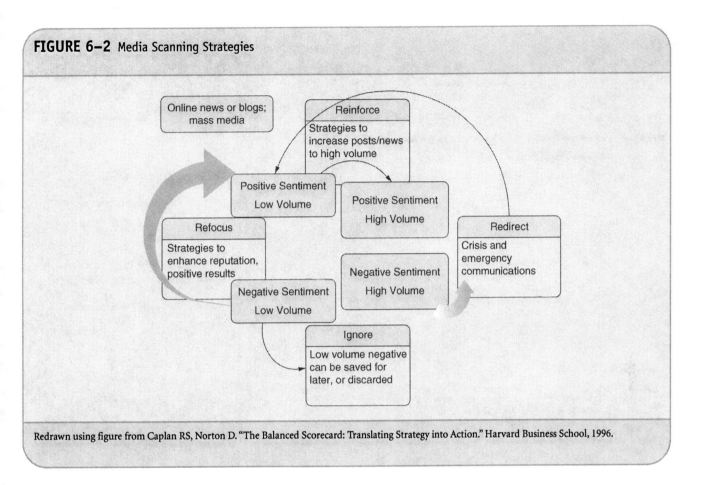

Redrawn using figure from Caplan RS, Norton D. "The Balanced Scorecard: Translating Strategy into Action." Harvard Business School, 1996.

there are some amazing free tools to help. However, separating actual news and expressions of opinion from multiple repetitions of the same item across a range of different media platforms is difficult. Twenty-four-hour news channels repeat the same story, or add barely noticeable differences to freshen it up. And, with blogs now also being tracked, getting an accurate sense of news coverage on an issue requires a lot of reading.

Because the amplification of the media (through repetition) can be so extreme, you might need to conduct an independent survey to see what the public is truly thinking about an issue. Almost all news agencies subscribe to **polling surveys** such as the *Gallup Poll** or *Harris Interactive*[†] for weekly national polling on critical issues. The CDC has worked closely with Harvard's Robert Blendon to conduct time- and region-specific surveys around critical health emergencies and preparedness.[‡] There is often a mismatch between how the media

portray public opinion, which can be shaped by a few people standing in front of a camera waving signs—shown over and over again, versus an entirely different majority opinion that is not making headlines.

New Media Tools

Probably the most accessible media tool that measures the online information-seeking behavior of the public on a particular issue is **Google trends**. **Figure 6–3** shows a trend analysis for "H1N1 vaccine" and "seasonal flu shots" in 2009. The figure shows that at the height of interest, nearly 8% of online searching was about the H1N1 vaccine. This compares with an unscaled peak in Google news reports on the same topic. What does 8% of online searching mean? For comparison, online searching for golfer Tiger Woods during the height of his 2009 scandal represented 75% of online searches. While 8% is probably a huge number for a public health topic, it is small when compared to the draw of a celebrity scandal.

Google trends can be customized to a state level, and possibly finer subdivisions, are in development. Google is also working on a "timeline" feature that pulls up news headlines by date ranges. It is still in development as of this writing.

*http://www.gallup.com/home.aspx
[†]http://www.harrispollonline.com/
[‡]http://www.hsph.harvard.edu/research/horp/project-on-the-public-and-biosecurity/

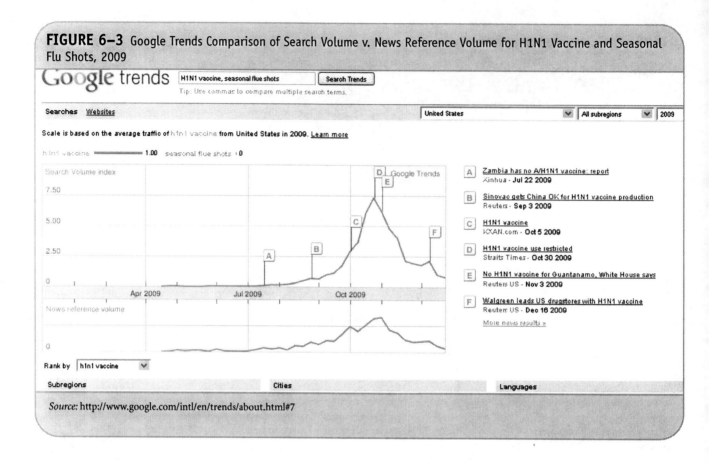

FIGURE 6–3 Google Trends Comparison of Search Volume v. News Reference Volume for H1N1 Vaccine and Seasonal Flu Shots, 2009

Source: http://www.google.com/intl/en/trends/about.html#7

By comparing the volume of media or blog postings on an issue, and whether they are positive or negative, you have a pretty good idea of how an elected official is going to interpret the same press. Together with the official's record, you can possibly assess whether the elected official wants to speak out on this issue or feels it is not important to his or her constituency. Finally, there is no law against calling and speaking to staff in order to prepare more effectively for a meeting. What you want to be able to say during your presentation when asked a question is "I thought you might ask about that and have prepared this analysis." You would rather not be in the position of having to say "I will have to get back to you on that," although it certainly can happen.

Preparing and Implementing a Policy Presentation

Research indicates that the vast majority of policymakers at national and state levels prefer face-to-face communication. Innavaer and colleagues reported factors that facilitate or reduce the use of information to make health policy decisions.[11] Primary facilitators were:

- Personal contact.
- Timely relevance.
- Inclusion of summaries with policy recommendations.

Primary barriers were:

- No personal contact.
- Research that lacked relevance.
- Mutual mistrust between scientists and policymakers.

In one-fourth of those surveyed to prepare this analysis, policymakers mentioned poor quality of health policy information as another barrier. Sorian and Bough found that among state policymakers, preferred ways of receiving information are summaries or brief reports, reports from similar states, and reports on states in the region.[12] In this study, state policymakers admitted they only read about 27% of health policy material they receive in detail. They "never get to" 35% of the material they are given. These findings underscore the importance of relationship building between public health communicators and policy- or decision-makers.

Crafting a Message

Developing an effective communication strategy is an important first step. The message needs to be direct, definitive, and defensible (backed up by the science).[13] It should be framed in a context that is easily understood by policymakers and is actionable, that is, capable of being implemented in reality. Public health practitioners often work in a context of prevention and treatment for which results are only achieved in 10 or more years. Elected officials work in an environment driven by election cycles and legislative calendars.

To narrow the message and make it compelling for policymakers, it is often useful to consider three questions that are usually most relevant to policy audiences:

- Is there a problem?
- Do we know what to do about the problem?
- How much will it cost to solve the problem?

And, while it might not be said, the policymaker will be balancing the answers to this question against his or her perceptions of the electorate. So, the last question that needs to be answered is,

- How does this help my constituency?

In addition, while you will need to be subtle about this, you also want to show the policymaker,

- Will this make me look good (to the media, to my electorate, to the powerful interests that shape my region)?

The Meta-Message

When crafting the message, it is useful to consider both the literal message and the **meta-message**. A meta-message is the larger context shaping the interpretation of a message. For example, the literal message about human papillomavirus (HPV) vaccine might be that a vaccine is now available that can protect females from the four types of HPV that cause most cervical cancers and genital warts.[14] A meta-message around the vaccine might include concerns related to teenage sexual activity or government involvement in parental decisions. In addition, meta-messages may present difficult conflicts for elected and appointed officials. Conflicting meta-messages around seatbelt policies might include benevolence, fairness, and personal rights. It is easy to see how clear public health messages get complicated by the contextual frame of reference surrounding a policy decision.

Framing

Framing also deals with the context of a message. When questions or answers are phrased in a way that misleads respondents and causes them to make an incorrect choice, this is referred to as **framing bias**. Choi has provided the following example of framing bias:[15]

Which operation would you prefer (a or b)?
a. An operation that has a 5% mortality rate
b. An operation in which 90% of patients will survive

People may choose the second option when they read "90%" and "survive," even though a 90% survival rate (which is a 10% mortality rate) is actually worse than a 5% mortality rate.

Another example of framing comes from the late 2009 release of the U.S. Preventive Services Task Force (see also Chapters 4 and 5) recommendation to begin routine biennial screening for breast cancer when a woman reaches the age of 50 years and leave decisions about screening before age 50 to the individual (see **Box 6–1**).

It was nearly impossible to craft simple messages out of the data supporting this recommendation. Depending on whether you wanted to support screening or eliminate it as a cost, you would likely frame the same data in very different ways:

- For example, you might site the NNI (Number Needed to Invite) data to say that screening of 1,904 women aged 40 to 49 years, and 1,339 women aged 50 to 59 years is needed to save one woman's life in each of these age groups. While both of these numbers attest to the relative inefficiency of screening (due to the absolute risk of one woman having cancer), you would say that it is less efficient for the younger age group.
- Or you could ignore the fact that the risk of dying from breast cancer is higher in the older age group and say that reductions in mortality risk are the same in either group, 15%.

Here is another set of data that give rise to two different frames for messages.[16] If 1,000 women between the ages of 40 and 69 undergo annual mammography for 10 years, approximately 80 women would develop cancer during this time frame. Forty women would be "cured" of cancer, and we could estimate that mammography is responsible for directly saving the lives of 12 of them.

- If for some reason you wanted to put an end to what you saw as "wasteful spending" on mammography, you might say that only half of the women with cancer were able to be saved at all and that most other women did not get the disease at all. Therefore, only 12 women out of the 1,000 who were screened for 10 years had any benefit. (Or, in this case, not even 2 lives saved by 10,000 screenings.) It's a very powerful argument if the focus is on cost-efficiency and not the individual lives saved.
- If on the other hand, you are trying to convince policymakers to support mammography screening—say, for uninsured or underinsured women—you might say: "The best chance of protecting women from breast cancer death comes with regular screening. While some women come to screening too late, we will be able to effectively treat half of the women who develop breast

Box 6–1 U.S. Preventive Services Task Force Recommendation for Breast Cancer Screening

- The USPSTF recommends biennial screening mammography for women aged 50 to 74 years.
  Grade: B recommendation.

- The decision to start regular, biennial screening mammography before the age of 50 years should be an individual one and take patient context into account, including the patient's values regarding specific benefits and harms.
  Grade: C recommendation.

- The USPSTF concludes that the current evidence is insufficient to assess the additional benefits and harms of screening mammography in women 75 years or older.
  Grade: I Statement.

- The USPSTF recommends against teaching breast self-examination (BSE).
  Grade: D recommendation.

- The USPSTF concludes that the current evidence is insufficient to assess the additional benefits and harms of clinical breast examination (CBE) beyond screening mammography in women 40 years or older.
  Grade: I Statement.

- The USPSTF concludes that the current evidence is insufficient to assess the additional benefits and harms of either digital mammography or magnetic resonance imaging (MRI) instead of film mammography as screening modalities for breast cancer.
  Grade: I Statement.

ADDITIONAL DATA ON BREAST CANCER

The American Cancer Society's most recent estimates for breast cancer in the United States (for 2009) are:

- 192,370 new cases of invasive breast cancer.
- 40,170 deaths from breast cancer.

Breast cancer is the most common cancer among women in the United States, other than skin cancer. It is the second leading cause of cancer death in women, after lung cancer.

The chance of a woman having invasive breast cancer some time during her life is a little less than 1 in 8. The chance of dying from breast cancer is about 1 in 35. Breast cancer death rates have been going down. This is probably the result of finding the cancer earlier and better treatment. Right now there are more than 2½ million breast cancer survivors in the United States (http://www.cancer.org/docroot/CRI/content/CRI_2_2_1X_How_many_people_get_breast_cancer_5.asp).

SOME SUPPORTING DATA FOR THE USPSTF RECOMMENDATION

The updated USPSTF recommendation endorses this approach for deciding at what age to start breast cancer screening. However, the current USPSTF is now further informed by a more recent systematic review,[a] which incorporates a new randomized, controlled trial that estimates the "number needed to invite for screening to extend one woman's life" as 1,904 for women aged 40 to 49 years and 1,339 for women aged 50 to 59 years. Although the relative risk reduction is nearly identical (15% and 14%) for these two age groups, the risk for breast cancer increases steeply with age starting at age 40 years. Thus, the absolute risk reduction from screening (as shown by the number needed to invite to screen) is greater for women aged 50 to 59 years than for those aged 40 to 49 years.

The current USPSTF statement is also informed by the Cancer Intervention and Surveillance Modeling Network (CISNET) modeling studies[b] that accompany this recommendation. The Task Force considered both "mortality" and "life-years gained" outcomes. In this case, given that the age groups (40 to 49 years and 50 to 59 years) are adjacent, the Task Force elected to emphasize the mortality outcomes from the modeling studies. Of the eight screening strategies found most efficient, six start at age 50 years rather than age 40 years. The frontier curves for the mortality outcome show only small gains but larger numbers of mammograms required when screening is started at age 40 years versus age 50 years.

The USPSTF reasoned that the additional benefit gained by starting screening at age 40 years rather than at age 50 years is small and that moderate harms from screening remain at any age. This leads to the C recommendation. The USPSTF notes that a "C" grade is a recommendation against *routine* screening of women aged 40 to 49 years. The Task Force encourages individualized, informed decision making about when to start mammography screening.

continues

The National Cancer Institute, on the basis of Surveillance Epidemiology and End Result data, estimates the lifetime risk for a woman to develop breast cancer at 12%.[c] The risk for breast cancer increases with age. The 10-year risk for breast cancer is 1 in 69 for a woman at age 40 years, 1 in 42 at age 50 years, and 1 in 29 at age 60 years.[d] The incidence rate of breast cancer has been increasing since the 1970s. However, recent data show this rate to be decreasing, both overall and on an age-adjusted basis. The incidence rate in 2003 was 124.2 per 100,000 women, a 6.7% decrease from the previous year.[e] Discontinuation of hormone replacement therapy may be largely responsible for this observed decrease,[e,f] although slowed growth or even a decline in screening mammography also may have contributed.[g] Breast cancer mortality has been decreasing since 1990 by 2.3% per year overall and by 3.3% for women aged 40 to 50 years. This decrease is largely attributed to the combination of mammography screening with improved treatment.[h,i,j]

References

a. U.S. Preventive Services Task Force. Screening for Breast Cancer: U.S. Preventive Services Task Force Recommendation Statement. *Ann Int Med* 2009;151: 716-726.

b. Cancer Information and surveillance Network (CISNET). Modeling various screening scenarios to inform clinical recommendations for mammography use. Accessed at http://cisnet.cancer.gov/breast/comparative.html on May 31, 2010.

c. National Cancer Institute. *Surveillance Epidemiology and End Results (SEER) Stat Fact Sheets: Breast Cancer.* Bethesda, MD: National Cancer Institute; 2009. Accessed at http://seer.cancer.gov/statfacts/html/breast.html on 25 September 2009.

d. Horner MJ, Ries LAG, Krapcho M, Neyman N, Aminou R, Howlader N, et al. (Eds.). *SEER Cancer Statistics Review, 1975-2006.* Bethesda, MD: National Cancer Institute; 2009. Accessed at http://seer.cancer.gov/csr/1975_2006 on 25 September 2009.

e. Ravdin PM, Cronin KA, Howlader N, Berg CD, Chlebowski RT, Feuer EJ, et al. The decrease in breast-cancer incidence in 2003 in the United States. *N Engl J Med* 2007;356:1670-4. [PMID: 17442911]

f. Kerlikowske K, Miglioretti DL, Buist DS, Walker R, Carney PA; National Cancer Institute-Sponsored Breast Cancer Surveillance Consortium. Declines in invasive breast cancer and use of postmenopausal hormone therapy in a screening mammography population. *J Natl Cancer Inst* 2007;99:1335-9. [PMID: 17698950]

g. Chagpar AB, McMasters KM. Trends in mammography and clinical breast examination: A population-based study. *J Surg Res* 2007;140:214-9. [PMID: 17418862]

h. Berry DA, Cronin KA, Plevritis SK, Fryback DG, Clarke L, Zelen M, et al. Cancer Intervention and Surveillance Modeling Network (CISNET) Collaborators. Effect of screening and adjuvant therapy on mortality from breast cancer. *N Engl J Med* 2005;353:1784-92. [PMID: 16251534]

i. Humphrey LL, Helfand M, Chan BK, Woolf SH. Breast cancer screening: a summary of the evidence for the U.S. Preventive Services Task Force. *Ann Intern Med* 2002;137:347-60. [PMID: 12204020]

j. Breast Cancer Surveillance Consortium. Evaluating Screening Performance in Practice. Bethesda, MD: National Cancer Institute; 2004. Accessed at http://breastscreening.cancer.gov/espp.pdf on 25 September 2009. [PDF file, 935 KB; PDF Help]

Source: USPSTF

cancer. And one out of three breast cancer survivors will be able to thank mammography for saving her life." By focusing on survivors, we have brought the denominator down sufficiently to dramatize the impact of screening.

• One final "statistic" comes with its own frame. "There are two kinds of women in the U.S. Those who have breast cancer, and those who think they are going to get it."* It is hard for anyone to deny the fear that women have of this dreadful disease, and that while screening is imperfect, it currently is the best prevention option at our disposal.

Finding Success Stories

On a more positive note, policymakers want to hear about solutions. And, nothing succeeds like success in describing what you want the policymaker to do. The three basic types of success stories[17] describe an issue, a planned intervention or its potential impact. In another use of the stream analogy, **upstream stories** tell about a project that is needed or just be-

ginning. Supporting data will come from early pilot program or from estimates based on available science. At this early stage, policymakers want to know about support for the program, funds leveraged and potential success. **Midstream stories** tell the progress of a program already in place. Policymakers now want to hear about utilization of funds, beneficiaries of the program, public support, and positive impact on their public image. If funds are needed to continue or expand the program, mid-stream stories help to make the case. After a long period in service, **Downstream stories** describe the impact a program has had on the population served. At this stage policymakers are interested in health impact, economic impact, sustainability, public support, and added value of the program. Downstream stories that address these issues may make the case for continued funding or expansion of the program to new populations. (See **Box 6–2** for an example.)

Selecting a Messenger

The credibility of the messenger is as important as the strength of the message. As mentioned earlier, it helps if this person is a

*Attributed to Bette Iacino, Communication Director for the Colorado Coalition for the Homeless, who was one of the founders of National Breast Cancer Awareness Month when she worked at the CDC.

Box 6–2 Success Story Example for Blood Pressure Control in Georgia

LOWER COSTS AND BETTER CARE ARE RESULT OF GEORGIA PROGRAM

Treating low income residents with high blood pressure reduces the expected number of adverse events such as stroke and heart attack and saves money.

Public Health Problem

- High blood pressure is a major cause of heart attack, stroke, kidney and heart failure.
- Lifestyle changes, such as healthy eating and increased physical activity, combined with medication when prescribed, can control blood pressure and prevent adverse events such as heart attack and stroke.
- People with less education and low incomes are not as likely as others to have their blood pressure under control, partly because they cannot afford regular care and medications.

Program

- The Georgia Stroke and Heart Attack Prevention Program provides services to low income patients with high blood pressure.
- Patients receive intense monitoring, health assessments, and lifestyle counseling and treatment that are based on established protocols for blood pressure treatment, and on the essential elements of health care described in the Chronic Care Model.
- Prescribed medicines are provided at low or no cost. Nurse case-managers monitor blood pressure, encourage regular clinic visits, and work with patients to help them take their medicine regularly.

Impact

- Program participants had better blood pressure control, lower treatment costs for those who received treatment, and lower overall costs per eligible patient according to an evaluation funded by the Centers for Disease Control and Prevention.
- The rate of expected adverse events such as heart attack or stroke was reduced by half in program participants, compared to people who received no preventive care. When compared to patients receiving usual care, the rate was cut by slightly less than half.
- For the 15,000 patients in the Stroke and Heart Attack Prevention Program costs were an average of $138 less per patient annually, compared with the cost of usual care. If these results included the costs of lost productivity and death, the program's demonstrated cost savings would likely be even higher.

Primary Contact
Jane Doe
Georgia Health Department
Phone: (404) XXX-XXXX

Source: Patricia Jones, Georgia Division of Public Health.

"voter" as well as a spokesperson for the issue. When representing a government agency, and speaking to a national official, this is of less importance. Whatever the information, it should be presented in a forthright, nonconfrontational manner, regardless of the prior stated positions of either the official or the spokesperson. Messengers are most effective when they have earned the respect of legislators and have a reputation for providing information that is accurate, timely, and in a manner that is free of rancor.

Agencies are frequently asked to provide testimony to a congressional subcommittee (e.g., testimony against the tobacco industry). If the message is intended to engage decision-makers in thoughtful review of health policy options, the outcome is less about awareness and more about action. The pressing question then becomes, "To whom will they listen?"

Knowing the preferences of policymakers and staff can facilitate the selection of trusted communicators. In a testimony scenario, the most compelling and effective messenger might not be a public health official, but instead, he or she could be a trusted community leader, constituent, business leader, adolescent, or even a celebrity, depending on the topic or issue. A comprehensive communication strategy may involve several layers of messengers, including health leaders, political insiders, and constituents.

Giving formal testimony at a congressional or state legislative hearing is not likely something you would be asked to do early in your career. However, it is possible to imagine that you may be the most qualified person to speak about an issue that is important to your organization. So, remember that you have this resource to help you! **Box 6–3** is an example of testimony

Box 6–3 Selections from Congressional Testimony of Richard Hamburg on Obesity in America, March 26, 2009

Original testimony by Richard Hamburg, Director of Government Relations, Trust for America's Health Before the House Agriculture Committee Subcommittee on Department Operations, Oversight, Nutrition, and Forestry.

The State of Obesity in America

Good afternoon. My name is Richard Hamburg, and I am the Director of Government Relations for Trust for America's Health (TFAH), a nonpartisan, nonprofit organization dedicated to saving lives by protecting the health of every community and working to make disease prevention a national priority. . . . Today I would like to discuss the scope of obesity in America, the potential factors that may be contributing to it, the health and economic impacts of obesity, and the importance of developing a national strategy to coordinate our response to obesity.

Scope of the Problem

Adult Obesity

Approximately two-thirds of American adults are obese or overweight. To examine obesity trends each year, TFAH publishes a report on obesity entitled *"F as in Fat: How Obesity Policies Are Failing in America."* The 2008 report, based on the Centers for Disease Control and Prevention's (CDC's) Behavioral Risk Factor Surveillance Survey (BRFSS) 2005–2007 data, found that adult obesity rates increased in 37 states in the past year. No state saw a decrease. More than 25 percent of adults are obese in 28 states, and more than 20 percent of adults are obese in every state except Colorado. A study published in the July edition of *Obesity* estimates that 86 percent of Americans will be overweight or obese by 2030.

Overall, approximately 23 million children are obese or overweight, and rates of obesity have nearly tripled since 1980, from 6.5 percent to 16.3 percent. Eight of the 10 states with the highest rates of obese children are in the South. According to a recent analysis from the National Health and Nutrition Examination Survey (NHANES), the number of U.S. children who are overweight or obese may have peaked after years of steady increases. According to researchers from the CDC, there was no statistically significant change in the number of children and adolescents (aged 2 to 19) with high BMI for age between 2003–2004 and 2005–2006. This is the first time the rates have not increased in over 25 years. Scientists and public health officials are unsure whether the data are due to recent public awareness campaigns (about obesity, increased physical activity, and healthy eating among children and adolescents), or just a statistical anomaly. We can expect to know more when the 2007–2008 NHANES data are analyzed. Even if childhood obesity rates have peaked, the number of children with unhealthy BMIs remains unacceptably high, and the public health toll of childhood obesity will continue to grow as the problems related to overweight and obesity in children show up later in life.

Impacts of Obesity

Health Impacts

Obesity and overweight are associated with a number of serious chronic conditions. More than 80 percent of people with type 2 diabetes are overweight. People who are overweight are more likely to suffer from high blood pressure, high levels of blood fats, and high LDL ("bad") cholesterol—all risk factors for heart disease and stroke. Obesity is a known risk factor for the development and progression of knee osteoarthritis and possibly osteoarthritis of other joints. Obesity may increase adults' risk for dementia and may increase the risk of developing several types of cancer.

The health impacts of obesity can start at a young age. Physical inactivity is tied to heart disease and stroke risk factors in children and adolescents. A number of studies have documented how obesity increases a child's risk for a number of health problems.

Economic Impact

These health impacts come at a great cost to our nation. According to the Department of Health and Human Services, obese and overweight adults cost the U.S. anywhere from $69 billion to $117 billion per year. One study found that obese Medicare patients' annual expenditures were 15 percent higher than those of normal or overweight patients. The cost of childhood obesity is also growing. Between 1979 and 1999, obesity associated hospital costs for children (ages 6 to 17 years) more than tripled, from $35 million to $127 million.

continues

The poor health of Americans of all ages is putting the nation's economic security in jeopardy. More than a quarter of U.S. health-care costs are related to physical inactivity, overweight and obesity. Healthcare costs of obese workers are up to 21 percent higher than nonobese workers. Obese and physically inactive workers also suffer from lower worker productivity, increased absenteeism, and higher workers' compensation claims.

National Security Impact

The problem of obesity and overweight has reduced the number of volunteers for military service who must meet height and weight requirements. At a time when military recruiters are struggling to meet the needs of our armed forces, we are finding more and more volunteers who are overweight and obese. In 1993, 25.6 percent of 18-year-old volunteers were overweight or obese; in 2006 that percentage rose to almost 34 percent. This problem continues during active duty. Each year between 3,000 and 5,000 service members are forced to leave the military because they are overweight.

Factors Contributing to Obesity Rates

How did this problem arise?

• We have placed kids in a less nutritious environment—it is not just too much food, but too much unhealthy food that kids are eating, and we have not harnessed the opportunities of the school to compensate for this.

• We have placed a particular burden on our poor and minority Americans, who are disproportionately overweight and obese, primarily because our poverty programs have not kept up with the rising cost of nutritious food; access to healthy foods is often limited in poor neighborhoods, and physical activity may be limited because of safety concerns or inadequate recreational facilities.

• We have also created a physical environment that reinforces a less active lifestyle, and we have not compensated for this in the level of physical activity we promote in the schools and in the workplace.

Recommendations

It is clear that obesity is a multifaceted issue with diverse causes and impacts across all sectors of society. Progress can be made by adopting some of the provisions referenced above [cut out of this selection but available in full testimony] in various reauthorization bills. However, to truly begin to mitigate and ultimately reverse this epidemic, we will need a sustained commitment over time to investing in population-based prevention strategies and coordinating our efforts to combat obesity.

Strengthening Our Investment in Community Prevention

Real prevention requires changing the communities in which we live and approaching this as a communitywide, not just an individual challenge. It will also be the most cost effective way to mitigate this epidemic. To truly tackle the obesity epidemic, we must make healthy choices easy choices for all Americans, regardless of where they live or what school they attend. We need a cultural shift, one in which healthy environments, physical activity and healthy eating become the norm.

Last July TFAH released *Prevention for a Healthier America: Investments in Disease Prevention Yield Significant Savings, Stronger Communities*, which examines how much the country could save by strategically investing in community disease prevention programs. The report concludes that an investment of $10 per person per year in proven community-based programs to increase physical activity, improve nutrition, and prevent smoking and other tobacco use could save the country more than $16 billion annually within five years. This is a return of $5.60 for every $1. The economic findings are based on a model developed by researchers at the Urban Institute and a review of evidence based studies conducted by the New York Academy of Medicine. The researchers found that many effective prevention programs cost less than $10 per person, and that these programs have delivered results in lowering rates of diseases that are related to physical activity, nutrition, and smoking.

The evidence shows that implementing these programs in communities reduces rates of type 2 diabetes and high blood pressure by 5 percent within 2 years; reduces heart disease, kidney disease, and stroke by 5 percent within 5 years; and reduces some forms of cancer, arthritis, and chronic obstructive pulmonary disease by 2.5 percent within 10 to 20 years, which, in turn, can save money through reduced healthcare costs to Medicare, Medicaid, and private payers.

Examples of Successful Interventions

Community and school-based approaches aimed at using reducing obesity in the United States have already shown to be successful. The Child and Adolescent Trial for Cardiovascular Health (CATCH) elementary school program in the town of Somerville, Massachusetts developed a comprehensive program called "Shape Up Somerville" to curtail childhood obesity rates. Another example of a coordinated approach to obesity reduction at the community level is the YMCA's Pioneering Healthier Communities. This project supports local communities in promoting healthy lifestyles. TFAH urges Congress to build upon these successes and to make a sustained investment in population-based disease prevention.

continues

Implementing a National Strategy to Combat Obesity
... TFAH supports the development of a *National Strategy to Combat Obesity*. This needs to be a comprehensive, realistic plan that involves every department and agency of the federal government, state and local governments, businesses, communities, schools, families, and individuals. It must outline clear roles and responsibilities. Our leaders should challenge the entire nation to share in the responsibility and do their part to help improve our nation's health. All levels of government should develop and implement policies to make healthy choices easy choices-by giving Americans the tools they need to make it easier to engage in the recommended levels of physical activity and choose healthy foods, ranging from improving food served and increasing opportunities for physical activity in schools to securing more safe, affordable recreation places for all Americans. The "National Strategy for Pandemic Influenza Planning" provides a strong example for how this type of effort can be undertaken . . .

Conclusion
Our country needs to focus on developing policies that help Americans make healthier choices about nutrition and physical activity. Thank you again for the opportunity to testify.

Source: Richard Hamburg, Director of Government Relations, Trust for America's Health Before the House of Agriculture Committee Subcommittee on Department Operations, Oversight, Nutrition, and Forestry. http://healthyamericans.org/assets/files/TFAHHamburgtestimony.pdf

provided by Richard Hamburg before a Subcommittee of the Congressional Agriculture Committee about obesity in America.

Delivering the Message

Table 6–3 provides suggestions of important factors to include in your presentation to elected officials.[13] In particular, it is important to develop a positive working relationship with the legislative staffer(s) of elected officials. Staffers tend to have a great deal of influence in shaping the activities and priorities of an elected official.

There are many modes by which to communicate the message to public health administrators and policymakers. These communications may occur in highly structured or less structured settings. The techniques and amount of preparation needed may differ depending on the setting. An example of a highly structured and formal setting is a legislative hearing. In such a hearing, a group of elected officials gather in a committee meeting room to hear testimony from experts (witnesses) in the public health field. The witness is usually given just a few minutes to present his or her position. Therefore, it is critical to be well prepared and have key pieces of information on hand. It is usual in these settings to be required to bring "posters" of data instead of projecting slides. No more than four should be prepared in a format that can be easily set on an easel (usually 2 feet by 3 feet) and read from a distance of 10 feet. It is often useful to prepare a one-page handout for each legislator that summarizes key points. **Box 6–4** shows some tips for preparing fact sheets for policy briefings.

Every profession has its own language, and public health is no different. When delivering your message, it is important to avoid jargon (this point is mentioned throughout this book) because it may confuse an audience and project an attitude of elitism. Not everyone will understand technical terms, and you cannot afford to lose one individual who might be a potential ally and advocate for your position. Do not use words that are in vogue (e.g., "infrastructure," "modality"). Such words are overused and may project the disagreeable impression of an overly academic or bureaucratic style. You should seek to express, not impress.

TIPS FOR FACE-TO-FACE MEETINGS WITH POLICYMAKERS

In preparing for an interaction with an elected official, try to develop a positive working relationship with his or her legislative staffer(s). These individuals often have a great deal of influence in shaping the activities and priorities of an elected official. When meeting with an elected official, specifically remember to:

- Make an appointment.
- Select a primary spokesperson if a group is meeting the official.
- Go with a specific purpose and be prepared.
- Be brief and cover only one or two topics.
- Have a few pieces of key data at your fingertips that support your position.
- Provide an illustration of the program or policy impact—a human interest story often works best.
- Know precisely what you want your elected official to do.
- Anticipate questions so that your answers are well-thought-out.
- Provide written data or a fact sheet.

TABLE 6-3 Ten Factors and Approaches for Effectively Communicating with Elected Officials

Factor/Approach	Rationale/Process
1. Develop familiarity with the legislative process	• Every legislative body has its own unique structure, calendar, and culture. • The process has numerous hearings, floor debates, amendments, conference meetings, and other opportunities within which to provide input.
2. Show knowledge of the issue	• Analysis needs to be done that clearly establishes what problem is being addressed and whether there is a legislative solution. • It is useful to answer three questions: Who will this help? Who will it hurt? How much will it cost?
3. Develop knowledge of the opposition	• Elected officials will want to be aware of formal and informal opposition to a given proposal. • It is critical that proponents know who these groups or individuals are, the reasons for their opposition, and the strength of opposition.
4. Develop an established relationship with legislators	• Efforts should be undertaken to have knowledge of key members, their constituencies, and their prior records on issues relating to yours. • It is important to have "get acquainted" meetings at a time convenient to the elected official and not during the actual session of the legislative body. • Periodically providing brief program updates or providing information for he/she to use in his/her district is a useful tool to supporting that relationship.
5. Maintain integrity	• It is essential that your integrity be assured in all dealings with elected officials. • If an answer to a specific question is not known, say so. • If a mistake is inadvertently made, immediately acknowledge it, and ask for the benefit of the doubt in future encounters.
6. Respect their role	• Elected representatives are generally doing their best to represent the citizens of their district or region. • Advocates should understand that rarely does a legislator represent an area that has universally accepted opinions.
7. Respect the role of their staff	• Legislative staff plays critical roles of gatekeeper and opinion shaper. • As with the individual elected officials, it is essential to have a professional working relationship with staff members as well.
8. Show a willingness to listen	• Perhaps the most essential product of conversations with elected officials and advocates is the listening regarding the position of the official or his/her other constituents who may be in support or opposition. • Active listening is a learned trait, and it is essential to success in this arena.
9. Be forthright in your position	• Let the legislative sponsor know of your support or opposition to avoid public disagreement or embarrassment. • A private meeting should be held in which you articulate your position and your rationale. • These interactions can help to build a greater appreciation and respect for your position.
10. Maintain a focus on "the long view" and "the big picture"	• Think about issues in the big picture rather than issue by issue. • While an elected official may not support your position on one issue, it is important to be able to come back to him/her on future occasions. • Remember that there will be other issues, and it is never advisable to "burn any bridges."

Box 6–4 Tips on Preparing Fact Sheets

- Summarize the problem in one or two sentences.
- Use current data and supporting statistics.
- Do not lie with statistics or use misleading graphs.
- Keep it simple, and gear it to the audience.
- Make it local, but also compare local data with state and national figures.
- Include the name, address, and telephone number of a contact person.
- Formatting:
  - Use headings.
  - Keep it to one page in length (front and back).
  - Include a professional-looking chart or graph (i.e., bar chart, trend line graph, icon array, pie chart).

Source: Revised from http://www.healthpolicyguide.org/advocacy .asp?id=5209

- Be cordial and always thank the official for his or her time.
- Follow-up with a brief thank-you note later.

In addition to the content and language, tone of voice and body language are also powerful communication tools. A few techniques to remember:

- *Shake hands and make eye contact.* When meeting an official, shake hands and greet him or her with eye contact. In a formal presentation, you should attempt to maintain eye contact with your audience. When you have a large audience, you should address the committee chairperson or other person in charge of the meeting. Avoid darting your eyes across the room or to your notes.
- *Sit upright in the chair.* Appear interested and involved. Be relaxed and confident and at ease with your subject and your audience.
- *Dress professionally.* Your look and the manner in which you present your message are clear reinforcements to your message. It is generally good practice to dress conservatively; wear simple, not ornate jewelry; select solid colors over flashy patterns; never wear a hat; avoid shaded or dark glasses unless medically required; use makeup sparingly. Most importantly, it is essential that you look professional and that physical appearance does not detract from the message.
- *Start with your message.* Give your conclusion early, and follow with supporting data and information.

- *Involve the audience.* Make your message relevant to the audience at hand. When presenting an abstract concept, such as the value of disease prevention, choose concrete examples that bring the concept home to the audience. For example, when testifying to the impact of premature mortality from chronic disease in a given city, you might frame the issue in the following way: "Last year, more people died from chronic diseases in [this state] than live in [a local city of a smaller size]."

TIPS ON LETTER WRITING

In addition to the preceding approaches to presenting information in written and oral form, there are several points to keep in mind when writing a letter to an elected official (**Table 6–4**). It is also important to select the signatory for the letter who will have the most impact with the recipient. Letters are likely to be more effective if they are tailored to the policymaker and come from the policymaker's known constituents.

TIPS ON ELECTRONIC COMMUNICATION

The explosion in information technologies over the past few decades has greatly enhanced the ability to communicate nearly instantaneously with persons who can influence public health programs. **Electronic communication** (usually e-mail) is more likely to be effective at the national level than at the state level,

---

TABLE 6–4 Pointers for Composing a Letter to an Elected Official

- Keep a letter to a single page.
- Do not use a form letter.
- Cover only one topic or issue.
- State the purpose at the outset.
- When possible, provide cost impacts.
- Identify yourself and your organization.
- Enclose applicable editorials, data fact sheets, or position papers.
- Ask your policymaker for a response.
- If applicable, provide a courtesy copy to your organization.
- Thank your policymaker for his or her cooperation.
- When applicable, describe legislation by its bill number.
- Be polite/give reasons for support.
- Include recipient's name and address on both envelope and letter.
- Write legibly or type.
- Send a note of appreciation if and when the issue is supported.

more likely to be used by staff than elected officials, and more likely to be used by younger than older individuals. In addition, state legislators are more likely to use e-mail with constituents and political insiders than with intermediary groups, including advocacy organizations, lobbyists, and the media.[18] E-mail from constituents, advocacy organizations, and political insiders are viewed differently by policymakers. Many advocacy groups have networks developed by which they can alert their members of key issues needing attention.

BARRIERS AND CHALLENGES IN COMMUNICATING WITH POLICYMAKERS

Several barriers and challenges are important to consider in relation to communicating directly with policymakers:

- Trends in the legislative arena (e.g., term limits) and other leadership changes (e.g., the rapid turnover in state health officers) will influence the timing and intensity of efforts to effectively communicate public health data.
- Social determinants of health are individual characteristics (e.g., income, education, race/ethnicity) that often have a powerful effect on one's health status or health outcomes (Chapter 5), yet the policy solutions to address these determinants are not straightforward.[19]
- Public health leaders and policymakers need to take a "long view" of health. Such a vision is needed because many of the "modern epidemics" such as cancer and HIV/AIDS are manifested over years and decades. Also, working in many populations requires a substantial commitment of time and energy to build the necessary trust between public health practitioners and community members.
- Effective methods of communication may also be affected by organizational "climate", the dynamics and structure of the organization. For example, a highly formal organization with a strong chain of command would imply that communication with higher-level administrators would be highly structured and channeled through one or more intermediate supervisors.
- Related to the preceding discussion of "climate," practitioners may be affected by a failure or restriction on trying to make an important policy change. For example, employees at the middle or lower levels within an organization may have official or unofficial restrictions on policy or advocacy efforts related to their programmatic area.
- Reliable data for small area analyses (e.g., a rural county or a legislative district) often do not exist, and this may lead to frustration among administrators and policy-

makers. Increasingly, public health agencies are aware of the need for more extensive and timely small area data.[20]

ADVOCACY

We have just described the most effective ways to communicate about public health directly with policymakers. But, there are many times when you might not have that option available to you. The issue about which you are concerned might not seem that important to an elected official or agency administrator. How do you bring this up on the radar? The primary method is through grassroots advocacy, done by working with a group of concerned citizens. This group then works through the media to amplify their voices so that they are heard. There are now a number of "cookbooks" for what used to seem like a mysterious process. For example, the American Public Health Association (APHA) has published a useful advocacy guide for its membership.* State and national organizations have developed many tools, including websites,† and advocacy tool kits.‡

The actual advocacy process is not that different than what we described earlier for presenting information to policymakers, or the persuasive communication process discussed in the next section. The principal difference is the amount of effort devoted to forming an effective coalition; in-depth study of the issue and potential solutions; and then creating events, or working directly with the news media (chiefly local news), to frame the discussion according to your objectives. Government agencies do not lead advocacy initiatives, although they may play key roles in providing data and information to organizations or groups striving to increase funding for programs within their jurisdiction.

Use of Media, New and Traditional

Search Engine Optimization

An interesting twist in the past few years has been the dominance of the Internet in this area. Where as advocacy results used to be measured in terms of TV and print news pick up, **search engine optimization (SEO)** has become a key strategy. In order for a search engine to find you, you obviously have to have a website, blog, or other online resource (e.g. a video posted on YouTube) that will pop up when a user types in the search terms. **Box 6–5** presents some tips on how to make searches by others lead to your online doorstep more often. The Internet and all of its applications have clearly become the medium of choice for advocacy as we move into 2010.

---

*http://www.apha.org/NR/rdonlyres/A5A9C4ED-1C0C-4D0C-A56C-C33DEC7F5A49/0/Media_Advocacy_Manual.pdf
†http://www.tobaccofreemaine.org/
http://www.dekidscount.org/
http://www.healtheducationadvocate.org/
‡http://www.aahperd.org/naspe/advocacy/governmentRelations/toolkit.cfm

Box 6–5 Search Engine Optimization

Ninety-five percent of all Internet users start their experience with a search engine. The tips presented in this box are paraphrased from an article posted on the *Online Digital Review*.[a] Most of these tips come from Danny Sullivan, the editor of *Search Engine Land*,[b] with additional points made by Robert Niles and the Knight Digital Media Center's News Entrepreneur "Bootcamp" held at the University of Southern California, May 2009.

1. Use Google AdWords' keyword tool to find the most popular keywords related to your website and your issue.
Before you begin tuning your specific key words and phrases, you need to discover what key words and phrases Internet readers are using in search engines to find content like yours. Google's various keyword tools can help you do that. The AdWords tool will show you the approximate number of searches conducted on Google for words and phrases that you enter, or for phrases associated with a URL of your choosing.

Google's Search-based Keyword Tool quantifies the popularity of various key phrases, with both search volumes as well as suggested advertising bid prices to "buy" those keywords through Google's text-ad program. That last bit of information can show you not only which key phrases will drive the most traffic to the site, but which will drive the most lucrative traffic to you, as well.

Use the tools to identify the best overall phrases for your site, and the ones that you will use in the site's title and on its home page and navigation. Then use the tool to build experience that will help you select the best key words and phrases to spotlight when writing and producing individual articles and blog posts on your site.

Google's home page provides guidance, as well, as Google now suggests various keywords and phrases -and reports their popularity-based on the partial search terms you type in its entry box.

2. Use keywords and phrases in your HTML title tag.
Once you've identified your keywords and phrases, use them in the most importance place where search engines will consider them. The search engines give the content of the title tag the greatest weight of any single element on the page, so your most appropriate key phrases better be there, Sullivan said.

If you are using a content management system (CMS), know which input field will populate the title tag (usually the headline). Use the resources described earlier to determine which words ought to make it into that headline. Imagine yourself as a reader, and ask what terms you would use on Google if you were searching for this story. Those terms had better be in the head and page title on your website.

Also, be sure to use powerful, popular keywords in the title, description, and tags of the videos you post on YouTube and elsewhere.

3. Write an engaging meta-description tag for each page.
Sullivan, and others, find little SEO use for the plethora of descriptive meta-tags that can be included in the head of a webpage. But the description tag still provides good value, because Google uses it to create the short blurb that it displays under a page's title on its search engine results pages (SERPs). A sharp description can help lure a visitor to your site over others, including ones that rank ahead of you on the page.

4. Switch from AP style to "SEO style" on references in body copy.
Keyword repetition and density on the page still play a role in where you end up in the SERPs (though not nearly as much as in the pre-Google era). You can help yourself, therefore, by moving away from rigid AP style rules on second references and place names to more SEO-friendly use of full names on some (but not all) subsequent references within a story.

5. Use keywords in your URLs whenever possible.
The search engines value the use of keywords in URLs as well. If you've got one in your site's domain, great. But keywords in the directory path or file name of the URL also provide a boost. Rather than use numbers or nonsense text in article URLs, opt for a CMS that uses real words, ideally keywords for which readers will be searching.

Sullivan also recommends that you configure your CMS to use hyphens instead of underscores to separate keywords in your URLs.

6. Never publish the same article under two or more URLs on your site.
Duplicate content penalties have killed news websites' positions in the SERPs in the past. You shouldn't publish the same article at multiple URLs on your site. It's fine to reference one piece with multiple tags and from multiple index pages, but they should all point to the same, single URL when referencing that story or blog post.

continues

Much of Google's decision on where to rank a page in the SERPs is based upon the number and quality of links to that individual page. Concentrate the inbound links to one story on a single URL. Posting that content on multiple webpage addresses simply dilutes the power of all those links across those multiple URLs.

7. Create standing pages as linkbait for popular ongoing stories and issues.
This extends the point made earlier. In an ideal world, you would concentrate all the inbound links to a story you are following to a single URL, driving it to the top of the SERPs for all related searches. But that's tough in a traditional news publishing environment where each day brings a new article with a new URL. Staff-written summary wikis and well-crafted index pages can provide a standing URL that others can link when referencing your coverage of a particular person or issue, boosting the search engine popularity of your work.

8. Never retire or change page URLs without providing a 301 redirect.
Search engines respond to a variety of responses from a Web server when a search engine requests a URL that no longer exists. A "404" or page not found response is the worst response your server can deliver. It should, instead provide a 301 redirect that tells the search engine to which new URL it should transfer the old URL's SERPs position.

9. Use bit.ly or other URL shorteners that use 301 redirects and provide click stats when posting to Twitter.
When you are using URL shorteners, you want to make sure that your site is getting the search engine "credit" for that link, and not the shortener itself. Sullivan suggested bit.ly as one of several services that use 301 redirects. After trying it, he was impressed with the click-through statistics it tracks for each URL.

10. Link to other great, original content and invite other publishers to link to yours.
The last advice might be the most important. Great on-page SEO ultimately will do little to move your pages up in the SERPs if other websites are not linking to you. Use your social media and offline promotional skills to let other influential online news publishers know about your work, and invite them to link to it. Tweet your posts and write them with enough flair that others will want to retweet.

Of course, the best way to encourage others to link to you is to practice what you ask, and to link to them and their best coverage.
Robert Niles, ODR (Annenberg, USC)

References
[a]http://www.ojr.org/ojr/people/robert/200905/1733/
[b]http://searchengineland.com/

Source: Robert Niles, ODR, Annenberg, USC

Traditional Media Advocacy

Heeding Tip O'Neill's advice, traditional media advocacy has focused on local TV, radio stations, and newspapers. As with policymakers, it is important to know the people responsible for researching, reporting, and presenting the news and feature stories in your area. Call ahead and make an appointment for an **informational interview.** You want to know what their "beat" is (e.g., health, food, beauty and fashion, science, environment, violence prevention, local interest, even entertainment, might all be relevant), so that you can frame a story for their audience. You need to also know their deadlines and news cycles. Reporters have one thing in common in that they want to bring important information to their audience. If you are supporting a national campaign, it is important to tell the media why this is important *in your area* by using local data, spokespersons, and visuals.

As with **earned media** (publicity gained by promotional efforts rather than paid, discussed in Chapter 11), you usually need an event in order to attract media coverage. If you want television

to come, there need to be good visuals and on-air interview opportunities. Similarly, for radio, be sure that you have an interesting soundscape-and that the event is not so noisy that you can't hold a quiet interview nearby. Print (newspapers or magazines) is different because you can send a report or announcement to the editor or reporter, who might only need to call you on the phone to check a few facts. Contact the reporters well in advance to build the relationship and give them time to arrange for someone to cover the event. Media that reach out to specific populations, such as Spanish or Asian language media, or African American radio stations, might take a particular interest in an issue that affects their audience disproportionately. Reporters or editors at these outlets might be willing to become champions for your issue and volunteer to be speakers or presenters or, in other ways, to add some pizzazz to a community event. This kind of give-and-take is also good because a larger crowd might come as a result of the local celebrity's appeal, and the media network would be happy to cover the event both for their own publicity and because there will be a larger crowd present.

*Media Relations Tools**

Boxes 6–6, 6–7, and **6–8** feature some key **media relations tools** that you need to interact with the media about your event or issue. These include:

---

*Much of the information in this section is based on the CDC's guide for partners to work with the media on folic acid campaigns. *Media Campaign Implementation Kit. A Guide to Media Outreach and Placement for Your Health Education Program.* Available free at http://www.cdc.gov/ncbddd/folicacid/documents/MediaCampaignKit.pdf

- Press release. This generally is for "hard news," which means a new finding, report, or release of data on your issue. [Box 6–6]
- Media alert. This is a kind of invitation to promote a special event. It highlights what you would put in a party invitation: the who, what, when, where, and why of your event. Assignment and calendar section editors can use this news alert. [Box 6–7]

Box 6–6 Media Tools: Sample Press Release

Violent Death among Children Linked to Household Firearms

For immediate release: February 19, 2002

Boston, MA—A new study from the Harvard School of Public Health (HSPH) found that in states and regions with higher levels of household firearm ownership, many more children are dying from homicide, suicide, and gun accidents. The differences in rates of violent death to children across states are large. The higher death rates in high gun states are due to differences in deaths from firearms. This elevated rate of violent death to children in high gun states cannot be explained by differences in state levels of poverty, education, or urbanization.

The article "Firearm Availability and Unintentional Firearm Deaths, Suicide, and Homicide among 5-14 Year Olds" is published in the February 2002 issue of *The Journal of Trauma* (www.jtrauma.com) and a table from the study appears on the journal cover.

Matthew Miller, M.D., ScD, associate director of the Harvard Injury Control Research Center at HSPH and lead author of the study, said: "In states with more guns, more children are dying. They are dying in suicides, in homicides, and in gun accidents. This finding is completely contrary to the notion that guns are protecting our children."

"The differences in violent death rates to children are large, and are closely tied to levels of gun ownership," he said. "The differences cannot be explained by poverty, education or urbanization."

This study focused on children aged 5 to 14, and compared data across all 50 states over a 10-year period (1988–1997). In one table, the authors compare the five states with the highest gun ownership levels with the five states with the lowest levels. While these states have equal numbers of children, they have very different rates of violent death. In the 10-year period, 253 children died from firearm accidents in the high gun states, compared to 15 in the low gun states. While the numbers of non-gun suicides were similar, 153 children killed themselves with guns in the five high gun states, compared to 22 who committed suicide in the five low gun states.

Children in the high gun states were also at much higher risk of being murdered with a firearm. During this 10-year period, 298 children aged 5 to 14 were murdered with guns in the high gun states, compared to 86 in the low gun states. The non-gun homicide rates were fairly similar (a little over 100 non-gun homicides in both sets of states).

Miller emphasized that, while no study that is a snapshot of the U.S. over a short period of time can prove causation, the strong and robust association between gun ownership and children's violent death is compelling.

These results are also consistent with international comparisons. The U.S. level of private firearm ownership is much higher than in other developed nations and U.S. children aged 5 to 14 are far more likely to be murdered, commit suicide, and die from gun accidents than children in other developed countries. Indeed, for children aged 5 to 14 in the United States, death from firearms is the third leading cause of mortality, following only motor vehicle crashes and cancer.

The study was supported in part by the Joyce Foundation, the Packard Foundation, the Robert Wood Johnson Foundation, the Open Society Institute, and the Centers for Disease Control and Prevention.

For further information, please contact:
Robin Herman
Director of Communications
677 Huntington Avenue
Boston, Massachusetts 02115
Phone: 617-555-1212
Email: rherman@hsph.harvard.edu

Source: Herman R. Harvard School of Public Health, Office of Communication, 2002

Box 6–7 Sample Media Alert

B.2. Local Event Promotion Media Alert
Note: You can adapt this sample media alert to fit your specific program or event. Try to keep the alert to just one page.

For Immediate Release
[Date}

Contact: [Your Name]
{Organization}
{Telephone Number]

"Before You're Pregnant" Women's Health Fair Set for [Date]
Media Alert

What: "Before You're Pregnant" Women's Health Fair

This event will feature free information, displays, booths, and activities for all women, showcasing pre-pregnancy advice.

Specal events will include a seminar with local expert [name] and a class on pre-pregnancy diet and exercise.

Who: Sponsored by [organization], with [supporting and contributing partners]

When: [Start time] to [Finish time] and Date

Where: [Location]

[Include directions if necessary]

Why: To help women navigate the maze of pre-pregnancy advice while encouraging them to think ahead about what they can do to ensure a healthy pregnancy and baby. What women do, or don't do, before getting pregnant can directly affect the baby. For instance, many women know that taking folic acid every day can prevent certain birth defects but few realize that it must be taken before conception to be effective.

Media Opportunity: Photography: Governor/Mayor elect/spouse will be on hand to open the day and meet participants.
Interviews: [expert names and affiliations] will be available [when] for interviews.

Source: CDC, Preventing Neural Tube Birth Defects: A Prevention Model and Resource Guide:30. http://www.cdc.gov/nchddd/folicacid/prevention-guide.html

---

- Backgrounder. This usually has more detailed information about your issue, event or campaign from which the media can pull out relevant facts. [Box 6–8]
- Optional items:
  - Fact sheets on different topics.
  - "Frequently asked questions" (FAQs) and answers.
  - Biographies of organizational leaders and spokespersons.
  - "Real-life stories" of individuals affected by the issue. If willing, these individuals can be spokespersons.

Special Tools

Advocacy groups will often conduct an assessment, or collect data, to point out the deficiencies in a program. Many efforts use a "report card" to highlight the problems and compare the targeted entity being evaluated to others in its class. We gave one example in Chapter 5 on Healthy Wisconsin. **Figure 6–4** shows another example of report cards used for advocacy pur-

poses. You would prepare a media or news release to announce the report, and work with the media in order to gain coverage of your issue.

Working with Youth

You might want to start on a local level and look into the resources for prevention that are available to your former school system, middle or high school. Community groups have been actively promoting tobacco-free schools, elimination of soda and fast-food contracts, and improved choices in school cafeterias. For example, California Project LEAN (Leaders Encouraging Activity & Nutrition) developed a guide to combat school district soft-drink contracts. While there have been some great success stories—such as when Los Angeles Unified, the second largest school district in the nation, banned soda and other sugary drinks—there is much work to be done in this arena. **Box 6–9** features examples of strategies from these efforts.[21]

Box 6–8 Sample Backgrounder

Note: Consider adding any local statistics on NTD rates or levels of folic acid awareness or consumption.

Q. What is folic acid and why is it so important?
A. Folic acid is a B vitamin that can be found in some enriched foods and in most multivitamin pills. Folic acid has been proven to reduce the risk of neural tube defect (NTD)-affected pregnancies when taken as a vitamin supplement one month before conception and throughout the first trimester. Folic acid is necessary for proper cell growth and development of the embryo. Although it is not known exactly how folic acid works to prevent NTDs, its role in tissue formation is essential. Folic acid is required for the production of DNA, necessary for the rapid cell growth needed to make fetal tissues and organs (such as the baby's brain and spine) in early pregnancy. **That is why it is important for a woman to have enough folic acid in her body both before and during pregnancy.** Getting enough only takes a small effort, but it makes a big difference.

Q. What serious birth defects can folic acid prevent?
A. Folic acid prevents NTDs, such as spina bifida and anencephaly. *Spina bifida*, a birth defect of the spine, is a condition that often has disabling consequences. With spina bifida, a person's legs may be paralyzed, and there are often problems with bowel and bladder control. Learning disabilities are common in children with spina bifida, and mental retardation sometimes occurs. *Anencephaly*, another type of NTD, affects the brain. All babies with *anencephaly* die before or shortly after birth.

Q. When do women need to start taking folic acid?
A. The U.S. Public Health Service recommends that **all women of childbearing age should consume 400 micrograms (mcg) of folic acid daily.** Women need to have folic acid in their system a month before getting pregnant and throughout the first few weeks of pregnancy. No one expects an unplanned pregnancy, but it happens every day. In fact, about half of all pregnancies in the United States are not planned. *That's why all women should get enough folic acid every day if there's any chance of getting pregnant.* Even if a women is not planning a baby until next month, next year or later, she should take folic acid because by the time she knows shes pregnant, the baby's brain and spine are already formed.

Q. Where can I get folic acid?
A. Take a vitamin . . . For many women, an easy way to be to get enough folic acid is to take a vitamin with folic acid in it. Most multivitamins contain 400 micrograms (0.4 milligrams) of folic acid. Vitamins containing folic acid can be bought at groceries, pharmacies, or discount stores that sell vitamins. If multivitamins cause an upset stomach, women may want to try taking them with food or just before going to bed. Vitamins containing only folic acid are also available, and they are smaller and easier to swallow.

And eat right. . . . Most of us get some folic acid in our diets every day. Folic acid has been added to some foods. Foods made from "enriched" flour or grain products now contain additional folic acid, examples are bread, pasta, rice, and cereals. Many breakfast cereals

Source: CDC, Preventing Neural Tube Birth Defects: A Prevention Model and Resource Guide:33. http://www.cdc.gov/ncbddd/folicacid/prevention-guide.html

Get Involved

Finally, through the Association of Schools of Public Health (ASPH),[*] the Trust for America's Health, national organizations such as the Campaign for Tobacco Free Kids,[†] as well as state and local organizations, you have many opportunities to become involved in promoting public health policy development.

CONCLUSION

Policy has had, and will continue to have, a vast impact on our daily lives and on public health indicators in part due to its long-term effects and relative low cost.[22] Effective communication of public health data to key policymakers is a challenging

*http://www.asph.org/document.cfm?page=1074
†http://www.tobaccofreekids.org/index.php

FIGURE 6-4 Examples of Advocacy Report Cards: A School Food Policy Report Card

To determine the progress states have made in improving the nutritional quality of school foods, the Center for Science in the Public Interest (CSPI) evaluated the school nutrition policies of all 50 states and the District of Columbia regarding foods and beverages sold outside of the school meal programs through vending machines, a la carte (i.e., foods sold individually in the cafeteria), school stores, and fundraisers. Each state policy was graded based on five key considerations: 1) beverage nutrition standards; 2) food nutrition standards; 3) grade level(s) to which policies apply; 4) time during the school day to which policies apply; and 5) location(s) on campus to which policies apply. These evaluation criteria are the same as those used in our June 2006 School Foods Report Card.

State School Foods Report Card 2007

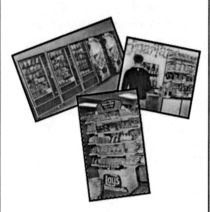

A State-by-State Evaluation of Policies for Foods and Beverage Sold through Vending Machines, School Stores, A La Carte, and Other Venues Outside of School Meals

Center for Science in the Public Interest
November 2007

State School Foods Report Card 2007

A−	Kentucky (1)[1], Oregon (2)
B+	Mississippi (3), Nevada (4), Alabama (5), Arkansas (6), California (7), Washington (7), New Mexico (8)
B	New Jersey (9), Arizona (10), Tennessee (10)
B−	Louisiana (11), Texas (12), West Virginia (13), Connecticut (14), Rhode Island (15), Florida (16)
C+	Hawaii (17)
C	Maine (18), Illinois (19), District of Columbia (20)
C−	Colorado (21), South Carolina (22)
D+	New York (23), Maryland (24), North Carolina (25)
D	Oklahoma (26), Virginia (27)
D−	Indiana (28), Georgia (29)
F	Alaska, Delaware, Idaho, Iowa, Kansas, Massachusetts, Michigan, Minnesota, Missouri, Montana, Nebraska, New Hampshire, North Dakota, Ohio, Pennsylvania, South Dakota, Utah, Vermont, Wisconsin, Wyoming (all ranked 30)

[1]The members in parenthesis give the state's mark as compared to the school policies in other states with being the strongest policy.

Source: CSPI, State School Foods Report Card 2007

Box 6–9 Strategies to Involve Teens in School Nutrition Advocacy

Hold a fun event to recruit students.

Case Study

Using a Contest to Create Student Interest
Francisco Bravo Medical Magnet High School

Francisco Bravo Medical Magnet High School in Los Angeles used a billboard contest to engage students in nutrition issues and to recruit student advocates. The *Food on the Run* community partner, California State University, Los Angeles, organized the contest in which students designed healthy billboard messages and then sponsored the production of the billboards. Students came up with messages that promoted fruit and vegetable consumption. English-language and Spanish-language concepts were chosen and made into billboards that were located in East Los Angeles. This activity educated students and the community about healthy eating and began to demonstrate to students how their direct involvement and planning efforts could facilitate change in their own communities.

Organizing a Team of Teens

Once you've found interested teens, you need to have an idea of how your advocacy team will work. Important logistics such as meeting times and locations should be determined early on, so that the group can focus on their advocacy ideas.

Gain buy-in from the school

A key to success is having support and buy-in from the school. Whether you are working as an outside entity, or within the school system, establishing a Memorandum of Understanding (MOU), or some kind of partnership agreement with the school is a helpful way to ensure some level of support.

Add legitimacy to your effort

Establishing ground rules or bylaws for the group and affiliating the group with other known associations can help build confidence that your group is an organized, legitimate entity for change. There are many ways to do this.

One example is to form a Nutrition Advisory Council (NAC) through the American School Food Services Association (ASFSA).

Case Study

Give Students A Voice
McKinleyville, Arcata, Eureka, and Zoe Barnum High Schools

"Teens are good consumers of information, but have little or no experience in providing information for their peers and the public. They are anxious to be a part of marketing to teens," said Joyce Houston, project director. The following outline describes how *Food on the Run* successfully partnered with a local radio stations to give student advocates a public voice.

Step 1: Researched the radio stations that target teens and their receptivity to partnership.
Step 2: Identified one media company that was connected with rock/pop and country music stations with broad teen appeal.
Step 3: Identified teen spokespeople to be used for radio interviews.
Step 4: Trained teen spokespeople on interview topics and interviewing techniques. Topics included: Calcium; Fast Food; Sports Nutrition; Healthy Snacks; How to Fit Physical Activity into Your Day; Physical Activities in Humboldt County; and How Physical Activity Decreases Stress.
Step 5: Each student was accompanied to the station by a health department staff member for moral support and back-up information.
Step 6: Educational incentives were presented to the radio DJs to encourage future discussion regarding healthy eating and increased physical activity.

The results of this campaign were very empowering. The teens were very effective in giving messages on the radio to their peers, and they loved being on the radio. This was a very exciting activity for everyone involved.

---

continues

Case Study

Healthier Vending Machines and Salads
Francisco Bravo Medical Magnet High School

Students determined they wanted healthier choices in the vending machines in addition to the high fat, high calorie, high sugar choices already available. They also noticed there were no fresh salads or fruit offered on a daily basis. After hearing of the successful addition of salads at a nearby school, *Food on the Run* advocates decided this would be a great option for their school as well.

Step 1: Student advocates established a relationship with the cafeteria manager and vice principal to discuss bringing the healthier offerings to campus.

Step 2: The vice principal contacted school vendors about obtaining samples of healthier options and the cafeteria manager developed two salads to taste test.

Step 3: The advocates sampled the items and voted on the healthy options to test with the general student body.

Step 4: The healthier options were introduced to the rest of the campus. The healthy vending machines and the bottled water machine sold more items than the regular machines. They became permanent on campus. The salads also proved to be very popular, and are now offered on a daily basis in addition to fresh fruit.

The keys to success included involving the key people from the school in the decision-making process and holding taste tests to determine student acceptability.

Source: California Project LEAN.

task. To produce change in our field, we need to communicate public health information to policymakers in a manner that is clear, articulate, and inspiring. Strategic use of scientific information and data in these communications can greatly enhance their impact. Although there is not a single "recipe" for every audience and setting, the set of principles and approaches outlined in this chapter should help form the basis for more effective communication with administrators and policymakers.

KEY TERMS

Advocacy
Downstream stories
Earned media
Electronic communication
Environmental factors
Framing
Framing bias
Google trends
Informational interview
Media relations tools
Media scanning
Meta-message
Midstream stories
Policymaker
Polling survey
Search engine optimization (SEO)
Upstream stories

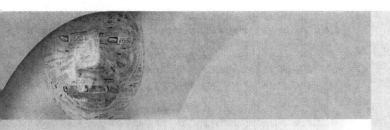

Chapter Questions

1. What are two (or more) factors that virtually every elected official has to juggle when developing or voting on policy that affects his or her constituency?

2. Why is it important to get to know a policymaker, as well as his or her staff, before presenting information to him or her?

3. What did Tip O'Neill mean by "All politics is local"?

4. Describe some ways you can anticipate the questions or concerns of a policymaker about your issue.

5. What are three things that are essential to an effective policy presentation?

6. What is meant by "framing" an issue, and do you consider it to be ethical?

7. Besides serving food, how else can you attract the news media to an event?

8. What is meant by "search engine optimization," and why is it such an important tool for advocacy?

ADDITIONAL RESOURCES

From the National Council of State Legislatures, both by T. Neal, 2005, www.ncsl.org:
- Learning the Game: How the Legislative Process Works
- Making your Case: How to Win in the Legislature

Brownson R, Chriqui J, Stamatakis K. Understanding evidence-based public health policy. *Am J Public Health.* 2009;99:1576-1583.

Brownson RC, Royer C, Ewing R, McBride TD. Researchers and policymakers: travelers in parallel universes. *Am J Prev Med.* 2006 Feb;30(2):164-172.

Jones E, Kreuter M, Pritchett S, Matulionis RM, Hann N. State health policy makers: What's the message and who's listening? *Health Promotion Pract.* 2006 Jul;7(3):280-286.

Nelson DE, Brownson RC, Remington PL, Parvanta C, Eds. *Communicating Public Health Information Effectively: A Guide for Practitioners.* Washington, DC: American Public Health Association; 2002.

Sederburg WA. Perspectives of the legislator: allocating resources. MMWR. 1992;41(Suppl):37-48.

REFERENCES

1. Center for Health Improvement. *Health Policy Guide: Bringing Policy Change to Your Community.* 2009. Available from: http://www.healthpolicy guide.org/advocacy.asp?id=23

2. Brownson RC, Fielding JE, Maylahn CM. Evidence-based public health: A fundamental concept for public health practice. *Ann Rev Public Health.* 2009 Apr 21;30:175–201.

3. Milio N. Evaluation of health promotion policies: tracking a moving target. *WHO Reg Publ Eur Ser.* 2001(92):365–385.

4. Schmid TL, Pratt M, Howze E. Policy as intervention: Environmental and policy approaches to the prevention of cardiovascular disease. *Am. J. Public Health.* 1995;85(9): 1207–1211.

5. IOM Committee for the Study of the Future of Public Health. *The Future of Public Health.* Washington, DC: National Academy Press; 1988 1207–1211.

6. Brownson RC, Royer C, Ewing R, McBride TD. Researchers and policymakers: Travelers in parallel universes. *Am J Prev Med.* 2006 Feb;30(2): 164–172.

7. The Library of Congress. *Membership of the 110th Congress: A Profile, 2008.* Congressional Research Report for Congress. Washington, DC: The Library of Congress; 2008 [updated 2008 November 20, 2008; cited]. Available from: http://opencrs.com/document/RS22555/2008-11-20

8. National Conference of State Legislatures. Full- and Part-Time Legislatures. Updated June, 2009. http://www.ncsl.org/default.aspx?tabid=16701

9. Tip ONeills autobiography, *Man of the House,* written with James Novak, 1987. As posted by Daniel Grays at http://www.geekbooks.com/all_ politics_is_local_6.html

10. Weissert CS, Weissert WG. State legislative staff influence in health policy making. *J Health Polit Policy Law.* 2000 Dec;25(6):1121–1148.

11. Innvaer S, Vist G, Trommald M, Oxman A. Health policy-makers' perceptions of their use of evidence: a systematic review. *J Health Serv Res Policy.* 2002 Oct;7(4):239–244.

12. Sorian R, Baugh T. Power of information: Closing the gap between research and policy. When it comes to conveying complex information to busy policy-makers, a picture is truly worth a thousand words. *Health Aff (Millwood).* 2002 MarApr;21(2):264–273.

13. Nelson DE, Brownson RC, Remington PL, Parvanta C, Eds. *Communicating Public Health Information Effectively: A Guide for Practitioners.* Washington, DC: American Public Health Association; 2002.

14. CDC. HPV vaccine. What you need to know. Atlanta, GA; 2007 [updated 2007; cited]; Available from: http://www.cdc.gov/vaccines/Pubs/vis/downloads/vis-hpv.pdf.

15. Choi BC. Twelve essentials of science-based policy. *Prev Chronic Dis.* 2005 Oct;2(4):A16; Choi BC, Pang T, Lin V, Puska P, Sherman G, Goddard M, et al. Can scientists and policy makers work together? *J Epidemiol Community Health.* 2005 Aug;59(8):632–237.

16. Fletcher SW, Elmore JG. Mammographic screening for breast cancer. *N Engl J Med* 2003;348:1672–1680

17. Stamatakis K, McBride T, Brownson R. Communicating prevention messages to policy makers: The role of stories in promoting physical activity. *J Phys Act Health.* 2010 Mar;7 Suppl 1:S99-107.

18. Richardson L, Cooper C. E-mail communication and the policy process in the state legislature. *The Policy Studies J.* 2006;34(1):113–129.

19. Woolf SH. Social policy as health policy. *JAMA.* 2009;Mar 18;301(11): 1166–1169.

20. Figgs LW, Bloom Y, Dugbatey K, Stanwyck CA, Nelson DE, Brownson RC. Uses of Behavioral Risk Factor Surveillance System data, 1993-1997. *Am J Public Health.* 2000;90(5):774–776.

22. Brownson RC, Chriqui JF, Stamatakis KA. Understanding evidence-based public health policy. *Am J Public Health.* 2009 Sep;99(9):1576–1583.

21. Agron P, Berends V, Purcell A, Robertson J, Takada E. Food on the Run: Lessons from a Youth Nutrition and Physical Activity Advocacy Campaign. Sacramento, CA: California Project LEAN; June 2004. Available at: www.CaliforniaProjectLEAN.org

CHAPTER 7

Speaking to the Public: Health Literacy and Numeracy

David E. Nelson and Claudia Parvanta

LEARNING OBJECTIVES

By the end of this chapter, the reader will be able to:

- Identify key principles of information processing theory that underlie literacy.
- Define basic literacy, health literacy, and numeracy.
- Describe the factors that affect health literacy.
- Define the current state of health literacy in the United States.
- Explain why health literacy is important to the public's health.
- Describe tools for assessing health literacy in research and practice.

INTRODUCTION: THE 3 Rs

Literacy refers to an individual's ability to make sense of information in any form in which it is presented. While it was once sufficient to sign your name to be considered literate, the definition has acquired a larger meaning of social competence. Primary education in the United States is still meant to ensure that, if nothing else, graduates leave with the basic abilities of Reading, wRiting and aRithmetic, the so-called 3 Rs. As we will see later in this chapter, too few high school graduates in the United States, let alone those with only an elementary education, possess adequate levels of basic, quantitative and health literacy to make sound financial, legal, medical, or other decisions. This is a social disparity that must be addressed outside of the health sector, although much of its impact is felt there. Health literacy goes beyond basic skills and really refers to a knowledge base, as well as to our ability to add information to that to make health-related decisions. So, it is important to first understand how we create that knowledge base in the first place.

HOW DO WE UNDERSTAND ANYTHING? INFORMATION PROCESSING THEORY

Humans are limited in how much information we can actually process. As infants we learn to separate out word units of sound (phonemes), and meaning (morphemes). We also learn to pay attention to other important sounds, as well as sights, smells, tastes, and textures. This is a gross oversimplification of an incredibly sophisticated process that most infants have mastered by 8 months of age, at least at a level that can be used for survival.[1]

As functional adults, our brains have developed to include our knowledge, attitudes, and beliefs. There are millions of bits of new information passing by our sensory apparatus daily-that is, all the sights, sounds, smells, tastes, textures we either recognize as "information" or ignore. On a higher level, there are thousands of words, numbers, and other organized packets of information that pass by us, some of which we process. But on top of our learned or inherent predilection to ignore most of the communication we receive on a daily basis, *individual* limitations also affect our ability to use complex information. The key to our not going crazy is simplification, and linking new information to what we already possess in our brains. Once we have managed to "learn" something, when we need to use it to make a decision our brain continues to use shortcuts. There is an extensive literature on the heuristics (shortcuts, logical rules) of decision making, including the well-known book by Kahneman, Slovick, and Tversky.[2] The basic idea is that we interpret anything new in terms of what we already know and we make inferences based on the way in which information has been presented to us.

In addition to our basic cognitive structures for taking in information and using it, our ability to pay attention to information is also affected by how much we care about it. The **Elaboration Likelihood Model (ELM)**[3] suggests that if you are already engaged in an issue, you will pay more attention to new information about it. On the other hand, if you are not engaged, you need peripheral stimuli to grab your attention. A very common example is that women who are hoping to get pregnant will pay a lot of attention to information (e.g., advertising) about pregnancy or baby care, while those still in the "fabulously single" mode do not look twice at ads for diapers. Conversely, the use of scantily dressed models to sell personal care products makes use of the ELM. Many men in particular do not generally spend a lot of time thinking about personal care products and would scan information about them (on TV, in magazines) superficially, if at all. Sexy models "grab their attention," and bring them to "elaborate" on some of the information presented by the advertiser. In this case, the peripheral cue is also an "outcome expectation" (a construct used in persuasion, addressed in Chapter 8).

In order to help people build health literacy, **Information Processing Theory** suggests that, before anything else, we should:

1. Keep our communications simple.
2. Make the message attention-getting (and this will vary with the recipient of the information).
3. Structure the appearance of the information into small chunks.
4. Use decision rules and heuristics to our advantage.[4]

These and other recommendations discussed in this chapter and in Appendix 7A will help us as health communicators to present information in ways that evoke more positive responses from recipients.

LITERACY

Basic Literacy and Its Components

The Educational Testing Service, well known as the ETS to those who have taken college entrance exams, has provided the framework for defining and assessing different forms of literacy in the United States. The most basic definition of *literacy*, used in the National Assessment of Adult (age 16 and older) Literacy, is "using printed and written information to function in society, to achieve one's goals, and to develop one's knowledge and potential."[5]

ETS further categorizes literacy as prose (the ability to read sentences and paragraphs), distinguished from "document literacy," the ability to interpret tables, forms, graphs, or other structured formats. Information that requires a mathematical operation for interpretation is considered to require

quantitative literacy (QL). QL is a subset of *numeracy*, which is "the knowledge and skills required for managing the mathematical demands of diverse situations."[5] The situations may include using measuring spoons, calculating a tip, or playing Blackjack—which do not necessarily require the use of a printed document. We discuss numeracy in more detail later, particularly the ability to understand mathematical or numerical information related to one's own health and health risks.

How Literate Is the U.S. Public?

Every 10 years the U.S. Department of Education surveys U.S. adults age 16 and over for their literacy abilities. The most recently completed survey in 2003 drew a nationally representative sample including 19,000 adults in homes and more than 1,000 inmates in state and federal prisons across the country. The **National Assessment of Adult Literacy (NAAL)**[5,6] measures literacy on a scale of 0 to 500. Scoring varies by the literacy task (prose, document, or quantitative), but roughly falls into the levels listed in **Table 7–1**.

Using this scoring procedure, in 2003 approximately 43% of Americans tested by the NAAL scored below level 3 for prose literacy. Projected nationally, this means that about 93 million Americans read at or below the *basic* level of literacy. The comparable percentage for document literacy was 34%. By comparison, for quantitative literacy an estimated 55% functioned at or below basic levels.[6]

HEALTH LITERACY

What Affects Health Literacy?

Health literacy is our ability to understand and use complex health information, so it is a multifaceted skill with many domains feeding into it. These domains include communication skills, knowledge or beliefs about health topics, cultural and linguistic factors, public health and healthcare system demands, and contextual factors.[7,8] Let's explore each of these domains in more detail.

Communication Skills

In the context of health literacy, communication skills are those needed to use language (spoken, written, signed, or otherwise communicated) for interaction with others, including basic reading, writing, listening, speaking and comprehension. Persons with limited reading ability will be less able to use written information on websites or printed health materials or to navigate a typical healthcare setting with its numerous signs. If they have trouble writing, they will be less able to fill in forms in medical settings, and reduced verbal ability will make it difficult for them to explain a health concern or raise questions to healthcare providers.

TABLE 7–1 NAALS Scoring for Adult Literacy

Level	Definition	Score	Abilities	Examples
1	Below Basic. Very roughly equivalent to reading at a 5th-grade level, or below.	0 to low 200s	Adults range from being nonliterate in English to being able to read very simple prose; locate easily identifiable information and follow written instructions in simple charts or forms; and perform simple addition in a very concrete and familiar context.	Signing one's name; finding an expiration date on a license or milk carton; totaling amounts on a bank deposit slip.
2	Basic. Roughly equivalent to reading at an 8th-grade level.	210 to high 200s	Adults are able to manage slightly more complex prose and documents. They may also perform most basic one-step mathematical functions of addition, subtraction, and multiplication.	Reading a pamphlet for prospective jurors to understand how people are selected for a jury pool; using a television guide to find programs by days and time slots; comparing ticket prices for two events.
3	Intermediate	Mid-200s to mid-300s	Adults understand and can interpret texts similar to newspaper articles, novels or basic reference books. They can use arithmetic operations to solve more complex problems, and consult charts or tables for specific information.	Consulting reference materials to determine which foods contain a particular vitamin; identifying a specific location on a map; ordering office supplies from a catalog.
4	Proficient	Mid-300s to 500	Adults who score at this level can read and synthesize complex and abstract prose. They can work with multiple pieces of information located in charts or tables, and complete multistep arithmetic operations to solve problem.	Comparing viewpoints in two editorials; interpreting a table about blood pressure, age, and physical activity; computing and comparing the cost per ounce of food items.

Source: National Center for Education Statistics (NCES), U.S. Department of Education. National Assessment of Adult Literacy (NAAL). A First Look at the Literacy of America's Adults in the 21st Century. NCES 2006-470. Available from: http://nces.ed.gov/NAAL/PDF/2006470.PDF.

Knowledge

In health literacy, knowledge runs the spectrum from learning about a specific topic (e.g., the warning signs of a heart attack or that a skull and crossbones on a bottle means "poison"), to a general understanding of cause-and-effect or a scientific method. The greater challenge in working with persons with low health literacy is not their inability to read, but the lack of an explanatory framework, or *schema*, to use as a starting place for explanation of a complex health topic. Health literacy experts suggest the use of "living room language," language that uses commonplace words and analogies to explain phenomena that are outside common personal experience. Use of ordinary language is closely related to, but does not completely overlap, the use of cultural explanations and experience.

Culture

Health is a culturally constructed phenomenon (see Chapter 10 for more on cultural competency). People learn how to define health and illness, who to seek out for care, what constitutes a symptom, what causes illness and what supposedly cures it, and how to describe physical symptoms from their families and larger social groups. Furthermore, willingness to use health technology, medicines, or therapies may be determined by religious or cultural rules—just as the practice of certain risk behaviors or adherence to medical advice will have cultural dimensions. Contrast the health-protecting behaviors of Seventh Day Adventists, who are asked not to smoke, drink, or engage in extramarital sex, to the high-risk behaviors of certain street gangs that require use of hard drugs, unprotected sex, or other tests of belonging. In terms of health literacy, knowledge (see earlier section) describes what a person *knows*, while culture reveals what a person *believes or values*. Someone might have learned in school about genetics and the value of screening for birth defects but would absolutely oppose screening if it would mean terminating a pregnancy. How people evaluate health information for themselves or their family, the form of health information they prefer, and whom they trust to convey health information, are all filtered through culture.

English Language Proficiency

The 2010 census of the U.S. population is ongoing as of this writing. Based on its findings in 2000, 47 million people, or 18% of the U.S. population 5 years old or more, spoke a language other than English at home. Of these, about half said

they also spoke English "very well." Spanish is by far the foreign language most frequently spoken, with 28 million speakers in 2000. Of these, half also said they spoke English "very well."[9] **Table 7–2** shows a breakdown of the languages most frequently spoken at home in 1990 and 2000.

The number of foreign language speakers is anticipated to *increase* in the 2010 census. Clients might be perfectly literate in their native language-and even have a high degree of health literacy. However, their abilities in English might be limited. To respond to the needs of clients with **limited English proficiency (LEP)**,[*] the U.S. Office of Minority Health developed a standard set of language access services that all healthcare

*In some provider settings, you might hear these clients referred to as "LEPs" or "LEP clients." This jargon refers to their limitations with the English language.

TABLE 7–2 Languages Most Frequently Spoken at Home by English Ability for the Population 5 Years and Over: 1990 and 2000

Language Spoken at Home	1990		2000					
				Number of Speakers				
					English-Speaking Ability			
	Rank	Number of Speakers	Rank	Total	Very Well	Well	Not Well	Not at All
United States . . .	(X)	230,445,777	(X)	262,375,152	(X)	(X)	(X)	(X)
English only . . .	(X)	198,600,798	(X)	215,423,557	(X)	(X)	(X)	(X)
Total non-English	(X)	31,844,979	(X)	46,951,595	25,631,188	10,333,556	7,620,719	3,366,132
Spanish	1	17,339,172	1	28,101,052	14,349,796	5,819,408	5,130,400	2,801,448
Chinese	5	1,249,213	2	2,022,143	855,689	595,331	408,597	162,526
French	2	1,702,176	3	1,643,838	1,228,800	269,458	138,002	7,578
German	3	1,547,099	4	1,382,613	1,078,997	219,362	79,535	4,719
Tagalog	6	843,251	5	1,224,241	827,559	311,465	79,721	5,496
Vietnamese[1]	9	507,069	6	1,009,627	342,594	340,062	270,950	56,021
Italian[1]	4	1,308,648	7	1,008,370	701,220	195,901	99,270	11,979
Korean	8	626,478	8	894,063	361,166	268,477	228,392	36,028
Russian	15	241,798	9	706,242	304,891	209,057	148,671	43,623
Polish	7	723,483	10	667,414	387,694	167,233	95,032	17,455
Arabic	13	355,150	11	614,582	403,397	140,057	58,595	12,533
Portuguese[2]	10	429,860	12	564,630	320,443	125,464	90,412	28,311
Japanese[2]	11	427,657	13	477,997	241,707	146,613	84,018	5,659
French Creole . .	19	187,658	14	453,368	245,857	121,913	70,961	14,637
Greek	12	388,260	15	365,436	262,851	65,023	33,346	4,216
Hindi[3]	14	331,484	16	317,057	245,192	51,929	16,682	3,254
Persian	18	201,865	17	312,085	198,041	70,909	32,959	10,176
Urdu[3]	(NA)	(NA)	18	262,900	180,018	56,736	20,817	5,329
Gujarathi	26	102,418	19	235,988	155,011	50,637	22,522	7,818
Amenian	20	149,694	20	202,708	108,554	48,469	31,868	13,817
All other languages	(X)	3,182,546	(X)	4,485,241	2,831,711	1,060,052	479,969	113,509

Source: Shin, HB, Bruno, R. *Language use and English speaking ability: 2000*. Census 2000 Brief. U.S. Department of Commerce, ESA. U.S. Census Bureau. Issues October 2003. Table 1, p. 4. http://www.census.gov/prod/2003pubs/c2kbr-29.pdf. Retrieved July 8, 2010.

providers are encouraged to employ, and that medical facilities receiving federal funding must provide per Title VI of the Civil Rights Act of 1964.* **Box 7–1** lists these standards.[10]

*Title VI of the Civil Rights Act of 1964 states, "No person in the United States shall, on ground of race, color, or national origin, be excluded from participation in, be denied the benefits of, or be subjected to discrimination under any program or activity receiving federal financial assistance."

The use of interpreters in a medical encounter is discussed further in Chapter 15. There are numerous resources for guiding public health facilities and personnel in how to implement **culturally and linguistically appropriate services (CLAS)**.†

†See, e.g., *The Providers' Guide to Quality & Culture.* Available at: http://erc.msh .org/ mainpage.cfm?file=1.0.htm&module=provider&language=English& ggroup=&mgroup=

Box 7–1 Recommended National Standards for Culturally and Linguistically Appropriate Services [CLAS] in Health Care

Competent Care

1. Healthcare organizations should ensure that patients/consumers receive from all staff members effective, understandable, and respectful care that is provided in a manner compatible with their cultural health beliefs and practices and preferred language.

2. Healthcare organizations should implement strategies to recruit, retain, and promote at all levels of the organization a diverse staff and leadership that are representative of the demographic characteristics of the service area.

3. Healthcare organizations should ensure that staff at all levels and across all disciplines receive ongoing education and training in CLAS delivery.

Language Access Services

4. Healthcare organizations must offer and provide language assistance services, including bilingual staff and interpreter services, at no cost to each patient/consumer with LEP at all points of contact and in a timely manner during all hours of operation.

5. Healthcare organizations must provide to patients/consumers in their preferred language both verbal offers and written notices informing them of their right to receive language assistance services.

6. Healthcare organizations must ensure the competence of language assistance provided to limited English proficient patients/consumers by interpreters and bilingual staff. Family and friends should not be used to provide interpretation services (except on request by the patient/consumer).

7. Healthcare organizations must make available easily understood patient-related materials and post signage in the languages of the commonly encountered groups and/or groups represented in the service area.

Organizational Supports

8. Healthcare organizations should develop, implement, and promote a written strategic plan that outlines clear goals, policies, operational plans, and management accountability/oversight mechanisms to provide CLAS.

9. Healthcare organizations should conduct initial and ongoing organizational self-assessments of CLAS-related activities and are encouraged to integrate cultural and linguistic competence-related measures into their internal audits, performance improvement programs, patient satisfaction assessments, and outcomes-based evaluations.

10. Healthcare organizations should ensure that data on the individual patient's/consumer's race, ethnicity, and spoken and written language are collected in health records, integrated into the organization's management information systems, and periodically updated.

11. Healthcare organizations should maintain a current demographic, cultural, and epidemiological profile of the community as well as a needs assessment to accurately plan for and implement services that respond to the cultural and linguistic characteristics of the service area.

12. Healthcare organizations should develop participatory, collaborative partnerships with communities and utilize a variety of formal and informal mechanisms to facilitate community and patient/consumer involvement in designing and implementing CLAS-related activities.

13. Healthcare organizations should ensure that conflict and grievance resolution processes are culturally and linguistically sensitive and capable of identifying, preventing, and resolving cross-cultural conflicts or complaints by patients/consumers.

14. Healthcare organizations are encouraged to make available regularly to the public information about their progress and successful innovations in implementing the CLAS standards and to provide public notice in their communities about the availability of this information.

Source: U.S. Department of Health and Human Services. Office of Minority Health. Healthcare Language Services Implementation Guide. Available from: https://hclsig.thinkculturalhealth.org/page/view.rails?name=Section+2:+Page+2,3.

This is important for routine health communication, but particularly important in the case of emergencies.

Complexity of Health Care

There are challenges and demands inherent in accessing healthcare services and benefits and navigating healthcare settings on both macro and microscopic levels. Challenges include whether individuals know the services available to them or whether they are eligible for different forms of care or insurance. Case-in-point, for a low-income woman who is pregnant to know she might be eligible for WIC (the federal special supplementary food program for Women, Infants and Children) benefits, she must know of the existence of this service in her community and be confident enough to contact the provider. Furthermore, many people are overwhelmed by the complexity of negotiating a simple appointment with a healthcare provider because they do not know where to start. They also frequently find it difficult to understand and complete written health forms. Written materials from Medicare and private health insurers are notoriously difficult to understand, even by college graduates.

Context

A specific setting or situation can make someone feel fearful or stressed. This might be because they are in an unfamiliar or intimidating environment, or they might possess a mental or physical impairment. These factors are especially present when people find themselves unexpectedly facing a serious illness or injury and have to interact with people and systems that can be difficult and often impersonal. Even persons with a high degree of literacy and education may become less able to process health information when they have been given bad medical news or when in a stressful setting, such as placing a loved one in a skilled nursing facility.

Patient–provider encounters have dominated much of the agenda of health literacy. Many of the tools that have been developed to enhance communication have focused on patient processing of medical information (see Chapter 15). At a different level the ability of the public at large to comprehend health information broadly and make decisions based on this information can have major effects on the health and economy of the entire nation. This impact is discussed in the next section.

Relatively Few Americans Are Proficient in Health Literacy

The definition of health literacy used by Healthy People 2010 and the Institute of Medicine (IOM) are similar: "The degree to which individuals have the capacity to obtain, process, and understand basic health information and services needed to make appropriate health decisions."[11] Some of the domains where health literacy is needed include actions that involve health promotion, health protection, disease prevention, health care and maintenance, and accessing needed services or navigating the healthcare system.[11]

The 2003 NAAL was the first time that health literacy was specifically assessed. Twenty-eight health-related prose, document, and quantitative tasks were embedded in the main NAAL assessment (out of a total of 152 NAAL tasks). On these health specific tasks, 36% of the participants scored *at or below basic* health literacy. Only 12% were judged to have *proficient* health literacy.

NUMERACY

Numeracy is the ability to think and express oneself quantitatively. Very few people truly understand the significance of numbers used in public health. Why is it hard to talk about numbers? Think about the statistical concepts conveyed by *confidence intervals; mean, median,* and *mode;* or $p = 0.005$ as opposed to $p = 0.05$, let alone more grounded (but equally hard to imagine) terms such as *parts per million.* These are not concepts that most Americans think about once they leave high school, if they learned them then. And, these concepts are particularly difficult to explain in common language. As discussed in Chapter 4, public health policies and interventions are derived from scientific findings. But, deciding whether to share numerical data with the public, choosing the data to present, and "styling" them for presentation are not simple tasks.[12]

Neuroscience has revealed that different regions of our brains are active depending on the type of mathematical calculations we perform. As with other forms of learning, actively used portions of our brain build up with repeated practice.[13] However, because of lack of practice our ability to use numbers is not being developed, as is reflected in the low math skills of many Americans. The 2007 Trends in International Mathematics and Science Study indicated that the United States ranks 9th in mathematics and 11th in sciences compared to other developed nations.[14] Significantly, we stopped comparing our final year of secondary school after 1998, when the math scores of our 12th-grade students ranked 19th of the 21 countries assessed, second to last. The United States definitely lags behind other leading countries in mathematical education. This may explain why so many Americans find numerical data to be overwhelming.

Where we find particular difficulty in communicating about numbers is in the area of risk and probability. For example, in one study, when asked whether "5%" or "1 in 20" sounded bigger, 81% of participants thought 1 in 20 sounded bigger in the context of prenatal diagnosis of chromosome abnormalities.[15] Many studies have demonstrated that people have difficulty understanding very small or very large numbers.[13] Small ratios present difficulties, and the magnitude of difference between 1 in 1,000 and 1 in 10,000,000 can be missed. Another challenge is that many people misinterpret probability estimates, believing, for example, that a risk of 1 in 250 of developing a disease is higher than if the risk were 1 in 20. Converting data to percentages and probabilities (e.g., 3 in 1,000; 0.3%; 0.003) and vice versa is especially problematic. Studies show that most people cannot make such conversions.

As mentioned previously, in the 2003 NAAL, 55% of U.S. adults performed at basic or below basic levels in the quantitative portions. Stated differently, this means that about 115 million adults will have trouble performing simple mathematical tasks (e.g., adding two numbers together, locating two numbers on a bar chart and calculating their difference or determining the cost of a meal based on selection of different-priced menu items). The differences in quantitative literacy by education level are especially striking: 64% of persons without a high school degree performed at a less than basic proficiency, compared to 3% to 4% for persons with a bachelor's or graduate college degree.[16] Even among persons with a college degree, it is worth noting that only about one-third performed at the proficient level.

In addition to numeric ability, there are several tendencies that influence people's understanding of data.[12] The **representative heuristic** (a heuristic is a rule or "mental shortcut") refers to the tendency of people to make overarching conclusions based on limited amounts of evidence. This might include their own experience, a vividly described anecdote about one person, or limited data from a study reporting on a new cancer treatment. **Anchoring** and **adjustment bias** refer to the way in which people "anchor" their understanding of data, based on their initial impressions or on a pre-existing belief. First impressions tend to be long lasting, thus the need to ensure that the first data released to the public are accurate.

Two other tendencies influence how people explain findings: A misperception of correlation as causation and failure to consider randomness as an explanation of apparent differences. As introduced in Chapter 4, when two types of data are found to be correlated, people tend to believe that they are causally related. While this sometimes is the case, often mere correlation is meaningless. For example, just because the number of houses of worship and crime increase at the same rate in a metropolitan area, it should not be concluded that church growth caused an increase in crime (or that crime causes churches to be built).

People rarely consider that chance alone might explain some scientific findings, believing that some type of "discoverable" cause exists. This occurs most often whenever some type of disease cluster is believed to occur, such as an increase in the number of cases of cancer in a defined population (e.g., in a community or employees in an occupational setting). These so-called clusters usually lead to speculation about the cause, which is often assumed to be external in nature (e.g., an occupational exposure or receipt of a vaccine). Even when well-conducted research studies demonstrate that chance is the likely explanation, many people refuse to accept such a conclusion.

THE IMPACT OF HEALTH LITERACY AND NUMERACY ON PUBLIC HEALTH

There is a great deal of research that demonstrates the negative effects of low health literacy.[8,9,17-21] Some of these effects are summarized in **Table 7–3**.

Two studies have shown that there is an independent association between low levels of health literacy and an increased risk of premature death,[19,20] with one study finding an increased risk of 50% among older adults.[20] Other research has shown that low health literacy is associated with increased risks of unnecessary visits to hospitals and hospitalizations and increased healthcare costs.

On the prevention front, persons with low health literacy cannot make the best use of disease prevention and health promotion information.[22] These persons are less likely to receive mammograms, flu shots, prostate or cervical cancer screening. Low health literacy is also related to low levels of health knowledge. It is difficult for people with low health literacy to compare evidence about health risks, such as tobacco or a sedentary lifestyle. They might be less aware, and less concerned, about environmental quality.[22] They often have poorer self-management of chronic or infectious diseases

TABLE 7–3 Low Health Literacy and Health-Related Outcomes

Higher mortality rates
Increased number of unnecessary hospitalizations
Decreased use of preventive health services
Lower levels of physical functioning and quality of life
Lower ability to effectively manage chronic diseases
Higher risk of medication errors
Lower ability to comprehend insurance coverage information
Higher healthcare costs

(e.g., asthma, diabetes, HIV), medication-related errors, and lower levels of physical functioning and quality of life. The effect of limited health literacy on decision-making during a public health emergency is still unknown.[22] A further challenge is that persons with limited health literacy can feel ashamed about their lack of skills and be unlikely to voluntarily report when they do not understand information presented to them. And there is always a human cost at the individual level that cannot be fully portrayed with findings from research studies (**Box 7–2**).[7]

People with low health numeracy are at a special disadvantage in making decisions about their medical care and in understanding the risks of certain health outcomes, death from cancer, for example. Inversely, people with high numeracy tend to be much better at navigating health concepts, issues, and priorities.[23]

In summary, a person's health literacy influences his or her ability to:

1. Adopt healthier behaviors.
2. Respond appropriately to health-related information.
3. Share information with healthcare providers.
4. Manage their own health care.
5. Navigate the intricacies of healthcare systems.[9]

The same can be said for health numeracy.[23] The implication of this research is clear: communicators need to be aware of the problem of low health literacy and shape health messages to the needs of audiences with low health literacy levels.

Most of the efforts directed toward health literacy are concerned with our encounters with the healthcare system, including provider-patient communication, interactions with

Box 7–2 A Tragic Example of the Impact of Low Health Literacy

A 29-year old African-American woman with three days of abdominal pain and a fever was brought to a Baltimore emergency department by her family. After a brief evaluation, she was told that she would need an exploratory laparotomy. She subsequently became agitated and demanded to have her family take her home. When approached by staff, she yelled "I came here in pain and all you want is to do an exploratory on me! You will not make me a guinea pig!" She refused to consent to any procedures and later died of appendicitis.

Source: Nielsen-Bohlman L, Panzer AM, Kindig DA (eds.). *Health Literacy: A Prescription to End Confusion.* Reprinted with permission from the National Academies Press, Copyright 2004, National Academy of Sciences.

insurers, use of prescription and nonprescription drugs, decisions about diagnostic tests, and so on. Within a larger public health framework, the combination of health literacy with other factors in the ecological model enables an individual to "produce health."[22]

Health literacy was assigned a central role in our nation's health objectives for 2010. Two primary objectives in health communication are presented. Objective 11-2 asks us to strive to, "Improve the health literacy of persons with inadequate or marginal literacy skills."[11] The objective goes on to say:

> Closing the gap in health literacy is an issue of fundamental fairness and equity and is essential to reduce health disparities. Public and private efforts need to occur in two areas: the development of appropriate written materials and improvement in skills of those persons with limited literacy. The knowledge exists to create effective, culturally and linguistically appropriate, plain language health communications. Professional publications and federal documents provide the criteria to integrate and apply the principles of organization, writing style, layout, and design for effective communication.[11]

TOOLS FOR ASSESSING HEALTH LITERACY IN RESEARCH AND PRACTICE

In clinical practice, it may be important to assess patients' health literacy abilities in order to:

- Comply with quality of care standards within a profession or facility.
- Avoid potential medication or self-care errors.
- Use different communication media (printed material, videos, computer screens).
- Know that a patient understands what he or she is being told.
- Rule out other complications, such as cognitive impairment, hearing or visual loss.

There are practical limits to assessment of health literacy in a healthcare context compared to a research setting. Research or survey participants have consented to the tests, which might take a considerable amount of time, and they have been assured of anonymity. Usually these participants are not suffering the additional stress of an illness, or the fear of a medical diagnosis or treatment. In practice, the act of being in a health provider's office or being interviewed by a public health worker is stressful. Patients resent the time required to fill in additional paperwork and most importantly, they fear exposure if they have difficulty reading or understanding.[24]

Tools for Assessing Health Literacy

The four most widely used instruments for assessing individual health literacy are the REALM, TOFHLA, NVS, and one- or two-question tests. Next we examine their characteristics and potential applications.

- **Rapid Estimate of Adult Literacy in Medicine (REALM).**[25] The REALM is a word-recognition test of 66 medical words and is one of the oldest and most widely used health literacy assessment tools. It starts with easy words (e.g., fat, flu, pill) and moves to difficult words (e.g., osteoporosis, impetigo, potassium). Patients are asked to pronounce each word out loud. The test makes no attempt to determine if patients actually *understand* the meaning. REALM can be administered in about three minutes, and it is available only in English. The number of correctly pronounced words is used to assign a grade-equivalent reading level.
    - Scores 0–44: skills ≤ 6th-grade level
    - Scores 45–60: skills 7th/8th-grade level
    - Scores > 60: skills ≥ high school level
    - Patients with scores ≤ 60 may be at risk for misunderstanding written information.
- REALM-R.[26] The REALM-R is a much shorter version of the REALM. The total list of words are these:

Fat	Osteoporosis	Anemia	Colitis
Flu	Allergic	Fatigue	Constipation
Pill	Jaundice	Directed	

Fat, flu, and *pill* are not scored and are positioned at the beginning of the REALM-R to decrease test anxiety and enhance confidence. Unlike the REALM, (which must be purchased), all materials related to the REALM-R may be downloaded for free from the American Society on Aging and American Society of Consultant Pharmacists Foundation website.*

- **Test of Functional Health Literacy in Adults (TOFHLA).**[27] The TOFHLA is the instrument of choice when a detailed evaluation of health literacy is needed for research purposes. It is available in both English and Spanish. The full-length form requires 20 minutes, and there is a short version requiring only 12 minutes. The full TOFHLA has two parts: multiple-choice questions that test document and numeracy and what are called "CLOZE" type (fill-in-the-blank) questions. A testing kit may be ordered from the distributor, Peppercorn Books.†

- **Newest Vital Sign (NVS).**[28] The NVS instrument is available in English and Spanish, and can typically be completed by patients in about three minutes. Many patients find the instrument acceptable as part of standard medical care, with more than 98% of patients agreeing to undergo the assessment during a routine office visit. The NVS can be obtained online at no cost from the Partnership for Clear Health Communication.‡

- **One- or two-question tests.**[29] Studies have found multiple-question tests are more effective than those with one single question. These questions have been tested together:
    - How often do you have problems learning about your medical condition because of difficulty understanding written information? (always, often, sometimes, occasionally, or never)
    - How often do you have someone help you read hospital materials? (always, often, sometimes, occasionally, or never)
    - How confident are you filling out medical forms by yourself? (extremely, quite a bit, somewhat, a little bit, or not at all)

One study showed that the question about filling out medical forms to be the most effective, while another study found that the question about getting help reading hospital materials to be the most effective.

Health Literacy in Clinical Practice

As of this writing, relatively few clinicians assess health literacy in their patients using any formal tests. A survey conducted for the Commonwealth Fund in 2008, found that 95% asked their patients if they had any questions; 67% used their "gut feeling"; 65% asked the patient to repeat information back; and 27% looked at the last grade of education completed by the patient.[30] While this is less than ideal, experts agree that sensitivity to patients' feelings about being judged as "uneducated" is more important that a finely tuned measure of health literacy. (For more on patient–provider communication, see Chapter 15).

A consensus on "universal precautions" for health literacy are:

- You can't tell by looking at someone.
- You should strive to communicate clearly with everyone.
- You should confirm understanding with everyone.

See **Box 7–3** for more specific recommendations for communicating with low literacy patients in a healthcare setting.[31,32]

---

*http://www.adultmeducation.com/AssessmentTools_1.html
†http://www.peppercornbooks.com/catalog/information.php?info_id=5
‡http://pfizerhealthliteracy.com/physicians-providers/newest-vital-sign.html

Box 7–3 Health Literacy Communication Guidelines for Patient Care Settings

❑ To assess with an instrument, or not. What are you trying to achieve?

1. Obtain accurate information from the patient.
2. See if the patient can read, process, and fully understand medical instructions.
3. Avoid liability; Adhere to a policy or regulation.
4. The key to requesting a formal assessment from a patient is, "Will you help me?" Ask the patient to help you find out what materials will be best for them in dealing with their illness.
5. Choose the tool (e.g., NVS, REALM-R, TOFHLA, one- or two-question test) that is best for your patients and practice.

❑ Basic strategies to improve communication

1. Explain things clearly in plain language.
2. Focus on key messages and repeat them.
3. Use a "teach back" or "show me" technique to check understanding.
4. Effectively solicit questions.
5. Use patient-friendly educational materials to enhance interaction.

These are explained below.

1. Explain things clearly in plain language.
   - Slow down the pace of your speech.
   - Use plain, *nonmedical* language:
     ° "Blood pressure pill" instead of "antihypertensive"
     ° Pay attention to patient's own terms and use them back
   - Avoid vague terms:
     ° "Take 1 hour before you eat breakfast" instead of "Take on an empty stomach."
2. Focus on key messages and repeat them.
   - Limit information:
     ° Focus on one to three key points.
   - Develop short explanations for common medical conditions and side effects.
   - Discuss specific behaviors rather than general concepts.
   - Review each point at the end.
3. Use a "teach back" or "show me" technique to check understanding.
   - Sample scripts:
     ° I want to make sure I explained everything clearly. If you were trying to explain to your husband how to take this medicine, what would you say?
     ° Let's review the main side effects of this new medicine. What are the two things that I asked you to watch out for?
     ° Show me how you would use this inhaler.
4. Effectively solicit questions.
   - Don't say: "Do you have any questions?" Or "Any questions?" (Too easy to say "No.")
   - Instead say: "What questions do you have?" Or, "What *else* would you like to know?" (Allows them to ask something even if you've covered it in a face-saving way.)
5. Use patient-friendly materials. Check that the handouts and instructions you plan to give the patient follows guidelines for:
   - Plain Language.
   - Layout.
   - Illustrations.

And try to choose materials that are focused specifically on their illness and treatment plan. (I.e., not overly comprehensive or requiring too much interpretation.)

Source: Weiss BD. *Health Literacy: A Manual for Clinicians.* American Medical Association and American Medical Association Foundation; 2003
Kripalani S, Weiss BD. Teaching about health literacy and clear communication. *Journal of General Internal Medicine.* 2006;21(8):888–890.

CONCLUSION

As you can see, health literacy and numeracy are crucial factors as you plan your communication efforts, and these factors demonstrate the importance of audience analysis before designing or implementing any communication intervention. Fortunately, research and practical experience have shown that there are many approaches you can use to help overcome the challenges of low health literacy and numeracy. We've hinted at some of these approaches here. In Appendix 7A we spell them out more thoroughly and suggest ways to address numeracy and data presentation challenges. So, if you want to learn ways to resolve many of the problems raised in this and previous chapters, read on.

KEY TERMS

Adjustment bias
Anchoring
Culturally and linguistically appropriate services (CLAS)
Elaboration Likelihood Model (ELM)
Health literacy
Information Processing Theory
Limited English proficiency (LEP)
Literacy
National Assessment of Adult Literacy (NAAL)
Neuroscience
Newest Vital Sign (NVS)
Numeracy
One- or two-question tests
Quantitative literacy (QL)
Rapid Estimate of Adult Literacy in Medicine (REALM)
Representative heuristic
Test of Functional Health Literacy in Adults (TOFHLA)

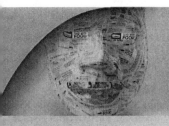

Chapter Questions

1. Define literacy, health literacy, and numeracy.

2. Why is low health literacy a critical communication consideration?

3. With what adverse health outcomes has low health literacy been associated?

4. What are the implications of low numeracy levels for communication?

5. What are the best available ways to assess health literacy in a healthcare setting?

REFERENCES

1. Teinonen T, Fellman V, Näätänen R, Alku P Huotilainen M. Statistical language learning in neonates revealed by event-related brain potentials. *BMC Neurosci.* 2009;10(21). Published online 2009 March 13. doi:10.1186/1471-2202-10-21. http://www.biomedcentral.com/1471-2202/10/21. Accessed January 12, 2010.

2. Kahneman D, Slovick P, Tversky A. *Judgment under Uncertainty: Heuristics and Biases.* Cambridge, UK: Cambridge University Press; 1982.

3. Petty, RE, Cacioppo, JT. The Elaboration Likelihood Model of persuasion. *AdvExperl Soc Psych.* 1986;19:123–205.

4. Glanz K, Lewis FM, Rimer BK. Eds. *Health Behavior and Health Education: Theory, Research and Practice,* 2nd ed. San Francisco: Jossey-Bass; 1997.

5. Kutner, M, Greenberg, E, Baer, J. *A First Look at the Literacy of America's Adults in the 21st Century. Report No.* NCES 2006-470. Washington, DC: National Center for Education Statistics, Institute of Education Sciences, U.S. Department of Education; 2006. Available at: http://nces.ed.gov/NAAL/PDF/2006470.PDF. Accessed January 12, 2010.

6. U.S. Department of Education Institute of Education Sciences National Center for Education Statistics. *National Assessment of Adult Literacy.* Demographics, Overall, Average Scores. http://www.nces.ed.gov/naal/kf_demographics.asp. Accessed January 12, 2010.

7. Nielsen-Bohlman L, Panzer AM, Kindig DA (eds.). *Health Literacy: A Prescription to End Confusion.* Washington, DC: National Academies Press; 2004.

8. U.S. Department of Health and Human Services. *Health Literacy Improvement.* Washington, DC: Office of Disease Prevention and Health Promotion, Department of Health and Human Services. Available at http://www.health.gov/communication/literacy/. Accessed: March 29, 2009.

9. Shin, HB with Bruno, R. Language Use and English-Speaking Ability: 2000, Census 2000 Brief. Report No. C2KBR-29. October 2003. http://www.census.gov/prod/2003pubs/c2kbr-29.pdf. Accessed January 12, 2010.

10. U.S. Department of Health and Human Services Office of Minority Health. *Healthcare Language Services Implementation Guide.* Available from: https://hclsig.thinkculturalhealth.org/page/view.rails?name=Section+2:+Page+2,3. Accessed January 12, 2010.

11. U.S. Department of Health and Human Services Office of Disease Prevention and Health Promotion. *Healthy People 2010,* 11 Health Communication. http://www.healthypeople.gov/document/HTML/Volume1/11HealthCom.htm. Accessed January 12, 2010.

12. Nelson DE, Hesse BW, Croyle RT. *Making Data Talk.* New York: Oxford University Press, 2009.

13. Houd O, Tzourio-Mazoyer, N. Neural foundations of logical and mathematical cognition. *Nat Rev Neurosci.* 2003;4:507–514.

14. National Center for Education Statistics. *Overview and Key Findings across Grade Levels.* Report No. NCES 1999-081. http://nces.ed.gov/pubs99/1999081.pdf. Accessed January 12, 2010.

15. Abramsky L, Fletcher O. Interpreting information: What is said, what is heard-A questionnaire study of health professionals and members of the public. *Prenat Diagn.* 2002;22:1188–1194.

16. Kutner M, Greenberg E, Jin Y, Boyle B, Yung-chen Hsu, Dunleavy E, White S. *Literacy in Everyday Life: Results from the 2003 National Assessment of Adult Literacy.* Report No. NCES 2007-480. Washington, DC: U.S. Department of Education; 2007.

17. Gazmararian JA, Curran JW, Parker RM, Bernhardt JM, DeBuono BA. Public health literacy in America: an ethical imperative. *Am J Prev Med.* 2005;28(3):317–322.

18. Sanders LM, Federico S, Klass P, Abrams MA, Dreyer B. Literacy and child health: A systematic review. *Arch Pediatr Adolesc Med.* 2009;163(2):131–140.

19. Sudore RL, Yaffe K, Satterfield S et al. Limited literacy and mortality in the elderly: The health, aging, and body composition study. *J Gen Intern Med.* 2006;21:806–812.

20. Baker DW, Wolf MS, Feinglass J, et al. Health literacy and mortality among elderly persons. *Arch Intern Med.* 2007;167(14):1503–1509.

21. DeWalt DA. Low health literacy: epidemiology and interventions. *NC Med J.* 2007; 68(5):327–330.

22. Centers for Disease Control and Prevention. *Scientific and Technical Information Simply Put,* 2nd ed. Atlanta, GA: Centers for Disease Control and Prevention; 1999.

23. Fagerlin A, Ubel PA, Smith DM, Zikmund-Fisher BJ. Making numbers matter: present and future research in risk communication. *Am J Health Behav.* 2007;31(Suppl 1):S47–S56.

24. Paasche-Orlow MK, Wolf MS. Evidence does not support clinical screening of literacy. *J Gen Intern Med.* 2008;23(1):100-102. doi: 10.1007/s11606-007-0447-2. http://www.ncbi.nlm.nih.gov/pmc/articles/ PMC2173929/. Accessed January 12, 2010.

25. Davis TC, Long SW, Jackson RH, et al. Rapid estimate of adult literacy in medicine: a shortened screening instrument. *Fam Med.* 1993; 25:391–395.

26. Bass PF III, Wilson JF, Griffith CH. A shortened instrument for literacy screening. *J Gen Intern Med.* 2003;18:1036–1038.

27. Parker RM , Baker DW, Williams MC, Nurss JR. The test of functional health literacy in adults. A new instrument for measuring patients' literacy skills. *J Gen Intern Med.* 1995;10:537–541.

28. Weiss BD, Mays MZ, Martz, W, Castro CM, DeWalt DA, Pignone MP, Mockbee J, Hale, FA. Quick assessment of literacy in primary care: The Newest Vital Sign. *Annals Family Med.* 2005;3:514–522.

29. Wallace LS, Rogers ES, Roskos SE, Holiday DB, Weiss BD. Screening items to identify patients with limited health literacy skills. *Journal of General Internal Medicine.* 2006; 21:874–877.

30. Barrett SE, Puryear JS, Westpheling K. *Health Literacy Practices in Primary Care Settings: Examples from the Field.* Commonwealth Fund pub. no. 1093 2008:5. http://www.commonwealthfund.org. Accessed November 12, 2009.

31. Weiss BD. *Health Literacy: A Manual for Clinicians.* American Medical Association and American Medical Association Foundation; 2003.

32. Kripalani S, Weiss BD. Teaching about health literacy and clear communication. *J Gen. Int. Med.* 2006;21(8):888–890.

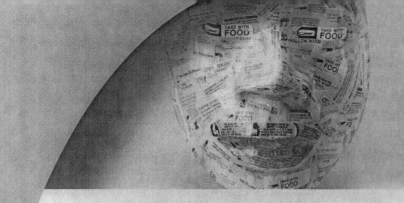

Summary
Informing and Educating People about Health

INTRODUCTION

The following is a summary of the information discussed in Chapters 2 through 7, and it builds on several of these chapters by providing tips to address the issues underlying health literacy, numeracy, and reaching lay audiences to inform them about relevant health topics. Summary topics include:

1. Key recommendations that are foundational to effective health communication.
2. How to communicate in clinical settings.
3. Extensive recommendations to improve communication when a population's health literacy is low.
4. Approaches to overcoming literacy limitations, which focus particularly on numeracy and presenting health data to lay audiences.

COMMUNICATION RECOMMENDATIONS

There are 11 key recommendations to improve communication meant to inform:

1. Get to know the intended users and the context for the information.
2. Conduct a needs assessment to gauge knowledge and skills.
3. Use information processing theory to your advantage.
4. Use the Elaboration Likelihood Model to your advantage.
5. Practice culturally competent verbal and nonverbal communication.
6. Pretest messages and materials.
7. Use plain language and easy-to-understand design layouts for written materials.

8. Supplement or replace written materials with visual or audio aids.
9. Conduct usability testing (especially for Internet websites).
10. Collaborate with others to share effective materials.
11. Keep it simple.

Get to Know the Users and the Context

We will discuss formative research extensively in Chapter 9. In developing materials to inform, we have focused on the abilities of the intended user to read and understand. This involves their comprehension of English, as a first or second language; their abilities to read tables, charts, or other graphical displays; and their general understanding of health as well as their worldview. In addition to their general abilities, you need to think about the challenges inherent in the context in which they will receive the material. Will it be a waiting room of a doctor's office? Will they likely be feeling under-the-weather, or stressed? Or, do you plan to distribute information in a noisy supermarket or at a pharmacy counter? These environmental factors also influence a person's abilities to process information.

Conduct a Needs Assessment to Gauge Knowledge and Skills

Using either a health literacy assessment instrument or some informal means, try to identify the intended user's strengths and weaknesses when it comes to using health information. For example, in a medical setting, if certain patients are comfortable with the Internet, they can be directed to online resources. Alternatively, they might better understand simple print materials or need everything in an audiovisual form. Any of these media might need to be produced in a different language for users. Such details about the patient users can be recorded in a few minutes by office staff in a healthcare provider setting and should become a part of patients' charts or electronic medical records.

Use Information Processing Theory to Your Advantage

There is a reason that phone numbers and Zip codes have 5 to 10 numbers. We seem to be able to remember seven (plus or minus three) numbers fairly easily. But, that's it. As we will discuss in Chapter 16, a "message map" is an effective way to organize your thoughts so that you sandwich your key message between two supporting messages—but provide no more than three. When giving oral instructions to someone, you can count on them being able to remember two or three things, but again, that is about all. So, prioritize your thoughts and give people only what they really need to make a decision now. You can give them more to read for later if you feel it is important to their welfare.

Use the Elaboration Likelihood Model to Your Advantage

Finding out how much someone cares about an issue is an invaluable tool. If an individual is deeply involved, then they will probably want the details. If this is of superficial importance to a person, he or she might say, "Just tell me what I have to do," and then likely forget that as well. Having materials that are culturally appropriate is helpful in two ways, because they make use of the ELM. The first way is that they demonstrate a level of attentiveness and caring on the provider's part and help make a patient, in particular, feel at ease. Second, they eliminate some of the distractions to processing the information that might be in the way if materials feature discordant models (e.g., giving pamphlets with older adults on them to adolescent patients; or materials featuring African Americans to Asian patients). So, having a stock of multicultural materials, at different reading levels, is really ideal, if possible.

Practice Culturally Competent Verbal and Nonverbal Communication

We will discuss this much more in Chapters 10 and 15. While it's nice to have print materials for different languages and cultural identities, it is even more important to realize that your verbal and nonverbal communication is also cultural. Being sensitive to differences among people, and knowing how to show respect and sincerity for different groups, is a wonderful skill. Such differences may be based on race, ethnicity, language, nationality, religion, age, gender, sexual orientation, income level, or occupational groups. So, your tone of voice, body language, gaze, a handshake, or touching the recipient's arm all send messages that might be read differently depending on the recipient's background. Your desire to become "culturally literate" is a starting point for acquiring a larger vocabulary. But numerous studies have shown that being polite (almost to what feels like an extreme) and practicing the Golden Rule will carry you farther than trying to learn lists of exotic words and practices.

Pretest Messages and Materials

We will discuss pretesting extensively in Chapter 9. Even straightforward messages should be checked with representatives of the intended audience before producing them in quantity. Techniques include focus groups, individual interviews, or giving people sample materials to critique while in the waiting room. It has become very simple to test materials in an online environment and rapidly receive feedback from specific audience segments.

Use Plain Language and Easy-to-Understand Design Layouts for Written Materials

There are some excellent resources available on how to prepare simplified materials for all audiences.[1-5] **Figure 7A–1** provides a readability checklist that summarizes key points to consider in reviewing health communication materials for educational purposes.[6-9]

Figure 7A–2 provides two examples of how to shorten sentence length and use plain language, both of which make the information much easier for users to comprehend.[10,11]

Supplement or Replace Written Materials with Visual or Audio Aids

For low health literacy audiences, and especially for audiences who have great difficulty reading English, strong consideration should be given to supplementing written materials with visual images, such as pictures or diagrams, to illustrate key points (e.g., instructions for washing hands). With technological advances in recent years, it is now possible to consider providing video or audio presentations to audiences, such as through online or handheld video or audio devices (e.g., iPods).

Conduct Usability Testing (Especially for Internet Websites)

Usability testing involves evaluating a communication product's ability to help support a task for the user of the product, such as decision making (e.g., healthcare treatments, receiving a newly developed screening test).[7] The most common usability example is for websites, but it can also be used for other

FIGURE 7A–1 Readability Checklist

READABILITY CHECKLIST FOR PARTICIPANT MATERIALS
Primary Review: Project Manager

✓	Check Material	Notes
	Reading level Most public health materials need to be between a 5th- and 8th-grade reading level, or run between 800 to 1050 Lexiles™.	Software tools, such as Microsoft Word™, allow you to use the Flesch-Kincaid method to assess a grade level equivalent and reading ease. A SMOG[7] test can be run for free at this website. The Fry[8] index can be calculated by hand. The Lexile Framework,[9] which is used extensively in primary education,[a] is a more precise measure where both the reader and the written material can be "matched."
	Common, everyday words • Jargon replaced or defined • Use examples and analogies	Use "living room" language, where possible. See PRISM Readability Toolkit for extensive glossary of alternative words for medical and health-related jargon. Instead of "5ccs" (of blood to be drawn), say, "We will use a needle to take about 1 teaspoon of your blood for the test."
	Active voice and first-person	"We will ask you questions about your health" is active. "You will be asked questions about your health" is passive. Pronouns such as "I," "We," and "You."
	Clarity of visual aids/drawings	Clear line drawings are easier to interpret than photographs. For statistical associations, "part to whole" icon arrays in a nonrandom arrangement[b] are the easiest for low literacy/numeracy users to interpret.
	Sentences are short and to the point. • Go for 15 words or fewer.	Break up sentences joined with conjunctions or semicolons. OK to begin a complete sentence with "And" or "But." Vary sentence length—some short, some a little longer.
	Paragraphs have one main idea with clear and descriptive headings	Start with a clear and concise topic sentence. Remove or move details that do not relate to the central topic. A paragraph of one or two sentences is fine.
	Large font, bold, or other emphasis, to ensure the headings stand out.	Meaningful headings that describe the content of different sections provide "road signs" that help the reader navigate your document more easily.
	User considerations	Include only the information that your audience really needs to know now. Use large font and/or age-appropriate or culturally sensitive language to meet the needs of special populations like the elderly, children, minorities, or people with chronic health conditions, etc.
	Clear organization and format • Lead with key information • Use **bold**, bullets, or <u>other emphasis</u> as needed (<u>no</u> *italics*)	Lead with the most important information, and sequence the information in a logical fashion that the audience can easily follow. Use bold, larger font, bullets, or graphics to emphasize critical information. *Do not* use justified margins or put entire sentences in all caps or italics. Put long lists of items into bulleted lists whenever practical. Use numerical lists whenever if the items need to be understood or completed in order.

continues

continues

[a] The Lexile Framework for Reading™ is a trademark of Metametrics Inc. Lexiles are well correlated with scholastic tests given through high school, but are not, as of yet, associated with standard adult literacy measures, such as the REALM. Blocks of prose text may be analyzed through a fee for service.

FIGURE 7A-1 Readability Checklist—continued

READABILITY CHECKLIST FOR PARTICIPANT MATERIALS
Primary Review: Project Manager

✓	Check Material	Notes
	Adequate white space and margins	Break up dense copy by using ample white space between paragraphs and headings. If document has space left over (e.g., print run requires 4, 8, 12, or 16 pages), add space between paragraphs or increase the font size of headers or text. Avoid decreasing margins to force text to fit on one page. Top and bottom margins should be at least 1 inch, and side margins should be at least 1.25 inches.
	Read aloud to ensure overall clarity and logical flow	This is one of the best ways to find errors and test for overall flow and clarity when you proofread. It can also help you troubleshoot—when you get stuck, try just speaking your thoughts.

Secondary Review: By Others

	Read by colleague unfamiliar with project	Someone unfamiliar to the project is more likely to notice text that is unclear.
	Read by primary user of document (e.g., research administrator, research nurse, health educator)	The person who will use the document most—such as the person who will administer informed consent—should always have a chance to review it.
	Pretested by intended user	Have at least 10 persons who represent the target beneficiaries use the material. Mark off where they experience difficulties, if any. If at least 8 of them can read it without difficulties, you may go on to the final review. If the score is less than this, revise based on where they have problems. Repeat the pretest until you get an 80% score.

Final Review: Project Manager

	Information correct	Call all phone numbers and check all links and e-mail addresses. Confirm that all names have been spelled correctly and that all titles are correct
	Final check	Whenever possible, set the material aside for a day or two and proofread it again after taking a break. This step, along with reading your document out loud, is a good way to find errors that may have been overlooked before. Be careful not to start "upgrading" the reading level.
	Production check	Work with the printer to ensure that the final product is clear, aligned, and free of smudges or other printers' errors.

Source: Based on PRISM Readability Toolkit. Ridpath, J.R., Greene, S.M., Wiese, C.J. *PRISM Readability Toolkit*, 3rd ed. Seattle: Group Health Research Institute; 2007. Version 4, updated June 2009. http://www.grouphealthresearch.org/capabilities/readability/readability_home.html

FIGURE 7A-2 Examples of Replacing More Complex Terms with Plain Language

Part A

Angina pectoris	Chest pain
Atrophy	Wasting away or shrinking
Cardiac	Heart
Demonstrate	Show
Etiology	Cause
Healthcare facility	Clinic or doctor's office
Lipid	Fat
Optimum	Best
Pulmonary	Lungs
Postpartum	After childbirth
Occupational	Work-related or job-related
Utilize	Use
Vascular	Blood vessels
Vertigo	Dizziness

Part B
Examples of Rewriting Complex Text to Be More Understandable by Lay Audiences

Changes to introductory language in a handbook published by the Health Resources and Services Administration:

Before

Title I of the CARE Act creates a program of formula and supplemental competitive grants to help metropolitan areas with 2,000 or more reported AIDS cases meet emergency care needs of low-income HIV patients. Title II of the Ryan White Act provides formula grants to States and territories for operation of HIV service consortia in the localities most affected by the epidemic, provision of home and community-based care, continuation of insurance coverage for persons with HIV infection, and treatments that prolong life and prevent serious deterioration of health. Up to 10 percent of the funds for this program can be used to support Special Projects of National Significance.

After

Low-income people living with HIV/AIDS gain, literally, years through the advanced drug treatments and ongoing care supported by HRSA's Ryan White Comprehensive AIDS Resources Emergency (CARE) Act.

Changes to a letter to consumers concerning potential Medicare fraud:

Before

Investigators at the contractor will review the facts in your case and decide the most appropriate course of action. The first step taken with most Medicare health care providers is to re-educate them about Medicare regulations and policies. If the practice continues, the contractor may conduct special audits of the provider's medical records. Often, the contractor recovers overpayments to health care providers this way. If there is sufficient evidence to show that the provider is consistently violating Medicare policies, the contractor will document the violations and ask the Office of the Inspector General to prosecute the case. This can lead to expulsion from the Medicare program, civil monetary penalties, and imprisonment.

After

We will take two steps to look at this matter: We will find out if it was an error or fraud. We will let you know the result.

Source: Part A adapted from Remington, P.L., Riesenberg, L.A., Needham, D.L., Siegel, P. Written Communication. In Nelson, D.E., Brownson, R.C., Remington, P.L., Parvanta, C., eds. *Communicating Public Health Information Effectively: A Guide for Practitioners.* Washington, D.C.: American Public Health Association; 2002:127–140.

Fagerlin A, Ubel PA, Smith DM, Zikmund-Fisher BJ. Making numbers matter: Present and future research in risk communication. *Am J Health Behav* 2007;31(Suppl 1):S47–S56.

Part B adapted from Advocacy Institute. *By the Numbers: A Guide to the Tactical Use of Statistics for Positive Policy Change.* Washington, DC: Advocacy Institute, no date.

communication-related tools or products. Unlike with formative evaluation, usability involves actually observing people in a structured manner while they use a communication product, and in some instances, asking them to provide oral or written feedback. This is done to help identify potential errors and to increase the functional ability of the product. As with formative evaluation, usability or a related type of performance testing can prevent unanticipated future problems and result in substantial cost savings.

Collaborate with Others to Share Effective Materials

An often overlooked aspect of health communication is the importance of collaboration. Let's face it: it can require extra work, time, and resources to communicate with diverse audiences. Close collaboration with other health departments, social service agencies, community groups, and educators may help you locate existing communication resources that may be readily available or adaptable to your intended audiences and vice versa. This may be especially pertinent for materials in a language other than English.

Keep It Simple

This tip requires practically no explanation, but to summarize, here are a few examples. Some of the most important, yet often overlooked, techniques are to limit the number of messages to just a handful, use short sentences that use active verbs, and stress action steps rather than lengthier descriptions. In clinical settings, speak slowly, avoid jargon, and use simple language. In written or visual presentations use a lot of white space. While "keeping it simple" sounds easy, public health and communication practitioners often have a knack for making information very confusing. How many PowerPoint presentations have you seen that have slide upon slide packed with so much text and bullet points that you get confused and ultimately stop paying attention? Think about these presentations when designing health communication messages and materials, and do just the opposite.

COMMUNICATION IN CLINICAL SETTINGS*

For those working in clinical settings, there are additional opportunities to communicate with persons with lower levels of health literacy.[12,13] These opportunities include:

- Asking patients or caregivers directly what they know or understand about the specific health situation.
- Speaking slowly, avoiding jargon, and using simple language.
- Asking open-ended questions. ("Tell me about your problem. What may have caused it?")
- Encouraging people to ask questions themselves. ("What questions do you have?")
- Applying the "teach-back" method to assess level of understanding. ("I just talked a lot about your health situation. Can you tell me in your own words what we just discussed?")
- Using an interpreter if a language barrier exists.
- Redesigning healthcare forms and instruction sheets so they are easier to understand.
- Improving the physical environment (e.g., using universally recognized icons on traffic signs or in health center corridors).

NUMERACY RECOMMENDATIONS

Communicating public health data is far more complicated than letting the numbers "speak for themselves." Selecting and presenting data is directly related to the communication purpose, audience, and context where communication occurs.[14] This means you need to put much thought into whether data should be communicated, what data you select, and how you present data.

Listed here are some considerations when determining what data to present and how to best present them:

1. Determine if data are needed to support your single overriding communication objective (SOCO).
2. Consider values and ethics.
3. Minimize the number of data items.
4. Select data that are more likely to be familiar and understood by audiences.
5. Explain unfamiliar statistical or epidemiologic terms.
6. Provide contextual information to assist with interpretation.

Determine if Data Are Even Necessary

You first need to consider whether it is even necessary to present numbers to audiences. Data generally serve to provide the rationale (reasons) behind scientific recommendations. You'll need to weigh whether data will assist in your efforts to communicate your SOCO. Sometimes numbers just confuse people. Generally speaking, messages with data generally resonate better with persons who:[14]

- Have higher levels of involvement with the issue at hand.
- Have lower levels of emotion (e.g., anger, fear).
- Have higher levels of education, including mathematical literacy.
- Are somewhat familiar with the topic or situation.

---

*These are discussed extensively in Chapter 15.

- Also, remember that in advocacy situations, data support a position, but do not speak for themselves.

Consider Values and Ethics

Values and ethics are critical, yet often overlooked, factors in the selection and presentation of data. Because data selection (or omission) is related to purpose, ethical rules, such as "greatest good for the greatest number," or "there are no just ends through unjust means" are calling the shots, even though the people preparing the data tables might think they are just crunching numbers. Public health professionals, because they are generally perceived as having high credibility, have an important ethical responsibility to be honest. If there is uncertainty about conclusions based on public health surveillance or research findings, be honest and convey this to audiences. Consider if you may be potentially misleading or manipulating people through the selection (and presentation) of data in your efforts to influence audiences toward a particular interpretation. The strategic use and misuse of data by the business and political community are daily occurrences in the United States, and public health professionals are subject to the same temptation, such as "cherry picking" data that support the desired point they wish to communicate.

Minimize the Number of Data Items

Many scientists, because of their familiarity with data and desire to use data to help prove their points, make the mistake of trying to communicate too many numbers to lay audiences.[14] As discussed earlier, numeracy levels are quite low for most of the population. In addition, people have limited ability to process and understand information presented to them, particularly information perceived as complex; this is referred to as cognitive burden or cognitive overload.

Thus, the "more is better" approach, when it comes to data, is a particularly *ineffective* communication strategy for most audiences; in fact, it is counterproductive when trying to persuade audiences.[14] Most people typically want public health (and other) experts to quickly get to their main conclusions and recommendations. The implication is clear: be cautious and use data sparingly when communicating with anyone but scientists. A general rule of thumb, particularly if data are being used for persuasive purposes, is to use only one or two numbers.

Select Data That Are More Likely to Be Familiar and Understood by Audiences

Closely related to minimizing the use of data is to select data measures for audiences that are likely to be familiar to them. Counts (frequencies) or whole numbers (such as 15 or 12,000)

are likely to be easily understood. In fact, Fagerlin, Ubel, Smith, and Zikmund-Fisher[15] indicate that when communicating health risk information (e.g., your chances of getting cancer if you are a smoker) to both patients and physicians, using frequencies is most effective at influencing the beliefs and decisions of these audiences. Proportions and percentages are not as effective when communicating health risk information. For other kinds of information, however, percentages (e.g., 40%) can be good choices, but it is important to avoid fractional percentages, such as 0.08%, because these can be misunderstood. To facilitate understanding, counts and percentages should be rounded (e.g., 9,000 rather than 9,136; 70% rather than 69.7%). If proportions are used, such as 1 in X, use the lowest possible denominator (e.g., 1 in 10 rather than 10 in 100). Also, when communicating lots of different information on health risks, it is best to use a consistent denominator (e.g., always say "out of 10" when talking about cancer risks associated with both smoking or red meat consumption).[15]

Explain Unfamiliar Statistical or Epidemiologic Terms

Many public health communicators mistakenly assume that statistical or epidemiologic terms are known or understood by lay audiences. Concepts such as statistical significance, probability, or relative risk are not likely to be familiar to most people. Terms should be defined in plain language, with additional background material made available for those interested in learning more.[14] Care should always be taken to explain the meaning of numeric representations and to remind the audience of how to put data into context.[14] Even the most common public health statistics, such as percentages or ratios, may be misunderstood without supporting explanation.

Provide Contextual Information to Assist with Interpretation

Data need to be presented with contextual information to help people understand what they mean. At a macro level, the news media regularly report unexpected (or shocking) new findings from research studies. An important role can be played by providing information about what these findings mean in light of prior research studies, particularly those based on research syntheses. A particular number means nothing unless it is put in perspective. Simply to report that there were X cases of a sexually transmitted disease in Illinois in 2008 provides little meaning unless further details are provided as to whether this represents an increase, decrease, or absence of change. Probability data in the form of comparative risk is particularly challenging.[14] If audiences, for instance, are familiar with games of chance (e.g., gambling odds), it may be possible to use gambling examples to help people better understand probability terms (e.g., your chance is about 50%—similar to flipping a coin). But there are commonly reports in the news media and elsewhere that people who eat food A or who are exposed to chemical B are at twice the risk for some type of cancer (a relative risk comparison). Such information often only presents part of the story, if, for example, the absolute risk of the cancer increased from 1 in 100,000 to 2 in 100,000. It is also concerning that low numeracy audiences are less likely than high numeracy audiences to be able to understand relative and absolute risk information, and research has shown that exposure to relative risk information has a tendency to increase one's beliefs about changes in individual health risk more than absolute risk information, even if the statistics are convening the same information.[15] Thus, communicators have an important responsibility to provide relevant contextual information when relaying numeric or mathematical data—such as relative and absolute risk statistics—to audiences, especially low numeracy audiences.

Tips for Presenting Data

Extensive details about how to present data to audiences are beyond the scope of this book. Basically, data can be presented one of two ways: through words or visual modalities.[14] Here are some straightforward approaches that will help improve your verbal and visual presentations:

1. Use metaphors and narratives in verbal presentations.
2. Display simple visual modalities in visual presentations.
3. Employ special presentation techniques to prevent cognitive burden.
4. Consider audiences risk perceptions when presenting messages about numeric data.
5. Understand the numeracy level of the audience.

Use Metaphors and Narratives in Verbal Presentations

As mentioned previously, one or two numbers can often be presented as part of communication efforts. However, there are other ways of communicating numbers through the use of words, particularly through the use of metaphors or narratives. A metaphor, in the context of data presentation, refers to the use of text to provide an analogy, such that "X is similar to Y." For example, anti-tobacco advocates often note that the annual number of deaths from smoking in the United States each day was equivalent to two jumbo jets crashing every day with no survivors.[16] Other public health metaphors are included in **Figure 7A–3**.[17–19] If employed, the metaphor should use an analogy familiar to the audience; it should be included

FIGURE 7A–3 Examples of Public Health Metaphors

Think of two twin towers falling from terrorist attack each day—that's cancer.

Only 3% of Canadians would prefer a U.S. private health insurance model to a single-payer model. Put in perspective, 16% of Canadians believe that Elvis Presley is still alive.

College students consume enough alcohol to fill 3,500 Olympic-size swimming pools on every campus in the United States.

Medium-sized buttered popcorn at the [movie] theater contains more artery-clogging fat than a bacon-and-eggs breakfast, a Big Mac and fries for lunch, and a steak dinner with all the trimmings . . . combined.

Source: References 17–19.

early in a communication effort; and no more than one metaphor should be included.[14]

Narratives refer to a vignette, anecdote, or some other type of short text description designed to illustrate a point; as a rule, narratives are longer than metaphors. Narratives can be a highly effective way of presenting information, including data, as they have the ability to "draw people in" (transport them) to a particular story; they have the additional benefit of potentially generating emotions.[14] Box 7–2 provided a poignant example of a narrative.

Display Simple Visual Modalities in Visual Presentations

There are many ways to present public health data visually, but the most common visual modalities are bar charts, line graphs, and pie charts because they are familiar and readily understood.[14] Icon arrays seem to be the best understood by persons with less numerical or health literacy ability, because they are generally more understandable by all (**Figure 7A–4**). Because of their versatility, bar charts are used most often because they do an excellent job of displaying relative magnitude (size) of numbers, such as counts or percentages. Line graphs are most widely used for showing data patterns, particularly trends over time. Pie charts are helpful for demonstrating relative size of a proportion (or small number of proportions) that total to 100%.

Employ Special Presentation Techniques to Prevent Cognitive Burden

When visual data presentation is used, there are several techniques that can prevent the problem of cognitive burden. First, limit the number of visuals whenever possible—rarely are

FIGURE 7A–4 Icon Array

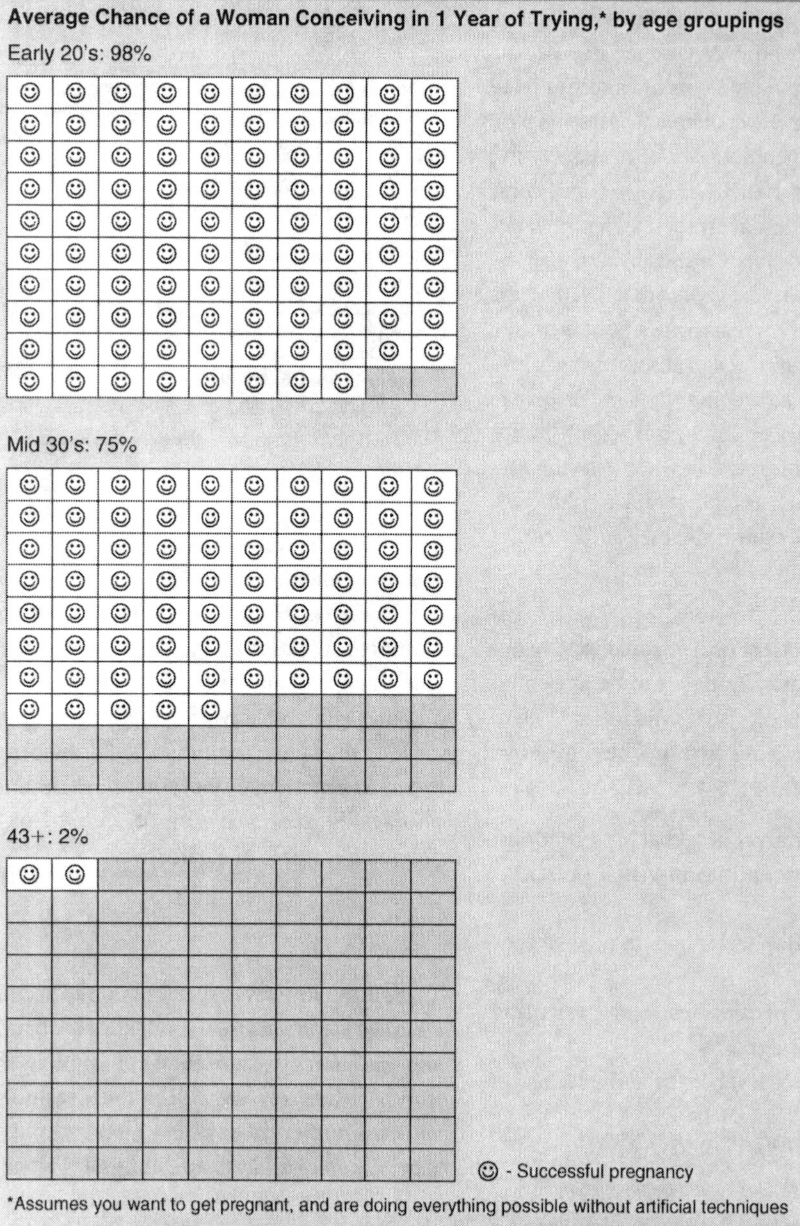

Average Chance of a Woman Conceiving in 1 Year of Trying,* by age groupings

Early 20's: 98%

Mid 30's: 75%

43+: 2%

☺ - Successful pregnancy

*Assumes you want to get pregnant, and are doing everything possible without artificial techniques

Source: Kristina Parvanta. Data from the US Department of Health and Human Services

more than a few visuals needed (often only one figure will suffice) when presenting data to lay audiences. Second, use short and simple titles, labels, and legends, and consider including text that mentions the key point (e.g., the number of hospital acquired infections declined 85% after implementation of prevention measures). Third, highlight key data points by using arrows or bolding the text. Fourth, only include a few bars, lines, or pie slices to avoid the problem of clutter, and maintain sufficient "white space" so that audiences quickly identify the major points.

Consider Audiences Risk Perceptions When Presenting Messages about Numeric Data

There are some other considerations to keep in mind when communicating specific kinds of numeric and mathematical information. The way that these data are conveyed can have very different effects on an individual's *risk perception*, or an individual's beliefs about the level of health risks associated with a particular behavior, exposure, or treatment. These tips are discussed in detail in a review of health risk communication research and interventions,[15] but we will summarize them here for you.

When presenting information about health risks and benefits, it is best to either use specific statistics—using terms that audiences with low numeracy can understand, of course (see earlier discussion)—rather than verbal explanations, or to use graphs or charts to provide visual comparisons of overtime risk or different outcomes of various health risks, behaviors, or treatments. These decisions depend on the goal of the communication project—that is, the message that the communicator wants the recipients to take away about their risk perception. The effect of the take-away message on a recipient's risk perception can also depend on the time span upon which health risk data are summarized. For example, an older audience might better understand lifetime risk statistics where as risks "over the next 10 years" might resonate more with younger audiences. Finally, positive and negative framing, or gain and loss framing, of messages can persuade audiences differently. Prevention messages are often more effective if they are framed positively (gain frame) than negatively (loss frame). For example, "Birth control pills are more than 99% effective in preventing pregnancy." However, messages about detection behaviors are often more effective if framed negatively, e.g., "Women who don't regularly perform self-breast exams have a lower chance of detecting cancer before it metastasizes." It is important to keep in mind that communication materials used in persuasion and behavior change should use both positive and negative framing of various messages in order to avoid biasing audiences risk perceptions and subsequent choices related to their own health. Message framing was discussed further in Chapter 6.

Understand the Numeracy Level of the Audience

When making any of these decisions on how to present data, a communicator must attend to the numeracy level of the audience.[15] As mentioned earlier, audiences with low numeracy will prefer, comprehend, and be more open to particular formats of mathematical information than audiences with high numeracy. Further research is still needed to de-termine the most effective ways of communicating data and health risks to these different audiences.[15] In the meantime, conducting formative audience research (see Chapter 9) before starting any sort of program or preparing materials to communicate data will be most helpful in reaching audiences at any health numeracy level, or health literacy level for that matter.

As you can see, health literacy and numeracy are crucial considerations as you plan your communication efforts with lay audiences. They demonstrate the importance of audience analysis. Fortunately, research and practical experience have shown that there are many approaches you can use to help overcome the challenges of low health literacy and numeracy. Keep these summary tips in mind when moving forward with any health communication intervention meant to inform lay audiences.

REFERENCES

1. Doak C, Doak L, Root J. *Teaching Patients with Low Literacy Skills.* Philadelphia, PA: J. B. Lippincott Company; 1996. Available from: http://www.hsph.harvard.edu/healthliteracy/doak.html. Accessed January 12, 2010.

2. Plain Language Action and Information Network. Plain Language.gov. http://www.plainlanguage.gov/. Accessed January 12, 2010.

3. Centers for Disease Control and Prevention. *Scientific and Technical Information Simply Put,* 2nd ed. Atlanta, GA: Centers for Disease Control and Prevention; 1999.

4. Maximus. *The Health Literacy Style Manual: Prepared for Covering Kids & Families.* 2005. Available at: http://www.coveringkidsandfamilies.org/resources/docs/stylemanual.pdf. Accessed January 12, 2010.

5. Ridpath JR, Greene SM, Wiese CJ. *PRISM Readability Toolkit,* 3rd ed. Seattle: Group Health Research Institute; 2007. Third edition, Version 4, updated June 2009 http://www.grouphealthresearch.org/capabilities/readability/readability_home.html

6. Ridpath JR, Greene SM, Wiese CJ. PRISM Readability Toolkit. 3rd ed. Seattle: Group Health Research Institute; 2007. Third edition, Version 4, updated June 2009

7. http://www.harrymclaughlin.com/SMOG.htm; http://wordscount.info/wc/jsp/clear/analyze_readability.jsp

8. http://www.ohiohealth.com/documents/university/fry%20directions%20and%20graph.pdf

9. www.lexile.com

10. Plain Language Action and Information Network. Plain language.gov. Available at http://www.plainlanguage.gov. Accessed March 29, 2009.

11. Remington PL, Riesenberg LA, Needham DL, Siegel P. Written Communication. In: Nelson DE, Brownson RC, Remington PL, Parvanta C, Eds. *Communicating Public Health Information Effectively: A Guide for Practitioners.* Washington, DC: American Public Health Association; 2002: 127–140.

12. Department of Health and Human Services. *Health Literacy Improvement.* Washington, DC: Office of Disease Prevention and Health Promotion, Department of Health and Human Services. Available at http://www.health.gov/communication/literacy/. Accessed: March 29, 2009.

13. Smith AK, Sudore RL, Perez-Stable EJ. Palliative care for Latino patients and their families: whenever we prayed, she wept. *JAMA.* 2009;301(10): 1047–1057.

14. Nelson DE, Hesse BW, Croyle RT. *Making Data Talk*. New York: Oxford University Press; 2009.

15. Fagerlin A, Ubel PA, Smith DM, Zikmund-Fisher BJ. Making numbers matter: Present and future research in risk communication. *Am J Health Behav* 2007;31(Suppl 1):S47–S56.

16. Advocacy Institute. *By the Numbers: A Guide to the Tactical Use of Statistics for Positive Policy Change*. Washington, DC: Advocacy Institute, no date.

17. Rose C. A discussion about cancer in America. In: *The Charlie Rose* [Television] *Show* Transcript; episode aired April 29, 2004.

18. Wallack L, Dorfman L, Jernigan D, Themba M. *Media Advocacy for Public Health*. Newbury Park, CA: Sage; 1993.

19. Wallack LM, Woodruff K, Dorfman L, Diaz I. *News for a Change: An Advocate's Guide to Working with the Media*. Thousand Oaks, CA: Sage Publications; 1999.

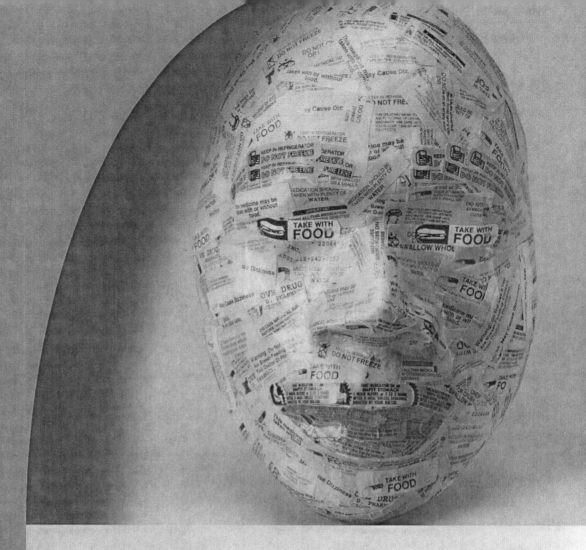

Being Persuasive: Influencing People to Adopt Healthy Behavior

CHAPTER 8

Persuasive Health Communications: The Role of Theory

Claudia Parvanta and Sarah Parvanta

LEARNING OBJECTIVES

By the end of this chapter, the reader will be able to:

- Understand the practicality of a good theory.
- Frame a fact for persuasive purposes.
- Grasp the fundamentals of social marketing.
- Describe the key theories of behavior change used most commonly in public health communication.

INTRODUCTION

Kurt Lewin* famously said, "There is nothing so practical as a good theory." His statement, so often attributed to other scientists, certainly reflects the essence of behavior change communication. Ed Maibach once called **self-efficacy** the "penicillin of the '90s,"[1] referring to how virtually every health intervention included this construct from Social Cognitive Theory. This chapter introduces the tools that every health communicator needs in his or her tool kit. If the Health Belief Model is a hammer, then the Transtheoretical and Precaution Adoption Process models are wrenches, Social Cognitive Theory is a screwdriver set, the Integrative Model is a Swiss Army knife, and Diffusion of Innovations is duct tape. Most behavior change interventions use one or more of these theories. While they might seem a bit frightening at first, with practice, you will

become as adept with them as you are with a screwdriver. As with tools, if you choose the wrong one your task become more difficult, like pounding nails with a wrench. In this and the following chapter, we help you select the right tool for the job by discussing each of the theories and showing you how to apply them appropriately in different health communication interventions.

We have already presented a few important theories that dealt directly with "informing" audiences. In Chapter 7 we introduced information processing theory as what we have learned about how people take in information, organize it mentally, and make sense of it. We also discussed the Elaboration Likelihood Model, which predicts that an individual will "elaborate," or think about new information more, if they are already concerned about or interested in the subject. If not, then other symbolic references valued by the intended user, such as spokespersons, models, settings, colors, language, are used to capture attention. These often cultural references are called **peripheral cues**, because they do not deal directly with the subject matter (which might, e.g., be smoking cessation or STD prevention), but more call out to the intended user—"Hey, look at me. I'm speaking to YOU." In addition to a person's health literacy and basic reading ability, these concepts guide how health communicators prepare information that is meant to "inform a decision." We use primarily "educational" approaches to present information that is clear, simple, and relevant to our intended user.

THEORIES OF PERSUASION

In this chapter we move on to the idea of **Persuasion Theory**. If a Precede–Proceed analysis of a problem in the ecological

---

Kurt Lewin (1890–1947) is considered by many to be the father of modern social psychology. He was early in emphasizing the importance of the environment together with personal characteristics, in causing behavior. Another relevant and famous quote, "If you want truly to understand something, try to change it."

framework in Chapter 2 leads us to conclude that health will be improved only if a change takes place, then we need to convince people to make that change. Using Rothschild's model[2] we need to determine how difficult and costly the change might be for those being asked to make it. Will we be trying to get a group of people to change a habit they view as an inalienable right, as throwing trash out of moving vehicles was viewed in the 1960s? Are we working with someone who is addicted to a substance, such as tobacco, but *wants* to stop using it? Are we trying to make people aware of a problem they don't even know they have, such as mothers in developing countries who are unaware that vitamins and minerals are necessary in their children's diets? Or, are we trying to motivate people to adopt a behavior that they know *is* beneficial, but for so many reasons, personal and external, is difficult to embrace? Examples include eating more fruits and vegetables, getting more exercise, practicing safe sex with a partner, etc. In most of these cases, information alone is not sufficient for people to change their behavior. They also need to feel that the change is important to them personally, that they have the ability to do it, that their loved ones and friends support it, and perhaps that they are part of a group making this change. They will probably need to make the change in small steps, think about it before they try it, and slide back a few times before they are able to maintain the change indefinitely. Most of all, they need to feel that the indirect rewards for making the change (e.g., peer approval, love, merit badges) or its direct benefits (e.g., appearance, energy levels, child health) outweigh the costs.

These needs represent **theoretical constructs**, with technical names that will be provided later. *Constructs* are pieces of a theory that can stand alone, much like atomic elements, but are most effective when used in combination with the other elements (or constructs) of a theory—for example, drinking water versus hydrogen or oxygen. Many of these theories come from the field of psychology and have been used successfully to persuade individuals to adopt healthier lifestyles. The overall framework for bringing these theories into public, or population level health, is social marketing. Social marketing is not a theory but a systematic approach to developing health interventions that have the best chance of being adopted by the intended users. Its processes are integrated into most other health communication or promotion efforts, although many practitioners may be unaware of marketing's place in what they believe to be health education campaigns, for example.

Before discussing social marketing and behavior change theories, we will review framing, first discussed in Chapter 6. There we described the selection and shaping of data for presentation to policymakers as well as for advocacy. Now we focus on framing messages for persuasive communication to change individual behavior.

MESSAGE FRAMING AS A PERSUASIVE COMMUNICATION TECHNIQUE*

Framing a message is giving it a context or even suggesting a point of view or an interpretation with which it is to be understood (also see Framing, Chapter 6). Whether consciously, or unconsciously, even as we speak, we "frame" information to make it more interesting, more palatable, or more frightening for our audience. The frame itself has been demonstrated to have a direct impact on how someone hears, processes, and acts on information. As such, it is an important technique for persuasive health communication, in addition to advocacy and politics.

In Chapter 6 we described "framing bias" in a negative light, as something that can be done to manipulate the reader's perception of the same numbers. For example, if we say that 1 in 20 people "die," many people think the death rate is worse than if we said 19 out of 20 people "survive." In persuasion theory, we can use our natural (though mistaken) tendencies to hear information this way to our benefit through "gain and loss" frames. **Gain-framed** appeals state the advantages of taking an action (e.g., you are 20% more likely to win if you buy four lottery tickets). **Loss-framed** appeals state the disadvantages of not taking an action (e.g., you are 80% more likely to lose if you don't buy four lottery tickets). Some research suggests that gain-framed appeals are more effective for promoting prevention behaviors for health maintenance, such as wearing sunscreen to prevent skin cancer. Loss-framed appeals seem more effective to promote detection behaviors for illness, such as performing breast self-exams to detect lumps.[3] An example of this conclusion comes from Rothman and colleagues[4] in which messages about using mouth rinse were tested among college students. See **Table 8–1**. As predicted by their hypothesis, the gain-framed appeal worked best in the prevention group, and the loss-framed appeal worked best in the detection group.

Other research has been less conclusive. Rothman and colleagues[3] note that one problem is that individuals define the behavior being "framed" differently. For example, some people might think HIV testing is a detection behavior, while others see it as a prevention behavior (i.e., preventing HIV transmission to a partner). Individuals also differ in the level of risk they attribute to performing a particular behavior and risk perception mod-

*Special thanks to Shawnika J. Hull, ABD, PhD, for her help with the discussion on message framing in this chapter. At the time of this writing, Dr. Hull was working on her dissertation at the University of Pennsylvania's Annenberg School for Communication.

TABLE 8–1 Examples of Gain and Loss Frames for Plaque-Fighting Mouth Rinse

	Gain-Frame	Loss-Frame
Prevention behavior (plaque-fighting mouth rinse)	"People who use a mouth rinse daily are taking advantage of a safe and effective way to reduce plaque accumulation."	"People who do not use a mouth rinse daily are failing to take advantage of a safe and effective way to reduce plaque accumulation."
Detection behavior (disclosing—or plaque detecting—mouth rinse)	"Using a disclosing rinse before brushing enhances your ability to detect areas of plaque accumulation."	"Failing to use a disclosing rinse before brushing limits your ability to detect areas of plaque accumulation."

Source: Rothman AJ, Martino SC, Bedell BT, Detweiler JB, Salovey P. The systematic influence of gain- and loss-framed messages on interest in and use of different types of health behavior. *Pers Soc Psychol Bull.* 1999;25(11): 1355–1369., p. 1361.

erates the impact of framed appeals.[5] This issue has generated a lot of controversy and you cannot apply gain and loss framing by a simple formula. Your framing should be tested during the formative research phase with target audiences to determine the most effective frame for a particular audience and behavior.

SOCIAL MARKETING

The concept of **social marketing** was introduced in Chapter 2. One definition, based on an article by Lefebvre and Flora is, "The design, implementation, and control of programs aimed at increasing the acceptability of a social idea, [or] practice [or product] in one or more groups of target adopters. The process actively involves the target population who voluntarily exchange their time and attention for help in meeting their needs as they perceive them."[6] The idea of social marketing is generally attributed to the psychologist, G.D. Wiebe, who is famously quoted as asking, "Can brotherhood be sold like soap?"[7] He suggested that the public would be likely to adopt a socially beneficial idea to the extent its promoters used commercial marketing practices. Later, Kotler and colleagues,[8] including Michael Rothschild,[9] Bill Novelli,[10] and Alan Andreasen,[11] applied marketing principles to a range of social issues and products. They found that as an offering becomes more tangible (i.e., the more it was actually like "soap"), the more the full dimensions of marketing (which include **p**rice, **p**lacement, and **p**roduct attributes) became relevant and concretely defined. In this case, communication is redefined as the fourth P (for **p**romotion) and is used to make consumers aware of a product and its benefits. But when offerings are less tangible—such as "brotherhood," or "reduce, reuse, recycle"—social marketing reduces to behavior change communication. There are numerous social marketing examples, including the "Friends don't let friends drive drunk" campaign, recycling and other green product ventures, and most of the subsidized health products marketed in developing countries (e.g., oral rehydration salts, contraceptives, insecticide-treated bed nets).

Social marketing is not considered a theory itself but there are theories that underpin social marketing. A few of these, such as exchange theory and rational decision making, come from the field of economics while most are derived from social psychology. More so than theory, it is the systematic, consumer data–driven approach of social marketing that has been so widely adopted in many health promotion efforts without ever calling the effort social marketing. Several critical components of social marketing are *market* (or audience) *segmentation*, *targeting*, *barriers* (or obstacles), *benefits*, and *competition*, as well as the *doer versus non-doer* comparative analysis.

Audience Segmentation

Segmentation is dividing something large into smaller pieces, such as an orange broken into slices. While we would like to help everyone who is affected by a particular health problem by providing "everyone" with the same prevention information, a one-size-fits-all approach works no better in public health than it does for clothing. We will be more effective if we can *reach* and speak to a particular group of people who are likely to be *interested* in what we have to say. As mentioned in our discussion of the Elaboration Likelihood Model, we can attract the interest of specific audience members by focusing on a topic in which they have already expressed interest, or by using demographic, cultural, media choice, place-based, or other references which they find meaningful. If we are going to be this precise in our communication, we need to focus our efforts on a fairly small group of people—referred to as our "target market" or "target audience." Thus, **audience segmentation** is a data-based method of identifying smaller target groups of people who share some relevant characteristics.

In an early article Slater,[12] cites Smith[13] as having developed the concept of segmentation for marketing products. Slater summarizes his contribution saying,

> Smith pointed out that marketers typically increased market share by product differentiation—attempting to increase demand by creating a supply of a product unique in some respect. Smith advocated, instead, market segmentation—identifying promising subgroups of consumers, learning what their needs and desires were, and developing products tailored to those subgroups.[12]

Slater goes on to describe nesting segmentation strategies from the broadest base of demographic and geodemographic variables to very specific antecedents of health or risk behaviors. He notes that few programs have the resources to pursue every unique audience segment directly.[12]

Many health communication segmentation strategies are limited by budget. As a result, **partner-based segmentation**—that is, working through intermediary groups who have the desired target audience in their constituency—is commonly used to simplify logistics and reduce cost. For the same reasons, **channel segmentation**, based on personal media preferences, is extremely popular. Since the expansion of the Internet, the potential for channel segmentation has increased dramatically. (In Chapter 10, we will discuss what is now an economic possibility: *message tailoring*, segmentation to an audience of one.)

For maximum impact, most programs use behavioral readiness, or other psychosocial indicators, to create segments. These will be described later in the Change Theories section.

The private sector subscribes to large marketing databases that divide up the U.S. public into very fine segments based on shopping, media choices, census tracts, and other data that are collected (increasingly without our knowledge) every time we use a credit card, place a phone call, or go online, let alone through direct surveys. Some of these, such as the Claritas Prizm system offered by Nielson[14] or Dun & Bradstreet's (D&B's) database of small businesses, are used by federal agencies in their public health communications efforts.

As a result, local health departments can sometimes work through government agencies to access some of these tools for market segmentation and analysis that might otherwise have been prohibitively expensive. It is difficult to predict if these intense consumer marketing database systems will still be relevant in the post-Internet world. Compared to even a decade ago, the internet provides better tools than local radio, direct mail, and phone calls (who likes *those*?!) to reach fine-grained, widely dispersed audience segments and at much lower cost.

Targeting

We have learned that **targeting** means focusing on one small group of people within a larger population that has critical features in common. The name is a bit unfortunate, because it does come from aiming at a target and firing. But, the idea is that if you aim at a bull's-eye on a target, and you come relatively close, it is better than just shooting randomly in the air. The metaphor works for aiming health communication interventions at a specific group of people. The people who are closest to this group will also likely be affected through word of mouth, or because they feel the information is also meant for them. In target marketing overage extends well beyond the specific targeted segment.

Targeting is just a shorthand way of saying that you are using demographic, cultural, or other factors in your communication strategy to reach specific audiences. Until relatively recently, the term *tailoring* was used for this approach. However, we reserve **tailoring** to refer to communications that are directed to an individual based on individually-collected information. These may be mass distributed, but they should still reflect individual interests and do not make the assumption that "birds of a feather flock together," as targeting approaches tend to do. (See Chapter 10 for more on tailoring.)

Benefits, Barriers, and Competition

An absolutely key contribution from marketing to the health communication field is the central position of the consumer's perspective of a product or service. An old advertising slogan coached salesmen to "Sell the sizzle, not the steak." Rarely do you see a hunk of raw meat used to promote a restaurant. Instead, you see meat sputtering over a grill. This strategy is used because a product's **attributes**, which are created by the manufacturer, are not equivalent to the benefits of the product as perceived by the consumer. So toothpaste marketers do not promote the chemical compounds making up their toothpastes' minty flavors, they promote the benefits of fresh breath directly and sex appeal indirectly. Soap, made of some combination of oils, surfactants, and perfume, is marketed as a product makes your skin soft and smooth, makes you smell nice and, yes, gives you more sex appeal.* It is the **benefits** of a product, service, or idea (not the chemical composition) that

---

*The more high tech a product is, the more it tends to actually speak about its attributes directly. The target market is often "nerdy" enough to like this and make consumer decisions on this basis. Automobiles are at the beginning of this list, as well as automotive supplies.

must outweigh the barriers to the product's use, or compete with something else being used in its place. The private sector has learned to ask the consumer about what he or she wants or likes in a product and public health communicators need to do the same.

Most **barriers**, like benefits, are in the mind of the consumer. The economic concept of price elasticity of demand (PED)[15] makes the point that barriers are not universal, nor are they necessarily stable for an individual. Cost is often seen as the most important barrier to acquisition of a product. But in fact, if consumers value a product sufficiently, they will pay just about any price for it. It is a little counterintuitive, but high price elasticity suggests that when the price of a good goes up, consumers buy less of it and when the price goes down, consumers will buy more. Low price elasticity implies that changes in price have little influence on product demand. It is beginning to appear that cigarettes have a relatively low price elasticity, whereas green vegetables and fruit have a higher one. The strategy of increasing tax surcharges on tobacco products did reduce adult smoking, but now seems to have less impact on younger smokers. On the other hand, the principle barriers to consumption of fruits and vegetables seem to be availability and price across many population segments. Many public health practitioners blame the obesity epidemic, in part, on the high price elasticity of fast food—with people consuming much more of it at cheaper prices.

Cost is far from the only barrier affecting an adoption of a health behavior. In many cases, the largest barriers are psychological, including pre-existing attitudes and perceived social norms (see the Integrative Model discussed later). For young people in particular, the idea of what their friends will think, or what they believe their friends are doing, is essential to a behavior change. Health communicators need to find and promote perceived benefits to offset the many perceived barriers to even an obvious health choice.

Finally, **competition** refers to what the intended user is doing now, or using now, instead of the behavior or product being promoted to improve their health. Sometimes this is just using brand X instead of brand Y. But, sometimes competition is using a rock instead of a hammer, our teeth instead of scissors, or sugary soda in place of low fat milk. What we have learned from marketing is that competing products or services may come from completely different domains. We might not be able to imagine that they compete with the healthy idea we are proposing to a target audience. This substitution of products or services from different domains is particularly important when introducing health concepts in developing countries. The habitual or preferential use of supernatural or ineffective natural products in place of contraceptives, vitamins, immu-

nizations, etc. has to be considered respectfully in every health communication strategy.

Doer versus Non-Doer Analysis

How do you find out what consumers need, what products they think are beneficial, or what prevents them from acting? And, how do you group consumers in a meaningful way? The simplest way is you ask those who are already using the desired product or performing the desired behavior about their choice. You also interview individuals who are not using the product, substituting something else for it, or doing nothing instead of the desired behavior. This is a **doer versus non-doer analysis**. This will be discussed more extensively in Chapter 9. You cannot do this kind of research if no one has adopted the healthy behavior. But it is very rare, even in the most unsupportive environment, that a few people have not found a way to live healthy lives on their own. The anthropological concept behind this marketing term is **positive deviance**.[16] An entire international health approach has grown up around identifying healthy individuals (or parents with healthy children) and finding out what they are doing *right*. The health communication strategy is then based on disseminating these healthy, and presumably (but not always) environmentally consistent, culturally appropriate behaviors to the larger population.

The fields of marketing and social marketing are large and their literature extensive.[17] The elements described have been selected because they are essential to health communication planning and cannot be overlooked, whether one is taking part in patient–provider communication, health education, or social mobilization. We will now delve deeper into what motivates individuals and groups to change behavior.

CHANGE THEORIES[18]*

Now we will look at some of the most commonly used behavior change theories in public health communication.† Behavior change theories are concerned with determining the predictors of behavior. These predictors are often made up of psychosocial constructs such as attitudes, beliefs, personal characteristics, and social and environmental factors.

---

*There is nothing that can beat the National Cancer Institute's (NCI's) Theory at a Glance for providing short, clear explanations of behavioral change theories. Most of the material in this section is drawn from this free resource, including all the figures in this section.
†See Edberg M. *Essentials of Health Behavior. Social and Behavioral Theory in Public Health*, Sudbury, MA: Jones & Bartlett; 2007. We will provide only a cursory overview.

Health Belief Model

The **Health Belief Model (HBM)** was one of the first in the field of public health to explain individual health behaviors, particularly individual decisions to participate in public health services such as free tuberculosis screening programs.[19,20] In the HBM, several sets of beliefs either motivate or discourage people to take on certain health behaviors:

- *Perceived susceptibility:* Your sense of personal risk for a health condition.
- *Perceived severity:* Your belief about how serious this condition is.
- *Perceived benefits of interventions:* Your perception of the effectiveness of taking action.

- *Perceived barriers or costs of interventions:* Your perception of the monetary, physical, or psychosocial costs to perform a behavior.
- *Cues to activate behavior change:* Specific messages or indicators that might prompt you to take action.
- *Self-efficacy to perform the behavior:* Your confidence about performing this specific action.

The HBM fell out of favor for a couple of decades, particularly when developing interventions for adolescents and young adults, who generally feel invulnerable to risk. However, the HBM appears to be coming into wide use again, particularly in developing interventions for older Americans. **Box 8–1** provides an example of HBM applied to colorectal cancer screening.[21]

Box 8–1 Example of HBM Applied to Colorectal Cancer Screening

The American Cancer Society[21] recommends that beginning at age 50, both men and women at *average risk* for developing colorectal cancer should use one of several recommended screening tests. The tests that are designed to find both early cancer and polyps are preferred if these tests are available to you and you are willing to have one of these more invasive tests.

Tests that find polyps and cancer
- Flexible sigmoidoscopy every 5 years.[a]
- Colonoscopy every 10 years.
- Double contrast barium enema every 5 years.[a]
- CT colonography (virtual colonoscopy) every 5 years.[a]

Tests that mainly find cancer
- Fecal occult blood test (FOBT) every year.[a,b]
- Fecal immunochemical test (FIT) every year.[a,b]
- Stool DNA test (sDNA), interval uncertain.[a]

Set of hypothetical factors from HBM that may influence a decision to have a colonoscopy to screen for colorectal cancer[c]
- *Perceived susceptibility:* Personal risk for developing cancer; particular concerns about colorectal cancer, or any cancer, based on family history.
- *Perceived severity:* Most people believe that cancer of any kind is very bad. Many people have known those who have died of colorectal cancer.
- *Perceived benefits of interventions:* An important message to stress about the colonoscopy is that polyps will be removed, and the chance of cancer virtually eliminated, if caught at an early stage. Another important benefit is that for someone found to have no polyps, and having no additional risk, the test is performed every 10 years.
- *Perceived barriers or costs of interventions:* Insurance to cover procedure; trusted physician; enema clean-out required; day of work lost; transportation home; fear of procedure [which is, in fact, done under anesthesia (twilight sleep) and painless]; and for many, men in particular, unpleasant perceptions of a rectal procedure.
- *Cues to activate behavior change:* Public messages that emphasize the higher death rate from colorectal cancer among African Americans are used to encourage their participation in colorectal cancer programs. Primary care physicians provide important cues when performing routine care for patients of appropriate age.
- *Self-efficacy to perform the behavior:* Arranging and organizing the appointment is the primary concern for self-efficacy. To overcome this and the obstacles previously listed, some programs use "patient navigators" to discuss what needs to be done and facilitate making an appointment.

[a]Colonoscopy should be done if test results are positive.
[b]For FOBT or FIT used as a screening test, the take-home multiple sample method should be used. A FOBT or FIT done during a digital rectal exam in the doctor's office is not adequate for screening.
[c]Based on ongoing research to promote colorectal cancer screening in African-American populations in Philadelphia. R. Myers, Principal Investigator, Thomas Jefferson University.
Source: American Cancer Society. Guidelines for the Early Detection of Cancer. Webpage. Available at: http://www.cancer.org/docroot/PED/content/PED_2_3X_ACS_Cancer_Detection_Guidelines_36.asp?siterea=PED. Accessed January 10, 2010.

Transtheoretical Model

The awkwardly named **Transtheoretical Model (TTM)**,[22] also known as **Stages of Change (SOC) Model**, indicates that individuals move through a specific process when deciding to change their behavior and then actually changing their behavior. These SOCs are:

- Precontemplation.
- Contemplation.
- Preparation.
- Action.
- Maintenance.

Different individuals may be at different stages along this process and thus must receive differently tailored interventions or communications according to their attitudes. For example, smokers who are in precontemplation have no intention of quitting smoking in the next six months, so information about cessation aids such as nicotine patches will not facilitate their cessation behavior. However, smokers in contemplation do plan to quit smoking in the next six months, and positively reinforcing this goal with enabling information should be more effective at this point. Descriptions of the other stages and appropriate health communication, education, and intervention strategies are listed in **Table 8–2**.[18]

The Precaution Adoption Process Model

The **Precaution Adoption Process Model (PAPM)**[23] looks quite similar to the TTM in that it consists of distinct stages between a lack of awareness and completed preventive action. According to its originators the stages are:

- Unaware of the issue.
- Aware of the issue but not personally engaged.
- Engaged and deciding what to do.
- Planning to act but not yet having acted.
- Deciding not to act.
- Acting.
- Maintenance.

PAPM asserts that these stages represent qualitatively distinct patterns of behavior, beliefs, and experience and that the factors that produce transitions between stages vary depending on the specific transition being considered.[23] The "deciding not to act" stage is unique to the PAPM, which was developed in reference to environmental hazards, hence *precaution adoption* in the name. It has been extensively applied to communicating about testing for radon in homes, installing smoke detectors, and the like. Now PAPM is being used increasingly in cancer screening communication.

Subsequent work[24] that combined the TTM with Social Cognitive Theory (see next section) eliminated the supposition that the TTM represents a smooth transition from one stage to the next, with different stages being influenced through quantity, not quality of message.

Social Cognitive Theory

Social Cognitive Theory (SCT)[25] hypothesizes that individual behavior is the result of constant interaction between the external environment and internal psychosocial characteristics and perceptions. This idea has been dubbed **reciprocal determinism**. There are many constructs included in SCT (**Table 8–3**). Self-efficacy ("I can do it") is one of them and has become an end

TABLE 8–2 Transtheoretical or Stages of Change Model Stages

Stage	Definition	Potential Change Strategies
Precontemplation	Has no intention of taking action within the next six months	Increase awareness of need for change, personalize information about risks and benefits
Contemplation	Intends to take action in the next six months	Motivate; encourage making specific plans
Preparation	Intends to take action within the next thirty days and has taken some behavioral steps in this direction	Assist with developing and implementing concrete action plans; help set gradual goals
Action	Has changed behavior for less than six months	Assist with feedback, problem solving, social support, and reinforcement
Maintenance	Has changed behavior for more than six months	Assist with coping, reminders, finding alternatives, avoiding slips/relapses (as applicable)

Source: National Cancer Institute. *Theory at a Glance, A Guide for Health Promotion Practice*, 2nd ed. NIH Publication No. 05-3896; 2005, p. 15. http://www.cancer.gov/PDF/481f5d53-63df-41bc-bfaf-5aa48ee1da4d/TAAG3.pdf.

TABLE 8–3 Social Cognitive Theory

Concept	Definition	Potential Change Strategies
Reciprocal determinism	The dynamic interaction of the person, behavior, and the environment in which the behavior is performed	Consider multiple ways to promote behavior change, including making adjustments to the environment or influencing personal attitudes
Behavioral capability	Knowledge and skill to perform a given behavior	Promote mastery learning through skills training
Expectations	Anticipated outcomes of a behavior	Model positive outcomes of healthful behavior
Self-efficacy	Confidence in one's ability to take action and overcome barriers	Approach behavior change in small steps to ensure success; be specific about the desired change
Observational learning (modeling)	Behavioral acquisition that occurs by watching the actions and outcomes of others' behavior	Offer credible role models who perform the targeted behavior
Reinforcements	Responses to a person's behavior that increase or decrease the likelihood of reoccurrence	Promote self-initiated rewards and incentives

Source: National Cancer Institute. *Theory at a Glance, A Guide for Health Promotion Practice,* 2nd ed. NIH Publication No. 05-3896; 2005, p. 20. http://www.cancer.gov/PDF/481f5d53-63df-41bc-bfaf-5aa48ee1da4d/TAAG3.pdf.

in itself for many behavior change interventions (e.g., teens avoiding high-risk behaviors or women negotiating condom use with their partners). **Vicarious (observational) learning** is another well-recognized construct in the SCT model, often used to teach people incremental behavior skills through role modeling.

Integrative Model

The **Integrative model (IM)**[26] represents an evolved version of Martin Fishbein's* *Theory of Reasoned Action (TRA).*[27] Ajzen developed the *Theory of Planned Behavior (TPB)*[28] as an extension of the TRA. Fishbein and Ajzen worked together to develop the IM, which they also referred to as the *Reasoned Action Approach.*[26] See **Figure 8–1** for an illustration of the IM.

The most important assumption of the IM is that the best predictor of behavior is the *intention* to perform the behavior. This model focuses on the antecedents (predictors) of an individual's intention to perform (or not perform) a behavior. The IM focuses on the following beliefs:

- **Behavioral beliefs** are expectancies about positive or negative outcomes related to performing the behavior. These lead to formation of **attitudes**.
- **Normative beliefs** are perceptions about what relevant others think about performing the behavior, or beliefs about what others are doing. Together, these beliefs determine a concept of *perceived normative pressure* related to the behavior.

- **Control beliefs** relate to whether or not there are barriers or facilitators to performing the behavior. These are directly associated with an individual's *perceived behavioral control,* or *self-efficacy,* when performing the behavior.

The IM also takes into account various background factors, which influence the constructs in the model differently. These background factors include race, gender, personality, education, income, past behavior, etc. Factors such as media exposure can also be included. This is where health communication messages fit in.

These components of the intervention work together. When performing research subject screening interviews, or initial surveys of the intended audience:

- Determine which of the direct antecedents of intention (attitude, perceived norms, self-efficacy) best predict intention.
- Elicit the beliefs underlying the attitudes, norms, and self-efficacy.
- Design your health communication message or messages to influence these antecedent beliefs.

Of course, if, during subject screening and surveys, you determine that your audience already intends to perform the behavior, you need not go through all the steps of the IM. In this case, it is not likely that their beliefs, attitudes, or self-efficacy are preventing them from adopting healthy behaviors. Instead, environmental factors, skills, or knowledge (factors that take *actual control* over the behavior) are likely precluding their behavior change. If environmental barriers exist, for example,

---

*This textbook includes a dedication to Dr. Fishbein, who passed away in 2009.

FIGURE 8-1 The Integrative Model

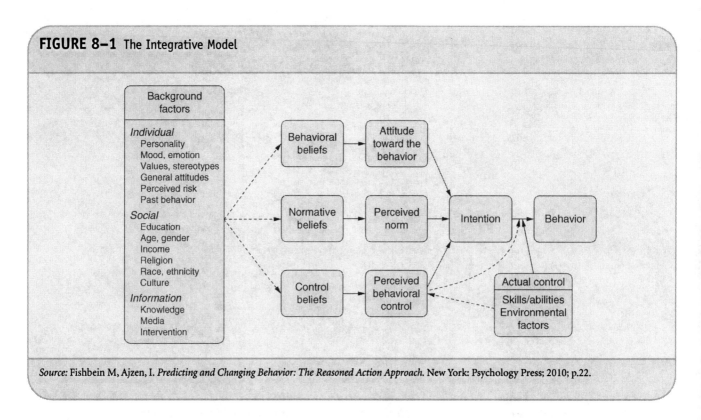

Source: Fishbein M, Ajzen, I. *Predicting and Changing Behavior: The Reasoned Action Approach.* New York: Psychology Press; 2010; p.22.

rather than designing your communication campaign to change intentions in a population, you might need to focus the campaign on changing policies (see Chapter 6) that affect the population's opportunities to perform the behavior.*

Diffusion of Innovations

All the preceding theories focus on individual behavior; **Diffusion of Innovations (DI)**[29] addresses change in a group. This can be a classroom, organization, or community. The theory describes how new ideas, or innovations, are spread within and among people, organizations, or communities. According to DI, innovations spread via different communication channels within social systems over a specific period of time. Health communicators should focus on specific aspects of an innovation, such as the *relative advantage, compatibility, complexity, trialability*, and *observability* of the innovation. The innovation should seem better than "the leading brand," be compatible with its specified audience, and be easy to adopt. People should also be able to "try it out" before committing to it, and the changes should be obvious enough for measurement.

Successful diffusion often relies on media communication as well as interpersonal communication and social net-

working. Messages should be targeted to the audience because some audiences are likely to adopt the innovation early, while other audiences will do so late. Still other audiences will *be* the innovators who diffuse the behavior change and will be receptive to very different kinds of message.

Malcolm Gladwell's popular book, *The Tipping Point*,[30] extends diffusion theory with the suggestion that the "innovators" in Rogers's terminology are indeed trendsetters who can create so much buzz around a new idea that it spreads very rapidly throughout a population. As discussed in Chapter 9, the strategy of targeting innovators is now being used for marketing segmentation. This is similar to the more traditional targeting of what Rogers called "early adopters" to lead the majority into adopting a behavior.

CONCLUSION

This chapter describes the theories used most often to predict persuasion and guide behavior change communication. There are two important take-away messages: (1) health interventions should be grounded in applicable change theories and audiences and (2) behaviors should be addressed systematically according to health marketing, targeting, and tailoring principles. In Chapter 9 we will discuss formative research that builds upon our theoretical understanding of health behavior. Chapter 10 shows how to apply these theories in communication practice strategies.

---

*This summary of the IM is based on the latest book by Fishbein and Ajzen, published in 2010. We are very fortunate to have received feedback from Dr. Fishbein about this summary in the fall of 2009.

KEY TERMS

Attitudes

Attributes

Audience segmentation

Barriers

Behavioral beliefs

Benefits

Channel segmentation

Competition

Control beliefs

Diffusion of Innovations

Doer versus non-doer analysis

Framing

Gain Framing

Health Belief Model (HBM)

Integrative Model (IM)

Loss Framing

Normative beliefs

Partner-based segmentation

Peripheral cues

Persuasion Theory

Positive deviance

Precaution Adoption Process Model (PAPM)

Reciprocal determinism

Segmentation

Self-efficacy

Social Cognitive Theory (SCT)

Social marketing

Stages of Change (SOC)

Tailoring

Targeting

Theoretical construct

Transtheoretical Model (TTM)

Vicarious (observational) learning

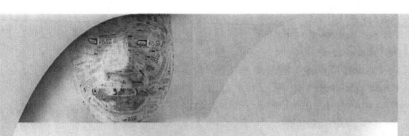

Chapter Questions

1. Describe different forms of segmentation. When would you choose various strategies?

2. What is the difference between targeting and tailoring?

3. List the four Ps of health marketing. How would you use these to describe a behavior to improve child nutrition in Bangladesh?

4. How is the Integrative Model different from Social Cognitive Theory or the Transtheoretical Model?

5. Pick a health behavior that is either a prevention or detection behavior, and develop either loss- or gain-framed messages to persuade people to adopt this behavior.

REFERENCES

1. Ed Maibach, Personal communication.

2. Rothschild ML. Carrots, sticks and promises: A conceptual framework for the behavior management of public health and social issues. *J Marketing.* 1999;63:24–37.

3. Rothman AJ, Bartels RD, Wlaschin J, Salovey P. The strategic use of gain- and loss-framed messages to promote healthy behavior: How theory can inform practice. *J Comm.* 2006;56:S202–S221.

4. Rothman AJ, Martino SC, Bedell BT, Detweiler JB, Salovey P. The systematic influence of gain- and loss-framed messages on interest in and use of different types of health behavior. *Pers Soc Psychol Bull.* 1999;25(11): 1355–1369.

5. Apanovitch AM, McCarthy D, Salovey P. Using message framing to motivate HIV testing among low-income, ethnic minority women. *Health Psych.* 2003;22:60–67.

6. Lefebvre, RC, Flora JA. Social marketing and public health intervention. *Health Educ Quart.* 1988;15,299–315.

7. Weibe GD. Merchandising commodities and citizenship on television. *Pub Opin Quart.* 1951;15(4):679.

8. Kotler P, Zaltman G. Social marketing: An approach to planned social change. *J Marketing.* 1971;35:3–12.

9. Rothschild ML. Marketing communication in nonbusiness situations or why it's so hard to sell brotherhood like soap. *J Marketing.* 1979;43:1–20.

10. Bloom PN, Novelli WD. Problems and challenges in social marketing. *J Marketing.* 1981;45:79–88.

11. Andreasen AR. *Marketing Social Change: Changing Behavior to Promote Health, Social Development and the Environment.* San Francisco: Jossey-Bass; 1995.

12. Slater MD. Theory and method in health audience segmentation. *J Health Comm.* 1996;1:267–283.

13. Smith WR. Product differentiation and market segmentation as alternative marketing strategies. In CG Walters & DP Robin (Eds.), *Classics in Marketing.* Santa Monica, CA: Goodyear; 1956:433–439.

14. Nielson. Prizm. http://www.claritas.com/target-marketing/market-research-services/marketing-data/marketing-segmentation/prizm.jsp. Accessed January 21, 2010.

15. Case KE, Fair RC. *Principles of Economics,* 5th ed. Upper Saddle River, NJ. Prentice-Hall; 1999.

16. PD Hearth website. http://www.positivedeviance.org/about_pdi/index.html.

17. Siegel M, Lotenberg LD. *Marketing Public Health. Strategies to Promote Social Change,* 2nd ed. Sudbury, MA: Jones & Bartlett; 2007.

18. National Cancer Institute. *Theory at a Glance, A Guide for Health Promotion Practice,* 2nd ed. NIH Publication No. 05-3896; 2005. Published online at: http://www.cancer.gov/PDF/481f5d53-63df-41bc-bfaf-5aa48ee1da4d/TAAG3.pdf.

19. Hochbaum BM. *Public Participation in Medical Screening Programs: A Socio-Psychological Study.* Washington, DC: U.S. Department of Health Education, and Welfare; 1958.

20. Rosenstock IM. Historical Origins of the Health Belief Model. *Health Education Monographs.* 1974;2:328–335.

21. American Cancer Society. Guidelines for the Early Detection of Cancer. Webpage. Available at: http://www.cancer.org/docroot/PED/content/PED_2_3X_ACS_Cancer_Detection_Guidelines_36.asp?siterea=PED. Accessed January 10, 2010.

22. Prochaska JO, DiClemente CC. Stages and processes of self-change of smoking: Toward an integrative model of change. *J Consult and Clinical Psych.* 1983;51(3):390–395.

23. Weinstein ND, Sandman PM. A model of the Precaution Adoption Process: Evidence from home radon testing. *Health Psych.* 1992;11(3):170–180.

24. Maibach EW, Cotton D. Chapter 3. Moving people to behavior change. A staged social cognitive approach to message design. In EW Maibach & EL Parrot (Eds.), *Designing Health Messages. Approaches from Communication Theory and Public Health Practice.* Thousand Oaks, CA: Sage Publications; 1995:41–64.

25. Bandura A. *Social Foundations of Thought and Action: A Social Cognitive Theory.* Englewood Cliffs, NJ: Prentice-Hall; 1986.

26. Ajzen I., Albarracin D, Hornik R. *Prediction and Change of Health Behavior: The Reasoned Action Approach.* Mawah, NJ: Lawrence Erlbaum Associates; 2007.

27. Fishbein M, Ajzen I. *Belief, Attitude, Intention, and Behavior: An Introduction to Theory and Research.* Reading, MA: Addison-Wesley, 1975.

28. Ajzen I. The Theory of Planned Behavior. *Organizational Behavior and Human Decision Processes.* 1991;50:179–211.

29. Rogers EM. *Diffusion of Innovations,* 4th ed. New York, NY: Free Press; 1995.

30. Gladwell M. *The Tipping Point. How Little Things Can Make a Big Difference.* New York: Time Warner Book Group; 2002.

CHAPTER 9

Formative Research for Strategy Development

Claudia Parvanta

LEARNING OBJECTIVES

By the end of this chapter, the reader will be able to:

- Describe what is meant by formative research.
- Explain when and why quantitative and qualitative methods are combined.
- Apply the behave framework to a formative research project.
- Analyze audiences, behaviors, benefits, costs, and motivating factors.
- Use social marketing to organize audience research.
- Design simple studies using each of the research tools presented.
- Describe high-tech formative research methods.

INTRODUCTION

This chapter presents a systematic approach to doing formative research and interpreting the results. Chapter 10 reviews how you use this information to develop and test materials and select media channels. In addition, we will discuss a **participatory approach** to message strategy development. Conceptual themes are generated through preliminary research, shared with members of the target audience or key intermediaries (such as community health workers), and used develop short skits or role-plays. There are many advantages to this approach, particularly when working in a cross-cultural setting.

Definition of Formative Research

Formative research refers to the information-gathering activities you conduct prior to developing a health communication strategy. Representatives of the target audience must guide concepts, messages, and materials as well as choice of media

channels to give your intervention the best chance of success. Formative research is done to *develop* an intervention. You may use both quantitative and qualitative methods to accomplish this goal.

Quantitative and Qualitative Methods

If you want to know how many people have a particular attribute or behavior you will need *quantitative* epidemiological data or behavioral survey results. This involves classifying and counting. For example, how many school children are obese? How many obese children say they hate sports and gym class.* As described in previous chapters, **quantitative research** is largely used to identify problems and precursors prior to intervention and to evaluate the impact of a communication intervention.

Qualitative research, on the other hand, provides the back story for the quantitative data and may point to the need for more quantitative studies. For example, by asking many individual or small groups of children why they hate exercising, you might learn that they feel ashamed of their bodies and are made fun of in school. They would exercise more if they could do it with other children who share their body shape, in a socially and environmentally safe environment. So do all obese children feel this way? That would require another quantitative survey, and you would most likely learn that a sufficient number feel that way, perhaps 60%, to justify a communication campaign focused on creating a safe social environment for overweight children to play.

---

*Hypothetical example.

Qualitative and quantitative research can be done independently, but more often are interwoven. For example, from quantitative data, we learn of issues that need to be probed further in qualitative research. Or, as in the example, qualitative research suggests behavior change hypotheses that need to be tested in a larger sample before devoting resources to a wide-scale campaign. The combination of quantitative and qualitative research is referred to as a **mixed-methods approach.**

Although **baseline evaluation** and formative research are both implemented in an early phase of an intervention, and may even be conducted simultaneously, they differ in magnitude and goals. Evaluation designs typically analyze a large number of samples and carefully control for confounding factors in order to detect a significant intervention effect (see Chapter 14). Formative research, on the other hand usually collects in-depth information from smaller groups of people with a view toward improving the design strategy for a planned intervention.

Sometimes it is efficient to mix these two methods. For example, if your **informed consent*** protocol allows for it, you may ask persons during an in-person or telephone survey if you may contact them again for a follow-up in-depth interview or focus group. (If this survey is part of your evaluation design, you will need to exclude these individuals from the data pool due to their additional contact with the researchers.)

Next we describe a widely used framework for behavioral change interventions, developed by the Academy for Educational Development (AED) with a core group of nongovernmental organizations (NGOs) working in developing countries.

WHAT DO YOU NEED TO RESEARCH: THE BEHAVE FRAMEWORK

The **BEHAVE framework**[1] provides four deceptively simple questions to be answered:

- Who are you trying to reach?
- What do you want them to do?
- What factors influence their behavior?
- Which actions will most effectively address these factors?

BEHAVE presents these questions in the form of a statement:

In order to help (*a specific target audience*) to (*perform a specific behavior*) we will focus on this

benefit (*something the target audience values*). We will approach this through these factors: (e.g., *self-efficacy, lowered barriers, enhanced health literacy, etc.*), and use these activities (means of reaching the audience: *media channels or other contact opportunities*).

If you cannot fill in these gaps, then you have to do formative research. You might be able to lay the groundwork with published literature and/or unpublished research reports from reliable sources, such as government agencies. But most likely you will need to conduct qualitative research with the target audience on location in order to collect the specific information you need to create a communication strategy.

Let's see what is required for each question.

Specific Audiences

Primary Audience

You start with a **beneficiary** in mind, the group of people most affected by the health problem. In some cases, this group is also the **primary audience,** defined as the group of people whose behavior you hope to influence through a communication intervention. Sometimes the beneficiaries—for example, infants and young children or persons with a mental disability—are incapable of acting for themselves. In that case, the primary audience is made up of those whose actions directly affect the health outcome. In this example, caregivers (mothers and others) are the primary audience whose behavioral change is sought to benefit the child or the person with the mental disability.

Your research should determine if there are subgroups in the primary audience who would benefit from specific forms of communication. This segmentation might be based on demographic variables such as age, sex, or number of children; geographic location; ethnic identity; or experience with a particular illness or disability. Other variables such as educational level or literacy abilities, language use, and media preferences might be used to identify subgroups in terms of how and where they can be reached through particular media channels. And finally, and perhaps most importantly, the relationship of the primary audience to the behavior in question provides very precise segments. These behavioral segments include current practice; readiness to adopt a new behavior; and other theoretically defined constructs such as needs for self-efficacy, perception of role models, types of rewards sought, or barriers blocking the way.

Secondary Audience

Your research might have uncovered the need to work with a **secondary audience** (or even *tertiary* audience) in order to reach or influence the primary audience. These people can be

---

*Research studies involving human subjects are examined and approved by an institutional review board (IRB) constituted for this purpose. IRB approval is based on a number of elements, all designed to protect human subjects from any type of abuse. A central issue during IRB review is evaluation of informed consent, i.e., are the participants full informed about the study and its risks, and are they capable of giving consent based on this information.

seen as allies to support a behavioral change, or they might need to be convinced to change their opinions, or even actions, before the primary audience will be free to act on its own. Very often, healthcare professionals act as effective **gatekeepers** in a community. They can help support a behavior change goal if they agree with it or prevent its adoption if they disagree. For this reason, it is often critical to use the advocacy approaches described earlier in this book before going forward with behavior change communications. Again, this secondary group can be further segmented according to demographics, attitudes, theory-based constructs, or need for training or educational outreach.

Behavior to Change

At the outset of our plan, we have an *ideal* behavior in mind. If we could convince the target audience to practice this behavior, we believe that the health problem would be greatly reduced. Let's take hand washing, for example, as shown in **Box 9–1**.

Box 9–1 Hand-Washing Exercise

This exercise demonstrates what might be involved in carrying out an ideal behavior in terms of time, supplies, and attitudes. Conduct yourself in a normal fashion in carrying out the requested steps.

Step 1: State Your Current Behavior

A. Frequency. Approximately how many times a day do you wash your hands?

[Write number down] _____

B. Steps. Go into a washroom and wash your hands. Keep track of everything you need to perform the behavior as well as the steps you take. Keep track of how long you spend doing this.

1. Resources needed to wash hands:

2. My hand-washing steps:
   (Your list might include the following: adjustment of clothing, removal of watch or ring, turn on tap, wetting hands, get soap, rubbing hands with soap and water, rinse, getting towel, etc.)

3. How long did I spend washing my hands? _____ seconds/minutes

Step 2: Identify Ideal Behavior

A. Frequency of behavior. Write down the number of times you do the following (approximately). You need to wash your hands:

Activity	Number of times a day
Prepare or help with meals	
Before and after eating	
After urinating or defecating	
After sneezing or coughing	
After touching or handling objects such as money, doorknobs, or anything with visible dirt	

Total number of times you would ideally wash your hands: _____

How does your current behavior compare with the ideal in terms of frequency?

B. Behavioral Steps

On the following page is a diagram from the Illinois Department of Health on how to wash your hands correctly to prevent spread of infectious diseases.

continues

PROPER HANDWASHING
ILLINOIS DEPARTMENT OF PUBLIC HEALTH

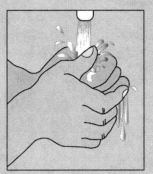

1. Wet hands with soap and warm water.

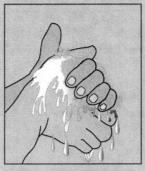

2. Rub hands for 20 seconds. Get under fingernails and between fingers.

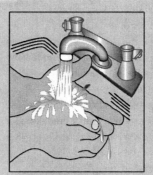

3. Rinse under warm running water.

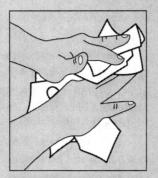

4. Dry hands on your own clean towel.

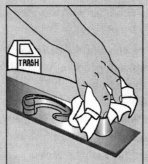

5. Turn off water with paper towel. Throw towel away.

Compare your own behavior to the ideal behavior. How is it different?

How much time would you need every day to wash your hands correctly? Do you always have access to water, soap, and disposable towels? What else can you do to properly clean your hands? Compare the responses of the women in the class to the men. Any differences? How would you formulate a behavioral objective based on this exercise?

Source: State of Illinois, Department of Public Health.

Over decades of social marketing, we have learned that "simple" behaviors, such as washing your hands, are comprised of several small steps and require multiple resources to complete. Any one of these steps (or resources) can be a limiting factor if people cannot perform the behavior without it. Inversely, once the limiting step is taken (or resource acquired) the remaining steps may follow in sequence without further input. We like to think of this step as a **behavioral lever**. Health promoters need to know exactly which steps of a behavior they are trying to change, and what factors can be used to predispose, enable, or reinforce that step.

Identifying a Behavioral Lever

Through observations and questions we determine what members of the primary audience are doing and create a start-to-finish sequence for the behavior to be changed. To show how this can work we introduce a new example, a development project to improve the nutritional status of children in rural Bangladesh by feeding them vegetables. In Bangladesh, similar to many other traditional countries, the men go to the public market to purchase items while the women remain within the home compound. **Table 9–1** shows the behavioral steps we observed that were necessary to achieve the desired outcome of feeding a child vegetables.

TABLE 9–1 Sequence of Steps to Feed Cooked Pumpkin to a Child

1. Woman sees pumpkins in market.
2. She thinks about cooking pumpkin.
3. She inventories other ingredients at home (oil, spices, possibly tomato sauce).
4. She asks husband to buy pumpkin, extra ingredients.
5. Husband brings pumpkin, extra ingredients home from market.
6. Woman cuts and cleans pumpkin.
7. She prepares cooking fire.
8. She cooks pumpkin according to her liking, with less spice.
9. She takes a portion of family pumpkin and sets aside for children.
10. She adds spice to remaining family portion.
11. She mashes child's portion.
12. She feeds mashed pumpkin to child.
13. She believes this was a good thing to do based on child eating pumpkin and not getting sick later.

From this example, the starting point of the behavioral sequence is that once thinking pumpkin is good for her child, and knowing the pumpkin is available, a woman *asks* her husband to purchase the vegetable in the market. So, if health communicators want more women to cook vegetables for their children in this setting, they need to begin by prompting more women to ask their husbands to bring something home.

Is this level of analysis going to be worth the effort? That takes us to the next level of behavioral analysis.

Behavioral Analysis Scale

AED also developed a **behavioral analysis scale**[2] that has been used extensively in international health communication programs. It appears in **Table 9–2**.

The scale includes the health impact of the behavior, its ease and costs of performance, and other factors that influence adoption. Any behavior can be rated using this scale. The score may help determine the advisability of a behavioral intervention. It is important that formative research provides sufficient information to complete a behavior analysis scale for the intended behavior change. **Box 9–2** shows our rating of the Bangladeshi example presented earlier.

Focus the Behavioral Objective through Stages of Change (or TTM)

You have selected what seems like an approachable and important behavior. How ready is your target audience to adopt it? As discussed in Chapter 8, Stages of Change (SOC) includes five distinct stages: precontemplation, contemplation, preparation, action, and maintenance. People at different points in

the process of change can benefit from different interventions, matched to their stage at that time. One important goal of your research is to map these theoretical terms onto everyday descriptions of behavior. The Bangladesh example continues in **Table 9–3**.

A specific message or media piece might be designed to encourage and facilitate individual change from one stage of behavior to the next. The reason for this specificity is that different stimuli motivate people to move from one stage to the next. For example, information alone might prompt movement from precontemplation to contemplation, but **observational learning** (seeing another perform the behavior with positive outcomes) or seeing a complex task broken down into simpler steps might be necessary to motivate trial. These stimuli are culturally determined. But, in general, the goal is to increase the number of positive feelings a person has toward a behavior and reduce the number of objections. Refer back to Table 8–2 for facilitators of change as you move through the stages.

Group Behavior Change

What if you are trying to change the behavior of a group? You have data that indicate that a few people practice the behavior regularly; some are starting to do it; and there is a big hump in the middle of people who have heard about it, but not tried yet it. Again, there's a tail at the end of people who haven't heard about it yet at all. You decide you want to focus on this **modal behavior** (the big hump in a distribution curve) and attempt to move these people up one step to preparation or trial. This group based behavioral staging relies on the Diffusion of Innovations theory[3]. Moving the majority might involve a trick,

TABLE 9–2 AED Behavior Analysis Scale

CATEGORY	CATEGORY
Health Impact of the Behavior	**Complexity of the Behavior (Ease/Difficulty)**
1. No impact on health problem	1. Unrealistically complex (difficult)
2. Little impact	2. Involves a great many elements
3. Some impact	3. Involves many elements
4. Significant impact	4. Involves several elements
5. Very significant impact	5. Involves few elements
6. Eliminates the health problem	6. Involves one element
Positive Consequences (Effects) of the Behavior	**Frequency of Behavior (Ease/Difficulty)**
1. None that mother could perceive	1. Must be done at unrealistically high rate to achieve any benefit
2. New perceptible consequences	2. Must be done hourly
3. Some consequences	3. Must be done several times each day
4. Significant consequences	4. Must be done daily
5. Very significant consequences	5. May be done every few hours
6. Major perceptible consequences	6. May be done occasionally and still have significant value
Cost of Engaging in (Performing) the Behavior	**Persistence (Duration)**
1. Requires unavailable resources or demands unrealistic effort	1. Requires compliance over an unrealistically long period of time
2. Requires very significant resources or effort	2. Requires compliance over a substantial period of time
3. Requires significant resources or effort	3. Requires compliance for a week or more
4. Requires some resources or effort	4. Requires compliance for several days
5. Requires few resources or little effort	5. Requires compliance for a day
6. Requires only existing resources	6. Can be accomplished in a brief time
Compatibility with Existing Practices	**Observability**
1. Totally incompatible	1. Cannot be observed by any outsider
2. Very significant compatibility	2. Is very difficult to observe
3. Significant incompatibility	3. Is difficult to observe
4. Some incompatibility	4. Is observable
5. Little incompatibility	5. Is readily observable
6. Already widely practiced	6. Cannot be missed
Similarity to Present Behaviors	
1. Nothing like this is done now	
2. An existing practice is slightly similar	
3. An existing practice is somewhat similar	
4. An existing practice is similar	
5. Several existing practices are similar	
6. Several existing practices are very similar	

Source: AED Tool Box, Question 15-3. USAID. http://www.globalhealthcommunication.org/tool_docs/29/a_tool_box_for_building_health_communication_capacity_-_question_15.pdf

explained below. Diffusion of Innovations describes how new ideas, products, or practices spread within a group. Innovations that are easy to use and understand, that can be tried without commitment, and that have visible results will diffuse more quickly than difficult changes requiring an outlay of money or time, and that have results that are slow to see. Rogers suggested that populations adopt innovations according to a bell-shaped curve, with about 5% to 10% being the vanguard, and 5% to 10% "lagging" way behind. Social marketing efforts often target new products to what Rogers described as **early adopters**

Box 9–2 Application of Behavioral Analysis Scale to Bangladesh Example

"Woman asks her husband to bring pumpkin home for her to cook for her children."

Scores run from lowest (1) to highest (6).

Health impact	4
Positive consequences	4
Compatibility	3
Frequency	6
Persistence	6
Costs	4
Similarity	5
Complexity	3

Average score: 4.4

It is recommended that we promote this behavior based on this analysis. From start to finish the process is somewhat complex and the people are not in the habit of cooking pumpkin daily or even weekly. However, even if pumpkin is cooked only once every two weeks and is included in the child's diet only three to five times every two weeks, it will have a very significant health impact.

(the second 20%), and great effort is spent trying to determine the psychographic makeup (personality, values, attitudes, interests, lifestyles) of this group.

Your formative research can both determine a diffusion spectrum for a group and describe the characteristics of each segment. The "doers" (see later) are ahead of an adoption curve, while the non-doers are everyone else, beginning with the majority in the middle. Your goal might be to target the early adopters of other, even completely unrelated, behaviors to get them to perform the new behavior (e.g., getting people who use fluoride toothpaste to try using sunscreen, or people who built latrines for their homes in Bangladesh to try feeding vegetables to their children). Your first goal is not to move the majority, but rather to move the innovators, the "doers," a much

TABLE 9–3 Bangladesh Example of Stages of Change for Target Behavior

Behavioral goal: Mothers will feed mashed cooked pumpkin (or a more preferred orange vegetable) to children 6 to 12 months of age at least once every other week while pumpkin is in season.

Precontemplation: Were aware of the positive effects of cooked vegetables, and that cooked pumpkin was being eaten by children in this age group with no ill effects.

Contemplation: Had thought about cooking/feeding pumpkin for their own 6- to 12-month-old child.

Ready-to-act: Expressed a commitment to cooking pumpkin for their child at their next opportunity, and knew how they would go about it.

Action: Cooked and fed pumpkin to their child at least once.

Maintenance: Cooked and fed pumpkin (or other seasonal orange vegetable) every other week for the past few months, and intended doing so indefinitely.

smaller audience. If you can get them to adopt the behavior, according to diffusion theory, there is a very strong chance that others will follow their lead. Hence, the trick mentioned earlier is that to move about 50% of the population forward, you might target your (paid) communication efforts on the leading 10% to 20%, relying on word of mouth, buzz, and other ways that information moves around a society to carry the rest. Gladwell described this process as **thought-leader** ("maven-based") **promotion**.[4] Some marketing database companies have commercialized segment analysis using this strategy.*

Identifying Benefits (and Barriers)

People perform a behavior when it *benefits* them. *Barriers* (or perceived costs) keep them from acting. You must identify a benefit that is really important, or several benefits combined, that can offset the barriers [one or several] to tilt the "scales" toward adoption of the behavior. The benefit is often implicit—that is, not actually perceived by the primary audience. How do you learn about what your intended audience perceives to be barriers and benefits?

Doer and Non-Doer Research

One way is to seek out the people who already perform a desirable behavior, the "doers," is described in Chapter 8. To conduct this kind of research, you can identify people using a Stages of Change (SOC) assessment. People who are maintaining or have tried and repeated the behavior would be the positives (doers) for the focus behavior.

You also want to interview people who have *contemplated* the behavior but not performed it. (You want to weed out simple lack of information as a reason for avoiding the behavior, because that is easily corrected.) How could comparing the doers and non-doers help you know what *really* influences the behavior? Can you determine the most important barriers to the non-doers and the benefits that have motivated the doers? You will next develop concepts based on these ideas. Put in a more positive light, your goal is to learn from doers what makes their behavior more fun, easy, and popular than not performing the behavior.[5] If we are talking about a soft drink or a videogame, a bunch of teenagers could probably tell us the features. But when working with a culture unlike our own, or when attempting to promote a behavior that seems the opposite of fun, easy, and popular—such as colon cancer screening—we need to use these terms as metaphors and work with Social Cognitive Theory (SCT) or the Integrative Model (IM).

Self-Efficacy

A seminal construct in both SCT and the IM is self-efficacy. Simply put, **self-efficacy** is an individual's belief that he or she can adopt a new behavior, such as quitting smoking. Self-efficacy is constructed from knowledge and skills (behavioral capability), expectations of what the outcome of performing the behavior will be, the value placed on getting these results (expectancies), and the reinforcement given to the individual to perform the behavior. The individual may directly build self-efficacy for a complex behavior by mastering a series of simpler steps or by observing others experience the behaviors and outcomes. This last concept, observational learning, also referred to as *modeling*, is the lynch pin for applying SCT to communications interventions. People can learn, rehearse, and gain mastery of behavior by watching role models, usually within a dramatic context, work through behavior change, and evaluate for themselves whether the modeled behaviors are desirable or not. Your formative research can be used to identify all of the elements comprising SCT constructs, including information for role models, role model stories, etc.

Communication Intervention

Where and when are the best ways to communicate with your intended audience? This is a question of space and time and takes into consideration the kind of media you think will also accomplish your purpose.

Settings

Settings include places where either the audience will need to go to make contact with your communication (e.g., a healthcare facility, shopping mall, bar or restaurant in town, a special event), or places where the media can be brought to them (such as radio or television programs, online environments, etc.). The time aspect is very important because a place that seems like a good setting for your audience might be impractical if they will not be attentive to your message or be unable to use the information they receive in a timely manner. Most people cannot remember phone numbers or other information given out during drive-time radio shows or on the back of busses, for example. The credibility of the setting to the audience is also important. For example, it has been popular to disseminate STD prevention information in the bathrooms of bars and restaurants. Younger people (who are the intended audience) find this setting more credible than warnings of their parents at home, for example.

Channels

It is easy to confuse *settings* with **channels**. Think of your home as a setting. There are many media channels that can come into your home, such as television, the Internet, direct mail,

---

*http://www.smrb.com/web/guest/core-solutions/tipping-point-segments

radio, etc. These are channels. But these channels can also be received in other settings, like the public library. How you react to the same message conveyed by the same channel might vary if you see it in the privacy of your home, or in a public setting like a library. The National Cancer Institute (NCI) describes several different channels, as noted in the following sections.[6]

Interpersonal Channels and Groups Interpersonal channels include healthcare providers, clergy, teachers, and others who will interact with the intended recipient in person. The strength of interpersonal channels is that people tend to trust the spokesperson and will possibly be ready to listen to what they say. Face-to-face channels are most effective when trying to help someone learn a skill; they need to trust the spokesperson in order to adopt a new attitude or belief. On the other hand, two-way discussion is necessary to cement a behavioral intention. Interpersonal approaches can be used with groups, particularly if discussion among group members is part of the communication strategy. To ensure the quality of health communication using interpersonal channels, it often is necessary to develop training and media supports. The major limitation of this channel is its reach.

Organizational or Community Channels Similar to other group communication channels, there is more formality and structure when dealing with business organizations, voluntary agencies, or religious groups. They can be a very effective partner for disseminating advocacy messages or health communica-

tion that is not too detailed. Bringing health communication into a trusted setting also reinforces the credibility of the message and lends a sense of community norms to the suggested behavior. Normally you would develop a whole "kit" to support working with partners such as businesses or other community groups to keep messages focused and align the timing of dissemination to coincide with mass media, if used.

Mass Media Media that reach large populations, either individually or in huge markets, have become even more diverse in recent years. Because there is so much to cover about this topic, Chapter 11 is devoted to new and traditional media choices to carry different forms of health communication. Mass media are known to be effective in raising awareness and knowledge, prompting health information seeking, and changing attitudes. When entertainment approaches are used (see Chapter 10), health communicators are often able to achieve vicarious learning, outcome expectancy, and self-efficacy through thoughtful use of role models demonstrating good behaviors and rewards or bad behaviors and negative consequences.

You will want to make sure your research provides the information for you to be able to select appropriate settings, channels, and media (**Table 9–4**).

Using Social Marketing to Organize Your Formative Research

If you are using a social marketing approach to develop a communication intervention, you will need all the information

---

TABLE 9–4 Criteria for Selecting a Communication Channel

Examples of channels: radio programs, TV shows, Internet websites, social media sites, print (mass media or micro media), outdoor advertising (billboards, buses), viral or buzz channels, intermediary distribution (e.g., doctor's office video, print materials).

- Which channels the target audience uses and can easily access.
- Which channels they say they like.
- Which channels are more effective for communicating audio or visual messages.

For any channel, ask the following:

- Is it a credible source of information or motivation for the target audience?
- Does the format lend itself to the content of the message?
- Can it provide the reach (coverage of the population) that you need?
- Will messages be seen or heard frequently enough to achieve your communication goals?
- Does it allow treatment of a subject in depth, or provide a "big idea" and "wow" factor?
- Do gatekeepers and other community leaders monitor the channel or provide direct or indirect oversight?

Logistical and budget considerations will be treated in depth in Chapter 13. Some media are much more costly to produce, while others cost more to air or disseminate. The calculus comes down to costs per view, client reached, or product sold.

described earlier and more. For example, in addition to benefits and barriers, you would think about how the costs of the behavior need to be offset by the benefits, how location (or place) influences behavior, in addition to promotional strategy. You will need to gather information to develop a new product, or present a behavior, so that its positioning is favorable to your target audience. You must be sure it has the right benefits, the price is right, it is convenient to do or obtain, and it is well promoted.

A tool based on the one developed by the Turning Point Collaborative* to identify social marketing research needs appears in **Box 9–3**.

RESEARCH METHODS

Typically, scientists learn a method (or two) in graduate school and then continue that method throughout their research careers. Social and public health scientists are no exception. Here we outline a spectrum of methods that can be used for formative research.

Anthropological Methods

Anthropologists study health behavior in its cultural context. Their work contains the richness necessary to begin developing hypotheses about behavioral antecedents and what might prompt behavior change. **Ethnography** is the study a group of people and their life-ways, typically over a long period of time. The term is used to describe what cultural anthropologists do and the body of research that they produce. Now, rather than taking years to research a problem, many programs have anthropologists train community members to conduct ethnographic research in a much shorter time frame (rapid assessment process, RAP),[7] or to conduct participatory[8] data collection with the target audiences. While it does take time and effort to learn how to do ethnography well, it has become standard to use rapid ethnographic concepts and methods in behavior change communication projects. These include a **positive deviance** approach, and techniques such as on-site observation, group and in-depth interviews, and various categorization tools (e.g., free listing, pile sorting). We review these methods and the kinds of information they produce next.

*Turning Point was a project funded by the Robert Wood Johnson Foundation and the W.K. Kellogg Foundation to improve public health management at the state level. States selected a management strategy to master and disseminate among others. Illinois, Maine, Minnesota, New York (Lead), North Carolina, and Virginia formed the National Excellence Collaborative in Social Marketing. They produced a tailored version of *CDCynergy*, and several supporting tools, with guidance from CDC's Division of Health Communication, AED, and the Florida Social Marketing Prevention Center. For more information, see http://www.turningpointprogram.org/

Behavioral Observations

Because most health marketing programs attempt to change a behavior, an important place to start is observing the behavior is in the setting where it is practiced. Sending trained observers into homes and communities to watch what goes on, usually over several hours for several days in a row, helps identify behavior patterns, alternative products, or obstacles to adopting new behaviors. It is important that the presence of the observer does not interfere with the routine behavior of the person or persons being watched. It can take a fairly long time for people to become comfortable with an outsider watching them. Even with the rash of reality television programs and video-cams documenting so much of what we do, the vast majority of people prefer their privacy. For this reason, observations are usually limited to short stints of time or very specific interactions (e.g., handwashing [Box 9–1]), at least in the United States. In other countries, health communicators often work with observers who are local health workers or educated *near peers* of the subjects in order to minimize the intrusiveness of observation.

Asking Questions: In-Depth Interviews

People are much more comfortable talking about what they do than having someone watch them do it. In-depth interviews are sometimes used to discuss highly personal topics, and usually at a stage of research where the program does not yet feel sufficiently informed to use a group format. The in-depth interview requires the interviewer to create a comfortable, nonjudgmental relationship with the person being interviewed. The researcher may use a topic guide or work from very open-ended questions.

Communications researchers typically conduct individual interviews either as a first step in the development of a focus group protocol (i.e., a group interview guide), or to interview **key informants**, such as gatekeepers. These informants work with members of the community, or influence them in some way, and hence have a great deal of pertinent information to share.

An individual, in-depth interview is easier to arrange than trying to organize a focus group, because it can be done in the respondent's home, office, or location of their choosing (even on street corners for the homeless). At times, individual interviews are the only choice, especially when preservation of anonymity is paramount.

Ethnolinguistic Techniques[9]

Ethnolinguistic techniques have been popularized by RAP and other rapid ethnographic tools as a quick way of understanding how another group of people organizes their world into different cognitive categories.

Box 9–3 Market Research Planning Worksheet
(Modeled after Turning Point Social Marketing Collaborative)

In order to help (primary target audience) to (perform key behavior):

Key Marketing Decision #1 Whose Behavior Needs to Change?	What Do We Already Know?	Information Needed
Identify the primary target audience.		
Who influences them? (secondary target audience)		
Other community influencers? (tertiary target audience)		

Key Marketing Decision #2 What Is the Target Audience Doing INSTEAD of the Recommended Behavior?	Existing Info	Information Needed
Are they using another product instead of the recommended product? What and how?		
How widespread is this practice; how long has it been practiced?		

Key Marketing Decision #3 What Are the Key Benefits of the New Behavior or Product?	Existing Info	Information Needed
What benefits would the primary audience gain from adopting the recommended behavior?		
Are there benefits to the secondary and tertiary audiences?		

Key Marketing Decision #4 What Costs and Other Barriers Must be Addressed?	Existing Info	Information Needed
What is the target audience asked to give up or exchange for the benefits? • What other barriers prevent them from performing the new behavior?		

continues

- Perceived risk
- Self-efficacy
- Availability
- Access
- Social norms
- Skills
- Policies

Key Marketing Decision #5 Where Should We Place the Product/Behaviors?	Existing Info	Information Needed
If the product is tangible, where is the best place(s) to make it available?		
If it is a behavior, where does it make the most sense to promote it?		

Key Marketing Decision #6 What Promotional Strategies Should We Use?	Existing Info	Information Needed
Are there time-limited opportunities that would support our program?		
Are there influential personalities to support the program? Who else is credible with the target audience(s)?		
What media channels are best for this kind of communication?		

Source: http://www.cdc.gov/communication/cdcynergy.html

Free Listing In **free listing**, a respondent is asked to list out all the examples of a particular kind of thing that they know about. For example, you might ask for a list of "appropriate foods for young children," "the most important qualities in a spouse or partner," or "flu symptoms." The researcher records these items, usually on separate index cards. After a number of respondents are asked, the researcher should have a fairly large stack of cards. (If your respondents cannot read, you will need to use pictures or find another way of representing their ideas.) Not all topics are suitable to free listing. People are often unaware of what they know or don't know and are not accustomed to analyzing their own behavior and are often unable to call up their "reasons" for doing something or not.

Pile Sorting and Ranking For **pile sorting**, you need to have individual items available on separate cards, with the item on the front and a number on the back. You ask respondents to sort the cards into piles. Often, you would begin by asking respondents to generate the categories themselves. For example, if respondents were given a stack of cards with pictures of food and asked to put them in piles, many American students would sort them into "foods I like" and "foods I don't like," followed possibly by the learned categories of "good for you" and " not good for you," or the original four or five food groups. Other people might sort the foods into those appropriate for breakfast, lunch, or dinner. Still others might divide them up according to another medical system, such as "hot and cold" foods in a humoral medical system. Once you feel you have a sufficient number of categories, you can then ask the respondents to sort the individual items according to those groupings.

Finally, you may ask people to **rank order** the individual items in a category. Here are some examples: flu symptoms, most unpleasant to least unpleasant; life partner qualities, most important to least important; breakfast food, most favorite to least favorite; etc.

The chief benefit of this method is that most people enjoy doing it, particularly if they get to work with illustrations and not words. It can be done fairly quickly, and it produces some interesting results in terms of what goes together in someone else's mind and what does not. You can use fairly simple statistics to determine the relevancy of categories and ranking of items, as well as more sophisticated multidimensional scaling analyses to assess the strength and weakness of associations and relationships of different categories and rankings.

Focus Group Discussions

Social marketing researchers love focus group discussions (FGDs) or interviews. By bringing a group of 8 to 10 people who share certain characteristics together, we can learn as much as if we conducted hundreds of surveys. At least, that is what qualitative researchers believe. **Focus groups** really give us a feeling for what people think, feel, and *say* they do. Focus group discussions are useful in developing hypotheses, exploring broad topics, and producing a large number of ideas. A well-moderated group creates a casual environment that enables people to talk freely about feelings, beliefs, and attitudes. Through such discussions, program planners and communicators become more sensitive to the values, concerns, and needs of target audiences.

Because only a relatively small sample of any target audience actually takes part in focus group discussions, even if many are conducted,* FGDs are exploratory, leading to hypothesis generation, not confirmation. Focus group participants need to be recruited and screened carefully so that participants are representative of the group you wish to study. For example, if you are using a doer versus non-doer analysis (see later discussion), you need to recruit practitioners of the behavior in one group and non-practitioners in the other. If you are interested in what young, Caucasian women have to say about a family planning product, that is who has to be in your focus group-not their mothers, not their boyfriends, and not people from other ethnic groups.

In the United States, the number of people you would invite to a casual dinner party is the ideal number for a focus group—no fewer than 6, and no more than 10, with 8 being the magic number. The group setting allows participants to question each other, and, while the moderator keeps the discussion on track, participants may bring up ideas the researcher never thought to ask. Perhaps it comes as a surprise but we have learned that participants often prefer discussing what might be considered embarrassing health topics with a group of people known to share their condition than alone with an individual investigator.

The group moderator must be able to create a comfortable environment in which everyone wants to participate. This trait, being a good conversationalist, is probably more important than any formal training in research or even the topic itself. The best focus group moderators are recruited from near peers of the target audience and trained in the technique and the topic guide.

While some researchers rely only on note taking, I have found it essential to record and transcribe focus group interviews. New qualitative analysis software can be used to code and analyze transcripts. If you are looking for verbatim quotations, you really need to get these exactly as they are said. And, if you use one of the more creative, interpretive methods, you might want to play a voice recording of respondents to a creative team for inspiration.[†]

There are many excellent resources on conducting focus group interviews.[10,11] The key elements are having a quiet location, a good audio recorder, refreshments, compensation for the participants, and, of course, an expert moderator and excellent topic guide.

Intercept Interviews

Maybe even more than focus groups, social marketers love central location **intercept interviews**. The researcher goes to the location where the intended audience would encounter information about a behavior or acquire a product and then invites the audience to participate in an interview. Shopping malls are used extensively in the United States for this kind of research, but so are health clinics, supermarkets, and parks—anywhere the location plays a part in the consumer's decision. The high-traffic volume of the intercept area allows the researcher to contact large numbers of respondents in a short period of time. Intercept interviews can be used to collect either quantitative or qualitative data, depending on the form of the study. Very often intercepts are done at the point in a study when a concept is

---

*And they shouldn't be. Whenever studies include more than four to six groups with the exact same audience segment, something fishy is going on.

[†]Again, it is critical that the informed consent for the focus group informs the participants exactly who will listen to or review what they say and that they understand the nature of the analysis or use of the recording. Participants must be allowed to withdraw from the group if they are not willing to be recorded or have anyone listen to the recording. Anyone listening to or using the recording should go through IRB training and be cleared for this purpose.

ready to be pretested with a larger number of people in the place where they would encounter the information. Finally, as discussed in Chapter 7, intercepts are also useful for evaluating the readability and acceptability of print materials in an environment that is typical for the intended user. It is one thing to take people into a quiet testing site; it is quite another for people to try to read something in a supermarket aisle. If the supermarket is where the target audience will encounter the information, then test it in the supermarket.

The procedure for the intercept interview involves approaching individuals, asking a few screening questions to determine whether they match the characteristics of the target audience, and then bringing the participant over to a testing site. A variation of this theme is the "exit interview," where participants who have already gone through an activity, such as a doctor's office visit or shopping trip, are invited to participate in the interview. While the advantage of this technique is the possibility of volume, many people do not want to be bothered. Researchers almost always offer incentives, such as gift cards or cash rewards, for central location intercepts.

The Doer versus Non-Doer Study[12] Combined with a Positive Deviance Study

Unlike the specific techniques mentioned earlier, a *doer versus non-doer study* is an overall approach to organizing your formative research, and you might implement it using some of the data collection techniques described previously. We recommend it highly as a shortcut to understanding why a particular behavior, product, or service might be attractive to a particular target audience and, conversely, what the most important barriers or obstacles are. In the following section, I have modified the instructions originally developed by Bill Smith of AED for this kind of analysis. When using a *positive deviance approach*, a critical first condition is that the doers and non-doers are nearly identical in terms of their socioeconomic and environmental conditions. It is also helpful to eliminate as many cultural differences as possible. In this way, when you find out how the doers have come to adopt a behavior, the chances are good that the non-doers will be able to emulate them. We discuss the seven steps in this process in some detail and provide some measure of the importance we attach to it.

Seven Steps

1. Clarify the behavioral goal.

Let's set the goal as helping middle-school-age children maintain a healthy weight. There are two ways to start this process: one based on behavioral doing and non-doing and one based on physical having (healthy weight) and having not.

- You may use a biological measure, such as body mass index (BMI), or weight for height, to identify middle school children who are in a healthy weight range for their age and height. Working with school authorities, and going through the proper research review procedures, you request to speak to all parents and compare the responses of parents with children who have a healthy weight to those who do not. Based on this first analysis, you develop a list of behaviors that seem to be associated with having a healthy weight. Suppose you find that middle school children who have a healthy weight eat fewer sugary snacks, watch less TV, participate in more physical activities and sports, and perhaps ride their bikes or walk to school. You might choose to focus on several or only one of these facilitating factors when comparing the two groups of children and their parents.

- A second way to start this process is to begin with what we already know about behaviors and environmental conditions that help middle school children maintain a healthy weight. These might include having healthy choices available in the school cafeteria for lunch; limiting school vending machines to water, low-fat milk, and low-calorie beverages; maintaining a regular physical education program; and encouraging children to walk or ride a bike to school instead of riding in a car or bus. Of these options, three are primarily under the control of the school administration, the cafeteria, the vending machines and the physical education program. This suggests that advocacy may be the best intervention to promote healthy decisions in these areas. The last option, having more children walk or bike to school, is a decision that will be made at home by the parents and the children.

2. Define the behavior and the audience.

The decision of walking or biking to school actually involves several people. First, the middle school child may not own a bike, feel too "tired" to walk or ride a bike, or be worried that either the bike or the act of walking isn't "cool" enough for his or her peers. Parents may worry that their child might be late for school or harmed by traffic, the bike might be stolen, or the child will be out in the dark on the way home. Which of these concerns are most valid in shaping a decision? In this case, we are going to start with the parents' concerns. We narrow our behavioral objective to the following two: parents will allow and encourage their child to walk or bike to school. The target audience is the parents of middle school children.

You might want to focus on conditions where bike riding or walking is more of a challenge, such as in urban environments. Or you might want to work with a population that typically does not engage in the recommended behavior, and seems to have a more of a problem with child obesity, for example urban African American or Hispanic families. So, you decide that you need to speak to city-living African American parents of middle school children and find out how they feel about children walking to school or riding bikes.

3. Determine how you will distinguish the doers from the non-doers.

The question you ask at this stage might seem pretty straight forward, such as, *"Do you allow your child to walk or ride a bike to school?"* But you realize that this is too vague a question, because how much walking or riding is necessary in order for it to actually contribute to a child's physical fitness? You might decide that the child needs to walk or bike to school at least three days a week. So, a doer would be defined as "always or almost always walks to school or rides his/her bike" or as "rides his/her bike more than twice a week." Again, working with the school authorities and using appropriate research reviewed protocols, you might be able to send questions home with children, identify children as they arrive at or leave school as walkers and bikers, and then do a phone, online, or in-person survey with their parents. Parents who do allow their children to bike or walk to school three days a week or more will be doers of the behavior. In the inner-city environment, and among the African-American population you have selected for focus, these parents represent a minority opinion. As such, they have "deviated" from the norm in a positive direction.

4. Develop the attitude questions.

We have reviewed the most essential theories that guide behavior change communication. In this case, we are going to focus on perceived consequences, self-efficacy (or enabling factors), and social norms. Now you need to think about how to phrase a question that captures these concepts so that you can ask about them. Keep in mind that you are asking doers why they do something, what positive feelings they have about it, and what makes it easier for them to do it. But you also want to know if they encountered obstacles, what they were, and how were they overcome. This personal story of change *will likely be a cornerstone of your message strategy*, particularly if you use a "role model" approach. You are asking the non-doers about what gets in the way now to their performing the behavior. But, you also want to know what they think might help them take a step toward performing the behavior.

Here are some suggestions to get at **perceived consequences:**

- What do you see as the advantages or good things that would happen if your child *(walked/rode a bike)* to school?

- What do you see as the disadvantages or bad things that would happen if your child *(walked/rode a bike)* to school?

Here is a probe for current doers:
- Thinking back about your decision to let your child walk/bike to school, did you have any worries? Can you tell me about how you compared the benefits to the disadvantages?

Here is a probe for current non-doers:
- When you compare the good and bad of walking to school, is there anything that would make you decide to let your child do it?

Here are suggestions to get at self-efficacy or enabling factors:
- What makes it difficult or impossible for you to let him/her *(walk/ride a bike)* to school?
- What makes it easier for you to let your child *(walk/ride a bike)* to school?

Here are suggestions to get at **social norms:**
- Who (individuals or groups) do you think would object or disapprove if you let your child *(walk/ride a bike)* to school?
- Who (individual or groups) do you think would approve if you let your child *(walk/ride a bike)* to school?
- Which of the individuals or groups in the preceding two questions is most important to you?

For any of these constructs, you may use free listing, pile sorting, and comparative tasks in order to get respondents to rank order the variables.

5. Organize the data collection.

As suggested earlier, you will be preparing a short questionnaire. Our experience has shown that asking the attitudinal questions in this order is helpful. You also need to avoid combining ideas-that is, DO NOT ask: "What good *and* bad things happen when. . . ." People will answer only part of the question, usually the bad side.

As you are doing formative research, drawing a statistically significant sample is not essential. However, again, you need a large enough number to differentiate what the doers tell you from the non-doers. If you can contact about 300 members of the target audience (parents of middle school children) you might be able to get 100 respondents in each group. You might have only 50 in the positive group and 250 in the negative group. Or, more realistically, 20 in the positive group and about 40 to 50 in the negative group. This is what you could anticipate in the way of a response from busy parents in a large city. Keep the questions open ended, and record as much of what people say as you can. You'll be using the behavior question as the initial screen. Once you have more than 20 parents in either group (doer, non-doer), you can seek out parents in the missing group until you have at least the same number. Continue then to ask either parent until you feel you have heard the same answers repeatedly from either group. This is called **saturation** in qualitative research.

If you are just looking for a general impression from the two groups, you may form groups of doers and groups of non-doers. But the better way to do this study is as previously described with individual interviews.

6. Tabulate the results.

In this step, you review all the answers and then list and count up the responses for each question. This is facilitated by using a coding sheet. You will have lists organized by doers and non-doers, with the most frequently mentioned answers at the top. In addition, make sure you have a way of collecting narratives of how a decision was made, how an obstacle was overcome, and what rewards were experienced immediately and possibly later on as a result of performing this activity. Someone may keep slipping back to their old behavior and then reinstating the new behavior; this is also important data to collect.

7. Interpret your results.

In looking at the key differences between how doers answered the questions compared to non-doers, focus on the five biggest differences. Also, look at where their responses are similar. Now let's discuss some tips to keep in mind.

Tips for Doer versus Non-Doer Analysis

- If doers and non-doers have similar percentages for any item, that item is *not* a likely determinant of the behavior for this audience.
- When doers' responses are radically different from non-doers' responses, that item *is* very likely a determinant of the behavior for this audience.
- Because this technique is not a statistical analysis, differences between the groups of respondents need to be large to mean anything. If you have 100 or fewer respondents in total, you will want to see a difference of at least 10%.
- Focus on what the doers tell you in terms of how they came to adopt the behavior. The concept of positive deviance suggests that because these strategies were developed under similar pressures and constraints as those faced by the non-doers, the behavior should be possible for everyone. Why did the doers choose to take the step? Can the non-doers be persuaded to follow their lead?

- Make sure you have collected the first-person stories from the doers and non-doers. These stories can be developed into compelling accounts and provide the creative energy for your message strategy and may contain answers to questions you had not thought to ask (see Chapter 15 for more on the value of story).
- Consider how the doers and non-doers answered the questions about approval and disapproval. You might need to reach out to a secondary audience in order to get their support of the behavior before focusing your attention on the parents you originally identified as your target audience.
- Finally, your research might reveal that structural differences actually exist between the two groups of parents-doers and non-doers. The doers might live in safer environments; they might be more economically prosperous and can afford bikes, or transportation fees, for their children; or, conversely, they might live in areas that do not provide school bus service and therefore have no choice but to have their children walk to school. In this case, you will need to address structural barriers before trying to promote individual behavior change through advocacy.

USING ROLE-PLAY

Take a look at **Box 9–4** for an update on the Bangladesh example.

We've chosen to use **role model stories**—in other words, fictionalized stories that show doers performing the behavior with positive outcomes. It's a great idea, but how do we get the material we need to write these stories?

Participatory Role-Play as Formative Research

As Marshall McLuhan observed, "the medium is the message."[13] These words seem even truer today if you compare

> ## Box 9–4 Recap of BEHAVE Framework for Bangladeshi Example
>
> In order to help (*a young mother*) to (*begin feeding her 6-month-old mashed pumpkin*), we will focus on this benefit (*child's health and energy*), and lower this barrier (*fear that vegetables cause diarrhea or illness*). We will approach this through these factors: (*self-efficacy for feeding skills, mother-in-law approval*) and use this means of reaching the audience: (*role model stories told by community agents with photo-novels*).

what is said in an e-mail, messaged in a Tweet, viewed on YouTube, or seen in a full-length movie. So much about *what* is said and, more importantly, *how* it is received is determined by the medium in which it is embedded. Extending this concept beyond the structural features of bandwidth, sound, film, and time limits, think about the difference between a child's bed time story, for example, Aesop's "The Ant and the Grasshopper," and the parental admonition to "do your homework before playing." We might refer to the latter as a *behavioral concept* or even a *key message*. But the *story* of the ant and the grasshopper, or a modern-day equivalent, engages children more and gets them to think about consequences and rewards. It enables vicarious learning, and it is memorable. In other words, it embodies many of the constructs in social cognitive theory by building a drama based on these recurrent human concerns.

There would be no way that a creative team could construct a story such as the ant and the grasshopper if all they were given were dry statistics about the target audience. Even with a creative brief (discussed in the next chapter), it is nearly impossible to put the flesh on the bones of a health message strategy unless some kind of "juicy" information is also collected in the first place. A way to jump-start the creative side of health communication planning is to engage the target audience, or those who are very close to them in a professional capacity (e.g., local health workers), in role-play. While engaging amateurs in the process is routine, the creative strategy can also be accelerated by bringing in actors early in the research interpretation process. They will see and hear things more related to what makes good drama, which is normally overlooked by health workers and health communication specialists. A concise resource is available to guide what is sometimes called **diagnostic role-play**, again produced by AED together with Save the Children in Malawi.[14] I started using this approach in West Africa in the late 1980s[15] and used it equally well in Bangladesh and in Atlanta, Georgia, much more recently.

In brief, the process begins as before with some kind of information gathering from the target audiences. Even before organizing focus groups, it helps to sit down with local health workers or other field personnel and engage them in a brainstorming session. While some field personnel are able to contribute valuable ideas just by speaking up, sometimes they are intimidated by the presence of the researcher or their superiors and keep pretty quiet. We have found that these same personnel are often more comfortable role-playing situations where they have observed that their constituents are blocked in adopting a healthy behavior. A set of preliminary behavioral issues might be available through existing ethnographic or other research. Field staff are often adept at playing out

scenes in which they have observed or could imagine how the behavior would be conducted in a family or community context. Characters and situations from these scenes can then be explored using rapid qualitative research in the community. The goal of this "pre-research" role-playing is not to eliminate in-depth research, but to focus it on real behavioral issues and more tightly defined target audiences.

We often use focus groups as the next step in this process. It is extremely helpful to make and keep an *audio* recording of each group, in addition to transcripts and notes. Again, it is essential that informed consent procedures make it clear that actors or health workers will be listening to audio recordings of the groups, or reading transcripts—although the identities of the focus group participants should remain anonymous—which is why *video recordings are not encouraged* for this kind of analysis.

The creative team, which again might be the field personnel, works with the researcher to review the communication objectives. They then listen to the audio recordings or read verbatim transcripts from the focus groups. When working with health personnel, it is often useful to summarize the focus groups themes and ask them to highlight statements in the transcripts that they feel present compelling quotations from participants. The group then role-plays dialogues that might emerge, inspired by these themes and quotations. This is the point at which videotaping works well-to capture the creative products of the team.

When working with professional actors or screenwriters, the audio portion carries the voices of the participants and adds a level of personality that will not transfer through a transcript. This can be quite inspirational to professional actors or screenwriters who are more attuned to drama than the average health worker, as said before. They often can create brief scenarios just by listening to the recordings and imagining "the rest of the story."

At this point you will have one of two products: video recordings of amateur role-plays or professionally written drama scenarios. (Perhaps you have both.) These materials can then be given to the production team to guide the next stage of creative development and then pretested with the target audience. This is discussed in Chapter 10.

Other Participatory Approaches

There are other participatory methods you can use to develop concepts and images for health communication. The most widely used today is "Photo Voice."[16*] In this approach,

---

*http://www.photovoice.org/

communities are given the tools to document their own lives, problems, and possible solutions through photography. It has been used extensively to put forward unheard voices for advocacy purposes. However, it is also a legitimate way of gathering how an affected group of people view their own situation, and it can be the precursor for a very compelling intervention to enable them to change their circumstances for the better.

ADVANCED FORMATIVE RESEARCH TECHNIQUES

Commercial marketers, and some public health communication researchers, are starting to use some very high-tech procedures to both collect data and analyze the results. To overcome some of the natural tendency of respondents to "please" the interviewer, respondents agree to be hooked up to a range of equipment that measures their direct, physiological response. Some of the responses measured include eye movements, heart rate, skin conductance, and brain waves (EEG) or functional magnetic resonance imaging (fMRI). **Box 9–5** describes how these measures are being used by communication researchers at Temple University in Philadelphia.

Participant responses to scaled questions are analyzed using a form of multidimensional scaling called **vector analysis**. These approaches tend to be used to test participant responses to preliminary concepts or draft materials.

Box 9–5 Use of Perceptual Mapping at Temple University Risk Communication Laboratory

The Risk Communication Laboratory at Temple University uses perceptual mapping methods that involve multidimensional scaling (MDS) and message vector modeling techniques to design risk communication materials. Advances in modeling and theory development allow us to produce dynamic models of complex cognitive and communication processes, critical for the development of optimally effective message strategies and decision aids. These models are graphically three-dimensional and can be displayed as multicolored simulations of cognitive processes. This allows us to study how framing effects, perceptions of risks/benefits, and attitudes toward risk contribute to both cognitive and affective dimensions of decision making for diverse populations. These messages are then tested for effectiveness using psycho-physiological measures, such as eye tracking, pupil dilation, galvanic skin resistance (sweating), body temperature, EEG brain responses, heart rate, and respiration rate.

Perceptual mapping uses multidimensional scaling (MDS) to yield a graphic display of how respondents perceive the relationships among a set of elements (e.g., medical treatments and their perceived risks and benefits).[a,b] The resulting maps . . . reflect how the key elements are conceptualized relative to each other and relative to "Self." The "Self" can be positioned in the model as an individual or as a group/sample average "Self." Using paper-pencil measures, respondents rate, on a scale of 0 to 10, the extent to which they associate elements with each other (based on similarities and differences or perceived association).[c] Unlike other "mental mapping" procedures that require the respondent to make complex overall judgments, perceptual mapping only requires the participant to judge the individual component associations; the software then puts these component parts together as a whole model. Thus, *this method is easy to use; even those with low literacy can use the method without having to use complex instrumentation or make complicated or abstract decisions.*

To construct the perceptual maps, computer software converts the scaled judgments into distances used in the mapping.[d] All distance matrix input data are assessed on a 0-10 scale and input values are "reflected" so that more important elements appear closer to the "Self," while those judged less important are farther away. In the last step, graphic arrays of the distances among the elements are plotted and displayed in two- or three-dimensions for visual inspection and interpretation. The percentage of variance accounted for by the analysis is provided as an index of the explanatory power of each map. The resulting maps display the elements (e.g., treatments, risks, benefits) relative to each other, and to "Self." Essentially, the maps provide a snapshot of the respondents' conceptualization of the situation, and reveal the relative importance of different elements to "Self." Looking at a perceptual map is like looking into the mind of the individual or group, to observe how they see their world and where they position themselves in relation to the elements affecting a specific decision or action.

The maps can then be used to determine optimum message strategies through vector analytic procedures.[e] For example, to optimally position a cancer screening concept in the perceptual space, a target vector . . . is used to start the mathematical vector resolution process. By specifying the target vector and the number of concepts to be used in the final message, the software creates all possible vector resolutions, using the specified number of concepts, then rank orders the solutions for best fit to the target vector. The "best fit" solution is then evaluated by the research team for conceptual consistency and practical utility. The decision aid is designed to include and illustrate, where needed, the concepts that were identified as critical for addressing the target population's concerns, knowledge, and perceptions of risks-benefits for that particular decision. This procedure allows us to accurately tailor the decision aid directly to the target population's conceptualization of the risks and/or benefits of carrying out the hoped for behavior.[f]

The Risk Communication Laboratory at Temple University is using these methods to develop targeted and/or tailored messages in a variety of public health areas. Current research has used these methods to assess healthcare attitudes about smallpox vaccination,[g] perceptions of a state health department disaster preparedness guide,[h] city health department HIV case managers' perceptions of barriers and resources,[i] statewide attitudes toward quarantine and vaccination for avian flu,[j,k] patient's perceptions of the environmental and emotional factors that trigger drug usage, development of a colorectal cancer screening decision aid for low literacy patients,[l-o] and development of a radiological terror event preparedness guide for low literacy adults.[p]

References

[a]Borg I., & Groenen, P. (1997). *Modern multidimensional scaling: Theory and applications.* New York: Springer-Verlag.

[b]Kitchin, R., & Freundschuh, S. (2000). *Cognitive mapping: past, present, future.* NJ: Routledge.

[c]Gordon, T. F. (1988). Subject abilities to use metric MDS: Effects of varying the criterion pair. In: Barnett, G. A., Woelfel, J. *Readings in the Galileo system: Theory, methods, and applications.* Dubuque, IA: Kendall/Hunt Publishing Co.

[d]Shiffman, S. S., Reynolds, M. L., & Young, F. W. (1981). *Introduction to multidimensional scaling: theory, methods, and applications.* New York: Academic Press.

[e]Woelfel J., & Fink, E. (1980). *The measurement of communication processes: Galileo theory and method.* New York: Academic Press.

[f]Gordon, T. F., Ruzek, S. B., & Bass, S. B. (2007, August). Using perceptual mapping, eye-tracking & pupilometer technologies with functional-MRI to design more effective health marketing strategies. Poster session at the Centers for Disease Control and Prevention Health Marketing and Media Annual Conference, Atlanta, GA.

[g]Bass, S. B., Gordon, T. F., Ruzek, S. B., & Hausman, A. J. (2008). Mapping perceptions related to acceptance of smallpox vaccination by hospital emergency room personnel. *Biosecurity and Bioterrorism: Biodefense Strategy, Practice, and Science,* 6 (2): 179-189.

[h]Gordon, T. F., Ruzek, S. B., Bass, S. B., & Kufs, L. S. (2006, September). Evaluation of the *Pennsylvania Disaster Preparedness Guide*: A pilot study using eye-tracking technology, heart-rate, and skin-conductance. Report prepared for the Pennsylvania Department of Health, Temple University Center for Preparedness Research, Education, and Practice, Philadelphia, PA.

[i]Matosky, M., Terrell, C., Gordon, T. F., Bass, S. B., & Ruzek, S. B., (2008, October). Using perceptual mapping to develop HIV medical case management. Paper presented at the American Public Health Association Annual Conference, San Diego, CA.

[j]Gordon, T. F., Ruzek, S. B., Bass, S. B., Hagen, M. Hanlon, A., Hausman, A. (2007, November). Mapping public perceptions of avian flu—a statewide survey: Using perceptual mapping to model perceptions and design health campaign strategy. Paper presented at the American Public Health Association Annual Conference. Washington, DC.

[k]Bass, S.B., Ruzek, S.B., Ward, L., Gordon, T.F., Hanlon, A., Hausman, A.J., & Hagen, M. (In Press). If you ask them, will they come? Predictors of Quarantine Compliance during a Hypothetical Avian Flu Pandemic: Results from a Statewide Survey. Disaster Medicine and Public Health Preparedness.

[l]National Cancer Institute Grant (5R 21CA 120122-02). Using perceptual mapping to develop a colorectal cancer screening decision aid for low-literacy African Americans. Principal Investigator: T. F. Gordon. 2007-2009.

[m]Gordon, T. F., Rovito, M., Ruzek, S. B., Bass, S. B., Ward, S., Lim, K., Myers, B., Wokak, C., Britto, J., & Abedin, Z. (2009, November). Improving colorectal cancer screening strategies for low-literacy African Americans: Using risk-benefit segmentation to define a typology of patients and mapping perceptions to design targeted decision aids. Paper presented at the American Public Health Association Annual Conference, Philadelphia, PA.

[n]Bass, S.B., Ruzek, S.B., Gordon, T.F., Wolak, C., Rovito, M., Britto, J., Parameswaran, L., Ward, S., Meyer, B., Lin, K. & Paranjape, A. (2009, November). Developing a computer touch screen interactive colorectal cancer screening decision aid for low-literacy populations: Lessons learned. Paper presented at the American Public Health Association Annual Conference, Philadelphia, PA.

[o]Bass, S.B., Gordon, T.F., Ruzek, S.B., Wolak, C., Ward, S., Meyer, B., & Lin, K. (2009, November). Perceptions of colorectal cancer screening in African Americans: Differences by gender and screening status. Paper presented at the American Public Health Association Annual Conference. Philadelphia, PA.

[p]National Institute of Biomedical Imaging and Bioengineering (R03 EB009561-01A1. Developing Radiological Risk Communication Materials for Low-Literacy Populations. Principal Investigator: SB Bass. 2009-2011.

Source: Thomas F. Gordon, PhD, Sarah Bauerle Bass, PhD, MPH. Risk Communication Laboratory, Department of Public Health, Temple University, Philadelphia, PA.

CONCLUSION

This chapter described the methods and approaches we use to conduct formative research. Chapter 10 will now show how to apply your findings to various communication strategies for different audiences.

KEY TERMS

Anthropologists
Baseline evaluation
BEHAVE framework
Behavioral analysis scale
Behavioral lever
Beneficiary
Channels
Diagnostic role-play
Early adopters
Ethnography
Ethnolinguistic techniques
Focus groups
Formative research
Free listing
Gatekeeper
Informed consent

Intercept interviews
Key informant
Mixed-methods approach
Modal behavior
Observational learning
Participatory approaches
Perceived consequences
Pile sorting
Positive deviance
Primary (target) audience
Qualitative research
Quantitative research
Rank order
Role model stories
Saturation
Secondary audience
Self-efficacy
Settings
Social norms
Thought-leader promotion
Vector analysis

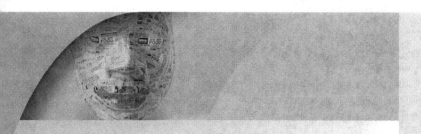

Chapter Questions

1. What is the purpose of formative research?

2 When are qualitative methods preferred to quantitative methods? What are mixed methods?

3. What is meant by a behavioral lever?

4. What does it mean to "start with the early adopters"?

5. How would you use a positive deviance approach to distinguish the doers from the non-doers for a behavior?

6. What is the difference between a setting and a channel?

7. Why do market researchers love central intercept studies?

8. Develop a role-play on a health topic, and map it into the BEHAVE framework.

REFERENCES

1. BEHAVE (not an acronym) was developed by the CORE Group, a coalition of nongovernmental organizations, including the Academy for Educational Development, devoted to international health. It can be accessed at http://www.coregroup.org/index.php?option=com_content&view=article&id=52&Itemid=1.

2. Roberts A, Pareja R, Shaw W, Boyd B, Booth E, Mata JI. Question 15-3. The Behavioral Analysis Scale. *Academy for Educational Development Toolbox for Health Communication.* HealthCom Project, USAID; 1995.

3. Rogers EM. *Diffusion of Innovations,* 3rd ed. New York: The Free Press; 1983.

4. Gladwell, M. *The Tipping Point, How Little Things Can Make a Big Difference.* New York: Time Warner Books; 2000, 2002.

5. Smith W. Marketing strategy—Fun, easy, popular. *CDCynergy,* video content. http://www.orau.gov/cdcynergy/demo/Content/activeinformation/videos/video18_bsmith_script.htm

6. National Cancer Institute. *Making Health Communication Programs Work.* NIH Publication No. 04-5145. 2004:28-34 Available at www.cancer.gov.

7. Scrimshaw N, Gleason G, Eds. *Rapid Assessment Procedures.* Qualitative Methodologies for Planning and Evaluation of Health Related Programmes. 1992 International Nutrition Foundation for Developing Countries (INFDC), Boston, MA. Accessible free from: http://www.unu.edu/unupress/food2/UIN08E/uin08e00.htm.

8. Chambers R. Participatory Rural Appraisal (PRA): Analysis of Experience. *World Development,* 1994;22(9):1253-1268.

9. Bernard HR, Ryan GW. *Analyzing Qualitative Data.* Thousand Oaks, CA: Sage Publications; 2010.

10. Debus, M. *Handbook for Excellence in Focus Group Research.* Healthcom Project, USAID. Washington, DC: Porter/Novelli; 1988.

11. Krueger RA. *Focus groups: A practical guide for applied research.* Newbury Park, CA: Sage Publications; 1988.

12. This section is adapted from Smith W. *Comparing Doers and Non-Doers. A Rapid Assessment Tool for Social Marketing Programs.* Washington, DC: Academy for Educational Development; 1998. Available from: http://www.soundpartners.org/files/A_Rapid_Assessment_Tool_for_Social_Marketing_P.doc

13. McLuhan M. http://www.marshallmcluhan.com/main.html

14. The Change Project and Save the Children/Malawi. *Guide to Diagnostic Role Play,* 2002. Academy for Educational Development. http://www.global-healthcommunication.org/tool_docs/45/guide_to_diagnostic_role_play_%28full_document%29.pdf

15. Fishman, C. Using African oral tradition to bridge the creative gap. In P. Koniz-Booher, Ed., *Proceedings of an International Conference on Nutrition Communication. Cornell University Monographs.* 1992:76-86.

16. Wang C, Yi W, Tao Z, Carovano K. Photovoice as a participatory health promotion strategy. *Health Promotion International,* 1998;13:75-86.

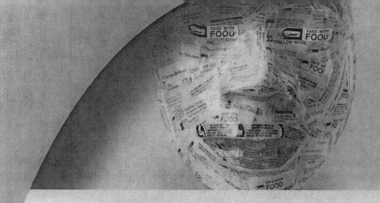

CHAPTER 10

The Strategic Health Communication Plan

Claudia Parvanta

LEARNING OBJECTIVES

By the end of this chapter, the reader will be able to:

- Describe eight principles of strategic health communication.
- Write SMART communication objectives.
- Use Intervention Mapping to match theories to practice strategies.
- Choose among, and provide examples of, practice strategies for a health communication intervention.

INTRODUCTION

Some people say that the essence of health communication is developing the strategic health communication plan that focuses on specific change objectives, audiences, messages, and media. For the past 30 years or more, the government has used a scientific, goals-oriented approach in its health communication in the United States as well as its international development efforts. Even today, though, too many small-scale efforts, with fewer resources than national agencies, begin their planning by saying, "We need a poster," "We need a brochure," or "If we could only get this on *Oprah*."* Making the job even tougher (for the health communication specialist), it is often a top executive who makes this proclamation.

Selecting a media format, channel, or spokesperson before analyzing audience research will not likely help a program meet a goal or be an effective use of resources. Performing these tasks too early is not strategic. So what is? The list in the next section

*This is a reference to the hugely popular Chicago-based television personality, Oprah Winfrey, whose television show is associated with the launch and success of many initiatives and products.

is based on a compilation by the Center for Communication Services at Johns Hopkins University,[1] which has been in the strategic health communication business for decades.

Principles of Strategic Health Communication

Strategic health communication can be defined by its characteristic. It is:

1. **Results-oriented.** While earlier health education campaigns focused on increasing knowledge, our efforts today strive for behavior change as well as the *health outcomes* associated with improved health behavior.
2. **Science-based.** We construct a framework for an intervention based on analysis of a problem and the best evidence for its solution, as well as theories about how to bring about change. As a result, every communication intervention tests one or more hypotheses about behavior change. And logic models—filled in with data collected before, during, and after its implementation—can be used to assess the value of the intervention.
3. **Functions on more than one ecological level.** As mentioned earlier, it is futile to try to change individual behavior when the larger social network or environment will not tolerate or support the change. Multiple approaches, tried together or phased, are more strategic. (Normally you would want to affect policy change and raise community awareness and support before focusing too strenuously on individual behaviors. Similarly, health professionals usually need to come on board with an idea before reaching out to consumers.)
4. **Participatory.** We have also learned from successful community programs as well as commercial ventures

that "stockholders are stakeholders." Or, the greater the number of people who have a vested interest in an outcome, the greater the likelihood of its adoption. Thus, while participatory methods and consultation with the target audience, gatekeepers, community influentials, and others might seem like it is the "polite" thing to do, it will facilitate attainment of a goal and is, therefore, also strategic.

5. **User-centered.** Learning from commercial marketing, we recognize that 'the customer is always right,' at least about what *they want*. We put the intended user of our information or product at the center of all decisions that we make and bring their views in through formative research, testing, and evaluation.

6. **Benefit-oriented.** As we have moved away from a strictly educational model, we have also learned to focus on the features of a behavior, product, or service that are most important to the intended user—in contrast to our earlier preoccupation with attributes.

7. **Distributed.** Our efforts today look for multiple means by which an intended user can obtain information or products to help them change their behavior. This might involve tiers of providers (and training systems). The emphasis is on self-efficacy or community empowerment. Again, learning from past success, *ground-up* and *widely available* are better than *top-down* and of limited *distribution*.

8. **Multichanneled, multimedia.** The most strategic communication is matched to where the intended user will most effectively receive it, where the user will be able to act on it, and where it appears in a format that someone can easily use. Blends of outlets and media are better than choosing only one channel or medium. Ideally, we can continue to engage in a dialogue with the user so that his or her input continues to shape the communication strategy or marketing offering. Additionally, research suggests that the more channels carrying a message, the more likely one user will receive and act on them. There seems to be a dose–response effect.

These eight points are a good summary of what makes a health communication plan strategic. (We will discuss an additional four points from the Johns Hopkins list in the following chapter on media planning and implementation.)

INTEGRATING STRATEGIC PRINCIPLES INTO A PLAN

Results Oriented

To begin, let's review our objectives for the Bangladesh project. See **Box 10–1**.

In the Bangladesh example, we decided to focus on the *secondary audience* first, in this case the husband or mother-in-law, before asking the primary target group, mothers of young children, to adopt the new behavior of actually preparing the pumpkin. Our new behavior change objective could be stated like this: *"Mothers-in-law will be supportive of feeding their grandchildren mashed pumpkin beginning at 6 months of age."*

How are we going to achieve this behavioral outcome? Luckily, we thought to explore this issue in our formative research. We conducted a doer versus non-doer analysis to see if the thinking and behavior of mothers-in-law who already supported the feeding was different from those who did not. We also analyzed the adoption sequence for the behavior, and how change theories—particularly Social Cognitive Theory and Diffusion—could be used to prompt movement up a behavior change continuum. **Table 10–1** shows our new, stage-based communication goals for mothers-in-law.

We can see through this assessment that before convincing the mothers-in-law in the community, *they* would need to feel that their sons, their peers, and the community in general, support this idea. So, we need to address a *tertiary audience* even before focusing our attention specifically on mothers-in-law *(secondary audience)* of the target moms *(the primary audience)*.

Thus, from a global goal of wanting to improve child nutrition—by getting mothers to prepare cooked vegetables—we had to both expand our view of the target audiences for the behavior and change the behavioral outcome that we are seeking. But, we weren't done quite yet.

Developing SMART Objectives

As part of a results orientation, we need to sharpen up our behavior change objectives using the **SMART approach:** **s**pecific, **m**easurable, **a**chievable, **r**elevant (or **r**ealistic), and **t**ime-bound.[2]

Here is our basic version of the behavior change goals we developed for the Bangladeshi case:

- "Mothers will feed their children mashed vegetables beginning at 6 months of age."
- "Mothers-in-law will be supportive of feeding their grandchildren mashed pumpkin beginning at 6 months of age."
- "The community will support feeding children mashed vegetables beginning at 6 months of age."

Let's look only at the objective involving the mother-in-law.

Specific. What action exactly are we trying to achieve? The "specific" part of an objective tells us what will change for whom in concrete terms. This part of our objective is halfway there in that we have identified the mother-in-law (MIL) and

Box 10–1 Bangladesh Project Update: Predisposing, Enabling, and Reinforcing Factors for Feeding Children Pumpkin

We analyzed pumpkin feeding behavior carefully to determine the lever for action (i.e., what needed to happen in order for the rest of a behavioral sequence to occur). We concluded that our **performance objective** (assuming there were no pumpkins in the home garden), was that a woman needed to ask her husband to bring a pumpkin home from the market place. This was a feasible behavior in the social ecological context. We identified important and changeable personal and external determinants of this behavior—the predisposing, enabling, and reinforcing factors. These appear in the accompanying table.

Performance Objective: Primary Audience (Mom)	Personal Determinants		
	Predisposing	Enabling	Reinforcing
Ask husband to bring pumpkin home	Believes feeding pumpkin is good for child.	Is able to make requests and negotiate with husband.	Husband's mother approves of action.
	Likes the taste of cooked pumpkin.	Has other ingredients at home.	Husband likes cooked pumpkin.
	Knows other women who have cooked pumpkin for children and family.	Has adequate fuel and cooking utensils to prepare.	Older children like cooked pumpkin.
	Respects these other women as having made the right decision.	Knows the steps to making cooked pumpkin.	Has made pumpkin before.
			Husband demonstrates his approval.

TABLE 10–1 Stages for Mother-in-Law (MiL) Supporting Preparation of Cooked Pumpkin for 6- to 12-Month-Old Children

Precontemplation
MiL is aware of the positive effects of cooked vegetables and that cooked vegetables were being eaten by children in this age group with no ill effects.

Contemplation
MiL had thought about discussing the issue with her daughter-in-law (DiL).

Ready-to-Act
MiL expressed a commitment to discussing this with her DiL and had discussed it with her son (DiL's husband).

Action
MiL suggested that son bring pumpkin home to cook and that DiL prepare it for family, including small child.

Maintenance
MiL approves of ongoing preparation of pumpkin or other cooked vegetables for family, including small children. Sometimes prepares and feeds them to children herself.

Sustainability (we added this!)
Begins planting pumpkins in home vegetable garden.

that her focus is on her daughter-in-law (DIL) feeding mashed pumpkin to a baby beginning at 6 months of age. This part of the objective is precise for when the child should start receiving vegetables. (We would write a different objective to state more precisely how much pumpkin and how often the mother should be feeding the child.) What we do not know is *how* the MIL will demonstrate her approval or support. We do not have a concrete, observable action. "Support" is an attitude that we need to translate into something tangible, such as a statement on an interview (e.g., "I believe my DIL is doing the right thing by feeding my grandchild mashed pumpkin.") Or, an action that we can see, such as helping in the preparation or feeding of this food or telling the DIL that she approves of her action. These latter actions could be observed through home visits, or again, reported on surveys (e.g., "My MIL says she approves that I feed my child mashed pumpkin," or "My MIL helps me prepare mashed vegetables for my children.")

Measurable. Can the phenomenon be measured, and do we have the ability to measure it? Having come up with a detectable action, we next have to devise a means of measuring or counting it using the resources at hand. If we are prompting adoption of a new behavior, we need an indicator that is categorical (i.e., yes it has happened; no it has not), or happens with enough regularity, that we have a good chance of detecting the change through limited observations. We might choose to use a baseline and follow-up survey to count how many MILs make positive statements about the new infant feeding behavior. Our objective will be to increase the number from the baseline (e.g., we start out at approximately 10% with inherent support of the behavior) to something that is a significant change. Given the evidence from past behavior change campaigns, we might set this at 50%. Projecting less of a change in an attitude, although measurable, might not affect the intended health outcome. Projecting more of a change might be completely unreasonable to expect, given the statistics of change, and the resources of our intervention. We will discuss this more in more detail in the Realistic/Relevant section.

Attainable/Achievable. Can the target population demonstrate this change within the proposed time frame? Do we have the resources available to prompt this level of change? As we described earlier, there are two parts to this parameter. One part is whether the person receiving the intervention will be able to adopt and demonstrate the proposed change by the time we plan to measure again. In our example, the seasonality of vegetables has to be taken into consideration, as well as the age of children in the community. While it is far fetched, it would be possible that setting a baseline and follow-up survey one year apart may be too long, or too short, to detect a behavior change

involving a plant with a short growing season, and for which the behavior is ultimately directed to 6-month-old infants. If the behavior change is one that requires considerable contemplation or preparation, again, more time might be necessary to detect adoption of behavioral "trial." We might need to pin the objective to an earlier stage in the behavior change continuum (e.g., contemplation, preparation) and determine how to observe and measure this (e.g., purchasing pumpkin, stating that they are considering buying or preparing pumpkin).

The second part of "achievable" has to do with the resources we will put into the communication campaign or intervention. We know from earlier chapters (and the health communication evidence base) that unless we are able to make at least 50% of the target audience aware of our message, it is unlikely that many people will move through the stages of contemplation, trial, and maintenance. We also know that new children will be born and move through the appropriate developmental stage for receiving mashed vegetables continuously. But, it is unlikely that their mothers or grandmothers will pay much attention to our messages unless their own child or grandchild is at this developmental stage. Therefore, we need to maintain the duration of our campaign, or find a more direct means of communicating with the new mother/grandmother, at the appropriate times. Do we have the resources to do this? If we do not, we should not set an objective that is unattainable given our resources. In the Bangladesh example, we planned to disseminate our information through garden group leaders visiting communities. How many visits could a volunteer make each month? How many women would she see? Thus, we would need to develop an objective that was limited in terms of percentage change in the short term, but that had a long enough time line in order to be attainable by the program within a year or two.

Realistic/Relevant. Will this objective have an effect on the desired health goal? Is it reasonable to expect this level of change? We determined that if everyone adopted the behavior, we would have an enormous reduction in the health problem. But, if things proceeded as they normally do, with no more than half of the population trying the behavior, we would end up with a relatively small impact on health, or no impact, unless we promoted this objective for several years. (We will discuss setting objectives using the RE-AIM approach to achieve genuine public health outcomes in Chapter 14.) This brings us to the last piece of a smart objective.

Time Bound. By when will this objective be accomplished? We should develop an ambitious, but reasonable time frame for the behavioral objective. As suggested earlier, if our resources are limited in terms of penetration of the target audience, we need to allow for more time. If the behavior in question is cyclical, or also constrained by environmental factors, these need to be taken into consideration.

Thus, our original objectives could be rewritten like this:

- "Fifty-percent of the women in surveyed communities, with infants 6 months to 2 years of age, will have fed mashed pumpkin to their infants at least three times from the project baseline survey (6 months to 2 years post-intervention)."
- "Fifty-percent of the mothers-in-law in surveyed communities will state they have encouraged or insisted that their DIL feed their infant grandchild mashed pumpkin beginning at 6 months of age from the project baseline survey (6 months to 2 years post-intervention)."
- "Fifty percent of fathers in surveyed communities, with infants 6 months to 2 years of age, will say they have brought pumpkin home for their wives to prepare for the children at least three times from the project baseline survey (6 months to 2 years post-intervention)."

These are the results we are trying to obtain. In addition, our background research tells us that these levels of behavioral adoption are possible and would begin to contribute to our overall goal of improving infant nutrition in this region. We will now look at a good way of matching our methods to our smart objectives, which can also be called "performance objectives," using Intervention Mapping[3] terminology.

Science Based: Mapping Theory to Practice Strategies

Intervention Mapping (IM) in its structure looks very similar to *CDCynergy*. But, IM uses the term *performance objectives* to define exactly what you hope the recipient of an intervention will do. IM is also more explicit in the rationale for choosing a theory-based method and practice strategy to bring about this performance objective. According to IM, **theory-based methods** are derived from empirical research on how change occurs in the behavior of individuals or groups. Individual studies use theory in different ways, creating theory-informed methods. One example of a theory-informed method is using "vicarious learning" (learning from another's experience) to promote constructs from Social Cognitive Theory. A **practice strategy** delivers this method in an intervention. For example, role model stories, a form of **Entertainment Education (EE)**, are practice strategies built upon the construct of vicarious learning from Social Cognitive Theory. Finally, practice strategies can be delivered through activities (or channels), in this case, plays mounted by community theater groups, photonovels, or radio or television soap operas. Specific media (the

play, the picture novel, the radio or TV script and production) will then be created to implement these activities. **Table 10–2** summarizes some examples of the distinctions between theoretical methods, practice strategies, and activities or channels.

Box 10–2 shows how we selected a practice strategy, EE, in Bangladesh.

Practice Strategies That Work

Entertainment Education. Since the mid-1970s, there has been extensive work done with Entertainment Education,[4] beginning with Miguel Sabido's development of *telenovelas* aired in Mexico based upon his analysis of the hugely popular Peruvian television soap opera named *Simplemente María*. The preponderance of EE was done in international settings* until relatively recently, when the CDC initiated its Hollywood, Health & Society program. (We will discuss creation of EE further in the following chapter in terms of media and channels.)

But why is EE such an effective way to use theory-based methods? If a picture is worth a 1,000 words, then a story is worth a 1,000 pictures—and at least a dozen theoretical constructs! See **Box 10–3** for how a group of behavioral scientists at the CDC have been working with EE.[5–9]

Many interventions in the United States now use an EE approach, particularly to reach a younger audience about risk behaviors. These are explored more in the next chapter on media. Creating Entertainment Education can also be a highly *participatory* form of intervention, with the target audiences directly involved in creation of the story lines and media products.

Elaboration Likelihood Model Application. Going back to our example of the national folic acid campaign, the CDC and the March of Dimes collaborated in the mid-1990s to prevent birth defects due to a lack of folic acid at the time of conception. While the designers did not specifically articulate that they were using the Elaboration Likelihood Model[10] (ELM; discussed in Chapters 7 and 8), their research identified two distinct audience segments: women actively contemplating pregnancy and women who felt they were "not ready" to think about having children. The "not ready" group included sexually active women, of any ethnic identity, between 18 and 24 years of age. Those who were consciously planning or hoping to have children were slightly older and included more women who spoke a language other than English at home. Using ELM, the "pregnancy contemplators" were motivated to pay attention and "elaborate" on persuasive messages pertaining to childbirth because they were highly involved with the issue. Those who

---

*Most of it sponsored through USAID in the service of family planning and, later, HIV programs.

TABLE 10-2 Theoretical Methods, Practice Strategies, and Activities

Theory-Based Method	Practice Strategy	Activity/Channels
Vicarious learning	Education entertainment	Role-model narrated stories, photo-novels, TV or radio serial drama.
Extended parallel process (fear + ease of solution)	Risk communication raising fear of outcome (e.g., skin cancer) and ease of solution (e.g., sunscreen).	TV, radio, and print public service announcements (PSAs) or commercial advertisin.
Elaboration Likelihood Model	Targeting on peripheral cues of image, music, channels, spokespersons.	Neighborhood outdoor advertising; targeted print, radio, or TV stations.
	Tailoring.	Personalized letters, materials, interactions; patient navigation.
Stage-based behavioral adoption	Motivational interviewing; goal setting and rewards.	In person, phone, or online counseling sessions between a trained counselor and client; group meetings (AA, Weight Watchers).
Norming (bring attention to actual normative behavior versus perception of minority behavior as norm)—particularly for youth	Education entertainment, buzz (viral) marketing.	Channel specific programming (e.g., MTV, VH1, YouTube, Facebook).
Agenda setting (media such as TV) influences public perception of subject proportional to air-time devoted to subject	Media advocacy, public relations.	Radio or TV appearances by leaders, personalities; organization of real or phony (e.g., astro-turf), grassroots demonstrations.
Self-efficacy for skills	Breaking complex behavior into steps: breaking it down.	Do-it-yourself episodes, youth media channels, online communities, rewards programs.
Diffusion of innovation; positive deviance	Target to early adopters.	Agricultural extension, online media, group "sensitization" through community organization partnerships.

were "not ready" would actually tune out information pertaining to pregnancy; even ads featuring cute babies made no impression on them. To reach these women, a "peripheral route" would be necessary that featured other cues (images, music, role models) and messages that resonated with their attitudes toward avoiding pregnancy. We will come back to their message and media strategy later in the textbook.

Social Marketing. As discussed previously, **social marketing** is more of an orientation to your audience and its perceived needs than a theory-based method. Social marketing is the epitome of a *user-centered and benefit-oriented* strategy. **Box 10–4** shows how the CDC used social marketing to organize the VERB campaign, its multipartner and multimedia campaign to reduce childhood obesity.

Marketing, in its unvarnished form, shapes a set of facts to match the interests of the intended consumer. When we are doing "social" marketing, we do attempt to be honest in how we present the benefits of a product or service. But, we still try to emphasize the positives and deemphasize the negatives according to what we have learned about our audience.

Branding. Like a cattleman's mark, a brand symbolizes "ownership" of a product. When a set of communication materials are branded, it usually means they carry the same format, color palette, logo, slogan, or other identifying marks to indicate where they came from. A brand has also taken on the meaning of a reputation, or even a "promise" made to a consumer

Box 10–2 Selection of a Practice Strategy for Bangladesh Project

Our formative research suggested that we needed to create *self-efficacy* on the part of young mothers and prompt widespread attitudinal change—even *create a norm*—for a new way of feeding infants in the community.

To accomplish all of our behavior change goals, the *theoretical approaches* that previous research suggested would work best in this context were Social Cognitive Theory and Stages of Change. Because we did not have a lot of time to devote to stimulating change across the population, we needed to enlist those members of the community who we could identify as "early adopters" of other beneficial behaviors. In Bangladeshi villages, it was easy to see who adopted new agricultural practices, such as making "green manure," or who built latrines in their compounds. We hoped these families might include role models for other new behaviors. Hence, we planned to work with Diffusion Theory, as well. The *practice strategy* that we selected, also based on evidence, was Entertainment Education (EE).

We liked the EE approach because we felt it posed the least risk in the relatively conservative culture, and we knew that entertainment was scarce in rural villages. We opted for *role-model stories* as the way to deliver our messages within an entertaining context. Because Bangladeshi culture requires most women to stay within the confines of their home or nearby gardens, and the local organization with which we were working had already established networks of trained gardening agents who visited homes, we selected these gardening agents as our *channel*. Finally, we knew that we were working with a largely nonliterate population. So we chose to create picture books that could be easily narrated by our garden agents to the men and women they encountered at home or in groups. The picture books were our medium. A page from a story book appears below.

Rachida's Story

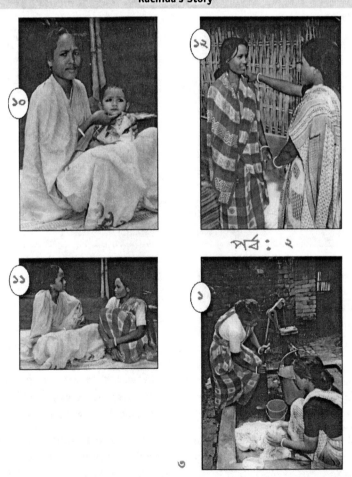

Source: C. Parvanta. Bangladesh Nutrition Education Evaluation Project.

Box 10–3 CDC's Use of Entertainment Education in an HIV Prevention Program

CDC has been managing the Modeling and Reinforcement to Combat HIV/AIDS (MARCH) program for about a decade.[a,b] They draw extensively on Bandura[c] and Bruner[d] as they explain the use of role modeling:

Role models can do several things. They can educate by providing basic information on how to change and by modeling the steps. They can also persuade and motivate by altering people's perceptions of the costs and benefits of a behavior. By showing the consequences of specific courses of action, models can illustrate how behavior may result in the achievement of desired goals or rewards and thus can influence people's expectations regarding the likely consequences of a behavior change. Anticipated consequences or outcomes can be powerful motivators.

To successfully change their behavior, people must not only want an outcome the behavior is likely to produce; they must also feel capable of performing the behavior and believe that by doing so they will obtain the desired outcome. Role models are particularly effective at enhancing belief in self-efficacy. When a man or woman sees a role model similar to him- or herself overcome an obstacle and achieve a desired reward, this provides information for social comparison, that is, "If he or she can do that, perhaps I can, too." Role models can demonstrate ways to think about a problem and cope with setbacks, as well as ways to achieve a goal. They can also help create an emotional stake in changing behavior, because we often want to emulate people with whom we have emotional bonds.

Role modeling is accomplished in many ways. In choosing Entertainment Education as a major component of our approach, we decided to emphasize its narrative, or storytelling, component. Scholars in disciplines from cognitive and social psychology to literary studies have argued that narrative forms govern thought: we process information by coding it into characters, scenes, and plots. In a sense, the MARCH projects can be thought of as a kind of narrative intervention that permits people "to understand the origins, meanings, and significance of [their] difficulties, and to do so in a way that makes change conceivable and attainable." One reason serial drama can educate is because it is closely aligned with the customs and norms of its audience and uses narrative forms with which they are familiar. Entertainment focuses on emotional as well as cognitive factors that influence behavior, and thus it keeps the attention of the intended audience.[e]

References

[a]Galavotti, C., Pappas-DeLuca, K. A., & Lansky, A. (2001). Modeling and reinforcement to combat HIV: The MARCH approach to behavior change. *American Journal of Public Health*, 91(10), 1602–1607.

[b]Petraglia, J., Galavotti, C., Harford, N., Pappas-DeLuca, K. A., Maungo, M. Applying Behavioral Science to Behavior Change Communication: The Pathways to Change Tools. *Health Promot Pract* 2007; 8; 384 originally published online Sep 5, 2007.

[c]Bandura, A. *Self-Efficacy: The exercise of control.* New York, NY: WH Freeman; 1997.

[d]Bruner, J. *Acts of meaning.* Cambridge, MA: Harvard University Press; 1990.

[e]Galavotti, C., Pappas-DeLuca, K. A., & Lansky, A. (2001). Modeling and reinforcement to combat HIV: The MARCH approach to behavior change. *American Journal of Public Health*, 91(10), 1603.

Source: Galavotti C, Pappas-DeLuca KA, Lansky A. Modeling and reinforcement to combat HIV: The MARCH approach to behavior change. *American Journal of Public Health.* 2001;91(10):1603.

who associates a level of quality with a particular brand. Many organizations have tried to implement this form of marketing communication for public health programs or initiatives over the past decade.[12]

truth® Campaign. The American Legacy Foundation launched the **truth® campaign*** in 2000 to prevent youth smoking. The campaign is "marketed as a popular youth brand that features risk-taking youth who may appear to be open to smoking, delivering facts and messages about the tobacco industry specifically. For example, many of the truth® advertisements focus on the marketing practices of the tobacco industry and their

efforts to obscure the health effects of smoking."[13] The national truth® campaign was built upon its successful originator in Florida. According to the Social Marketing Institute, the Florida TRUTH anti-smoking campaign built a new *product* and *branded* it.

The product/action was being cool by attacking adults who want to manipulate teens to smoke. The campaign reduced the *price* of the behavior (attacking adults) by selecting adults everyone agreed had been manipulating them. They created *places* where kids were found by means of a statewide train caravan and the founding of local "truth® chapters." And, of course, they used *promotion*—but promotion that went beyond the traditional media ads to having kids directly confront the tobacco industry and publicize this teen "rebellion"

---

*The truth® brand is always written in lowercase letters with a trademark sign.

Box 10–4 Social Marketing and VERB

VERB™—A Social Marketing Campaign to Increase Physical Activity Among Youth
Faye Wong, MPH, RD; Marian Huhman, PhD; Carrie Heitzler, MPH; Lori Asbury; Rosemary Bretthauer-Mueller; Susan McCarthy, MPH; Paula Londe

Abstract
The VERB campaign is a multiethnic media campaign with a goal to increase and maintain physical activity among *tweens*, or children aged nine to 13 years. Parents, especially mothers aged 29 to 46, and other sources of influence on tweens (e.g., teachers, youth program leaders) are the secondary audiences of the VERB initiative. VERB applies sophisticated commercial marketing techniques to address the public health problem of sedentary lifestyles of American children, using the social marketing principles of product, price, place, and promotion. In this paper, we describe how these four principles were applied to formulate the strategies and tactics of the VERB campaign, and we provide examples of the multimedia materials (e.g., posters, print advertising, television, radio spots) that were created.

Introduction
In response to increased concern about the health of our nation's youth, Congress appropriated $125 million in 2001 to the Centers for Disease Control and Prevention (CDC) to develop a national media campaign to change children's health behaviors. The CDC's response to this broad mandate was to focus on the sedentary lifestyle of young adolescents and to develop VERB™, a multiethnic campaign launched in June 2002 to increase and maintain physical activity among *tweens*, or children aged nine to 13 years. These children are between childhood and adolescence and are beginning to make their own lifestyle decisions. Parents, especially mothers aged 29 to 46, and other sources of influence on tweens (e.g., teachers, youth program leaders) provide the secondary audiences for the VERB initiative.

During the past 20 years, the combination of decreased physical activity and unhealthful eating has resulted in a doubling of the percentage of overweight children and adolescents.[a] Recent reports indicate that five of every eight children aged nine to 13 do not participate in any organized physical activity during their non-school hours, and almost one fourth do not engage in any free-time physical activity.[b] More than one in seven children aged six to 19 years are overweight,[c] and type 2 diabetes, a disease traditionally restricted to adults, has been reported among adolescents.[d]

Social Marketing Framework
VERB uses a social marketing framework that applies sophisticated commercial marketing techniques to address the public health problem of sedentary lifestyles among American children. The first year of the campaign consisted of national advertising, plus extra marketing activities in nine CDC-selected communities. The CDC based its selection of the nine communities on a variety of factors, including the size of the media market, racial and ethnic diversity, geographic diversity across the United States, existing infrastructure, and population size. Six of the nine communities received even more local advertising so that the CDC could evaluate whether the added media made a measurable difference in behavioral outcomes. These six evaluated communities were called "high-dose" communities.

Nine Communities Receiving Extra Marketing Activities

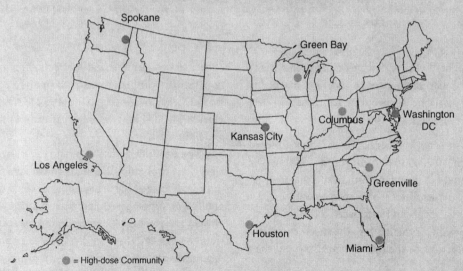

continues

Before campaign planners launched or named the campaign, they conducted extensive research on tweens and parents to gain an understanding of their attitudes, beliefs, and behaviors related to participation in physical activity. Research included numerous in-person focus groups, interviews, and ethnographic inquiries among multiethnic groups across the country. Additional audience research was conducted separately with African American, Hispanic/Latino, American Indian, and Asian American tweens and parents to gain deeper insights into their physical activity views and practices. The understandings gained contributed to the creation of VERB, a "for tweens, by tweens" brand that embraces the characteristics valued by tweens. VERB is not an acronym but is the word *verb* as a part of speech, meaning an action word. The tag line is, "It's what you do." (Formative research reports for the VERB campaign are available from http://www.cdc.gov/youthcampaign/research/resources.htm.)

Campaign planners applied the four *Ps* of commercial marketing—product, price, place, and promotion[e]—along with findings from the audience research to develop VERB as a social marketing campaign. In this paper, we describe how the four *Ps* helped to formulate the strategies and tactics of the VERB campaign.

Product

In social marketing, *product* is the desired behavior for the targeted audience. The VERB campaign's product is physical activity—a voluntary action that requires personal choice and internal motivation if it is to be performed repeatedly. The VERB "sales package" includes the intangible benefits of physical activity (e.g., enjoyment) in addition to tangible objects or services that support behavior change.[f]

For tweens, choosing to be physically active means giving up something they may like doing better. In today's world, numerous activities compete for tweens' attention, and tweens and their parents must overcome many barriers to become physically active, including lack of transportation, safety concerns, cost, and perceived lack of time.[b] Children report spending more than 4.5 hours daily watching television, playing video games, or using the computer; parents report their children's screen time to be almost 6.5 hours daily.[g] The VERB campaign's goal is to win or gain a greater market share of time tweens spend on sedentary activities.

The campaign's strategy is to influence participation in physical activity by associating it with the benefits that tweens value, such as spending time with friends, playing, having fun, having an opportunity to be active with parents, and gaining recognition from peers and adults. In addition, VERB offers tweens something else they value: the opportunity to explore and discover the world around them. Early VERB advertising stimulated curiosity about the brand and enticed tweens to identify and try the activities or VERBs (e.g., swim, run, jump) that most appealed to them.

Price

Price represents a balance of product benefits and costs to a consumer. When contemplating the purchase of a tangible product such as a tennis racquet, for example, a consumer balances the potential benefits of playing tennis against the price tag.[e,f] When the product is behavior change, the concept still holds: what are the benefits and costs of changing behavior?[h] For physical activity, the costs can be financial (e.g., price of dance classes), psychological (e.g., the tween does not "feel good enough" to participate in physical activity or organized sports), environmental (e.g., the neighborhood does not have sidewalks), or related to time (e.g., both parents work, leaving tweens with no time for supervised physical activity). VERB messages are designed to convince tweens and their parents that physical activity has the "right price"—that benefits outweigh costs.

Audience research yielded numerous insights into how tweens and parents view the benefits of physical activity; the CDC thus had information to show how the benefits of physical activity exceed those of non-active pursuits. The VERB campaign weaves these benefits throughout its messages, strategies, and tactics to make physical activity appealing and inviting to tweens.

Place

Place is where the target audience either performs the behavior or accesses programs or services; place must be readily available to enable the desired action.[e,f] A VERB place is where tweens can be physically active in a safe environment. As interest or demand rises, parents and communities need to increase the supply of accessible places and opportunities for tweens to be active every day. If the supply side is inadequate or inaccessible, tweens cannot act on their interest and intent to be more active. For VERB, a place may be a backyard, youth-serving organization, community-based organization, church, park or recreation department, school, public or private sports organization, business, government agency, or any other place that can provide facilities and year-round or periodic event-based opportunities for tweens to be physically active and have fun.

Partner organizations such as parks, schools, and youth-serving organizations can reap the benefits of tweens' affinity for the VERB brand and interest in becoming more active. Keeping VERB a "cool brand for tweens" is a critically important goal for partners as they collaborate on the campaign. (More information on keeping VERB "cool" is available from the VERB Coolness Tip Sheet.)

Promotion

Promotion is not simply the placement of advertisements—communication messages and activities are included as well, and those in charge of promotions must consider multiple ways to reach the target audience to promote the benefits of the behavior change, including its product, price, and place components.[f,g] The following sections provide descriptions and examples of the VERB campaign's messaging strategies, advertising and marketing strategies, and campaign tactics for reaching tweens and parents.

Messaging Strategies

Advertising and promotions do more than merely sell the features of a product; they depict a lifestyle that consumers aspire to achieve. By association, consumers perceive the product as providing the means to a desired outcome. In commercials, for example, a soft drink is more than a drink; it is a social experience. Running shoes are more than footwear; they make a statement about an individual's lifestyle. In the VERB campaign, commercial strategies for marketing to youth are applied to public health and used to "sell" physical activity to tweens, creating a distinct brand culture for VERB.

VERB aims to sell physical activity to consumers, but boys and girls cannot simply go to a store to buy it. Rather, tweens must develop a positive disposition to physical activity through a positive association and relationship with the VERB brand. To make the product of physical activity compelling and cool to tweens, VERB messages diverge from the "just-the-facts" delivery that is central to many public health campaigns. Rather than say, "Engage in moderate-to-vigorous physical activity for at least 60 minutes each day," the campaign asks tweens to discover new activities they like to do.

The fact that the campaign's brand name, VERB, immediately connotes action increases the audience's comprehension of the brand. To inspire tweens to do their own VERBs (physical activities), the campaign does not simply *tell* tweens that physical activity is for all tweens, it *shows* them with appealing visuals. Casting for television and print ads includes children of varied racial and ethnic backgrounds, body weights, and ability levels—including children with disabilities—to convey a sense of "kids like me do this" and "I can do that." VERB shows tweens playing backyard games in addition to participating in organized physical activities such as team sports.

If tweens are inspired by a VERB commercial and motivated to be active, parents will more likely support their participation. Had the campaign's strategy primarily focused on asking parents to encourage their children to be active, however, tweens might not have embraced VERB as their own brand. The campaign would have taken on a parenting agenda rather than becoming something for tweens. Notably, VERB features positive "can do" messages, not negative adult-delivered or adult-enforced "must do" or "don't do" messages.

Parents and others who influence tweens are asked to support, recognize, and praise children for being active; to encourage them to try new activities; and to be physically active as a family or group. VERB gives tips on how to communicate to tweens and engage them in being active in creative, positive, and fun ways. At the same time, facts on the health risks of inactivity and excessive screen time and on the benefits of being physically active are messages for adults. The messages are further tailored for different audiences, especially ethnic audiences, to address the specific parenting priorities learned through audience research.

All VERB campaign messages and the way they are presented in ads (i.e., television, radio, print) are tested with tween-aged focus groups to ensure they are motivating, clearly understood, and resonating positively. The messages are tested primarily with mothers to ensure they are acceptable and not offensive or inappropriate.

Advertising and Marketing Strategies

The VERB campaign strives for high brand awareness and affinity among tweens. The theory is that when tweens are positively bonded with VERB, they will be more receptive to messages about physical activity. In the first year of VERB, marketing efforts were dedicated to creating and introducing the VERB brand to tweens. As a previously nonexistent brand, VERB initially had no value to tweens. To sell VERB successfully to tweens as "their brand for having fun," the campaign associates itself with popular kids' brands, athletes, and celebrities, and activities and products that are cool, fun, and motivating.

Communications for parents and tweens are separated from each other to maintain tweens' positive affinity for the VERB brand and to avoid associating physical activity with something adults say "they have to do." Tweens' interests and trends evolve rapidly, whether the subject is music, clothing, electronics, or the enjoyment of being active. It is all about being "cool" to their friends and doing what's popular. The delicate balance of keeping the VERB brand cool for tweens while relying on parents and other adult influencers' support to help them be active is an ongoing campaign challenge.

VERB is distinct from traditional public service announcement (PSA) campaigns because advertising placement is purchased. In the first year of VERB, the campaign averaged 115 weekly gross rating points* (GRPs) in the national television media market with 50 percent more GRPs in the high-dose communities. The purchase of media enables the campaign to control when and where advertising

*Gross rating points is a measure of estimated exposure to advertising. Reach is defined as the proportion of the target audience that has an opportunity to be exposed to the ad. Frequency is the number of times an average target audience member is estimated to have an opportunity to view the advertisement in a given time period, usually weekly or monthly. Multiplying reach times frequency produces the GRP measure. Because GRPs are the product of reach and frequency estimates, a GRP estimate reflects many different possible exposure patterns. For example, if 10% of a population could be reached five times in a week, the weekly GRPs for that advertisement would be 50 (10 × 5); if 50% of the population could be reached once in a week, the GRPs would also be 50 (50 × 1).

continues

appears and to concentrate ad placement in delivery channels that reach the most tweens; popular delivery channels include kids' television networks (e.g., Nickelodeon, Cartoon Network) and teen magazines (e.g., *Teen People*, *Seventeen*). Furthermore, it assures that tweens are sufficiently exposed to the advertising to recognize and develop a personal relationship with the brand and to understand the campaign's messages to become active and have fun doing it. Having the funding to purchase media placements allows VERB to compete with commercial youth marketers to capture the attention and brand loyalty of tweens.

Campaign Tactics

VERB employs a broad mix of campaign tactics to reach tweens and their parents. The campaign is designed to surround tweens at home, in school, and in the community to give VERB visible presence in tweens' everyday lives.

Paid media advertising. The primary vehicle for reaching into the home is paid advertising in general market and ethnic media channels. VERB commercials air on age-appropriate television and radio channels such as Cartoon Network, Nickelodeon, The WB, ABC Saturday Morning Disney (including Radio Disney), Telemundo, and BET. Print advertising is placed in youth publications such as *Sports Illustrated for Kids*, *TIME for Kids*, *Teen People*, and *Seventeen*. Examples of parent publications include *Family Circle*, *Parent Magazine*, *Ebony*, and *Indian Country Today*. Spanish and Asian in-language advertising and advertorials appear in publications such as *Korea Times*, *World Journal*, and *Los Padres*. (An inventory of current VERB advertising is available from http://www.cdc.gov/youth-campaign/advertising/index.htm.)

Added-value opportunities. In addition to paid media placements, the campaign negotiates added-value opportunities from media partners. VERB's media partners donate their talent and properties or placements to help promote VERB's physical activity messages to tweens. For example, media partners have produced VERB PSAs using their television talent, such as the stars of The WB's *Gilmore Girls* and *7th Heaven* and properties such as Disney's *Kim Possible* and Cartoon Network's *Courage the Cowardly Dog*. The PSAs are aired in prime time during these shows. For parents, The WB produced VERB PSAs featuring Reba McEntire and CBS produced VERB PSAs featuring Deion Sanders. Other examples include VERB sponsorship of Nickelodeon's *Wild and Crazy Kids Show*, *Sports Illustrated for Kids' Road Show*, and *Teen People's Break for the Beach*. These added-value PSAs and sponsorships increase the "cool factor" and marketing reach of the VERB campaign among tweens.

Activity promotions. Several times a year, VERB features promotions that invite community-based organizations and schools throughout the United States to participate. For example, in 2003, VERB proclaimed the day of the summer solstice (the longest day of the year) as the "Longest Day of Play" and created a promotion with Radio Disney to motivate tweens to be active all day long. During fall 2003, when the clocks were turned back one hour from daylight saving to standard time, VERB featured its "Extra Hour for Extra Action" (EHEA) promotion, which included a kit of innovative and fun VERB materials for teachers and youth-serving organizations to use in activating tweens. Participating EHEA schools and organizations were eligible to apply for a small grant to support physical activity at the end of the three-week promotion.

Schools. School is a natural venue for reaching tweens; it also gives youth a prime opportunity to discover their interests and develop skills. For example, working with youth publications like *Weekly Reader* and *TIME for Kids*, VERB distributes custom-developed materials to middle schools throughout the country. Primedia's *Channel One* allows VERB advertising to reach tweens through schools. In-school vehicles include book covers, day planners, and customized lesson plans that incorporate physical activity into the classroom and encourage tweens to try many different VERBs.

Community-based events and grassroots marketing. VERB participated in existing community events, including cultural festivals such as the Harvest Moon Festival (Los Angeles, Calif), Calle Ocho (Miami, Fla), and the Gathering of Nations Pow Wow (Albuquerque, NM). At these grassroots community events, VERB hosted an "activity zone," a dedicated space for tweens to try out different activities such as kicking a soccer ball, dancing, performing martial arts, or other activities. Another community-based tactic is the use of "street teams," teams of five to eight college-aged men and women hired to engage tweens in being physically active at events and tween hangouts, including malls, parks, and community centers. Street teams create buzz about VERB and build affinity for the brand as tweens tell their friends and siblings about their fun experiences and show off their VERB premiums. The street teams distribute VERB-branded premiums to tweens, such as foot bags, T-shirts, temporary tattoos, and Frisbee disks.

Contests and sweepstakes. To increase the value of the product and reward tweens for being active, many media partners sponsor VERB contests and sweepstakes. For example, *Channel One* sponsored a pedometer-based middle-school competition, *Make Every Move Count*. The schools that accumulated the most steps won an "Action Pack" of physical activity equipment and materials to support their physical activity programs. In addition, *YM (Your Magazine)* featured the VERB *Move It to Groove It* contest, where tween contestants competed to win a video dance party for their entire school.

Public relations. VERB continuously communicates with the news media, stakeholders, and partner organizations to offer information on the importance of youth physical activity to parents and other influencers and to spotlight current campaign activities, such as events and promotions. The campaign maintains good relationships with key members of the tween/teen and parent news media to keep them current on the campaign and to serve as resources for information about youth physical activity, childhood overweight, and related topics. News media materials are tailored to meet specific needs, media tours are conducted in key markets, and special news media coverage is arranged when appropriate.

Community partnerships. In the first year of VERB, the campaign developed local partnerships in the nine cities that received extra marketing activities to bring the VERB brand to life and to establish a foundation of support in those locations. Now, the goal of VERB is to recruit organizations across the country to become site partners (organizations that can provide opportunities for tweens to be physically active) or outreach partners (organizations that can reach parents or influence the environment to support tweens' participation in physical activity). The campaign is actively reaching out to organizations that have a network of affiliates or chapters across the country and also is contacting regional, state, and local organizations. (More information on VERB partnerships is available from http://www.cdc.gov/youthcampaign/partners/index.htm.)

Corporate partnerships. VERB also is seeking partnerships with corporations to extend the reach and appeal of the campaign to tweens. For example, VERB is successfully negotiating partnerships with professional sports leagues for its ProVERB initiative; those who have made commitments include the National Football League, National Hockey League, Major League Soccer, and Women's Tennis Association. These sports leagues will provide content for the VERBnow.com Web site for tweens, donate athlete-signed merchandise for prizes, and provide opportunities for VERB sponsorship of their grassroots sports clinics.

Web sites. In partnership with AOL, VERB has created http://www.VERBnow.com, a Web site designed exclusively for tweens that includes the VERB Recorder, where tweens can report their participation in physical activity and become eligible to win prizes for being active. A parent site, http://www.VERBparents.com, includes in-language pages (Spanish, Chinese, Korean, and Vietnamese) in partnership with ethnic media partners. In addition, http://www.cdc.gov/VERB was created for partners and stakeholders to access information about the VERB campaign and to view advertising.

Summary

The VERB campaign is a public health and marketing partnership based on the social marketing principles of product, price, place, and promotion. It brings together a diverse array of public health, marketing, and community experts to engage tweens in being physically active every day by playing, having fun, and trying new VERBs, or new ways to be physically active. A lifestyle or behavior change such as increasing physical activity is difficult to achieve and even more difficult to sustain. One can speculate, however, that success in changing behavior among tweens is more likely to be achieved when the following conditions are met: consumers have an in-depth understanding of the product and price associated with it, they have easy access to appropriate places where they can perform the behavior in everyday life, and product promotion portrays benefits in a positive, appealing fashion and reaches audiences through channels they value.

Rigorous multiyear evaluation of the VERB campaign will determine its effectiveness in motivating tweens to be more active. To ensure objectivity, the CDC has retained an evaluation contractor. The outcome evaluation is designed as a nationally representative longitudinal study of more than 6000 tweens and their parents across the country, half of whom are from the six high-dose communities. A baseline survey was conducted before the campaign's launch in June 2002. Two follow-up surveys, one conducted in 2003 and one to be completed in 2004, will measure the effectiveness of the campaign. The evaluation methodology, a longitudinal dose-response analysis, controls for numerous baseline factors and allows evaluators to measure changes in physical activity specifically attributable to the VERB campaign.

Acknowledgments

The authors acknowledge and thank former CDC VERB campaign strategists Michael Greenwell, Suzanne Gates, and Claudia Parvanta; former campaign team members Jami Fraze, Victor Medrano, and Enbal Shacham; and current campaign staff Bill Wood, Wanda Price, Juanita Mondesire, Lula Anna Green, Heidi Melancon, Dana Robinson, Cynthia Mitchell, and Judy Berkowitz. We also

continues

thank the VERB campaign contractors Frankel (Chicago, Ill); Saatchi & Saatchi (New York, NY), Publicis Dialog (Chicago, Ill), Garcia 360 (San Antonio, Tex); G&G Advertising (Alburquerque, NM); A Partnership, Inc. (New York, NY); PFI Marketing (New York, NY); and Westat (Rockville, MD).

Author Information
Corresponding author: Faye Wong, MPH, RD, VERB Campaign, Division of Adolescent and School Health (DASH), National Center for Chronic Disease Prevention and Health Promotion (NCCDPHP), Centers for Disease Control and Prevention, 4770 Buford Hwy NE, Mail Stop K-85, Atlanta, GA 30341-3717. Telephone: 770-488-6427. E-mail: fwong@cdc.gov.

Author affiliations: Marian Huhman, PhD, Lori Asbury, Rosemary Bretthauer-Mueller, Susan McCarthy, MPH, Paula Londe, VERB Campaign, DASH, NCCDPHP, CDC, Atlanta, Ga; Carrie Heitzler, MPH, VERB Campaign, Division of Nutrition and Physical Activity, NCCDPHP, CDC, Atlanta, GA.

References

[a]Ogden CL, Flegal KM, Carroll MD, Johnson CL. Prevalence and trends in overweight among US children and adolescents, 1999-2000. *JAMA* 2002;288:1728–1732.

[b]Centers for Disease Control and Prevention. Physical activity levels among children aged 9-13 years—United States, 2002. *MMWR Morb Mortal Wkly Rep* 2003;52 (33):785–788.

[c]Centers for Disease Control and Prevention, National Center for Health Statistics. National Health and Nutrition Examination Survey; NHES 11/111 (1963-70) NHANES I (1971-74), NHANES II (1976-80), NHANES III (1988-94). Hyattsville (MD): National Center for Health Statistics; 2003. NHANES 1999 available from: URL: http://www.cdc.gov/nchs/about/major/nhanes/ Databriefs.htm.

[d]Goran MI, Ball GD, Cruz ML. Obesity and risk of Type 2 diabetes and cardiovascular disease in children and adolescents. *J Clin Endocrinol Metab* 2003;88:1417–1427.

[e]Andreasen AR. *Marketing social change: Changing behavior to promote health, social development, and the environment.* San Francisco (CA): Jossey-Bass; 1995. 368 p.

[f]Turning Point Social Marketing Collaborative, Centers for Disease Control and Prevention, Academy for Educational Development. *CDCynergy: Social marketing edition*, version 1.0 [CD ROM]. Atlanta (GA): CDC, Office of Communication; 2003.

[g]Woodard EH. *Media in the home 2000: The fifth annual survey of parents and children.* Philadelphia (PA): The Annenberg Public Policy Center of the University of Pennsylvania; 2000.

[h]Kotler P, Roberto N, Lee N. *Social marketing: Improving the quality of life*, 2nd ed. Thousand Oaks (CA): Sage Publications; 2002.

Source: Wong F, Huhman M, Heitzler C, Asbury L, Bretthauer-Mueller R, McCarthy S, et al. VERB™—A social marketing campaign to increase physical activity among youth. *Prev Chronic Dis* [serial online] July 2004. Available from: http://www.cdc.gov/pcd/issues/2004/jul/04_0043.htm. Accessed December 25, 2009.

in the popular media. The campaign routinely carried out surveys of its target audience that allowed the campaign to discover important micro-market segments (South Florida Hispanics), where impacts were lagging: "[F]rom 1998 to 2000, the percent of Florida middle school students who smoked cigarettes in the past 30 days fell from 18.5 to 8.6 percent while the percentage for high school students went from 27.4 to 20.9."[14]

We will discuss truth® much more in the next chapter on media strategy and implementation.

Media Literacy. As just mentioned, the truth® campaign uses branding, as well as a highly ironic multimedia strategy,[15] to empower young people to see the deceptions and misrepresentations used by the tobacco industry. Underlying this approach is essentially an education/empowerment strategy called media literacy. Shepherd defined **media literacy** as, "an informed, critical understanding of the mass media. It involves examining the techniques, technologies and institutions involved in media production; being able to critically analyze media messages; and recognizing the role audiences play in making meaning from those messages."[16] Media literacy is used chiefly with middle school students to enable them to evaluate advertising that explicitly targets them.

Other Practice Strategies That Are User-Centered, MultiChannel, and MultiMedia

Demographic Targeting. For about half a century, **targeting**, or communicating with audience segments comprised of members who share selected characteristics, was the most strategic communication method that we had. We have grown up with targeting in mass media to the point that we are fairly oblivious to it. For the past 100 years of advertising, consumer product ads (e.g., laundry detergent, hand soap, food to be eaten at home, clothing) featured women and were directed to women, while "big ticket" items and "spontaneous purchases" (e.g., cars, televisions, sporting events, fast food), have been predominantly targeted to men. (Watch prime time television and keep count.)

As a media channel strategy, targeting is still widely used by both commercial and social marketing. In the United States, there are radio, television, Internet, and print media that reach out *exclusively* to children (of all ages), and a spectrum of adults from first-time parents to seniors. There are media segmented by gender identity, ethnic identity, and language (there are approximately 50 different in-language media). And this says nothing about special interest media (*Aikido* to zippers). But how different are the message and creative strategy carried by these different media and channels?

In the early days of advertising, little was done to actually change the "creative" (images, copy, sound) that went out to different media. According to Davis, the publishers of *Ebony* magazine (which launched in 1945) started the trend of matching creative to how its readers saw themselves:

> Through its advertising policy, *Ebony* advocated the use of black models and encouraged advertisers to treat the black market as separate and unique because blacks had a psychological need for "self-identification"…By 1968, *Ebony* was running full-page ads in *Advertising Age* and the *New York Times* pointing out the quality consciousness and spending habits of black consumers, while describing the size and wealth of the black market.[17]

The effectiveness of *ethnic target marketing* made itself clear to commercial advertisers. Whether selling niche products, (e.g., cosmetics or hair care designed to meet the needs and desires of this market), or mass-market products, a return on investment supported this form of targeting. Public health was another story, with program managers questioning whether segments were large enough, and could be reached effectively, by using different media and channels. More often than desired, a "generic" campaign was created because differentiated media, from production to dissemination, were too expensive.

Probably the largest public health campaign that has effectively reached out to distinct ethnic groups by using a targeted "partnership" strategy is the National Diabetes Education Program (NDEP). NDEP worked with representatives of minority serving organizations to create media strategies and products that would resonate most with these distinct audiences. **Figure 10–1** features a set of photographs used in targeted print ads.

An extensive set of materials for different ethnic groups can be accessed from the program website.[18]

Behavioral Targeting. There are times when demographic distinctions are less important than behavioral intention, or having an illness or condition. For example, the folic acid campaign segmented women according to their desire to become pregnant versus being not ready to think about children. This attitude crossed ethnic lines, and the first wave of campaign materials featured multicultural women in the same television or print ads. Women who have recently learned they have breast cancer similarly pay little attention to the ethnicity of the person on the cover of a brochure and prefer to see and hear from women of any background who have survived the disease.

But, because people tend to pay less attention to prevention than to treatment and cures for a disease or condition they have, communicators use more peripheral cues of ethnicity, shared attitudes, age, and other indicators that a particular media piece is meant for a particular audience. Many nutrition, smoking cessation, and physical activity campaigns have been developed that use stage-based segments, or *behavioral/ attitudinal profiles*, to identify audience groups. Until the advent of the Internet, there was something of a shot in the dark as to how these media were disseminated, except through interpersonal channels (see the later discussion). For the most part, mass media campaigns featured different versions of creative to appeal to these different behavioral segments—but the channels were the same.

Target Marketing on Steroids. Can you give the Post Office direct mail with instructions to deliver it to the households that are making plans to become gym members? The answer is, yes you can send letters directly to aspiring gym members—sort of, if you've preaddressed the envelopes. And, that's where the new targeting services come in. You might find it quite frightening to know how much is known about us based on our Internet use, credit cards, magazine subscriptions, and even supermarket scanner swipes. For the direct-mail question, it is possible to use a service to pull households that have made inquiries into gym membership by means of the Internet or direct mail. One could, theoretically, send information supporting this positive step to those households. But, it is questionable as to whether this strategy would be worth the expense.

An example of a major marketing database is Mediamark Research & Intelligence (MRI),[19] which annually interviews

FIGURE 10–1 National Diabetes Education Program. Print Advertising for Different Ethnic Groups.

All ads featured this heading: Managing Diabetes. I made a plan. It wasn't easy, but I did it. So can you. It's not easy, but it's worth it.

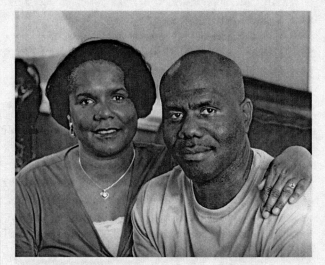

Brenda and her husband, Javier

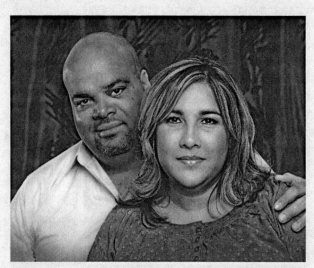

Haywood and his wife, Ellen

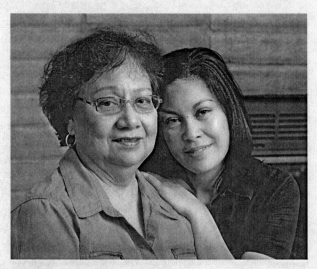

Sorcy and her daughter, Rinabeth

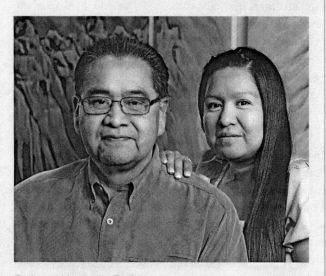

Rudy and his cousin, Faylinn

Source: National Diabetes Education Program (NDEP) is jointly sponsored by the National Institutes of Health (NIH) and the Centers for Disease Control and Prevention (CDC) with the support of more than 200 partner organizations.

26,000 consumers in-person, at home. According to the MRI website, their *Survey of the American Consumer™*

collects information on adult consumers' media choices, product usage, demographics, lifestyle and attitudes. Usage of nearly 6,000 product and service brands across 550 categories are measured, along with the readership of hundreds of magazines and newspapers, Internet usage, TV viewership to the program level, national and local radio listening, Yellow Pages usage and Out-of-Home exposure.

It is important to know about the availability of commercial marketing databases and surveys, as well as state and local data-gathering activities. For example, in Philadelphia, the Public Health Management Corporation (PHMC),[20] a nonprofit organization, conducts a biannual survey of more than 13,000 residents (children, adults, and seniors) living in the five-county southeastern Pennsylvania region. The survey investigates health topics including reported health status, access to and use of health care, personal health behaviors, health screening, health insurance status, and so forth.

The bottom line is that before conducting new survey research on a particular topic in a particular area, it is important to find out if another organization is doing so. After assessing whether the rigor and parameters of the organization's methodologies suit a program's needs, it will probably be less expensive—and yield better-quality results—to license the data or add a question to an **omnibus survey** (a survey, like that conducted by the PHMC, that allows organizations to purchase additional questions for specific analyses.)

In sum, targeting is a *mass* media strategy. When we use targeting, we try to create materials that appeal to audience segments that share characteristics. The goal is that our intended audience will recognize themselves in these materials and respond positively, but we know that we will not reach everyone we planned to reach. At the same time, people whom we did not expect to identify with the messages and materials will also find them useful. Targeting is a good, but imperfect way of refining our message, media, and channel strategy to improve reach and impact.

Tailoring. **Tailoring** takes a completely different tack away from reaching groups. With tailoring, we use information technology to simulate a conversation with an individual whom we have gotten to know pretty well. We plan to put the tailored material virtually into the person's hands by means of a direct channel, such as the mail, an in-person interaction, the Internet, or phone (or any personal communication device). Rimer and Kreuter define tailoring as a process for creating individualized communications by gathering and assessing personal data related to a given health outcome in order to determine the most appropriate information or strategies to meet that person's unique needs.[21] An example of a tailored piece appears in **Box 10–5** from the Center for Excellence in Cancer Communication Research at the University of Michigan.

As we have mentioned before, tailoring can be an extreme actualization of the ELM if several noncentral elements, such as demography and cultural references, are included in the tailoring factors. In addition to these, most tailored materials include theory-based elements such as an adoption readiness stage, self-efficacy and outcome expectations, and message frames. Finally, the central information pertaining to the intervention of most relevance to this individual is included. According to a recent review by Lustria et al., "Tailored interventions have led to positive outcomes across a variety of interventions, such as binge drinking,[22] nutrition and diet,[23] and smoking.[24] Moreover, recent reviews[25] and meta-analyses[26] have reported incremental benefits for tailored versus nontailored interventions in the literature as a whole."[27] **Box 10–6** provides a full explanation of tailoring from the second Center for Excellence in Cancer Communication Research at Washington University in St. Louis, Missouri.

Interpersonal Communication. **Interpersonal communication** is defined as person-to-person or small group interaction and exchange. It is essential for when a dialogue, or two-way communication, is necessary to diagnose a problem, help someone make a plan or decision, or direct someone to an appropriate resource. Persons who routinely use interpersonal communication are healthcare providers, but peer group facilitators and hotline call respondents also need to learn, and apply, best practices in interpersonal communication. Both verbal and nonverbal communication skills are important. These are addressed in Chapter 15.

Interpersonal communication is often part of multilevel, multimedia communication interventions, where individual behavior change is necessary to achieve a health outcome. Because of the burden of chronic disease, public health has directed considerable resources to creating effective counseling and other interpersonal approaches to help participants reduce or eliminate tobacco use, improve diets, increase physical activity, or seek screening services for cancer (mammograms, colorectal cancer screening, PSA tests). Similarly, interpersonal approaches have been used extensively in publicly funded programs to counsel women on prenatal care and to promote breastfeeding and optimal infant feeding practices (e.g., Women, Infants and Children, or WIC[28]). In addition, interpersonal communication is central to patient–healthcare provider interaction, including newly emerging fields of patient navigation, or hotline response. Hence, there are numerous situations in which interpersonal communication would be the lead strategy in a health communication plan, either alone or in combination with some mass media support.

Box 10–7 features an interpersonal counseling success story from the Well-Integrated Screening and Evaluation for Women Across the Nation (WISEWOMAN) program. It has been funded by the CDC to promote chronic disease prevention in women.

Patient Navigation. A last practice strategy to touch on in this chapter is **patient navigation**, which relies on interpersonal communication, although often delivered over the telephone. Patient navigators are specially trained health educators,

Box 10–5 Sample of a Tailored Message Page and Tailoring Elements

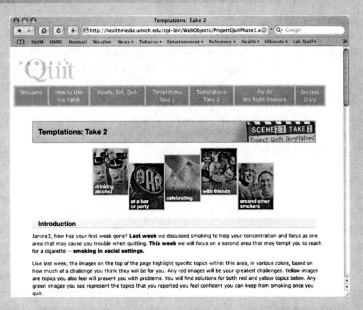

Characteristics that cause text/images to appear (Based on participant survey responses):

Red images = Very low self-efficacy

Yellow images = Low self-efficacy

Name, Quit date

Main barrier to quitting

Overall confidence about quitting

<u>Confidence about specific barrier to quitting</u>

Smoking weak spots (environmental)

Motivation to quit (Others)

Current smoking environment

<u>Lifestyle habits—regular physical activity</u>

You feel confident overall that you can quit for good, but <u>you are having doubts about keeping from smoking specifically during social times.</u> Let's take a closer look at what may work for or against you as you prepare to deal with the social scene without smoking.

Potential Concerns:
Bars and bowling alleys. Stay away from them or limit your time there significantly.

What Can Help:
You told us that people in your life would be disappointed if you continued to smoke. Look to them for support and encouragement when you are struggling.

A normal day for you doesn't include being around many, if any, smokers. This will definitely be a plus in the first few weeks.

<u>Since you exercise regularly, make it a social event. Get a group together for a game of volleyball, basketball, or a hike in the woods.</u>

Source: Example based on Centers for Excellence in Cancer Communication Research tailoring example, Victor Strecher, Principal Investigator, http://chcr.umich.edu/how_we_do_it/tailoring/examples/tailoring_efficacy.pdf. Strecher, V. CHCR. University of Michigan

Box 10–6 What Is Tailoring?

By Matt Kreuter, Principal Investigator

Tailored communication is intended to reach one specific person, based on characteristics that are unique to that person, related to the outcome of interest, and have been derived from an individual assessment. New communication technologies have made it not only possible but practical to collect individual-level data from large populations and use that information to customize educational and behavior change materials to individuals' unique needs.

Tailored health communication greatly reduces the burden of search and retrieval imposed by generic materials, and provides information that is truly individualized, not just superficially labeled with the recipient's name.

In contrast to other communication approaches, tailored communication can identify and address the specific informational and behavioral needs of any one person.

The process of tailoring health messages is a lot like the process an actual tailor uses in making custom-fit clothing. A tailor takes a customer's measurements; asks about preferences for fabric, color, and style; and uses this information to create a suit to fit that one customer. Likewise, a tailored health communication program measures a participant's needs, interests, and concerns, and uses that information to create messages and materials to fit that one person.

Tailored materials address only those factors known to be important to an individual recipient. For example, most smoking cessation materials address the benefits of quitting in some way or another. These benefits may include improved health, reduced disease risk, saving money, gaining control over your life, and improved physical appearance. But not every smoker will value each of these benefits. For some, the sole motive for quitting may be financial. For others, improved appearance. And even for those motivated by health benefits, there will be some who want to quit because they have been diagnosed with a smoking-related condition, others who want to prevent such illness, and still others who want to quit to protect the health of non-smokers in their family. If it is indeed important to address the benefits of cessation in quitting materials, it makes sense to frame these benefits in the terms most salient to an individual smoker. Tailored materials can do this.

The tailoring approach of conducting individual assessments and providing individualized feedback is not new, nor is its use unique to health educators. It is commonly employed by successful real estate agents, physicians, teachers, brokers, and salespersons, all of whom identify a client's needs through observation and inquiry, and use that information to customize solutions. In cancer prevention, individual counseling for behavior modification such as improved nutrition, increased physical activity, and smoking cessation is also based on this approach. In many ways, the interpersonal contact, interactivity, and immediacy of feedback that can be provided in one-on-one counseling makes this approach more desirable than a computer tailored print communication program. But the impact of counseling on the health of populations can be limited by cost and by the relatively limited number of individuals who can be reached by a small cadre of trained professionals. A skilled counselor can do everything a tailored message program can do except be available at all times to simultaneously serve multiple and diverse members of mass populations.

Why tailor health communication materials?

According to Petty and Cacioppo's elaboration likelihood model, people are more likely to actively and thoughtfully process information if they perceive it to be personally relevant. The model is based on the premise that under many conditions, people are active information processors—considering messages carefully, relating them to other information they've encountered, and comparing them to their own past experiences. Studies have shown that messages processed in this way (i.e., "elaborated" upon) tend to be retained for a longer period of time and are more likely to lead to permanent change. The rationale for using tailored communication follows from this theory, and can be summarized as a five-part logic sequence:

• By tailoring materials, superfluous information is eliminated.
• The information that remains is more personally relevant to the recipient.
• People pay more attention to information they perceive to be personally relevant.
• Information that is attended to is more likely to have an effect than that which is not.
• When attended to, information that addresses the unique needs of a person will be useful in helping them become and stay motivated, acquire new skills, and enact and sustain desired lifestyle changes.

We would expect, therefore, that compared to generic materials, tailored materials might elicit greater attention, comprehension, likelihood of discussing the content with others, and likelihood of behavior change. Several well-designed randomized studies,

continues

including those we have conducted, have reported findings consistent with these expectations. For example, tailored messages—though imperfect as described previously—are significantly more likely than generic messages to be read and remembered, saved, discussed with others, and to have generated a simple response. In addition, tailored messages are more likely to be perceived by readers as interesting, personally relevant, and having been written especially for them. These outcomes are, of course, central to many public health education efforts.

In addition to the theoretical rationale for tailoring, there is also a strong *public health* rationale supporting its use. Because tailored materials can be computer-generated, they have the potential to reach large populations at relatively modest costs. As a result, the traditional public health approach of using mass media to disseminate health information could eventually be supplanted with what may be termed "micro-mass media" or "mass customization"—allowing the fine-tuning of message content to individuals' needs, but on the scale of mass communication. This combination of broad reaching, assessment-based, low cost, individualized communication has led to some to characterize tailoring as a "promising approach" for population disease prevention.

Tailored health communication has shown promise in helping certain adult populations change a range of cancer-related behaviors including cigarette smoking, dietary fat consumption, fruit and vegetable consumption, physical inactivity, and mammography. Tailoring has also been shown to help change a person's inaccurate perceptions of their own cancer risk. In the first ever review of tailoring studies, Skinner and colleagues concluded that tailored print materials have the ability to attract notice and readership, influence behavior change, and support other interventions with shared objectives.

Source: Health Communications Research Laboratory, Washington University in St. Louis. http://hcrl.wustl.edu/content/what.html. Used with permission. Kreuter, M. CECCR, WUSt. L.

Box 10–7 Example of a Success Story from North Carolina WISEWOMAN Program Using Interpersonal Practice Strategy

A New Leaf Helps North Carolina Women Cope with Emotional Addiction to Tobacco

Tobacco use is an integral part of North Carolina's culture. Many North Carolina women grew up watching their mothers and fathers smoke, or worse, lighting cigarettes for parents. Today, 27% of the women who are active participants in North Carolina's WISEWOMAN program are smokers. They often use tobacco to try to cope with stresses in their lives. Sally, for example, is a WISEWOMAN participant who started smoking in her early 50s to relax. She was having personal problems and thought smoking would help her escape feelings of depression and anxiety.

Coordinators working in WISEWOMAN clinics talk to women every day who are physically and emotionally addicted to tobacco. They encourage these women to quit by telling them about the state tobacco cessation QuitLine and giving them brochures on women and smoking. Perhaps most importantly, they rely on the lifestyle intervention *A New Leaf . . . Choices for Healthy Living* as they coach women through the difficult process of quitting.

The first time a woman visits a WISEWOMAN clinic she gets a copy of *A New Leaf*. The manual is written for WISEWOMAN participants and is designed to be a workbook the women can use to improve their health. A WISEWOMAN staff member goes through the *New Leaf* manual with each woman to identify her current health practices and attitudes, help her make lifestyle changes one step at a time, and increase her confidence in making these changes.

WISEWOMAN staff members use *A New Leaf* to determine how ready and willing a woman is to make a lifestyle change that will improve her health. If she is a smoker, staff will use the smoking assessment tool, which is part of the manual, to find out why she smokes, when she smokes most, and any special barriers to quitting.

"*A New Leaf* is a great tool," WISEWOMAN coordinator Lori Green says. "It helps us find out if there are things going on in a woman's life that influence her smoking. Maybe she's worried she will gain weight if she quits, or maybe she's depressed, like Sally (not her real name), and smoking helps her forget about her problems for a few minutes." WISEWOMAN Health Educator Belinda Branson uses *A New Leaf* manual to help North Carolina women set a quit date, deal with triggers to smoking, and understand how their bodies will change when they quit smoking.

"These women are dealing with a number of issues: low income, unemployment, lack of health care, and multiple health problems," Director Carolyn R. Townsend adds. "We try to be someone they can talk to about what they are struggling with. We provide information about resources that might be of help to the women."

A New Leaf also offers a list of quitting tips. It advises WISEWOMAN staff on how to help women set a quit date and deal with triggers to smoking. It also explains how a woman's body will change when she quits smoking, what will happen the first day, the first month, and the first year after she quits. "Sharing this information with women who smoke—even if they are at the pre-contemplative stage—it helps motivate them to quit," Lori says.

Importance of Success

Since 2000, the North Carolina WISEWOMAN program has helped 14% of its enrollees who smoke to quit using tobacco. Sally quit smoking in April 2003 and is still enrolled in the WISEWOMAN program.

Lessons Learned

- Women can get physically and emotionally addicted to tobacco. Identify ways to help them address both types of addiction.
- Women who are struggling to quit smoking need someone to talk to about the emotional issues that may play a role in their habit. Using a structured tool can give staff a consistent way to help women set healthy goals and quit smoking. Be someone they can trust and offer them a safe time to talk about their problems.
- A well-developed lifestyle intervention that addresses the social influences of smoking can assist women in their efforts to stop smoking.

Success Story 10	*A New Leaf* Helps North Carolina Women Cope with Emotional Addiction to Tobacco
Location	North Carolina
Focus	Help women quit smoking by addressing their physical and emotional addiction to tobacco.
Strategy	WISEWOMAN staff members have used the lifestyle intervention *A New Leaf . . . Choices for Healthy Living* to guide women through the process of quitting smoking. They lead each WISEWOMAN participant through the manual step by step to help her make healthy lifestyle changes.
Early Successes	The assessment tools in the *New Leaf* manual help each WISEWOMAN participant identify the emotional issues related to her smoking and the barriers to quitting. WISEWOMAN staff members support women who are trying to make lifestyle changes by helping them set realistic goals for improving their health and quitting smoking. Since 2000, the North Carolina WISEWOMAN program has helped 14% of its enrollees who smoke to quit using tobacco.
Story Developed By	Carolyn R. Townsend, RN, BSN, MPH WISEWOMAN Project Coordinator North Carolina Department of Health and Human Services Division of Public Health

For program contact information visit http://www.cdc.gov/wisewoman

Source: Townsend CR. Success Story 10. http://www.cdc.gov/wisewoman

nurses, or social workers who provide help directly to patients or caregivers in how to work through the many barriers of the healthcare system. The concept is particularly tied to health literacy, as well as the idea of a "medical home," where we are beginning to recognize that there are so many obstacles to all but the most tenacious individuals in getting their healthcare needs met. See **Table 10–3** for examples of obstacles and how patient navigators assist clients.[29]

CONCLUSION

This chapter has discussed key characteristics of strategic health communication and how to integrate them into various practice strategies. The next chapter shows how to select channels and develop media that support these strategies. This is followed by the logistical steps to deliver the communication program.

TABLE 10–3 How Does a Navigator Help Patients Overcome Barriers?

Types of Barriers	Specific Barriers to Care	Solutions to Barriers
Financial/Economic	Lack of or inadequate insurance	Guide patients to sources of financial support
	Inability to afford medication or healthcare items	Answer questions about forms for financial and other types of assistance
Education	Low level of health literacy or health education	Help complete paperwork
	Difficulty completing forms and follow-up	Explain the healthcare system
	Fatalistic feelings about cancer	Educate patients on diagnoses and medical procedures
Logistic	Child-care responsibilities	Help with arranging child care or elder care
	Conflicts between clinic and work schedules	
Transportation	No car or no access to public transportation	Help patient find resources for transportation
	Difficulty arranging reliable transportation	
	Living far from treatment facilities (rural areas)	
Language and Culture	Cultural beliefs regarding treatment such as fear or mistrust of the healthcare system	Help patient to access culturally appropriate, supportive care
	Difficulty speaking or reading English	Direct patient to language interpretation services
	Difficulty communicating desires and needs	Communicate with providers about unique patient needs
Healthcare System	Lack of coordination between services	Coordinate appointments for timely delivery of diagnostic and treatment services
	Information for care not available when needed	Ensure that medical records arrive at scheduled appointments
Emotional	Delayed or refusal of care due to fear, stress, or financial burden	Provide health information about specific diseases or treatments
		Direct patients to support groups or counseling services

Source: Colorado Patient Navigator Training Program, Copyright 2008. http://www.patientnavigatortraining.org/course1/module1/overcome_barriers.htm

KEY TERMS

Entertainment Education (EE)
Interpersonal communication
Intervention Mapping (IM)
Media literacy
Omnibus survey
Patient navigation
Performance objective

Practice strategy
SMART approach
Social marketing
Tailoring
Targeting
Theory-based methods
truth® campaign

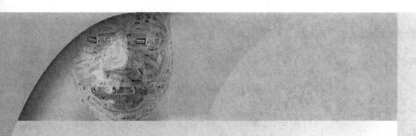

Chapter Questions

1. Why are the principles for strategic health communication listed in the order in which they are?

2. Which do you think is the most difficult of the SMART objectives to achieve?

3. What are the theory-informed methods that underlie Entertainment Education?

4. Describe three strategies for targeting.

5. What sorts of information would you be able to include in a tailored message page?

6. What are the pros and cons of interpersonal communication strategies?

REFERENCES

1. O'Sullivan GA, Yonkler JA, Morgan W, Merritt AP. *A Field Guide to Designing a Health Communication Strategy.* Baltimore, MD: Johns Hopkins Bloomberg School of Public Health/Center for Communication Programs; March 2003. Available at: http://www.jhuccp.org/pubs/fg/02/index.shtml. Accessed January 12, 2010.

2. http://www.cdc.gov/dhdsp/state_program/evaluation_guides/smart_objectives.htm

3. Bartholomew LK, Parcel GS, Kok G, Gottlieb NH. Planning health promotion programs: An intervention mapping approach; 2003. Slides downloaded from the University of Texas, Health Science Center. Available at: www.cpcrn.org/pubs/Intervention%20Mapping%20Presentation.ppt. Accessed November 2009.

4. Singhal A, Cody MJ, Rogers E, Sabido M (Eds.). *Entertainment-Education and Social Change: History, Research, and Practice.* Mawah, NJ: Lawrence Erlbaum; 2004.

5. Galavotti C, Pappas-DeLuca KA, Lansky A. Modeling and reinforcement to combat HIV: The MARCH approach to behavior change. *American Journal of Public Health.* 2001;91(10):1602–1607.

6. Petraglia J, Galavotti C, Harford N, Pappas-DeLuca K, Maungo M. Applying behavioral science to behavior change communication: The pathways to change tools. *Health Promot Pract.* 2007;8:384, originally published online Sep 5, 2007.

7. Bandura, A. *Self-efficacy: The exercise of control.* New York, NY: WH Freeman; 1997.

8. Bruner, J. *Acts of meaning.* Cambridge, MA: Harvard University Press; 1990.

9. Galavotti et al. Modeling and reinforcement to combat HIV, 1603.

10. Petty RE, Cacioppo JT. *Communication and Persuasion: Central and Peripheral Routes to Attitude Change.* New York: Springer-Verlag; 1986.

11. Wong F, Huhman M, Heitzler C, Asbury L, Bretthauer-Mueller R, McCarthy S, et al. VERB™—A social marketing campaign to increase physical activity among youth. *Prev Chronic Dis* [serial online] July 2004. Available at: http://www.cdc.gov/pcd/issues/2004/jul/04_0043.htm. Accessed December 25, 2009.

12. Kirby SD, Taylor MK, Freimuth VS, Parvanta CF. Identify building and branding at CDC: A case study. *Social Marketing Quarterly.* 2001;7:16–35.

13. Davis KC, Matthew L, Farrelly C, Messeri P, Duke J. The impact of national smoking prevention campaigns on tobacco-related beliefs, intentions to smoke and smoking initiation: Results from a longitudinal survey of youth in the United States. *Int J Environ Res Public Health.* 2009 February;6(2):722–740.

14. http://www.social-marketing.org/success/cs-floridatruth.html. Accessed October 14, 2009.

15. See, for example, Do you have what it takes to be a tobacco company executive. Available at: http://www.thetruth.com/?utm_source=google&utm_medium=cpc&utm_term=truth_campaign&utm_content=Brand&utm_campaign=Brand.

16. Shepherd R. Why teach media literacy, *Teach Magazine,* Quadrant Educational Media Services, Toronto, ON, Canada; Oct/Nov 1993.

17. Davis JF. Ebony advertising in 1968: Mirror of key events in contemporary black America. Available at: http://faculty.quinnipiac.edu/charm/CHARM%20proceedings/CHARM%20article%20archive%20pdf%20format/Volume%209%201999/253%20davis.pdf. Accessed October 15, 2009.

18. www.ndep.nih.gov

19. http://www.mediamark.com/

20. http://www.phmc.org/site/index.php?option=com_content&view=article&id=66&Itemid=20

21. Rimer BK, Kreuter MW. Advancing tailored health communication: a persuasion and message effects perspective. *J Commun* 2006;56:S184–201.

22. Chiauzzi E, Green TC, Lord S. My student body: a high-risk drinking prevention web site for college students. *J Am Coll Health* 2005;53:263–274.

23. Oenema A, Brug J, Lechner L. Web-based tailored nutrition education: results of a randomized controlled trial. *Health Educ Res* 2001;16:647–660. Brug J, Steenhuis I, van Assema P, de Vries H. The impact of a computer-tailored nutrition intervention. *Prev Med* 1996;25:236–242.

24. Strecher VJ, Shiffman S, West R. Randomized controlled trial of a web-based computer-tailored smoking cessation program as a supplement to nicotine patch therapy. *Addiction* 2005;100:682–688.

25. Kroeze W, Werkman A, Brug J. A systematic review of randomized trials on the effectiveness of computer-tailored education on physical activity and dietary behaviors. *Ann Behav Med.* 2006;31:205–223. Richards KC, Enderlin CA, Beck C, McSweeney JC, Jones TC, Roberson PK. Tailored biobehavioral interventions: a literature review and synthesis. *Res Theory Nurs Pract.*2007;21:271–285.

26. Noar SM, Benac CN, Harris MS. Does tailoring matter? Meta-analytic review of tailored print health behavior change interventions. *Psychol Bull.* 2007;133:673–693. Sohl SJ, Moyer A. Tailored interventions to promote mammography screening: a meta-analytic review. *Prev Med.* 2007;45:252–261.

27. Lustria, M.L.A., Cortese, J., Noar, S.M., Glueckauf, R.L. Computer-tailored health interventions delivered over the web: Review and analysis of key components. *Patient Education and Counseling.* 2009;74:156–173.

28. http://www.fns.usda.gov/wic/

29. Table from the Colorado patient navigator training site: http://www.patientnavigatortraining.org/

CHAPTER 11

It's a Multimedia World

Claudia Parvanta and Sarah Parvanta

LEARNING OBJECTIVES

By the end of this chapter, the reader will be able to:

- Define a spectrum of traditional and new media options available to health communicators.
- Describe the state of traditional media use in the United States.
- Use a systematic and data-based approach for selecting media channels to reach a target audience.
- Describe examples of several government and foundation-led health communication efforts using new media.
- Choose among multiple media options and approaches for a health communication plan.

INTRODUCTION

McDonald's Restaurant has its own Facebook profile page,[1] and just before the end of 2009, the Golden Arches had more than 1.3 million Facebook friends out of 300 million Facebook users.[2] On this page, "friends" can play games and read about the restaurant's newest menu options. McDonald's is still evaluating whether this new form of advertising drives more customers to the ubiquitous restaurants. But the message is clear: marketing and communication efforts today depend on new media technology to attract audiences, especially young people, who consume multiple forms of new media every day. These new media forms include, but are not limited to, Facebook, MySpace, Twitter, blog sites, mobile phones and their many "apps," YouTube, the world of wikis, virtual reality gaming, and more.

THE STATE OF TRADITIONAL MEDIA

In the face of our expanding multi-media world, what's happening to **traditional media**, such as television, radio, magazines, and newspapers? Don't believe the death knell tolling in the blogosphere. The following sections describe each of these forms of traditional media, how they have been used in the past, and how they are still being used today even in very different or less prominent ways.

Television (TV)

According to the Neilson Company, there are 292 million Americans with televisions.* As of December 18, 2009, the average American spent nearly 31 and a half hours each week tuned into the TV. Still paling in comparison to the good old 'tube,' Internet use *averages* only a little over four hours. Believe it or not, Millennials (those who were 13 to 24 years of age in 2009), spent less time online per week (about 2.5 hours) than Generation X (25 to 41years old) at about 5.5 hours, and the younger end of the Baby Boomers (50+) topped them all at 6.5 hours.[3] People who get their news from nightly television network news has declined to 28%, again, varying greatly by age, and local news viewership is about 54%.[4] But, we're still talking about half of the adults living in any media market watching the local news. This is good news for health communicators, because local news media buys are much less expensive than network programming.

Radio

An amazing 91% of Americans who are 12 years old or more listen to the radio at least once a week. In a survey conducted

---

*Neilson provides television ratings that the industry uses to assess the popularity, and hence, advertising potential, for TV shows. There are 305+ million people in the United States, which includes a large number of children. Thus, you can pretty much count on every American having access to a TV.

by Arbitron,* 21% of the listening public said that AM/FM radio has a "big impact" on their lives. The number tuning into radio online is increasing (17% to 20%, depending on age group), but the online site is still controlled by a specific radio station. Listening format varies greatly by geographic location (or market), making radio one of the most customizable media available short of tailoring (discussed in Chapter 10). The most popular formats in the United States are "news, talk, information," with a 12.6% share of all listenership, followed immediately by "country," with 12.5% share. All other forms—for example, adult contemporary, rock, classics, urban—fall into single-digit percentages of listeners. But, we're still talking about millions of people tuning in every day.[5]

Magazines

Some think that magazines must surely be on the decline. This is not true, according to Mediamark Research & Intelligence (MRI).[†] As reported in the *Media Daily News*, women's magazine readership[‡] is up from the start of the decade, reaching 337 million in 2009. Men, who consume far fewer magazines than women, still purchased 115.5 million in 2009. General-interest magazines did fall substantially during this period, including the *National Enquirer* and *Reader's Digest*. So, on average, the American magazine reading public actually increased by 8% from 2000 to 2009.[6]

Newspapers

According to a recent press release from Scarborough Research,[7][§] in 2009, "Three_quarters (74%) of U.S. adults, or nearly 171 million people, read a newspaper—in print or online—during the past week." This American consumer research agency went on to report the following:

> While our data does show that print newspaper readership is slowly declining, it also illustrates

that . . . the reported pending death of the newspaper industry is not supported by audience data. . . . In an average week:

- 79% of adults employed in white collar positions read a newspaper in print or online.
- 82% of adults with household incomes of $100,000 or more read a printed newspaper in print or online.
- 84% of adults who are college graduates or who have advanced degrees read a printed newspaper.

What does this mean?

Traditional media still provide the most powerful channels to reach large numbers of audiences quickly. New media channels are born (and die) like fruit flies, but their ability to reach specific segments in highly credible and interactive ways cannot be matched by traditional media. Together they provide a wide array of outlets to mix and match for health interventions, particularly those directed to younger audiences. For example, **Figure 11–1** shows the mix that the National Institute on Drug Abuse (NIDA; part of the National Institutes of Health) is using to communicate with teens.[8]

Advertising agencies emphasize their digital strategies for commercial sponsors and have the "analytics" and metrics to back it up. But, health communication planners have not yet developed a strategic approach to combining traditional and new media in ways that enable them to predict and measure outcomes. Early efforts, such as those undertaken by the NIDA, CDC, NCI, and other federal agencies will start providing the critical return on investment data necessary to guide the next wave of media strategy in health communication.

In a presentation made at the Advertising Council,[9][||] Greg Cangialosi described an adoption curve for social media. He points out that it requires two paradigm shifts to fully embrace the new media. The first is the transition from using new media as a broadcast vehicle—in other words, from using social media as additional one-way promotional venues to engaging in two-way dialogue with others. Having developed a more participatory relationship with online users, the next big transition requires "sharing value" with this online community—in other words, the networks and discussions are not just there to sell yourself or your idea to others in more effective ways, but to encourage collaboration with others to produce even better ideas, products, etc.

---

*Arbitron Inc. (NYSE: ARB) is an independent media and marketing research firm serving the media—radio, television, cable, and out-of-home—as well as advertisers and advertising agencies. They can be accessed at www.arbitron.com.

†MRI, now a subsidiary of the German GfK Group, conducts *The Survey of the American Consumer™*, which collects information on adult consumers' media choices, product usage, demographics, lifestyle, and attitudes. MRI interviews 26,000 consumers face-to-face, in their homes, to provide this information.

‡Titles such as *Allure, Better Homes & Gardens, Bon Appetit, Cosmopolitan, Elle, Entertainment Weekly, Essence, Family Circle, Fitness, Glamour, Good Housekeeping, Harper's Bazaar, House Beautiful, Marie Claire, Martha Stewart Living, People, Seventeen, Southern Living, Vanity Fair, Vogue,* and *Women's Day* were all higher. What might be considered traditional homemaker's books, such as *Ladies' Home Journal, Redbook,* as well as the *Soap Opera Digest* and *Weekly* decreased in readership substantially during this period.

§Surveying more than 220,000 adults annually, Scarborough is a joint venture between Arbitron Inc. (www.arbitron.com) and The Nielsen Company (www.nielsen.com). For more on how to write press releases that get picked up and quoted, see Chapter 6.

||The Advertising Council is the best-known nonprofit organization devoted to development and placement of public service media in the United States. Its legacy includes Smokey the Bear's "Only you can prevent forest fires," the "Tearful Indian" campaign against pollution, the crash test dummies for motor safety, "A Mind Is a Terrible Thing to Waste" (for the United Negro College Fund), and more recently, "Buzzed Driving Is Drunk Driving." You may find them online at www.adcouncil.org.

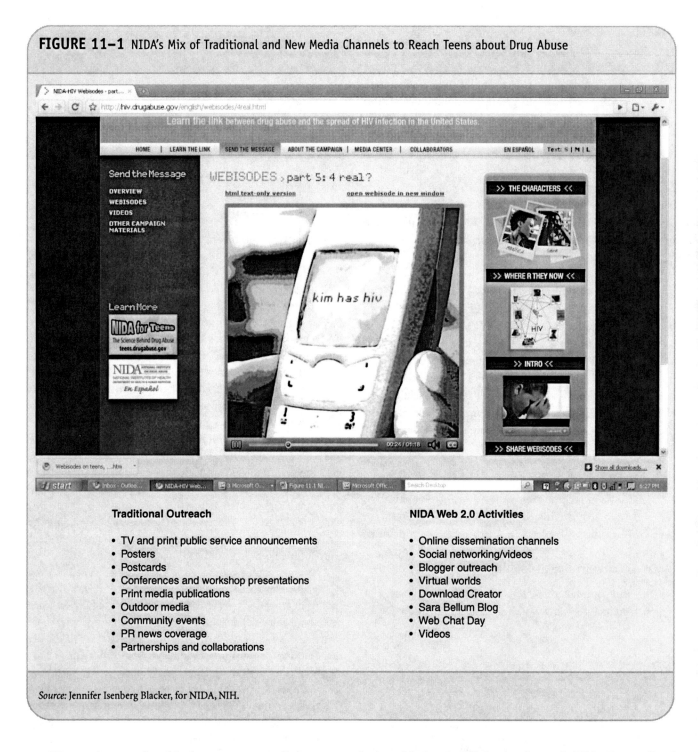

FIGURE 11–1 NIDA's Mix of Traditional and New Media Channels to Reach Teens about Drug Abuse

Traditional Outreach

- TV and print public service announcements
- Posters
- Postcards
- Conferences and workshop presentations
- Print media publications
- Outdoor media
- Community events
- PR news coverage
- Partnerships and collaborations

NIDA Web 2.0 Activities

- Online dissemination channels
- Social networking/videos
- Blogger outreach
- Virtual worlds
- Download Creator
- Sara Bellum Blog
- Web Chat Day
- Videos

Source: Jennifer Isenberg Blacker, for NIDA, NIH.

We promise to update this chapter as new media become dominant. With that said, let's begin a discussion on how to use traditional media options for public health communication.

USING TRADITIONAL MEDIA AND CHANNELS FOR PERSUASIVE HEALTH COMMUNICATION

In Chapter 10 we discussed matching practice strategies, such as entertainment education, risk communication, or viral marketing with theories of behavior change. In Table 10–1, we lined these up with the activities and media channels that were most supportive. So, for example, if you plan to use the Transtheoretical Model or Precaution Adoption Process Model to motivate adoption of a behavior in small steps, once you are past the level of awareness, in-person channels tend to be more effective. While most of these involve face-to-face encounters with trained counselors or peers, there has been some success doing the same thing in the virtual online world. Because all behavior change theories begin with recognition or awareness on the part of the target audience, just about any mass media will be more cost-effective than in-person channels in achieving that goal.

So you have thought about the best theory-informed practice strategy for your target audience. How do you select the most effective channels to reach them? Again, you look at the behavior of your target audience to answer that question. What does their typical day look like?[10] **Table 11–1** shows an hypothetical "typical day" for a young woman (age 20 to 29) who holds a full-time job in an urban setting of a major metropolitan setting in the United States. There are many opportunities when communication could potentially reach her through numerous channels.

TABLE 11–1 "Typical Day" Channel Opportunities Analysis*

Time of Day	Location, Activities	Communication Channel Opportunities
Wakeup	Home, dressing.	Radio, morning TV news.
Morning commute	Public transportation.	Bus, subway posters, billboards, podcast downloads, radio, magazines.
Office, 9 a.m., to 5 p.m.	Work. Breaks. Lunch. Not allowed external media.	Worksite print: posters, brochures. Worksite health promotion in-person. Online possibly. Magazines possibly.
	Work. Breaks. Lunch. Allowed external aural media.	Same as above. Plus radio, Internet sound, podcast downloads.
Evening commute	Public transportation.	Bus, subway posters, billboards, podcast downloads, radio, magazines.
Evening activities—alone or with friends, family	Gym workout 3 times per week.	Cable TV, radio, podcasts, magazines. Onsite print: posters, brochures. Trained health coaching.
	Church or educational gatherings 1 time per week.	Special event: live interaction. Print support: brochures, flyers.
	Grocery shopping 2 times per week.	In-store promotional media: cable TV, radio, print. Checkout line: magazines.
	Home, dinner preparation 4 times per week.	Radio, podcasts.
	Home, relaxation 7 times per week.	Internet, TV (network, cable), videos, radio, magazines.
Weekend events— usually with others	In-town entertainment: shopping malls, sporting events, concerts, plays, movies 1 time per week.	Outdoor/mall advertising, site specific print, cable TV. Entertainment education placement, video spots.
Personal care and related	Hair, nail salons 1 time per month.	Cable TV, magazines, brochures, posters.
Seasonal opportunities— Usually with others	Location-based activities, e.g., swimming pool, ice skating rink, parks.	Radio, podcasts, limited outdoor and print.

*For an average, single American woman (20 to 29), working full-time, Northeast, urban.

You can get this information by either following your target audience around, surveying them, or through media research companies such as the ones mentioned earlier. It will vary greatly depending on how you have segmented your audience. For example, if you wanted to reach boys of about 12 years old, in addition to school being their "8 a.m. to 2 p.m." activity, there's a very good chance they will spend seven or more hours a day consuming media, either alone, online, or with friends. A new study released by the Kaiser Family Foundation says:

> [W]ith technology allowing nearly 24-hour media access as children and teens go about their daily lives, . . . 8–18 year-olds devote an average of 7 hours and 38 minutes (7:38) to using entertainment media across a typical day (more than 53 hours a week). And because they spend so much of that time "media multitasking" (using more than one medium at a time), they actually manage to pack a total of 10 hours and 45 minutes (10:45) worth of media content into those 7½ hours.[11]

Many of the media referred to in the study (e.g., music downloads, gaming videos, mobile phone communication with friends) are not commonly used for public health programming, but this is likely to change.

After working out the various options for your audience and channels, then use **Table 11–2** to estimate the channels' cost against its efficiency and credibility.[12] In this example, we assume we need to pay for the media placement. We will discuss earned media (i.e., free public service placement) next.

A note of caution: Media buying has always been an art reserved for practitioners of advertising and public relations. If you are able to work in a media-related business, even as an intern, try to work in the media buying (traffic) department first. The primary rule is that there are no rules. Prices are always negotiable and depend on volume, time (duration) commitment, the organization's prestige and reputation, and many other factors. If you are a huge and powerful customer (such as Procter & Gamble, Verizon, AT&T, General Motors, Johnson & Johnson)[13] and spend billions of dollars on advertising, you—and your advertising agency—are treated very differently than even Coca-Cola, which spent a paltry $752 million in 2009 and weighed in as the 55th-ranked advertiser. So where do you stand with your possible $100,000 to $250,000 to spend on your communications? Or is it more like $1,000 to $10,000? Let's take a look at possible media channels for a health communication campaign that is not being bankrolled by corporate giants, or even a federal agency. Table 11–2 presents the best estimates as of January 2, 2010, for various media channel options in an urban setting. None of these estimates include the cost of developing, testing, and producing the final media—only the costs to disseminate them through a specific channel.

EARNED MEDIA

Did I hear you say "free" was looking really good to you right about now? The term **earned media** is an old school term meaning that you do not pay to disseminate your information—it is "picked up" by the news, local programming, or run as a public service announcement (discussed later). With new media, this may be as simple as posting a really great video on YouTube, or using Twitter and Facebook advantageously. With traditional media, which are managed, there are editorial hurdles to clear. So, it isn't called *free media* because you will need to invest a lot of effort to get your material on air. We will discuss how you might be able to earn some media coverage in a moment. But, it is important for you to realize that your "adversaries" in chronic disease prevention who purvey fast foods loaded in calories and/or fats, or tobacco, or even beer, for example, will outspend you $100,000 to $1, at a minimum. Is health promotion like politics, where the candidate who spends the most wins? Are we doomed in our effort to promote healthy behavior? As the Millennial Generation, we are counting on you to come up with new ideas, using new media, to reverse this trend. Let's first take a look at the more traditional options that are still at your disposal.

Public Service Advertising/Announcements

In Chapter 6, we discussed how to work with the news media to get an important event covered for advocacy purposes using **public service announcements (PSAs)**. In a similar vein, there are numerous organizations that will partner with you to develop and disseminate health communication campaigns, usually consisting of audio and video spots as well as print ads through their own channels, and sometimes at their own cost. You normally need to pay for the costs of initial production. In other words, if you want to put something on television, you will need broadcast-quality footage; on the radio, broadcast-quality sound; and in print, something better than a black and white photocopy.

What does it take to put this together? If you are planning a national campaign, and have more than a million dollars to spend over several years, you might want to work with the Advertising Council. Putting this in context, a government agency, or a national organization would likely be able to marshal $750,000 a year for communication costs. This is far, far less than the billions of dollars being spent in the fast-food and tobacco industries.

If the Advertising Council adopts your issue, they will identify a high-quality partner to produce your media products at cost (this is what you are paying for), and then find media channels that will disseminate the material for free. **Box 11–1** features a case study of the ongoing AdCouncil's "Buzzed Driving is Drunk Driving" Campaign.[14]

TABLE 11–2 Example of Paid Media Channels to Reach Young, Single, Working Women (Ages 20–29) in Urban Setting

Channel	Target Audience Reached[a]	Cost in U.S. Dollars	Cost per Thousand (CPM)	Credibility Rating (1–5) 1 low 5 high Estimated	Best Bets for This Audience x = good X= great
Television: 30-second spot average prime time		$200,000		2	
Oprah M–F, 4 p.m.[b]	100,000				
One 30-second advertisement. National market. Local markets considerably less.		$250,000–$300,000	$2,500	3	
American Idol (finals)[c]	980,000	$750,000	$76	3	
CBS *Crime Scene Investigation* shows (4+)[d]	1,000,000	$230,000	$230	4	
Desperate Housewives (M) 9pm.	5,000,000	$229,000	$45.80	3	x
Radio: average for week rotator (12–15 or more 30-second spots in various segments)		$90–$1,200	$0.09	3+	X
Magazines (*Elle,*[e] *Glamour, InStyle*): 1 full-page ad, once. Prices decrease with multiples.	1,050,000	$128,000	$122	4+	X
Bus: varies hugely on market. Side of bus "King" ad. (e.g., Philadelphia);1 bus. 1 ad. Bus shelter/bench ad	3,000 5,000		$3.04 $5.00	3+	X
Local cable (varies greatly)		$300–$3,000	$30	2	
Print materials: variable rates depending on quality and number (e.g., FedEx Office rates[f]). Color, 2-side, highest quality paper, tri-folded B&W, 2 side, standard paper, tri-fold.	1,000		$1,230 $160	4	?
Online: average rate $0.60 per click. Other rates quoted.	Very variable. Can be enormous.		$600	5	

Total national population of age/sex in 2009: approximately 20 million.

[a]See http://media.onsugar.com/static/imgs/WhyYWomen.pdf for excellent new media-use profile of target audience: Generation Y Women (compared to Generation X).

[b]Nationally 7.4 million people watch *Oprah* daily—about 2.6% of American households. Four percent of American women (about 5.7 million) watch her daily, compared with 1.2% of men (1.7 million people). Overall, 2% of all 18- to 49-year-olds watch *Oprah.* About 0.5% of 20- to 29-year-old women watch *Oprah,* or 100,000 nationally.

[c]*American Idol,* at its peak, pulled in 28 to 30 million viewers. But, only about 7% are in the 18 to 24 age group. Ratings researchers indicate that the average age for *Idol* is creeping up, with a mean of 40 at the end of 2009.

[d]Neilson says that 15 to 20 million viewers watched these programs in 2009, approximately 50% in the 18 to 49 age group. This is an estimated 10% of the target audience.

[e]http://www.hfmus.com/hfmus/media_kits/fashion_beauty_design/elle/magazine_advertising/rates

[f]www.fedex.com/us. Brochure printing-FedEx office. Tri-fold brochures. Accessed January 2, 2010.

Box 11–1 Advertising Council Case Study: "Buzzed Driving Is Drunk Driving" Campaign

Drunk driving kills someone in America every **41 minutes.**

Background

Drunk driving is one of the most frequently committed crimes in the United States. Drunk driving kills someone in America every 41 minutes, representing nearly 40% of all traffic fatalities. In 2005, nearly 15,000 people died in highway crashes involving a driver or a motorcycle operator with a blood alcohol concentration (BAC) of .08 or higher.[a] Thousands more were injured. Since its debut more than 20 years ago, the Ad Council's "Friends Don't Let Friends Drive Drunk" campaign has played a significant role in improving the safety of our roads. In large part due to the PSA campaign, more than two-thirds of Americans (68%) say they have tried to stop someone from driving impaired.[b] Alcohol-related crashes dropped dramatically, reaching a low point in the late 1990s. In conjunction with stepped-up law enforcement, this long running PSA campaign has changed the social norm. "One for the road" was transformed into "Friends don't let friends drive drunk." It has been one of the Ad Council's most well-known and successful campaigns.

Despite these successes, crashes involving alcohol consumption started rising again in 2000. Younger drivers age 21–34, predominantly men, are responsible for nearly 60% of alcohol-related traffic crashes. In response to these trends, the Advertising Council and its longtime partner, the U.S. Department of Transportation's National Highway Traffic Safety Administration (NHTSA), decided to refocus the Drunk Driving Prevention campaign. Rather than targeting the intervener, the new campaign would target those most likely to drive impaired. Mullen, the Massachusetts-based advertising agency, was recruited on a pro bono basis to provide strategic direction and guide creative development for the campaign.

[a]*Fatality Analysis Reporting System* (FARS), NHTSA, 2005
[b]Ad Council national tracking survey

Reaching the Audience
Strategic and Creative Development of the Campaign

Strategic Development

The team set out to study the nature of the problem and the mindset of the target audience. First, they reviewed the data on major trends in drunk driving. Drawing on several research studies, including an exhaustive study by the firm Porter Novelli, a demographic and psychographic profile was developed of those most likely to get behind the wheel impaired. In June 2003, the team conducted a series of focus groups with the target audience in New Jersey and Chicago.

Through this research, the mindset of the target audience became clearer. These young men age 21–34 are mostly well-meaning "average Joes" who don't intend any harm but continue to drink and drive. Many have driven impaired multiple times in the past without getting into trouble. They tend to feel either invincible or just overly optimistic about the control they have over their lives. Throughout the research, one theme kept coming up. The most common excuses for impaired driving were "I'm just buzzed" or "I just had a few." "Buzzed" is part of their vernacular and can signify anything from feeling slightly tipsy to being falling-down drunk. And even when they may have had more than a few drinks in a short period of time, before getting behind the wheel they tend to shrug it off by saying they just had "a few."

With this understanding of the target audience, the team set the following objectives for the campaign:

• To inspire discussion about the dangers of driving "buzzed"
• To prevent impaired driving by defining the feeling of being "buzzed" as a reason not to get behind the wheel

Creative Development

Mullen produced a compelling advertising campaign that adhered closely to the strategy. Multiple ads were developed for television, radio, billboards and other out-of-home venues, the Web, newspapers and magazines. Television spots depicted various scenarios featuring young adults who were clearly drunk, and then contrasted them with onlookers who were impaired but

continues

not obviously drunk. The ads concluded with the lines, "It's easy to tell if you've had way too many. But what if you've just had one too many? Buzzed driving is drunk driving." Radio ads took a similar approach, describing embarrassing scenarios where it is obvious someone has had too much to drink. Print ads gave recipes for making drinks such as a margarita, but added ingredients such as "1 false sense of security." The print ads conclude with the lines, "Never underestimate 'just a few.' Buzzed driving is drunk driving."

TV Spot:
"Karaoke"

Man sings while spilling his drink and stumbling.
Voiceover: It's easy to tell if you've had way too many. But what if you've just had one too many? Buzzed driving is drunk driving.

Through a special agreement, the Outdoor Advertising Association of America (OAAA) committed to placing more than 8,000 "Buzzed Driving" billboards and 100 vinyl bulletins nationwide, with a concentration in areas with higher rates of impaired driving fatalities.

   The Ad Council's PR team led several other activities to get the word out through the press. A localized "Bites and B-Roll" package, featuring sound bites and video footage, was distributed to TV stations. Local NHTSA spokespersons were made available for interviews. The Ad Council also developed Web streaming video packages customized for local viewing. Finally, in partnership with the North American Precis Syndicate, the Ad Council distributed a mat release (a prepackaged newspaper article) to more than 10,000 suburban daily and weekly newspapers.

Television Bureau of Advertising: Project Roadblock
The Ad Council partnered with the Television Bureau of Advertising (TVB) to create a "roadblock" of the TV PSAs during the month of December. The TVB worked hard to encourage its network of local broadcast TV stations to donate airtime to the PSAs in December, particularly during the week between Christmas and New Year's. Through different forms of outreach, the TVB secured commitments from more than 600 television stations in nearly 200 markets.

2006 Redistribution and Roadblock
The ads were redistributed in July 2006, including one new TV spot in Spanish. In December 2006, the TVB again led a "Project Roadblock," leading to an even higher level of commitment from local TV outlets.

Evaluating Ad Effectiveness
As with all Ad Council campaigns, the ads required approval from the Ad Council's Campaign Review Committee, a peer review group consisting of top executives in the advertising industry. In addition, in August 2005 boards and scripts of the ads were presented to a series of focus groups of the target audience in Boston and Chicago. Feedback from the focus groups was largely positive. Young male respondents found the PSAs clear and relevant. Finally, a quantitative copy test of the produced TV PSAs was conducted in November 2005, prior to the campaign launch. The study, fielded by Lightspeed Research, was conducted online among 305 men age 21–34 nationwide. After viewing an ad, respondents were asked a series of evaluative questions about it. The results echoed the earlier qualitative feedback. A large majority of respondents said that the ads were clear, memorable and motivating. About 7 in 10 (69%) agreed that "this ad makes me think twice about driving when I feel 'buzzed' from alcohol."

Campaign Launch
The first phase of the campaign launched in December 2005—appropriate timing, since drunk driving crashes spike during the Christmas–New Year's week. The Ad Council distributed the ads to more than 28,000 media outlets nationwide. A range of ads was produced in a variety of media formats, including television, radio, print, Web, out-of-home and alternative media. As with all Ad Council PSA campaigns, media is not planned or bought; instead, the campaign relies on media outlets to donate time and space for the ads. In addition, the Ad Council's Media team marketed the campaign to media companies through several forms of outreach.

Press Coverage
News reports about the 2005 campaign launch extended the campaign's reach to 49 million people, generating more than $6 million in publicity value. The campaign was also covered by 932 local broadcast news programs on 336 television stations in 168 markets. It was featured on such high-profile programs as ABC's *Good Morning America* and CNN's Headline News channel. Additionally,

the "Buzzed Driving" campaign was highlighted in radio segments throughout the country. ABCNews.com was among several high-traffic news Web sites that featured the campaign. Among print outlets, press coverage generated more than 300 newspaper articles in 24 states, reaching a circulation of over 16.5 million readers.

Tracking Survey Results

The Ad Council fielded a benchmark tracking survey immediately prior to the campaign launch in December 2005. Follow-up surveys were fielded in January 2006 and January 2007, immediately following the December TVB roadblocks. Each survey included a national sample of 800 adults, including 500 general market adults and 300 men age 21–34. To qualify, respondents had to be frequent drivers and drink alcohol at least occasionally. The survey tracked awareness, relevant attitudes, and self-reported behaviors over time.

Results from the January 2006 survey, immediately following the launch, demonstrated the campaign's impact in the short term. Results from the second follow-up survey, one year later, were even more impressive:

- Awareness of the campaign: Approximately one-third of all adults (35%) recalled seeing or hearing the campaign's ads.
- Four in 10 men age 21–34 (41%) were aware of the campaign.

Creating Change
Evaluating Campaign Impact

Campaign Evaluation
As with all Ad Council campaigns, multiple tools are used to assess the campaign's effectiveness and impact.

Estimated Donated Media
In terms of support from the media community, the campaign has been a top performer at the Ad Council. From late 2005 to late 2006, the campaign garnered nearly $80 million (estimated) worth of donated media. Radio garnered a large share of media donations, but support in other media was also strong. Of particular importance, the TVB roadblocks in December 2005 and December 2006 were responsible for a total of $6.8 million of TV support during those concentrated one-month periods. In December 2005 alone, the TV spots aired more than 21,100 times on 638 stations in 179 markets.

ESTIMATED DONATED MEDIA TOTALS
December 2005–December 2006
Medium Donated Media ($)
Radio $42,387,000
Broadcast and Cable TV $15,409,000
Out-of-Home $12,115,600
Interactive $5,474,900
Newspaper and Magazine $1,416,000
Alternative Media $392,700
Public Relations (News stories) $2,746,300
Total $79,941,500

Data Sources
TV: SIGMA, a product of Nielsen Media Research
Radio: Verance and Mediaguide monitoring services
Newspaper and Magazine: Burrelle's clipping service
Out-of-Home, Alternative, and Interactive: Self-reporting by media companies
Public Relations: PR Trak

- Opinion of the campaign: Of those aware of the campaign, approximately 9 in 10 men age 21–34 (89%) called the advertising extremely/very/somewhat effective.
- Importance of the issue: There was a significant increase in the proportion of men age 21–34 who called themselves "extremely concerned" about the issue of drunk driving, from 22% in 2005 to 29% in 2007.

continues

- Behaviors over the holiday season: A growing number of respondents reported that they thought twice about drinking and driving during the holiday season. In early January 2007, 10% of all adults, and 17% of men age 21–34, said that in the past few weeks they had decided to NOT drive after they had been drinking. These results were even higher than similar results measured in January 2006.
- Ad effectiveness: Those who were aware of the "Buzzed Driving" campaign were significantly more likely to report that they had "recently" refrained from driving after drinking (74% ad aware vs. 55% not ad aware); "recently" stopped an impaired friend or family member from driving (48% ad aware vs. 35% not ad aware); and "recently" discussed the risks of impaired driving with friends or family members (68% ad aware vs. 46% not ad aware). While the PSAs cannot claim to be the sole motivating factor behind these behaviors, it is likely they played a large role.

Source: The Advertising Council, Inc., www.adcouncil.org. *Buzzed Driving Is Drunk Driving.* Drunk Driving Prevention Campaign Case Study.

If your budget is much more modest, you can work with the best professional content producer you can find (including your friends taking media production classes) to create a set of video, radio, and print spot ads. If you are at a university, speak to the local health department or to community-based organizations (including local chapters of national organizations such as the American Cancer Society, the American Heart Foundation, etc.) to assess their needs. Most likely, they already work with local media production companies and would be interested in partnering with you to create new health promotion materials for their target audiences. As was often the case at CDC when this book's lead author worked there, an arrangement can be reached where you provide the research for free, and the company pays for production and disseminates through its channels. Perhaps, you would also do the evaluation for them, again, for free. This kind of win–win is a great academic–community partnership that advances public health! And, you might be able to identify a grant to cover your costs, as well.

There is only one major glitch with the whole PSA world these days: digital cable TV changed the rules of fair play.[15] The Federal Communications Commission (FCC) was established by the Communications Act of 1934 as the government agency charged with regulating interstate and international communications by radio, television, wire, satellite, and cable. When analog television used the airwaves to broadcast, the FCC required that stations provide a standard number of hours of public service content in return for this usage. Public service television includes children's educational programming, as well as coverage of issues deemed important to the health and welfare of the community. In September 2004, the FCC extended children's television rules to digital television, which requires that stations broadcast at least three hours per week of educational television programming in digital format and that parents are able to identify educational shows. Other rules that pertain to new forms of broadcast include:

- Direct broadcast satellite providers must reserve 4% of their channel capacity exclusively for noncommercial programming of an educational or informational nature.
- Cable providers are required to set aside channel capacity for local public, educational, and governmental (PEG) access programming, but the amount of local programming is not federally mandated.[15]

So, apart from children's educational shows, there are no longer set requirements for how much air time a cable TV station must devote to public interest programming. As a result, it is all a matter of how much unsold inventory a station has available for a particular day. As was true for advocacy, you need to work closely with the people responsible for selecting and running public interest pieces in your local TV and radio markets, the public service directors. You have more clout than you might realize. **Figure 11–2** provides an overview of how TV and radio public service directors select content.[16]

You will see that the interests of local nonprofit organizations and the credibility of the agency sponsor, as well as local associated news coverage, all are important factors, but so is the production quality of the materials. Unfortunately, you are competing for a very small portion of time on the air, as the last chart shows in Figure 11–2. While a local PSA beats out one from a national organization, television broadcasters are likely to devote less than 6% of their unsold air time to them; radios about 13%. But these figures are estimates and averages, so you might be able to have some great success with your local stations, particularly with radio. Other national cable stations, such as MTV and BET, tend to run more PSAs. They might be particularly good choices for reaching specific audiences.

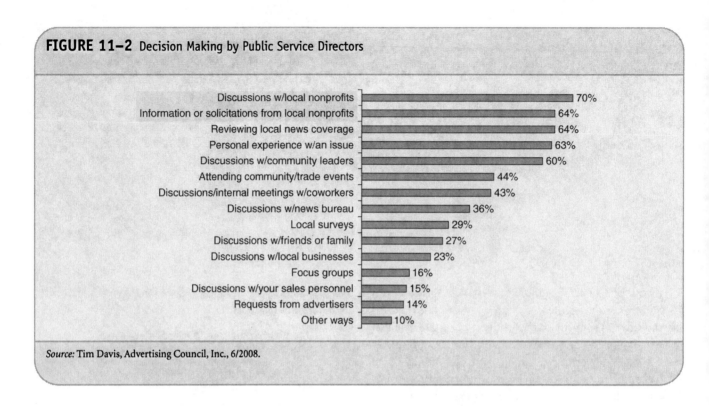

FIGURE 11–2 Decision Making by Public Service Directors

Discussions w/local nonprofits	70%
Information or solicitations from local nonprofits	64%
Reviewing local news coverage	64%
Personal experience w/an issue	63%
Discussions w/community leaders	60%
Attending community/trade events	44%
Discussions/internal meetings w/coworkers	43%
Discussions w/news bureau	36%
Local surveys	29%
Discussions w/friends or family	27%
Discussions w/local businesses	23%
Focus groups	16%
Discussions w/your sales personnel	15%
Requests from advertisers	14%
Other ways	10%

Source: Tim Davis, Advertising Council, Inc., 6/2008.

Entertainment Education

Perhaps you've decided that the best possible strategy for communicating your health issue is to embed it in a dramatic story. We discussed educational entertainment (EE) in Chapter 10. Just to review, Singhal and Rogers define **entertainment education** as "the process of purposely designing and implementing a media message to both entertain and educate … [and] a communication strategy to bring about behavioral and social change."[17(p.5)] Entertainment education interventions could be nationally broadcast soap operas or prime time shows with storylines about drunk driving or locally broadcast radio series with storylines about HIV or domestic violence. These storylines can be developed to influence psychosocial constructs of known behavior change theories, such as self-efficacy or social norms. EE has been implemented through various media channels, including the Internet,[18] and even theater,[19] in addition to radio[20] and, of course, television. Hollywood, Health & Society (HHS) is an agency that has been working extensively on television-based entertainment education initiatives in the United States and internationally. Sandra Buffington, the director of HHS, describes how this agency is working with Hollywood to incorporate accurate health information into the storylines of television shows that we watch everyday in **Box 11–2**.

If you are able to create a dramatic format for your topic, or convince a known dramatic show to incorporate your issue,

you have earned a lot of valuable media. Of note, the extremely popular program *House* has featured a storyline on addiction and mental health for which it was nominated for a Prism award in 2006 and 2007. The Prism award is given by the Substance Abuse and Mental Health Association.[21] In 2009, *House* featured a National Alliance on Mental Illness PSA[22] on stigma at the end of the show. It discussed how friends can help someone in recovery and displayed a website and phone number in conjunction with the story. This kind of package is about the best you could dream of for a health communication intervention using traditional media.

THE CONVERGENCE OF OLD AND NEW MEDIA: THE INTERNET WEBSITE

We've been making an assumption that anyone reading this book understands the importance of having a website. Your website, either for a project or an organization, is the cornerstone of your health communication campaign, as well as your face to the virtual world. What does your website say about you? Look at the website in **Figure 11–3**, hosted by NIDA.[23,24]

Your website is limited only by your imagination, and to some extent, your resources and local policies or regulations. A lot can be done with open-source software, although sites including interactive or animated features will require more sophisticated programming skills to develop and maintain. Websites that are created using Web 2.0 technologies (such as

Box 11–2 Entertainment Education: Working with Hollywood to Improve Public Health

By Sandra de Castro Buffington, Director, Hollywood, Health & Society, USC Annenberg Norman Lear Center

At Hollywood, Health & Society (HHS), we think of entertainment as more than just a leisure activity. We think of entertainment as the way messages grab and hold our attention. HHS works to educate audiences about important topics, like health. At HHS, we harness the power of media and entertainment education to improve the health and well being of individuals and communities worldwide. This, in short, is the mission of our organization. HHS was created by the Centers for Disease Control and Prevention (CDC), and the University of Southern California's Annenberg Norman Lear Center in an effort to provide health information to Hollywood so that it could communicate this information accurately to the public. More about our organization can be found at www.learcenter.org, but here is a brief glimpse of some of the projects and activities going on at HHS.

Our role with the entertainment industry is to provide a systematic and sustained program of outreach to Hollywood's writers and producers. We serve as a resource to them, and advise them on how to incorporate health messages into their storylines, including messages about HIV/AIDS, swine flu, breast cancer, childhood immunizations, malaria, and other health topics deemed important by the CDC, the Health Resources and Services Administration, National Institutes of Health, California Endowment, Bill & Melinda Gates Foundation, and other health agencies.

As part of these efforts, we work with CDC and our other donors to create tip sheets for writers and producers on health and safety topics. Tip sheets include basic information and case examples for storylines, and additional resources on the topic. We provide a forum for health experts to hold briefings and consultations to provide information about current health issues that might become part of a storyline on a TV show or series. We also create public service announcements, and use new media in multi-platform pro-social campaigns to refer viewers to credible sources of health information and to field questions from the public, normally after a program that has featured a particular topic, using a 1-800 phone line, web links or other Interactive online media.

We reward Hollywood's writers and producers who make a concerted effort to represent and convey health topics and messages accurately within media entertainment storylines. The HHS Sentinel for Health Awards recognize exemplary TV health storylines. As HHS Director, I presented 11 awards on September 23, 2009 at the Writers Guild of America, West. The NBC drama *ER* received first place in the primetime drama category for a storyline involving a grandmother's anguish as she makes the difficult decision to allow her grandson's organs to be donated, giving meaning to his tragic death and a second chance at life to others. The same *ER* episode also earned first place for a primetime minor storyline about the use of a safe surgery checklist in the operating room, and ABC's *Desperate Housewives* took first place in primetime comedy for a storyline about childhood obesity. In daytime drama, the CBS soap opera *As The World Turns* took first place for a storyline about alcoholism, and NBC's *Law and Order: SVU* took home a Sentinel Award in the new global health storyline category for a show about HIV/AIDS deniers, whose disbelief in the existence of the HIV virus results in tragedy.

Research is also a primary component of the HHS mission. We evaluate TV viewing habits, TV content, and the impact that TV storylines have on audiences. For example, the Kaiser Family Foundation (KFF) and HHS consulted on an episode of *Grey's Anatomy*. KFF surveyed 1,500 regular viewers of the episode one week before, one week after, and six weeks after a particular episode dealing with HIV/AIDS and pregnancy, which had more than 17.5 million viewers on U.S. prime time television, according to the Nielsen Ratings. Viewers were asked what are the chances that a pregnant woman who has HIV and receives proper treatment will give birth to a baby without HIV. Correct answer: Over 90%. Before the *Grey's Anatomy* episode, only 15% of these viewers gave the correct response. One week after the *Grey's* episode, 61% of viewers got the answer right, and even six weeks after the episode, 45% of viewers still got it right.

Another example of our work and the impact of health messages on TV is an evaluation of episodes of *House* dealing with Chlamydia and Bacterial Vaginosis. HHS posted web links on the *House* website to refer viewers to CDC's credible sources of information on these topics. Monitoring hits on the CDC web site, we saw a large spike in searches for information on these specific health topics in the hours during and directly after these episodes aired.

These findings indicate that health information in entertainment television can have significant impact on public health awareness. Furthermore, repetition of the information is the key to maintaining public awareness at peak levels. In short, entertainment education is a means to present health information that can save lives, improve health, and enhance the well being of people in the United States and abroad. HHS is committed to continue working with Hollywood to this end, as the TV industry has an important opportunity serve public health just by doing what it does best: entertaining.

FIGURE 11–3 Screenshot of NIDA Website

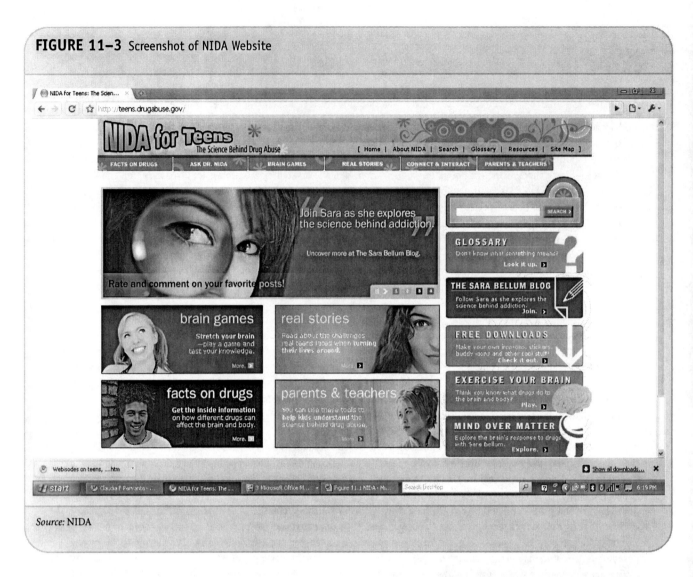

Source: NIDA

blogs, wikis, and social networking sites) often use their membership to generate at least a portion of the site's content. This is generally referred to as user-generated content (UGC), user-created content (UCC), or **consumer-generated media (CGM)**. Some websites are hybrids of both UGC and content provided by the website administrator.[25] An excellent resource to guide the development of websites and related Internet-based tools for health communication is available from the National Coalition of STD Directors.*

USE OF NEW MEDIA

How do you work with new media channels effectively to accomplish health communication purposes? Looking back at Figure 11–2, the first question is who is going online or en-

gaging in new media channels, and when are they doing so? You already know the answer to the first question, because it is chiefly Generation Y, as well as your younger siblings, the Millennials. You are mostly the children of the Baby Boomers—about 70 million strong, or 20% of the U.S. population. You were born between the mid-1970s and the first decade of 2000. **Figure 11–4** shows data from a survey conducted in 2008 comparing Generation Y women (18 to 28 years old) to older respondents in their use of online media.[26(p.7)]

What is Generation Y using online? At least half are going to user-generated sites in contrast to company-generated sites. These include social media sites such as Facebook, Twitter, wikis, blogs, and YouTube, to name a few in existence today. As Dr. Sylvia Chou suggests (see Box 11–4 later in this chapter), social media level out the health information and acquisition playing field, which currently gives an unfair advantage to the socioeconomic "haves" over the "have-nots," further aggravat-

*http://www.ncsddc.org/.

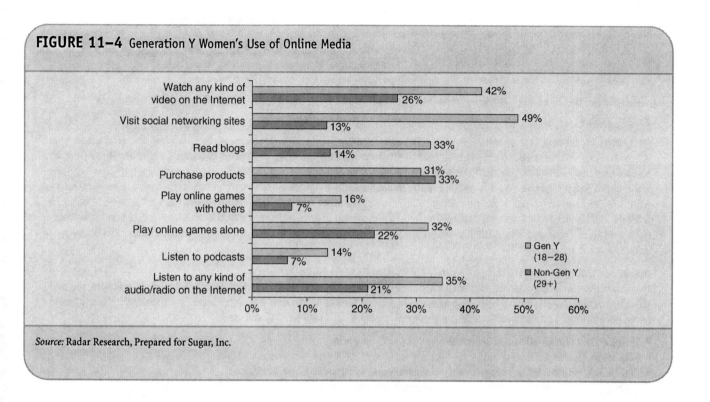

FIGURE 11–4 Generation Y Women's Use of Online Media

Source: Radar Research, Prepared for Sugar, Inc.

ing public health disparities between these groups. At the same time, and possibly of some concern, Generation Y users do not draw a sharp distinction between experts and lay opinion.[26] They are just as likely, in fact more likely, to believe something written in what they deem to be a reliable blog as something appearing in *The New York Times*.

Realizing that social media are all about conversation, you use them to improve relationships with key audiences. Questions that social media strategists ask include:

- Am I reaching the people whom I want to reach?
- Are we having a dialogue? (Is the conversation one-sided?)
- Am I participating in conversations where I have not been involved previously?
- What are people saying about me?
- Are people continuing to talk about me after I leave? In a favorable way?

If it sounds like you and your friends discussing a party you went to, that is the idea.

The following sections present less of a "how-to" and more of a "learn-by-example" set of guidelines of how several government agencies, as well as their multimedia providers, are using new media in health communication campaigns.

Digital Media: A Full Spectrum

In **Box 11–3**, program managers from the CDC describe how that agency is using a range of digital media to reach out to consumers.[27–52]

In **Box 11–4**, Dr. Sylvia Chou describes how the National Cancer Institute (NCI) is thinking about social media based on data collected through its Health Information National Trends Survey (HINTS).

Additional examples demonstrate how public health agencies are strategically using two of the most popular social networking sites, MySpace and Twitter, to improve public health.[53]

Twitter

Twitter is "a real-time short messaging service that works over multiple networks and devices"[54] connected to the Web. Individuals, businesses, organizations, sports teams, and television shows use this site to communicate with one another and "follow" the activities, thoughts, and news that users post on a daily basis, or even from one moment to the next. Twitter was launched in March 2006,[55] and in September 2009 alone, it had more than 23.5 million hits from unique users.[54] Ogilvy Public Relations Worldwide is an agency dedicated to working on public health initiatives. Ogilvy provides advice to public

Box 11–3 Social Media at CDC*

Authors: Ann Aikin, MA; Holli Hitt Seitz, MPH; Janice R. Nall, MBA; Jessica Schindelar, MPH

BACKGROUND

The Centers for Disease Control and Prevention (CDC) strives to collaborate "to create the expertise, information, and tools that people and communities need to protect their health—through health promotion, prevention of disease, injury and disability, and preparedness for new health threats."[27] One science-based and customer-centered communications approach at CDC has been the use of social and interactive media in public health campaigns and emergency response. We define social media as media, usually electronic, through which users can interact with other users. Another closely related concept is Health 2.0, "the use of social software and its ability to promote collaboration between patients, their caregivers, medical professionals, and other stakeholders in health."[28] These media help CDC provide accessible, accurate, relevant, and timely health information and interventions that work to protect and promote the public's health.

USE OF SOCIAL MEDIA IN HEALTH COMMUNICATIONS AND HEALTH MARKETING

To encourage information sharing, collaboration, and interactivity, CDC utilizes a variety of social media to help reinforce and personalize messages, expand reach to engage new audiences, and further health communications practice. Increasingly, many health communicators and social marketers also use these new media in this manner.[29] Social media can

- Increase the dissemination and potential impact of CDC's science;
- Help reach diverse audiences;
- Provide innovative ways to engage users, tailor messages, and encourage participation;
- Encourage transparency and increase timely access to information;
- Facilitate interactive communication and community; and
- Empower people to make healthier and safer decisions.

The goal for these efforts is to provide CDC content, tools, and services when, where, and how targeted users want them. By expanding CDC communications activities to include social media channels (such as Twitter, Facebook, and YouTube) and providing information in multiple formats (including text messages, widgets, and podcasts), we can strategically reach large audiences, increase access of information, and reinforce important health messages. In deciding which tools to utilize for a specific campaign, intervention, or emergency response, we look to three factors—communications objectives, audience(s), and key messages. Then, we develop a plan based on a careful and regular review of research from a number of organizations. This research helps us to better understand which social media tools will work best to reach our target groups for specific health communications objectives. For example, if we are seeking to reach underserved populations, or those disproportionately affected by health disparities, we might utilize mobile technologies, eGames, targeted social networking sites, online videos, and other forms of traditional communications. Likewise, we might choose different activities based on our communications needs. For instance, if we are trying to raise awareness of a health issue we would develop a different plan than if our goal is to induce long-term behavior change.

As social media become more widespread, portable, and easy to use, it is likely that messages will be passed along virally. We also recognize that many health information seekers turn to friends and relatives for information,[30] so we encourage users to engage with us and share credible health messages within their expanded social network. An individual can become a health advocate in a number of ways, including posting a button on a social networking site, sharing a widget on his or her blog, commenting on our Facebook page, or reposting our Twitter updates.

SOCIAL MEDIA TOOLS

Mobile

Mobile technology, including cell phones, personal digital assistants or PDAs, mobile games, and other technical applications available on mobile devices, offer tremendous opportunities for improving the health, safety, and preparedness of people in the United

---

*Disclaimer: The findings and conclusions in this case study are those of the authors and do not necessarily represent the views of the Centers for Disease Control and Prevention.

continues

States and globally. CDC encourages the use of mobile technology to communicate health messages, collect data, foster engagement, and increase participation. According to a June 2009 report from Pew Internet & American Life Project, The Social Life of Health Information, "Mobile access is changing the behavior of Internet users and, in particular, changing the behavior of health care consumers. The mobile Internet draws people into conversations about health as much as online tools enable research."[31]

Likewise, mobile technology, and text messaging in particular, also shows promise for rapidly disseminating and retrieving information in emergency and risk communications responses. Because timely messages and expanded reach are important factors in emergency risk communications, text messaging may become one of the most powerful and relevant methods for communicating to and among selected target audiences during times of public health crisis. Mobile devices are becoming increasingly ubiquitous[32] and can help reach important audiences, like African Americans,[33] Hispanics,[34] deaf persons, teens, and people on the go, including moms, migrant workers, or others in transition.

In collaboration with health and technology partners, CDC developed a number of innovative mobile projects to exchange vital health information and engage users to participate in improving their health. CDC leverages mobile platforms by providing mobile Web content, text messages, mobile applications, and the like. For instance, CDC offers a number of text messaging programs on a variety of topics, including HIV testing locations, MRSA skin infections, and emergency messages. The following three mobile examples provide a context for the range of mobile possibilities, from text messaging to mobile applications.

Kenyan Text Messaging System to Encourage Blood Donation

CDC is collaborating with the government of Kenya to develop an opt-in text messaging system to communicate with blood donors and encourage blood donation. The program addresses several specific needs to increase repeat blood donation and recruit in times of crisis. The participants receive text message reminders when they are eligible to donate again or in times of critical shortages when the need arises to recruit a specific blood type. Likewise, the program addresses a critical need in Kenya to use a communications channel people can access. In Kenya, cell phones are less expensive and more accessible than personal computers, the Internet, and phone lines. With a population of 39 million people,[35] 11.3 million of them are current cell phone subscribers, with estimates of 100% mobile penetration in Kenya by 2013.[36] In contrast, 3.4 million Kenyans are estimated to be Internet users.[35]

Mobile Text Messaging Pilot

In September 2009, CDC launched a pilot project to explore using text messages to share important health information about H1N1 flu and other important and timely health topics, like second-hand smoke and food safety. As a pilot project, CDC will collect participant feedback on the text messages and the overall project to learn user preferences in message content, timing choices, channel input and other factors that will help us better deliver health information via text messages. The text messages in this pilot contain short health tips or quiz questions with links to the CDC mobile Web site and a phone number to call for additional information for those who have questions or want to learn more.

Mobile Diabetes Management Research

The Georgia Institute of Technology partnered with CDC to study the use of a glucometer-integrated mobile phone for improving management of diabetes. Study participants can use the phone to record their blood sugar and ask questions in the grocery store or while eating a meal. The glucometer readings and answers to questions are made available on a collaborative Web site for discussion with a participant's diabetes educator. This two-year research study will compare the success of this program to the success of traditional diabetes management programs.

Blogging

Blogs, short for "Web logs," are regularly updated online journals that almost anyone with an Internet connection can use. Some blogs target a small audience, while others have a readership comparable to national newspapers. They may have only one author or a team of regular authors, but most blogs share a similar format in that the entries are posted in a reverse chronological order and may allow reader comments on posts.[37] Of the various types of user-generated media, blogs, in particular, are important because they cut across many segments of society and have continued to increase in number and popularity.[38] CDC is home to blogs on topics ranging from zoonotic diseases to injury prevention and control. CDC blogs allow programs to share information in a way that encourages readers to comment and engage with the content.

CDC also hosts "bloginars," webinars created specifically for bloggers, as a tool to reach out to bloggers and provide them with information about outbreaks or public health events. Each bloginar typically features a presentation by a subject matter expert or experts and a presentation of relevant social media products as well as provides participants an opportunity to interact with the presenters and ask questions. Bloginars also include promotion of social media tools designed specifically for bloggers, such as online graphics, widgets, or online video. Bloginars provide bloggers with accurate, credible information they can use to write blog entries about current topics of interest.[39]

CDC used blogger outreach during the 2009 outbreak of *Salmonella Typhimurium* and associated recalls of peanut butter and peanut-containing products. The bloginar, attended by 35 bloggers and media outlets, featured two subject matter experts who updated attendees on the current state of the outbreak at the time and outlined steps attendees could take to deal with the product recalls.

Microblogging

Microblogging allows users to post brief text updates, usually through a website that aggregates these messages for viewing by friends or the public. Microblogs may also include a social networking component allowing users to connect to other users to view updates.[40] The use of microblogging sites, particularly the microblog Twitter, has grown significantly in popularity, and microblogging is proving itself as a medium for seeking and sharing information.[41] In fact, "as of December 2008, 11% of online American adults said they used a service like Twitter...Nearly one in five (19%) online adults ages 18 and 24 have ever used Twitter and its ilk, as have 20% of online adults 25 to 34."[42]

CDC currently participates in the microblogging site Twitter. Twitter users can post updates, or "tweets," that are limited to 140 characters or less, and can "follow" other users' updates. CDC "encourages the strategic use of Twitter to effectively and inexpensively reach individuals and partners with timely health and safety information."[43] For example, during the 2009 H1N1 flu response, the CDCEmergency Twitter profile drew more than 1 million followers, and continues to provide regular updates to followers about emergency preparedness and response topics.

Online Video

Online video sharing is a popular and powerful activity for exchanging information. Using video-sharing sites, like YouTube or Google Video, to disseminate health and safety messages helps provide an engaging experience for consumers. With people watching more than 100 million clips a day on YouTube alone,[44] these online video sources can be a powerful mechanism to assist CDC in distributing current and accurate science and health messages. Currently CDC hosts videos on its YouTube channel, CDC Streaming Health, and on CDC-TV, a video-sharing site hosted on CDC.gov.

One of the most popular CDC videos provides a basic overview of H1N1 flu, also known as swine flu, highlighting the symptoms and what to do if you get sick. In five months, this one video generated more than 2 million views and has earned a 4.5-star rating based on more than 6,200 reviews. This video can be shared with friends and easily embedded on social networking profiles, blogs, or other Web pages. You can visit www.youtube.com/CDCstreaminghealth or www.cdc.gov/CDCTV to watch, share, and embed CDC videos.

Podcasts

Podcasting offers an opportunity for CDC to share information on a variety of subjects while allowing listeners to select specific topics of interest to them.[45] A podcast is a digital audio or video file that can be saved for playback on a portable media player or computer. CDC offers a library of podcasts developed to deliver health and safety information in a convenient and enjoyable format. CDC podcasts can be listened to or viewed directly from the CDC Web page, or copied to a personal computer or a mobile device, such as an iPod or other portable player.

CDC podcasts (available at www.cdc.gov/podcasts) include several series, such as "A Cup of Health with CDC," a weekly series that features a discussion about a topic from the *Morbidity and Mortality Weekly Report*. CDC also produces the "Kidtastics" podcast series specifically for kids and narrated by kids. The Kidtastics series, available in English and Spanish, features health information on topics such as hand-washing, flu, and food safety. CDC has also produced a variety of podcasts on 2009 H1N1 flu that have been viewed or listened to hundreds of thousands of times since the start of the outbreak.

Social Networking Sites

Social networking sites are online communities where people can interact with friends, family, coworkers, acquaintances, and others who share similar interests. Social networking sites provide an immediate and personal way to share information with individuals or groups within a personal network.[45] Most social networking sites provide multiple ways for their users to interact that may include chat, messaging, video, file-sharing, blogging, and discussion groups. Popular social networking sites are used daily by millions of people and are becoming a part of everyday online activities.

CDC has used social networking sites to effectively and inexpensively reach users with personalized and targeted health information. CDC currently participates in several social networking sites, including MySpace and Facebook. As of December 2009, the CDC Facebook page (http://www.facebook.com/CDC) had gained more than 52,000 fans since its launch in May 2009. Each week, featured articles and events from CDC.gov are posted to the CDC wall, with many articles eliciting comments and discussion from fans.

continues

Virtual Worlds

A virtual world is an online environment in which users can create a virtual persona, or avatar, and interact with other avatars in the online environment. In recent years, virtual worlds have become increasingly popular and numbers of participants are growing. CDC participates in two different virtual worlds, Second Life and Whyville, in order to evaluate the potential for engaging audiences in modeling healthy behaviors and lifestyle choices.[46]

In Whyville, a virtual world for "tweens" (adolescents aged 8 through 12), CDC has conducted a "WhyFlu" campaign to raise awareness among Whyville members about seasonal flu. Educating tweens empowers them to pass along vaccine-related information to others in their households who would benefit from being vaccinated. For several years, CDC has collaborated with Whyville to promote virtual vaccinations for seasonal influenza. Whyville citizens had the opportunity to be virtually vaccinated, protecting them from catching the "WhyFlu," which causes red spots to appear on an avatar's face and causes the avatar to sneeze while chatting. During the six-week activity for the 2008–2009 flu season, almost 9,000 Whyvillians were vaccinated, and Whyvillians virtually washed their hands 385,000 times collectively to help stop the spread of WhyFlu.[47]

Widgets

A widget is an online application, or software created to perform a task, that displays featured content from one website on another blog, social networking site or other Web page. Widgets are automatically updated, so CDC widget users can access up-to-date, credible health and safety content in other sites or blogs where they connect with friends or go for information. CDC provides a number of widgets, available at http://www.cdc.gov/widgets/, on a variety of topics, including smoking and tobacco use, body mass index, and everyday health tips.

Because widgets can easily be added to Web pages, users of those pages interact with them and help increase the reach of CDC's content far beyond the CDC website. It is also very easy to share widgets, making it easier for the widget to go viral, and further increase reach. The U.S. Food and Drug Administration (FDA) and CDC experienced this during the peanut butter and peanut-containing product recalls. The FDA and the CDC, in partnership with the Department of Heath and Human Services, developed a widget to

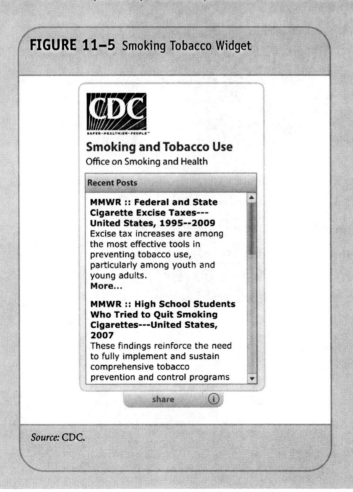

FIGURE 11–5 Smoking Tobacco Widget

Source: CDC.

help identify recalled products. This widget was embedded on thousands of sites and interacted with more than 28 million times as of June 2009.[48]

Content Syndication

Content syndication is a technical application that provides automatically updated CDC.gov content on partner websites. This tool allows federal public health agencies, state and local public health departments, nonprofit organizations, academic institutions, and commercial organizations to easily gain direct access to CDC's health information without having to monitor and copy updates or maintain similar content on their own. Partners report liking this service because it provides them with content they want on their website, it is low maintenance, and their visitors stay on the site, rather than leaving to view the information on CDC.gov. CDC can measure the number of page views on the syndicated pages, so we can monitor the content being viewed via syndication.[49]

eCards

Electronic greeting cards, or eCards, are online greeting cards that can be used as communication tools to encourage healthy behaviors. The Greeting Card Association estimates that 500 million eCards are sent worldwide every year.[50] CDC has more than 200

FIGURE 11–6 Injury Prevention Card Outside and Inside

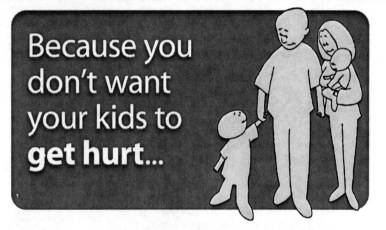

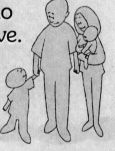

Learn about all you can do to protect the ones you love.

Visit www.cdc.gov/safechild to learn how you can help prevent the leading causes of child injury.

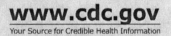**www.cdc.gov**
Your Source for Credible Health Information

Source: CDC.

continues

free eCards, or Health-e-Cards, that can be used to encourage healthy living, promote safe activities, remind people of check-ups, or celebrate a health- and safety-related event.

eCards are an effective and inexpensive way to share personalized and targeted health information by allowing users to send a personal message as well as health messages to their friends and family.[51] Most CDC Health-e-Cards provide a link to a CDC.gov Web page for more information, and some of the cards have generated an 80% click-through rate. There are also a number of viral components to eCards—these cards can be easily sent to multiple people at one time enabling us to take advantage of the sender's established email networks. All of CDC's Health-e-Cards can be viewed at www.cdc.gov/eCards.

Buttons and Badges

Buttons are Web graphics that usually include an image, a short message, and a URL for more information and often include HTML code that allows them to be shared and posted on a website. They are used to spread health messages and information about campaigns and causes online. Badges are small graphic images similar to buttons that include a message and link to a Web page. However, badges are often posted on an individual's social network profile or personal blog to show support for or affiliation with a cause or issue. Unlike buttons, badges typically include messages that show a personal action was taken, for example "I got tested" instead of "Get tested."[52]

CDC has created buttons and badges to promote action and awareness for a number of health topics, campaigns, and health observances. For example, buttons created for World AIDS Day can be shared with partners for placement on websites, as well as individuals who may post them on a personal blog or social networking profile, like MySpace. Additionally, as of December 2009, buttons created for the 2009 H1N1 flu response had generated more than 175,000 click-throughs to related CDC and Department of Health and Human Services (HHS) websites.

FIGURE 11–7 World Aids Day Button

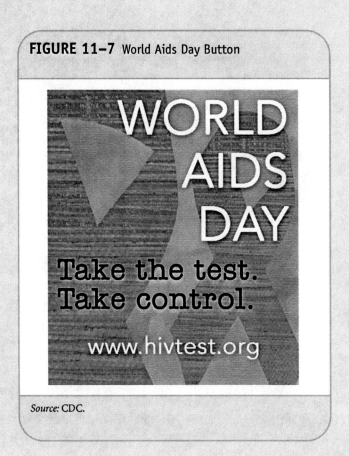

Source: CDC.

Strategy, Challenges, and Opportunities

Social media use at CDC is part of CDC's overall communication strategy that also uses traditional media channels and a strong Web presence. Our intent is to reach target audiences through the media channels they are regularly using and lead them back to CDC.gov for more information. Similarly, we create a number of portable communications products, which can easily be shared with users existing social networks. As a part of this strategy, all social media products are closely tied to the CDC.gov website and provide links, when appropriate, to specific CDC Web pages on health topics. Products may also direct users to CDC-INFO, CDC's comprehensive contact center, where users can e-mail or talk via a toll-free number with a customer service representative 24 hours a day, seven days a week, in English and Spanish.

With the tremendous potential of social media comes a number of challenges and opportunities. One of the most critical challenges is managing multiple health messages in multiple social media channels and encouraging user engagement without losing control of the message. We accomplish this in a number of ways, including moderating and sometimes responding to comments submitted to blogs, instituting and enforcing a comment policy on Facebook, and monitoring multiple social media channels. We also address this challenge by creating low-risk social media products, such as buttons, podcasts, and widgets.

As social media grow as a medium for health communication, the need for cohesive metrics, evaluation, and research in the area becomes increasingly important. While robust metrics can be collected fairly easily with many social media tools, evaluating a multichannel campaign can still present some challenges, because many of the tools do not collect the same metrics, which can make it difficult to compare activities. Additionally, the metrics are often available in different places in multichannel campaigns. For example, in evaluating the 2009 H1N1 flu response, CDC reported metrics from CDC.gov, YouTube, Facebook, Twitter, and several other social media sites. Therefore, to account for all of the activities, one must go to each site and collect different metrics and then create an integrated report.

Moreover, metrics reporting does not provide a full measure of success. When using social media, there is an opportunity to evaluate much more than simple metrics, such as use of information, engagement with content, and meaningful participation. In looking at Twitter, for example, CDC can easily monitor the number of followers on our Twitter accounts and the number of messages posted around an activity. These metrics provide some information, but do not tell us much about engagement. To measure engagement, CDC can monitor click-through rates to CDC.gov content from the Twitter message. CDC can also report the number of retweets, or the number of messages shared on Twitter. Additionally, we can follow conversations on Twitter through the use of a hashtag—a tag used in Twitter to help those interested in a topic find tweets related to the topic.

From a health communications perspective, more research is needed to build the science around the social and interactive aspects of these media and how this relates to trust, messaging, and behavior change. As we continue to advance social media research at CDC, furthering our understanding of the most effective methods for using Health 2.0 strategically to improve message reach, clarity, repetition, consistency, and other important communication attributes will remain an important priority. Additionally, evaluating campaigns, interventions, and emergency response efforts with strong social media components will likely help us improve reach to key audiences, induce behavior change, reduce health disparities, empower users to make informed health decisions, and share health information.

These challenges are all tempered by the tremendous opportunity to shape health behavior in innovative ways and share critical health and safety information when, where, and how our users want it. Whether through a tweet about an impending hurricane, a widget database of recalled food products, or a MySpace button that encourages someone to get tested for HIV, social media provide the opportunity to disseminate important, credible health information in a timely manner.

RESOURCES

CDC.gov hosts several, valuable sources of information on social media efforts at CDC, including the following key resources:

- The social media overview page at http://www.cdc.gov/socialmedia. This page provides a comprehensive overview of social media activities at CDC, including an overview of our tools, campaigns, and presence in social media channels.
- The eHealth Data Briefs page at http://www.cdc.gov/healthmarketing/ehm/databriefs/. The eHealth data briefs contain data highlights and demographics information on many eHealth tools at CDC so programs can better understand our users and the most powerful ways to reach them.
- The eHealth Metrics Dashboard at http://www.cdc.gov/metrics. This dashboard provides data and analyses on CDC's eHealth activities and includes customer satisfaction scores, eHealth products, top search keywords and referrers, Web campaign metrics, and most popular pages. The dashboard is updated quarterly.

Box 11–4 What Social Media Use in the United States Means to Health Communication

By Wen-ying Sylvia Chou, PhD, MPH Cancer Prevention Fellow, Health Communication and Informatics Research Branch, National Cancer Institute

Internet use and social media are catalysts in the rapidly changing communication landscape, underscoring the importance of understanding how these new (and some not-so-new) forms of communication impact how we as health communicators move forward. So, our research team aimed to "identify the characteristics of current social media users . . . [to] inform health promotion/communication efforts aiming to effectively utilize social media."

We used data from the Health Information National Trends Study (HINTS). "HINTS is a nationally representative cross-sectional survey on health-related communication trends and practices" (http://hints.cancer.gov/). Nearly _ of more than 7,000 U.S. adults who took this survey reported having accessed the Internet in 2007. Of those, 5% said they participated in an online support group, 7% blogged, and 23% used a social networking site (e.g., MySpace, Facebook, etc.). Results showed that, "While racial/ethnic and health status-related disparities exist in Internet access, among those with Internet access, these characteristics do not affect social media use" as much as might be expected. Explained differently, "social media are penetrating the U.S. population independent of education, race/ethnicity, or health care access." Results also showed that different age groups are accessing and using social media differently, with younger people being the heaviest uses of this form of online communication.

So what does all this mean for us as health communicators? Namely, "health communication programs utilizing social media must first consider the age of the targeted population to help ensure that messages reach the intended audience." For example, given the popularity of social media among young Internet users, health marketing efforts using social media would likely have the broadest reach among young folks; however, social media penetration in older population is expected to increase. Furthermore, "[a]mong the three forms of social media considered in this study, social networking sites by far attract the most users, making them an obvious target for maximizing the reach and impact of health communication and e-health interventions."

"If we can enable broader and more equitable Internet access (e.g., increasing broadband access or wireless mobile access), thus reducing the Digital Divide, the potential for impacting the health and health behavior of the general U.S. population through social media is tremendous." The "Digital Divide" is a phenomena currently taking place, in which the disparity of access to Internet and other new technologies is growing larger between people of low versus high socioeconomic status, and people of low status, therefore, have less access to health information on the Internet than people of high status, ever increasing the health disparities between these groups as well. Social media might not enable targeted communication messages, but it may have the capacity to reach a wider audience than the traditional media have been able to reach, providing additional new opportunities to narrow this health disparities gap.

As part of health communication research efforts, we need to identify the role of new and emerging forms of social media through diverse methods, like different data sets, survey items, and multiple measurement tools, including ethnography. We can also use social media strategically as part of multifaceted interventions to reach people in their own familiar environments. It's important to note that we can't completely assume the results of our study are generalizable to the entire population because there were low response rates and this is a cross-sectional study (i.e., we did not test effects over time). "In order to track the public's use of new media, future research should track different age groups' social media adoption while identifying new forms of social media. Given that the younger age groups are likely to continue their use of social media, we would expect to see a persistent increase across the middle-age population in the near future."

Indeed there seem to be key opportunities and implications for social media-based health communication efforts in this growing digital age. This is an exciting and important new field that would interest many students in public health communication.

Source: Chou, WS, Hunt YM, Beckjord EB, Moser RP, Hesse BW. Social media use in the US: Implications for Health Communication. *J Med Internet Res* 2009;1(4):e48.
Note: This is a summary of findings reported in the longer article by Dr. Chou and her colleagues. All quotes in this summary have been taken directly from their article.

health and health communication practitioners on the benefits of using Twitter and best practices for using this new medium to reach the public, as shown in **Box 11–5**.

MySpace

MySpace is another social networking site where users (individuals, rock bands, campaigns, agencies, etc.) can have public or private profile pages where they can post photos, video clips, messages, and more to share with MySpace "friends," other users, and sometimes nonusers.[56] MySpace reported having more than 65 million unique users in the United States as of June 2010, and more than 100 million users worldwide.[57] The New York City Department of Health and Mental Hygiene has created its own MySpace page as part of a campaign to improve mental health among teens. This campaign is described in **Box 11–6**.

Box 11–5 Twitter Best Practices for Nonprofits and Health Communicators

By Sarah Marchetti, Digital Influence Strategist, Ogilvy Public Relations Worldwide

As a part of a "Twitter Best Practices" series, Ogilvy Public Relations Worldwide recently developed a simple methodology to help health communicators to engage on Twitter. Twitter is a micro-blogging service that asks the simple question, "What are you doing?"; however, it might be better interpreted as "What would you like to share?". Users must answer this question in 140 characters or less.[55]

Health communicators can use Twitter to join/start the conversation around an issue, educate interested parties, raise awareness, "call to action," and increase positive share of voice for an organization. Twitter followers can also serve as "instant focus groups" for testing messages and getting feedback. To do these things, there are three steps a health communicator should follow to get started on Twitter: Follow, Create, and Engage.

1. *Follow:* Follow other nonprofits/health advocacy organizations, industry thought leaders, and, of course, people interested in your cause/issue to find people interested in your subject area. Follow people who follow you and search for mentions of your campaign or organization.
2. *Create:* Provide value to your followers by tweeting useful information and links. Consider the unique value of your issue and campaign. Set a tone around the issue, brainstorm topics, and constantly be on the lookout for news.
3. *Engage:* Twitter is a conversation tool, not a broadcast tool. Participate in the conversation around your issue. Use @replies (replies to another Twitter user using their handle name, which is like a screen name) to participate in the discussion. Create conversations by responding to people who respond to your tweets.

Remember these best practices when using Twitter for your health communication initiatives and campaigns.

Twitter Do's. For an effective Twitter campaign, do:
- Create a strategy for engaging in Twitter. Know what you want to achieve before you start.
- Create a descriptive bio for your Twitter page so people know what kind of tweets they will see from you if they follow you.
- Listen to what people are saying about your issue/organization on Twitter using the Twitter Search function.
- Provide value for your followers.
- Use Twitter to start a conversation.
- Be dedicated to Twitter. Having more than one employee on Twitter will ensure an ongoing presence for your organization.
- Ask questions and get feedback from your followers.

Twitter Don'ts. Be sure not to:
- Just Tweet. Instead, follow others to join in or start a conversation.
- Use Twitter to broadcast information. It is a conversation tool.
- Be boring!
- Panic if someone says something negative about your organization. Thank them for providing feedback and try to address their issue.
- Take on all the responsibility for Twitter yourself. Having a colleague or two to help you makes using Twitter easier.

Source: Sarah Marchetti, Digital Influence Strategist, Ogilvy Public Relations Worldwide.

Box 11–6 Reaching Teens: Why a Government Health Agency Joined MySpace

By Sabira Taher, MPH, Campaign Manager, Health Media and Marketing, New York City Department of Health and Mental Hygiene

FIGURE 11–8 NYC Health Logo

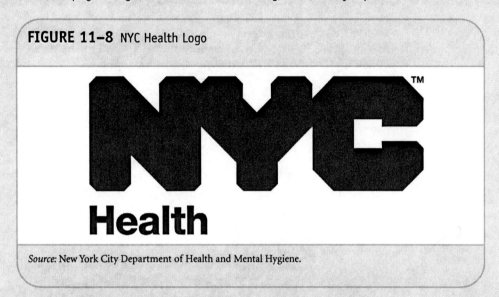

Source: New York City Department of Health and Mental Hygiene.

At the New York City Department of Health and Mental Hygiene (NYC DOHMH), we provide information to millions of New York City residents about important health topics. We use our homepage (http://www.nyc.gov/html/doh/html/home/home.shtml) and various outreach programs to reach the public. Despite these activities, we were anxious to find an effective way to reach teens—a population especially vulnerable to various risks associated with mental health including depression, drug use, and unplanned pregnancy. Results from formative research and previous marketing efforts also taught us that teens are unresponsive to traditional print media on the subject of mental health. We eventually launched a mental health awareness campaign for New York City teens on MySpace—an online social networking site they spend much of their time on already.

FIGURE 11–9 NYC Teen MindSpace Logo

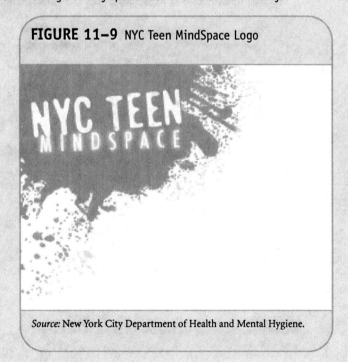

Source: New York City Department of Health and Mental Hygiene.

Nine out of 10 teens ages 12 to 17 go online, and most of them (65%) use social networking sites. A good number of these users go online to look for health information that they don't otherwise feel comfortable talking about with their parents or peers like drug use, sexual health or depression. Furthermore, many of them would like to see more informational messages directed at teens online.[58]

Given this information, we knew we could reach teens on social networking sites. Still, we faced a dilemma. Should we choose MySpace or Facebook as our platform? Both sites are very popular with teens. Three important facts informed our decision: (1) MySpace continues to dominate the teen market even as Facebook gains popularity; (2) MySpace still has traction in urban areas; and (3) MySpace is still home to marginalized teens.[59] These details supported our use of MySpace as a place for teens where they could find and interact with our mental health information. We called our page: "NYC Teen Mindspace," http://myspace .com/nycteen_ mindspace.

NYC Teen Mindspace is filled with teen friendly information about mental health. The content is emphasized primarily through multiple vignettes that portray New York City teens going through experiences that affect their emotions and behaviors. For example, Anaya finally decides to have sex with her boyfriend but they didn't use a condom. As a result, she deals with the stress of not knowing whether or not she is pregnant.

Our creative team developed characters like Anaya to reflect the diverse mental health needs of teens living in New York City. Video blogs for each character present their struggle with specific mental health issues and conclude with the characters seeking social supports to "talk it out" with someone they trust. Users of the site can interact with the content through quizzes and polls,

FIGURE 11–10 "Anaya's Story" Banner Ad

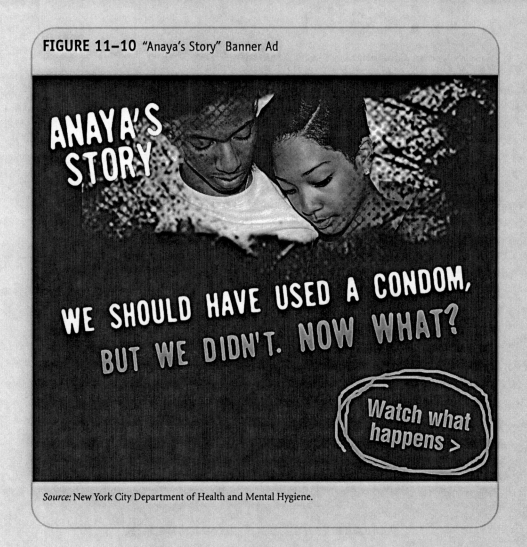

Source: New York City Department of Health and Mental Hygiene.

continues

quick facts, and downloadable emblems they can share with their friends. We also provided teens with an e-mail function and 1-800 number to LifeNet (www.mhaofnyc.org/ lifenet.html), a free, confidential help-line operated by the Mental Health Association of New York City in collaboration with the NYC DOHMH.

In its current state, the NYC Teen Mindspace page lacks user-generated content features—something we understand is the cornerstone of online social media. The agency took this path for two reasons: (1) We were dealing with minors. (2) We would be asking teens to contribute to a discussion about their own mental health. Both of these issues posed liability concerns for the agency with respect to how crisis situations would be handled online. Therefore, we opted to pre-produce all of the content ourselves. It turned out that creative development for the video blogs cost more compared to social media campaigns that rely heavily on user-generated content. However, our content experts found this an acceptable trade-off when we took into account the additional staff necessary to manage, vet, and update new content on a regular basis.

We rolled out two waves of marketing efforts to get New York City teens to visit the page. In year 1, we created and paid for banner ads on MySpace, geo-targeting New York City teens. To increase traffic in year 2, we expanded banner ad activities to include Teen.com and Wild Tangent Games Network in addition to MySpace, again geo-targeting New York City teens. We also aired promos on a local radio station with a large teen audience. On-air we advertised the benefits of visiting NYC Teen Mindspace and prize giveaways for visiting the page.

In any public health communication intervention, it is important to evaluate efficacy and eventually outcomes. Using an Internet-based campaign provides a unique opportunity to use Key Performance Indicators (KPI) previously established to measure campaign efficacy. For example, we measured audience reach and engagement using ideal website analytics including total visits, page views, and clickstream tracking. We found the following:

NYC Teen MindSpace Analytics

	Page Views (Organizational and Character Pages)	Banner Impressions*	CTR**	Quizzes and Polls Taken	Total "Friends"
Year 1	20,469	14,717,182	0.047%	2,463	310
Year 2	47,163	2,377,834	0.34%	6,647	997

*Banner Impressions are the number of times banner ads are displayed.
**CTR stands for click-through rate.

These numbers indicate a clear growth of NYC Teen Mindspace's popularity and reach between its first and second year. Still, in our opinion, MySpace Web analytics are lacking, and we do not have all of the KPI necessary for a comprehensive evaluation of online media. Furthermore, we could not survey NYC Teen Mindspace friends for statistical evaluation (i.e., to collect demographic information and to measure recall and increased awareness as a result of the campaign) due to human subjects testing concerns for minors.

Through youth advisory panels, we convened during the formative research phase and usability lab sessions we conducted with teens at the end of year 1, we learned that teens responded positively to the NYC Teen Mindspace characters. Teens believed their profile pages were realistic and that their complicated issues were presented well. E-mails sent by the teens to LifeNet indicated that the video blogs and widgets helped teens identify and work through their own emotional and behavioral issues.

What we also learned from other research is that the teen segment and new media users in general like to see content refreshed on a regular basis. We have continued to update the NYC Teen Mindspace page with new mental health issues, characters, and blogs to keep the campaign fresh and appealing over the long run.

Other lessons we have learned are: (1) New media campaigns need to be integrated into strategic health communications that incorporate outreach efforts and traditional media for sustainability. (2) Successful social media campaigns also require a paradigm shift within health agencies on how teams of health communication experts use their time and expertise to oversee these initiatives. (3) Lastly, cost is something to always keep in mind. The more user-generated content features we incorporate, the less we need to spend on creative development and marketing. On the flip side, as we increase the level of interactivity, the cost of backend management and timely responses goes up. It is a media paradox worth exploring, though. Never before has the NYC DOHMH been so successful in reaching teens on the subject of mental health awareness. We must be doing something right.

Sources:

Lenhart A, Macgill A, Madden M, Smith A. *Teen and Social Media Report.* Pew Internet and American Life Project. 2007. Available at: http:// www.pewinternet.org/. Accessed July 27, 2009.

Boyd DM. Taken Out of Context: American Teen Sociality in Networked Publics. Doctoral dissertation, University of California–Berkeley School of Information. 2008. Available from: http://www .danah.org/. Accessed July 27, 2009.

Viral Approaches

As you can see, social networking sites comprise some of the newest approaches to marketing healthy behaviors to the public. Not only are "friends" on Facebook or MySpace, for example, able to share information about themselves with one another, like where they are going on vacation or the newest photos from their favorite sporting events, but they can share info from public health sites like NYC Teen MindSpace, spreading the information to numerous other individuals and audiences with the click of a mouse. In this way, these sites are examples of viral marketing approaches. **Viral marketing** has been defined as "the process of encouraging individuals to pass along favourable *(sic)* or compelling marketing information they receive in a hypermedia environment: information that is favourable or compelling either by design or by accident."[60(p.144)] Traditional forms of viral marketing with which you might be familiar are the marketing campaigns for movies like, for example, *Paranormal Activity*, which encouraged audiences to demand that this low-budget film be shown in more movie theaters.[61] The buzz, or word-of-mouth communication, about the movie skyrocketed, and so too did its exposure and ticket sales.[62] Thus, in this day and age, where new media like text messaging, e-mail, and social marketing sites allow us to communicate with one another at a moment's notice without the requirement of face-to-face or even spoken contact, the potential for viral marketing in public health campaigns is indeed promising.

The Legacy Foundation, which created the "Campaign for Truth" described in Chapter 10, is one of the originators of viral marketing for health communication. In **Box 11–7**, Amy Struthers describes a smaller-scale campaign that aimed to increase health behavior by strategically generating a "buzz" around it.

Box 11–7 Starting the Buzz

By Amy Struthers, Assistant Professor of Advertising, College of Journalism and Mass Communications, University of Nebraska-Lincoln

In the fall of 2006, 20 college students in a capstone advertising class at a large midwestern university partnered with the Nebraska Department of Health and Human Services (DHSS) to explore the communications issues surrounding teen obesity. The students were charged with creating an innovative integrated marketing communications strategy and a suite of creative materials that zeroed in on one goal: to increase consumption of fruits and vegetables and the amount of physical activity among high school students.

Students conducted primary as well as secondary research, gathering both qualitative and quantitative data, in a search for the type of insights that they could use to help create campaign concepts. The college class conducted surveys, focus groups, and interviews with many teens across the state, and after analyzing the data, summarized what they felt was one significant insight about the teen audience that could provide the foundation for a campaign: "I want to be an individual like everyone else." This insight guided development of the integrated marketing communications campaign called *Whatcha doin?*

The *Whatcha doin?* campaign encourages teens to make individualized, independent choices regarding a healthy lifestyle, which is attainable at every moment in the "right now" in which teens live: youth can choose their own way to stay active and get their fruits and vegetables.

A key strategic component of the *Whatcha doin?* campaign is a form of marketing known as **buzz marketing**. Unlike the more organic and spontaneous concept of word of mouth, which typically relies on self-selected or volunteer members of a community, the term "buzz marketing" as used here implies a careful strategy with a clear marketing goal driving a suite of activities to engage the target audience.

While health promotion itself is a difficult message to sell, marketing communications experts recognize that the teenage target audience is one of the more complicated populations to target when selling health-related messages. In 2004, teens reported spending in excess of 8.5 hours per day of exposure to recreational media content, often using two or more media simultaneously, with more than a quarter of their media exposure time spent in media multitasking, simultaneous media usage including Internet, cell phones, television, and videogames.[63]

With age, adolescents begin to seek alternate information sources beyond media advertising. They rely on opinions of their peers and look to social norms rather than relying solely on their parents or on traditional mass media advertising in broadcast (television and radio) or print (newspapers and magazines).[64] This points to the viability of using structured, planned, word of mouth from peer to peer, or *buzz marketing*, to convey public health messages. Important personal relationships validate shared information and lend a level of credibility to the message that media savvy youth find lacking in anything that sounds like a sales pitch.

continues

Buzz marketing involves identifying, recruiting, and training members of a target audience to be a sort of internal sales force for a product or idea. In some cases, opinion leaders or trendsetters are selected, while other campaigns look for people who are very connected with their peers. By infusing these "buzz agents" with the brand message, they become a powerful communications channel, spreading the information to their communities, much as a carrier might communicate a virus; this is why buzz marketing is considered a form of *viral marketing*.

The idea for *Whatcha doin?* is to utilize teens themselves in spreading the message that a life filled with fruits, vegetables, and physical activity is "cool." Student organizations in both public and private high schools are recruited. A key feature of each of the groups is a committed teacher adviser, willing to assume responsibility for the team within the school structure while in fact giving the team as much independence as possible. These teachers have been identified in a variety of ways: through contact with school principals, through their subject area, or through personal contact with members of the *Whatcha doin?* network of community partners. The student organizations involved to date in the *Whatcha doin?* campaign have ranged from Student Councils to health classes to Key Clubs and DECA Clubs to physical education classes. Some buzz agent teams have been as large as a 20-person student council at an urban school in the state's capitol city; other schools have had teams as small as a four-student subset of the Key Club chapter at a science focus program school and a two-student team of a Family, Career and Community Leaders of America (FCCLA) chapter in a rural community of 300.

The campaign has been built around a handful of major tenets. The first is that this is a marketing campaign selling a concept; it is not an informational or educational effort. The assumption is that the target audience already believes they have all the information they need about nutrition and exercise; buzz agents are given no training or information about the health implications of fruit and vegetable consumption or participation in physical activity. Instead, they are provided with ideas of how to build awareness of the *Whatcha doin?* brand and to catch the attention of their target audience in an "under-the-radar" fashion.

A second campaign tenet is that, in order to engage the target audience, the message must not be explicit; instead, intrigue and stealth are used to pique curiosity over time. The campaign consists of phases, each lasting multiple weeks, starting with the "stealth phase." Activities build anticipation, a fundamental story telling technique. To build the anticipation, student buzz agents, or "Buzzers," slowly roll out the campaign using materials provided that visually establish the campaign look and feel without actually revealing the message.

FIGURE 11–11 Footprints for *Whatcha Doin?*

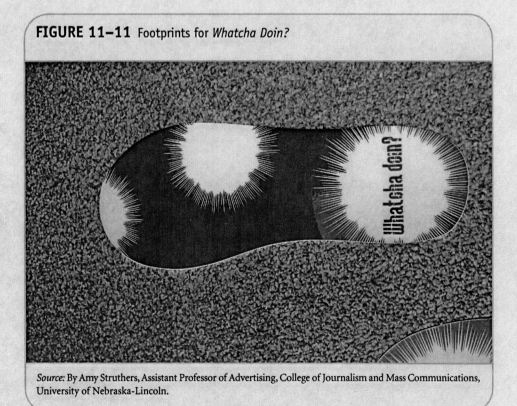

Source: By Amy Struthers, Assistant Professor of Advertising, College of Journalism and Mass Communications, University of Nebraska-Lincoln.

A third tenet is randomness. The teen zeitgeist of "randomness" is exploited in planned frequent small activities around each school that are branded with the campaign logo and color palette, have some relation to fruit and vegetable consumption or physical activity, and seemingly come out of nowhere. An example might be a couple breaking into a dance routine in the school hallways during passing time, wearing campaign T-shirts, while never saying or explaining anything. Teams are encouraged to think low-cost and close to the ground. The state campaign team also gives these buzz agents props to help increase the buzz, such as branded stability balls. Such props begin to crop up in classrooms, media centers, dining areas, and counseling offices building buzz among students who increasingly want to know what's going on.

The buzz agents are in charge of such props, as well as acting as keepers of "the secret." This empowerment of the buzz agents is a fourth tenet of the campaign. Within careful brand guidelines, and instructed to maintain clear communication with their teacher advisers, their school administration, and their custodial staff, the *Whatcha doin?* buzz agents relish the ownership of the message. They become invested, engaged participants in developing visible ways of communicating with their peers about fruits, vegetables, and physical activity. They love the idea of having the secret and watching their peers try to figure out why someone, for example, has just silently distributed fresh fruit kabobs to the class.

A fifth tenet is the emphasis on one-to-one messaging with support from selected mass media only near the end of the campaign's last phase. This means that there is never an all-school "reveal"—no assemblies where announcements make the message clear through presentations or lectures. Instead, the culture of random acts becomes gradually more pervasive, with the acceptance on the part of the campaign team that not everyone will grasp the message.

Whatcha doin? utilizes traditional media as a way to lend support to the buzz agents only after months of nontraditional buzz tactics. Traditional media that have been used have included television commercials on local cable during high teen viewing times and programs, billboards, movie slides, and a website (www.whatchadoin.org). The television commercials are the result of annual video contests, also a final component of the campaign. Students make and star in their own 30-second spots, submitted to the state team through the website. All submissions are posted there, and the top three selected by a panel of judges representing both the state and the creative advertising industry run on cable television the following school year. Billboards draw visuals from the brand and from the top video spots and take advantage of geographical targeting to appear only in areas around high schools.

FIGURE 11–12 Crime Scene Tape for *Whatcha Doin?*

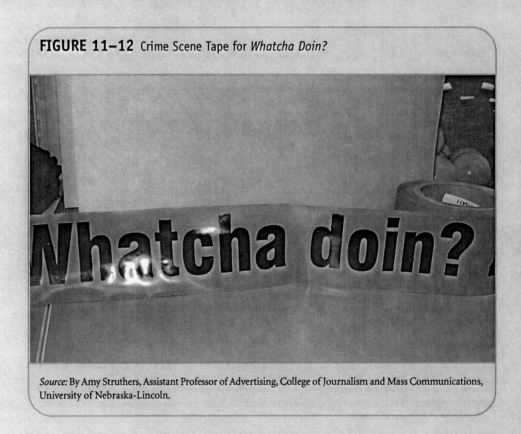

Source: By Amy Struthers, Assistant Professor of Advertising, College of Journalism and Mass Communications, University of Nebraska-Lincoln.

continues

The *Whatcha doin?* campaign launched as a pilot program for the 2007/2008 school year in four public high schools. Since that time, the campaign has been implemented in 15 public and private high schools across the state of Nebraska. Extensive evaluation activities indicate that buzz marketing may be effective in conveying a public health message to teens.

The concept of bringing together buzz marketing, teens, and important public health messages holds much potential to be beneficial to educators, public health marketers, and college students and advertising agencies attempting to break into the teenage target market. With a buzz marketing campaign, not only will students learn the campaign's message from each other, but also they will be engaged with the message rather than only viewing it in varying forms of traditional media.

FIGURE 11–13 *Whatcha Doin?* Carrot Man

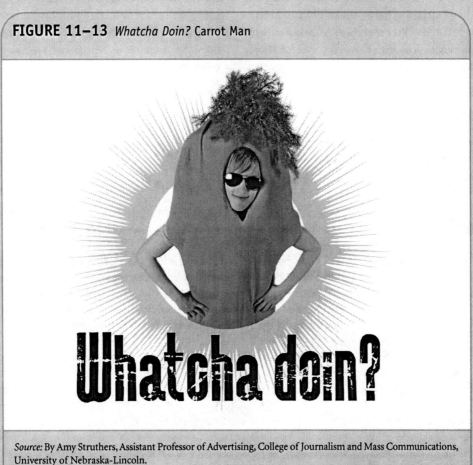

Source: By Amy Struthers, Assistant Professor of Advertising, College of Journalism and Mass Communications, University of Nebraska-Lincoln.

HEALTH COMMUNICATION RESEARCH: UNDERSTANDING MEDIA EXPOSURE

This chapter has unwrapped many of the ways in which health communicators can use media, both old and new, for public health promotion. However, we're missing a critical piece to the puzzle: the piece in which we empirically understand how people are exposed to the many health messages laced throughout media programming, and how this exposure affects their health behaviors. Buffington explains that evaluation of audience exposure to EE programming, as well as subsequent knowledge acquisition from such exposure, comprise important research components of the many Hollywood Health & Society (HH&S) activities. However, it's also important to understand how audiences receive and react to health messages already existing in the media, campaign-related or otherwise, before we can begin to understand how our own campaigns might affect these audiences. For example, researchers at the University of Pennsylvania's Annenberg School for Communication have been conducting research to understand how people purposefully *seek* out and/or incidentally come across, or *scan* for, information about cancer in the media,[65] termed seeking and scanning behavior (SSB). They are also studying how SSB is related to cancer prevention and screening behaviors in the general population[66] and how SSB affects the experiences of cancer patients specifically.[67] A culmination of such research could eventually inform the development of cancer communication campaigns,

and perhaps even health policy related to cancer prevention and control.

In a separate branch of health communication research, Dr. Jane Brown at the University of North Carolina, along with her colleagues, has studied teen exposure to sex in the media. Dr. Brown's "Teen Media" research holds something in common with the SSB research going on at Annenberg in that Teen Media provides crucial understanding about how teens are using the media to learn about health behaviors, either purposefully or incidentally, and how this exposure might be related to their own health behaviors, specifically sexual behaviors. (See **Box 11–8**.)

Box 11–8 Teen Media: Using Health Communication Research to Study Sex, Drugs, and Rock 'n' Roll

By Jane D. Brown, PhD, James L. Knight Professor, University of North Carolina School of Journalism and Mass Communication

I research 'sex, drugs, and rock 'n' roll,' or at least how they are portrayed in media used by millions of teens in the United States, and now around the world. One example of this research is the Teen Media study (www.unc.edu/depts/jomc/teenmedia/), which I helped lead from 2001–2007.

In the Teen Media study, we first conducted pilot surveys with early adolescents (12 to 14 years old) to find out which media they were using. The final list of media "vehicles" that we collected and analyzed for sexual content included 71 television shows, 94 movies, CDs by 67 music artists, 32 magazines, 34 Internet sites, and 3 newspapers. More than 3,000 teens from central North Carolina were then asked via self-administered questionnaires mailed to their homes to report how frequently they used each of these kinds of media. About 1,000 were then interviewed in their homes using laptop computers and were asked about their sexual health behaviors when they were 12 to 14 years old and then again two years later.

The analysis of content found that music contained dramatically more sexual content (40%) than any other medium. Next were movies (12% sexual content), followed by television (11%), magazines (8%), Internet sites (6%), and newspapers (1%). Of the six media, exposure to music and movies was most strongly correlated with teens' sexual behavior (from kissing to intercourse) when they were 12 to 14 years old.[68]

A measure called the Sexual Media Diet (SMD) based on the combination of media consumption and content was then created to assess each teen's exposure to sexual content across four kinds of media (movies, music, TV and magazines). A compelling finding of the Teen Media study was that white adolescents with the highest Sexual Media Diets when 12 to 14 years old were 2.2 times more likely to have had sexual intercourse when 14 to 16 years old than those who had the lowest Sexual Media Diets.[69]

In one of our papers,[70] we suggest that the media may encourage teen sexual behavior by providing "sexual super peers," appealing models who engage in unprotected sexual behavior without negative consequences. We tested this super peer hypothesis with a subsample of the adolescent girls in the study and found that earlier maturing girls were more interested in sexual media, were more exposed to sexual media, and perceived more sexual permission from media than later maturing girls. Thus, the girls who sexually matured earlier than their agemates may have been seeing the characters and stars in the media as friends who could provide information about sex that the girls' real-world friends could not provide.

The Teen Media study is important to health communication because it provides statistical support for a relationship between exposure to sex in the frequent entertainment content in the media and sexual behavior in a specific audience. Our work also demonstrates the importance of knowing as much about the audience as possible. Studies such as Teen Media could guide subsequent interventions to focus on adolescents who are seeing more sexual content in the media. Adolescents need to know that they are getting an incomplete message about sexual behavior since the media rarely include information about the three C's of sexual health: commitment, contraceptives, or consequences. Research such as this suggests a need for health communication interventions that can provide alternative messages about early sexual behavior as well as media literacy education so young people can become more thoughtful media consumers.[71]

CONCLUSION

Exemplars of new media use for public health communication featured in this chapter illustrate an important consideration in today's age of health communication: if McDonalds has a Facebook profile page, public health campaigns should have a page too. A Facebook profile *per se* might not be necessary, but some sort of attractive, dynamic, user-friendly presence in the new media social club could potentially help many health communication campaigns connect with younger audiences. The "old hands" at health communication must be willing to face the challenge of using new media, particularly acquiring the technological ability required (hire someone), and being adequately tuned in to which new channels will reach and attract diverse audiences.

The next generation of health communicators will indeed have a leg up on knowing how to integrate communications with the multimedia world because they have been using these kinds of new media most of their lives. Take advantage of your familiarity with new media. Know that you can get your messages out on TV, but it might also be effective to send eCards reinforcing those messages, or launch a Twitter site where at-risk audiences can ask questions and get involved in improving their own health. It's a multimedia world indeed. Make it work.*

KEY TERMS

Buzz marketing
Consumer-generated media (CGM)
Earned media
Entertainment education (EE)
Public service announcements (PSAs)
Traditional media
Viral marketing

---

*To quote Tim Gunn from the television show *Project Runway*.

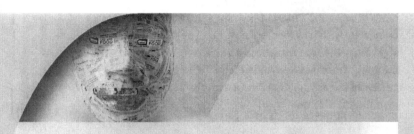

Chapter Questions

1. Describe two forms of new media that the CDC is using to promote public health.

2. How is MySpace being used to market health among teens in New York City?

3. Define entertainment education and how it is being used in Hollywood.

4. Why would we need to research how people use the media in order to develop health communication campaigns?

5. How would you launch a campaign using buzz or viral marketing?

6. Why would or wouldn't the *Oprah* show be a promising way to reach women under 35?

7. If you had $1,000 to spend on a campaign to prevent drunk driving among college-age men, what media and channels would you use? How would you spend your money?

REFERENCES

1. McDonald's. McDonald's Facebook® Web page. Available at: http://www.facebook.com/McDonalds. Accessed January 12, 2010.

2. Facebook. Press Room. Available at: http://www.facebook.com/press/info.php?statistics. Accessed January 12, 2010.

3. The Neilson Company. Television, Internet and Mobile Usage in the U.S. The Neilson Company: A2/M2 Three Screen Report. Volume 6, 3rd Quarter, 2009. Updated December 18, 2009. Available at: http://blog.nielsen.com/nielsenwire/wp-content/uploads/2009/12/Three-Screen-Rpt_US_3Q09REV.pdf. Accessed January 12, 2010.

4. Spectrum Science. The Communications Atmosphere: A Changing World. Picking Paths that Maximize Resources. Downloaded from: www.slideshare.net/.../spectrum-science-communications-presentation.

5. Arbitron, Inc. *Radio Today.* 2009 Edition. Available at: www.arbitron.com/radiotoday. Accessed December 30, 2009.

6. Sass E. Magazine audiences increase 8%, 2000–2009. *Media Daily News;* September 25, 2009. Available at: http://www.mediapost.com/publications/?fa=Articles.showArticle&art_aid=114355. Accessed December 30, 2009.

7. Scarborough Research. Scarborough Writes a Refreshing Headline for the Newspaper Industry: Three-Quarters of Adults are Reading Newspapers, in Print or Online. November 17, 2009. Available at: http://www.scarborough.com/press_releases/Scarborough%20Newspaper%20Audience%20Readership%20NAA%20November%202009%20A.pdf. Accessed January 12, 2010.

8. Jennifer Isenberg Blacker, on behalf of the National Institute on Drug Abuse. Web 2.0: How the National Institute on Drug Abuse (NIDA) Has Embraced This Interactive Social Networking Platform to Reach Youth with Its Messages. Talk presented at: Third National Conference on Health Communication, Marketing and Media; August 11, 2009.

9. Cangialosi G. Marketing in the social web. Presentation in: Viral Marketing: Creating Content That Catches Fire. Best Practices briefing, The Advertising Council, April 2009. Available at: http://www.adcouncil.org/files/seminar_series/viral/GregCangialosi.pdf. Accessed January 12, 2009.

10. This approach is based on the Johns Hopkins Field Guide to Designing a Health Communication Strategy. O'Sullivan GA, Yonkler JA, Morgan W, Merritt AP. *A Field Guide to Designing a Health Communication Strategy.* Baltimore, MD: Johns Hopkins Bloomberg School of Public Health/Center for Communication Programs; March 2003. Available at: http://www.jhuccp.org/pubs/fg/02/index.shtml. Accessed January 12, 2010.

11. Kaiser Family Foundation, Generation M2: Media in the Lives of 8- to 18-Year-Olds, 2010. Available at: http://www.kff.org/entmedia/mh012010pkg.cfm.

12. Table 11–2 developed by author based on numerous sources of data cited in table.

13. These were the top five spenders on all forms of advertising in 2009, according to *Advertising Age,* Marketer Trees 2009 Update (www.adage.com).

14. The Advertising Council, Inc. *Buzzed Driving Is Drunk Driving:* Drunk Driving Prevention Campaign Case Study. Available at: www.adcouncil.org. Accessed August 26, 2010.

15. Kohlenberger J, Taglang K. Citizen's Guide to the Public Interest Obligations of Digital Television Broadcasters. The Benton Foundation. Available at: http://www.benton.org/public_interest_obligations_of_dtv_broadcasters_guide. Accessed January 4, 2010.

16. Davis T. How PS Directors Fill Space. Based on Ad Council PSD Panel Survey. Presentation made to: The Advertising Council Inc., www.adcouncil.org. August 2007.

17. Singhal A, Rogers EM. The Status of Entertainment-Education Worldwide. In: Singhal A, Cody MJ, Rogers EM, Sabido M (Eds.). *Entertainment-Education and Social Change.* Mahwah, NJ: Laurence Erlbaum Associates; 2004:3–18.

18. Jibaja ML, Kingery P, Neff NE, Smith Q, Bowman J, Holcomb JD. Tailored, interactive soap operas for breast cancer education of high-risk Hispanic women. *J Cancer Educ.* 2000 Winter;15(4):237–242.

19. Stephens-Hernandez AB, Livingston JN, Dacons-Brock K, Craft HL, Cameron A, Franklin SO, Howlett AC. Drama-based education to motivate participation in substance abuse prevention. *Substance Abuse Treatment, Prevention, and Policy.* 2007;2(11). doi:10.1186/1747-597X-2-11. Available at: http://substanceabusepolicy.com/content/2/1/11/. Accessed January 12, 2010.

20. Rogers EM, Vaughan, PW, Ranadhan MA, Swalehe NR, Svenkerud P, Sood S. Effects of an Entertainment-education Radio Soap Opera on Family Planning Behavior in Tanzania. *Studies in Fam Plan.* 2003;30(3):193–211.

21. Prism Awards. Available at: http://www.prismawards.com/. Accessed January 12, 2010.

22. National Alliance on Mental Illness. Available at: http://www.nami.org/. Accessed January 12, 2010.

23. National Institute for Drug Abuse. NIDA for Teens. Available at: http://www.teens.drugabuse.gov/. Accessed January 4, 2010.

24. National Institute for Drug Abuse. Available at: www.drugabuse.gov. Accessed January 4, 2010.

25. National Coalition of STD Directors. *National Guidelines for Internet-based STD and HIV Prevention: Accessing the Power of the Internet for Public Health.* Washington, DC: Author. March 2008;9.

26. *Why Y Women?* Prepared for Sugar, Inc. Radar Research, 2009. Available at: http://media.onsugar.com/static/imgs/WhyYWomen.pdf. Accessed January 4, 2010.

27. Centers for Disease Control and Prevention. About CDC: Vision, mission, core values, and pledge. Available at: http://www.cdc.gov/about/organization/mission.htm. Accessed October 14, 2009.

28. Sarasohn-Kahn J. The Wisdom of Patients: Health Care Meets Online Social Media. 2008. Available at: http://www.chcf.org/documents/chronicdisease/HealthCareSocialMedia.pdf. Accessed September 18, 2009.

29. Thackeray R, Neiger BL, Hanson CL, McKenzie JF. Enhancing promotional strategies within social marketing programs: use of Web 2.0 social media. *Health Promotion* Practice. 2008;9(4):338–343.

30. iCrossing. iCrossing's How America Searches: Health and Wellness. 2008). Available at: http://www.icrossing.com/research/how-america-searches-health-and-wellness.php. Accessed September 18, 2009.

31. Fox S, Jones S. The Social Life of Health Information. Available at: http://pewinternet.org/~/media//Files/Reports/2009/PIP_Health_2009.pdf. Retrieved October 14, 2009.

32. CTIA. Competition and Consumer Choice are Hallmarks of U.S. Wireless Industry. Available at: http://www.ctia.org/blog/index.cfm/2009/6/16/Competition-and-Consumer-Choice-are-Hallmarks-of-US-Wireless-Industry. Accessed October 12, 2009.

33. Horrigan, J. Mobile access to data and information. 2008. Available at: http://www.pewinternet.org/Reports/2008/Mobile-Access-to-Data-and%20Information.aspx. Accessed October 14, 2009.

34. eMarketer. Minorities Lead Mobile Content Adoption. Available at: http://www.emarketer.com/Article.aspx?R=1007220. Accessed October 14, 2009.

35. Internet World Stats. Internet Usage Statistics for Africa. Available at: http://internetworldstats.com/stats1.htm. Accessed October 14, 2009.

36. IT News Africa. 100% mobile penetration for Kenya, Tanzania by 2013. Available at: http://www.itnewsafrica.com/?p=2379. Accessed October 14, 2009.

37. Centers for Disease Control and Prevention. Social media at CDC: Blogs. Available at: http://www.cdc.gov/SocialMedia/Tools/Blogs.html. Accessed October 12, 2009.

38. Technorati. State of the Blogosphere. 2008. Available at: http://technorati.com/blogging/state-of-the-blogosphere//. Accessed September 18, 2009.

39. Centers for Disease Control and Prevention. Social media at CDC: Bloginars. Available at: http://www.cdc.gov/SocialMedia/Tools/Bloginars.html. Accessed October 12, 2009.

40. Centers for Disease Control and Prevention. Social media at CDC: Micro-blogs. Available at: http://www.cdc.gov/SocialMedia/Tools/MicroBlogs.html. Retrieved October 12, 2009.

41. Giustini D, Wright M. Twitter: An introduction to microblogging for health librarians. *J Canadian Health Libraries Assoc.* 2009;30(1).

42. Lenhart A, Fox S. Twitter and Status Updating. Available at: http://www.pewinternet.org/Reports/2009/Twitter-and-status-updating.aspx. Accessed September 18, 2009.

43. Hurley, C. Y,000,000,000uTube. Available at: http://youtube-global .blogspot.com/2009/10/y000000000utube.html. Accessed October 14, 2009.

44. Centers for Disease Control and Prevention. Social Media at CDC: Podcasts. Available at: http://www.cdc.gov/SocialMedia/Tools/Podcasts .html. Accessed October 12, 2009.

45. Centers for Disease Control and Prevention. Social Media at CDC: Social Networking Sites. Available at: http://www.cdc.gov/Social Media/ Tools/SocialNetworking.html. Accessed October 12, 2009.

46. Centers for Disease Control and Prevention. Social Media at CDC: Virtual Worlds. Available at: http://www.cdc.gov/SocialMedia/Tools/Virtual Worlds.html. Accessed October 12, 2009.

47. Centers for Disease Control and Prevention. Social Media at CDC: Seasonal Flu 2008–2009. Available at: http://www.cdc.gov/SocialMedia/ Campaigns/SeasonalFlu/index.html. Accessed October 13, 2009.

48. Centers for Disease Control and Prevention. Social Media at CDC: Widgets. Available at: http://www.cdc.gov/metrics/socialmedia/widgets.html. Accessed October 12, 2009.

49. Centers for Disease Control and Prevention. Social Media at CDC: Content Syndication. Available at: http://www.cdc.gov/SocialMedia/Tools/ ContentSyndication.html. Accessed November 29, 2009.

50. Greeting Card Association. Greeting Card Association, About Greeting Cards Webpage. Available at: http://www.greetingcard.org/about.php?ID=2. Accessed December 14, 2008.

51. Centers for Disease Control and Prevention. Social Media at CDC: eCards. Available at: http://www.cdc.gov/SocialMedia/Tools/eCards.html. Accessed October 13, 2009.

52. Centers for Disease Control and Prevention. Social Media at CDC: Buttons and Badges. Available at: http://www.cdc.gov/SocialMedia/Tools/ ButtonsBadges.html. Accessed October 12, 2009.

53. Chou, WS, Hunt YM, Beckjord EB, Moser RP, Hesse BW. Social media use in the US: Implications for Health Communication. *J Med Internet Res.* 2009;1(4):e48.

54. Compete, Inc. Site profile for: Twitter.com. Available at: http://site analytics.compete.com/twitter.com/. Accessed January 12, 2010.

55. Twitter. About Twitter. Available at: http://twitter.com/about#about. Accessed January 12, 2010.

56. MySpace. About us. Available at: http://www.myspace.com/index.cfm? fuseaction=misc.aboutus. Accessed January 13, 2010.

57. MySpace. Fact Sheet. Available at: (http://www.myspace.com/press room?url=/fact+sheet/). Accessed January 13, 2010.

58. Lenhart A, Macgill A, Madden M, Smith A. *Teen and Social Media Report.* Pew Internet and American Life Project. 2007. Available at: http:// www.pewinternet.org/. Accessed July 27, 2009.

59. Boyd DM. Taken Out of Context: American Teen Sociality in Networked Publics. Doctoral dissertation, University of California–Berkeley School of Information. 2008. Available at: http://www.danah.org/. Accessed July 27, 2009.

60. Dobele A, Toleman D, Beverland M. Controlled infection! Spreading the brand message through viral marketing. *Bus Horiz.* 2005;48(2): 143–149.

61. *Paranormal Activity.* (2009). Official Movie Site & Trailer. Available at: http://www.paranormalactivity-movie.com/press.html. Accessed January 13, 2010.

62. Cieply, M. Film on a Tiny Budget Earns Big Money. *New York Times.* October 25, 2009. Available at: http://www.nytimes.com/2009/10/26/ movies/26box.html. Accessed January 13, 2010.

63. Roberts DF, Foehr UG, Rideout V. Generation M: Media in the Lives of 8-18 Year-Olds. A Kaiser Family Foundation Study. Report No. 7251. Kaiser Family Foundation, 2005 March. Available at: http:// www.kff.org/entmedia/ upload/Generation-M-Media-in-the-Lives-of-8-18-Year-olds-Report.pdf. Accessed January 13, 2010.

64. Moore RL, Stephens LF. Some communication and demographic determinants of adolescent consumer learning. *J Cons Res.* September 1975; 2(2):80–92. Available at: http://www.jstor.org/stable/2488749. Accessed January 13, 2010.

65. Niederdeppe J, Hornik RC, Kelly BJ, Frosch DL, Romantan A, Stevens R, et al. Exploring the dimensions of cancer-related information seeking and scanning behavior. *Health Comm.* 2007;22(2):153–167.

66. Kelly BJ, Niederdeppe J, Hornik RC. Validating measures of scanned information exposure in the context of cancer prevention and screening behaviors. *J Health Comm.* December 2009;14(8):721–740. DOI: 10.1080/ 10810730903295559. Available at: http://dx.doi.org/10.1080/10810730903 295559. Accessed January 13, 2010.

67. Nagler RH, Bourgoin A, Freres D, Parvanta S, Gray SW, Fraze T, Hornik R. Effects of information seeking on cancer patients' concerns about long-term risks. Presented at the American Public Health Association Conference, November 2009.

68. Pardun CJ, L'Engle KL, Brown, JD. Linking exposure to outcomes: Early adolescents' consumption of sexual content in six media. *Mass Comm and Society.* 2005;8:2,75–91.

70. Brown JD, Halpern CT, L'Engle KL. Mass media as a sexual super peer for early maturing girls. *J Adoles Health.* 2005 May; 36(5):420–427.

71. Brown JD (Ed.). *Managing the Media Monster: The Influence of Media from Television to Text Messages on Teen Sexual Behavior and Attitudes.* Washington, DC: The National Campaign to Prevent Teen and Unplanned Pregnancy, 2009.

CHAPTER 12

Developing and Testing a Media Strategy

Claudia Parvanta

INTRODUCTION

At this stage of the process you are ready to take your ideas to "the drawing board," so to speak, and develop your final message and media strategy. This chapter is all about ensuring quality and quality control as you move from your formative research to your final communication materials and dissemination plans. What kind of quality are we aiming for? The next section describes the characteristics of effective health communication.[1]

CHARACTERISTICS OF EFFECTIVE HEALTH COMMUNICATION

Accuracy

From the beginning we have stressed that being accurate and up-to-date are essential to public health communication. Putting this together with consistency and clarity (discussed later) is more difficult than one might think. Some health information changes rapidly, such as the number of cases of H1N1, how much we know about an evolving pathogen, the ability of a particular antibiotic to treat an infectious outbreak, the spread of the particles from a dirty bomb, and so on. Particularly in emergency health communication, staying up-to-date is the key threat to accuracy. But in both emergency and nonemergency situations, a more subtle threat has to do with the way scientific information is presented to the public. Using statistical concepts and other technical terms may increase accuracy but decrease the public's ability to understand the information. A health communicator needs to work side-by-side with a subject matter expert. This often requires negotiation to develop information that is simple enough for the general public to understand yet maintains its scientific authenticity.

Clarity

Clear messages are simple. According to the Health Communication Unit at the University of Toronto, every message should include a " 'What,' a 'So What,' and a 'Now What' (a clear indication of what the message is about, reasons the audience should care and clear next steps for the audience)."[2] Effective health messages contain almost no technical terms or jargon and eliminate information that the audience does not need to perform the action called for in the communication. It is again often difficult to pare down extraneous information. You might want to use a **message map** to develop clear, accurate, and consistent messages. (For message mapping in emergency communication, see Chapter 16.)

In addition to a message being simple, it should state clearly what the recipient should do upon receiving the information. In commercial applications, this is called "asking for the sale." If a salesperson does not ask the customers to buy the product, there's a good chance they will not. The same is true in health communication. There are ways to subtly ask for a response. For example, using a narrative format (and

Social Cognitive Theory), someone who has performed a recommended action can speak about the experience, describe his or her satisfaction with the outcome and then suggest that audience members also "give it a try." Asking for a response does not have to be as heavy handed as selling a car.

Lastly in this category, if the purpose of the material is to demonstrate how to do something, such as mix a medication or put on a condom, it is important to use illustrations (in this case, usually line drawings) that depict the process clearly, simply, and sensitively. Pretesting with the intended users as well as gatekeepers will result in a product that prevents disease and death without outraging the larger community. Chapters 6 and 7 discuss other issues to be considered when developing materials so as to be understood by the widest range of users.

Consistency

Consistency is important on several levels:

- In terms of *accuracy*, everything that one organization says about a particular issue should adhere to a playbook, a set of terms and information that have been vetted and standardized. Often organizational inconsistencies crop up in the middle of an emergency or during a presentation when attentive audience members point them out. The likelihood of inconsistency increases with the range of information that has been published in medical articles and textbooks and with the speed at which findings come to light. While it might seem like an imposition of authority, often the only way to avoid inconsistency in a large organization is to have everything reviewed and cleared centrally.

   The CDC has an elaborate clearance system that checks versions for timeliness and accuracy. In addition, it performs cross-clearance when topics, such as "skin cancer, Vitamin D and sunlight," require the sign-off of several scientific experts.* And, of course, there is also legal clearance for such things as vaccine information sheets (VIS), informed consent forms, and other documents where the CDC could be held liable if it does not explain a medical or research procedure to the public accurately and completely.†

- All materials, messages, and activities that are part of one communication effort should reinforce the others. The key tool to maintain this consistency is the *communication strategic plan* that culminates in a *creative brief.*
- Consistency is the essential element of brand identity. You should use the same logo, slogan, and other graphic identity elements in all the materials used for one campaign or emanating from one organization. The latter is particularly important if the name of the organization adds to the credibility and weight of the message. If the organization is not as essential to the message (e.g., the 'Pink Ribbon' has superseded any one organization's role in communicating about breast cancer awareness. The 'Red Dress' for women's heart disease is making similar headway in consumer recognition), then organizational branding is less important than establishing a consistent unifying look for an entire campaign.

While we do not discuss branding extensively in this textbook, it is key to remember that a "brand is a promise made by an organization to the consumer."‡ Anything marked with a brand needs to back up that promise. If, as a public health organization, your promise is to protect the health of the people that you serve, it makes sense to brand everything you do with your organization's logo, slogan, and other graphic elements.

Credibility

Credibility is closely linked to the accuracy and consistency of a message but also relies heavily on the spokesperson who delivers the information. While celebrities are good for calling attention to a message, most people do not really feel they can identify with the celebrity life style. Your research will probably show that "persons just like me"—that is, persons who match the target audience profile—are the most credible spokespersons. Very often, these are real people who have experienced a problem and are willing to make a testimonial. But, there is no hard-and-fast rule. The Harvard School of Public Health has been surveying the American public for years about public health risks. They find that during emergencies, national leaders such as the director of the CDC are considered to be credible spokespersons, but, generally, private physicians and clergy have more credibility. Politicians tend to rank quite low in terms of credibility.[3]

---

*In this case, both the Skin Cancer branch of the Cancer Division, and the Maternal and Child Nutrition branch of the Nutrition and Physical Activity Division were consulted.

†Contrary to our perception of industry, the legal department at the CDC has been one of the strongest advocates for, and experts in, clear and simple communication to the public. For example, they long required readability testing at below an eighth-grade level for VIS, informed consent, and related documents.

‡This idea is everywhere, with no clear first reference. According to Tom Asacker in his blog, "A brand is the customer's *evolving* expectation of value; value the way he or she subjectively intuits it. It is NOT your slow-to-change, inside-out declaration or "promise." http://www.acleareye.com/sandbox_wisdom/2009/06/a-brand-is-a-promise.html. Accessed October 26, 2009.

One reliable way to build credibility into your communication effort is to partner with organizations and persons who already are credible to the target population. The National Diabetes Education Program minority workgroup initiative is a very successful example. Working through trusted national organizations, well-known authorities and community leaders can offset some of the suspicion that minority audiences, in particular, feel toward government-led public health efforts as well as research programs. Specifically,

- Communication researchers have examined how to move past the legacy of distrust earned by the 40-year-long (1932–1972) Tuskegee syphilis experiment[4] in which the U.S. Public Health Service intentionally withheld treatment from 399 African American men in the late stages of syphilis. President Bill Clinton publically apologized to the eight remaining survivors on May 16, 1997, in this manner:

    The United States government did something that was wrong—deeply, profoundly, morally wrong. It was an outrage to our commitment to integrity and equality for all our citizens . . . clearly racist.

Young African Americans today, even if they do not know exactly what happened, will say, "You know, Tuskegee...," as a reason for not wanting to participate in clinical trials or as a reason for distrusting public health efforts to enroll them in programs. In a 1997 qualitative study, Freimuth et al.[5] found that African Americans maintained a level of distrust of medical research. They did not understand or feel protected by informed consent procedures and, while viewing medical research as necessary, they were very cautious in selecting studies in which to participate. Fueled by such distrust, the rumor that white supremacists intentionally infected Africans with HIV/AIDS periodically raises its head and has complicated treatment here and abroad.[6] However, in a more recent (2005) review of 20 trials, with more than 70,000 participants, African Americans, and those of African origins (in studies conducted outside of the United States) were no less likely to participate than non-Hispanic Caucasians. Freimuth et al. emphasized that, "efforts to increase minority participation in health research should focus on ensuring access to health research for all groups, rather than changing minority attitudes." While the meta-analysis supports this conclusion, our own experience has been that minority individuals, even while agreeing to participate in clinical trials and other forms of data collection, continue to mention the Tuskegee study as a reason "*other blacks* might resist doing this."

- Tribal nations (Native American Indians) also espouse an historical distrust of the U.S. government that extends beyond the Indian Health Service. It has proved crucial to involve Native American medical specialists and Tribal leaders in health communication efforts that address Native Americans as a focus population. The National Diabetes Education Campaign is a successful example of this approach.
- Finally, people can be quite suspicious of profit motives, not only from the private sector, but from what they assume are government attempts to save money at their expense. This came up during the anthrax attacks of 2001, when the CDC determined that the antibiotic doxycycline was as effective as ciprofloxacin in eliminating the risk of anthrax. Postal workers perceived they were getting lesser care with doxycycline, although CDC's primary motivation was to maintain the efficacy of ciprofloxacin as an antibiotic of last resort.[7]

Thus, the credibility of the U.S. government, a state or local health agency, or even a large teaching hospital cannot be assumed to be high in a particular population in the absence of recent supporting data. Credibility can be enhanced by partnerships with national and community groups that are considered credible.

Having said this, U.S. Department of Health and Human Services sites such as the CDC and NCI are considered widely to provide the most credible *health* information on the Internet. Much work has gone into examining what makes a site credible not only in terms of its content, but its layout. **Box 12–1** features a recent article from Usability.gov on what makes a website credible.

Relevance

We have spent a lot of time discussing what makes health communication relevant and meaningful to different groups of people. The most effective messages make use of the information you have gathered about your target audience. In addition to personal factors (psychological state, and readiness to adopt a behavior, etc.) there are many environmental factors that make information more or less relevant. Here are some examples: images of rural settings may not play well in urban environments and vice versa; time of year matters and needs to be matched up in visual imagery; some groups are more sensitive to style of dress and other cultural artifacts that might find their way into your materials. Pretesting with the intended audience will help you prevent mismatches that distract from the message and use the good matches strategically to help the audience identify with and elaborate on the message.

Box 12–1 Website Credibility

By Beth A. Martin

PART 1: INTRODUCTION

The perception of credibility goes a long way in reassuring users that they've reached a Web site that provides useful information (content) and that there's substance behind that content. In fact, Lightner (2003) found that information quality and information quantity, along with security, ranked first in overall importance in a survey of online shoppers.

So, how do you optimize the credibility of your Web sites?

Credible Web sites should be perceived to have high levels of trustworthiness and expertise, according to Fogg et al. (2001). Perceptions of both factors can be enhanced if designers:

- Ensure the site looks professionally designed
- Arrange the Web site in a logical way
- Keep the site is as current as possible
- Provide an archive of past content (where appropriate)

Show Expertise

Expertise, according to Fogg et al. (2003) includes aspects such as "knowledgeable, experienced, [and] competent." Other aspects of expert sites include:

- Links to/from other Web sites show the site is well-respected
- Credentials of the author(s) are valued
- Articles contain citations and references
- News stories are few but contain details

In addition, including a statement that it is the official site for a topic is a strength for government Web sites.

Show Trustworthiness

Users assess trustworthiness by determining how "well-intentioned, truthful, [and] unbiased" a Web site is. This can be done if designers:

- Provide a useful set of frequently asked questions (FAQ) and answers
- Provide links to outside sources and materials
- Ensure the site is frequently linked to by other credible sites

Federal Web sites must also comply with requirements for Web content. Many of the recommendations support credibility, especially trustworthiness, because sites must communicate ownership and make clear what their policies are. (See Part 2 of this box.)

References

Fogg, BJ. (2002). *Stanford guidelines for web credibility. A research summary from the Stanford Persuasive Technology Lab.*

Fogg, BJ, Marshall, J, Laraki, O, Osipovich, A, Varma, C, Fang, N, et al. *What makes Web sites credible? A report on a large quantitative study.* CHI 2001 *Conference Proceedings* 2001;3(1):61–66.

Lightner, NJ. What users want in e-commerce design: Effects of age, education and income. *Ergonomics* 2003;46(1–3):153–168.

Nielsen, J. (2003, November 10). The ten most violated homepage design guidelines. *Alertbox.*

PART 2: BUILDING TRUST

By Susanne Furman, PhD

Wang and Emurian discuss the implications of their work in online trust for web interface design. They suggest the following framework of trust-inducing features.

Wang & Emurian: Trust Inducing Features

Dimension	Features
Graphic Design: Graphic design factor—first impressions	• Three-dimensional, dynamic, and half-screen size clipart • Symmetric use of moderate pastel color of low brightness and cool tone • Use of well-chosen, good-shot photographs
Structure Design: Overall organization and accessibility of information	• Easy-to-use navigation (consistent) • Use of accessible information (e.g., no broken links) • Use of navigation reinforcements (e.g., tutorials) • Page design techniques (e.g., white space, visual density)
Content Design: Informational components, either textual or graphical	• Display of brand-promoting information (e.g., prominent display of company logo) • Up-front disclosure of all aspects of the customer relationship (e.g., company security, privacy, financial or legal concerns) • Display of seals of approval or third-party certificate • Use of comprehensive, correct, and current product information • Use of a relevant domain name
Social-cue design: Embedded social cues, such as face-to-face interaction and social presence	• Including of representative photograph or video clip • Use of synchronous communication media (e.g., IM, chat lines)

Conclusion

Trust, whether it is building online trust or the lack of online trust, is one of the most formidable barriers for people engaging in online relationships, interactions, and transactions. Degree of trust is dynamic and a function of actions and consequences over time. There is still a level of risk even with an interface that is designed to induce trust. The beauty of a Web site (i.e., aesthetics) impacts first impressions and also enhances trust. Designing interfaces to optimize trust will continue to foster customer trust.

References

Wang, YD, Emurian, HH. An overview of online trust: Concepts, elements, and implications. *Computers in Human Behavior*; 2005;21:105–125.

Part 1 Source: http://www.usability.gov/newsletter/pubs/122006news.html. Accessed October 29, 2009.
Part 2 Source: http://www.usability.gov/articles/092009news.html#wang.

You won't always get it right. The Health Communication Unit (Toronto) makes the wise comment that you should put the information that is most critical for convincing your audience to adopt the recommended behavior at the beginning of the message. "That way, audiences who lose interest or become otherwise distracted will still have the opportunity to process some key points."[8]

Correct Tone and Appeal

The tone of the message is how you use the aesthetic elements—imagery, lighting, and sound—to provide an atmosphere that reinforces the message appeal. Think of the music in *Jaws*, the documentary style of *The Office*, or the shaky camera in *The Blair Witch Project* to grasp the idea. If you are trying to be "authoritative" by using cultural icons of authority as spokespersons, you also must ensure that all the aesthetic ele-

ments support the authoritative image. As mentioned in other chapters, entertainment education (particularly when concepts and messages are embedded in television programs) presents an entire package, including tone and appeal. The characters (and actors), storylines, music, and even sponsors of a show may either support your message or work against it. Therefore you try to have an advance agreement with the writers and producers to review the final show before release. (Assuming you are not your own writer and producer!)

- The tone of the messages should support the topic, the desired response, and the target audience. For a long time, public health "campaigns" were uniformly urgent, figuratively (or literally) banging a drum to get everyone on the "band wagon." Social mobilization is popular in many countries and still uses this approach to rally a massive population in response to a short-term event, such as a National Immunization Day.

- Fear appeals, warning people of dire consequences if they do not take the proposed action, often go hand-in-hand with urgent, large-scale campaigns. In an essential meta-analysis, Witte and Allen found that "strong fear appeals and high-efficacy messages produce the greatest behavior change, whereas strong fear appeals with low-efficacy messages produce the highest levels of defensive response," that is, backfire.[9] Witte's extended parallel processing model suggests (and it hadn't been obvious before) that if you scared people too much, and didn't show them how to overcome the obstacles preventing them from taking action, they would freeze up and avoid the subject.

Fear was used extensively in the early days of HIV prevention. The epitome was probably the Australian "Death goes bowling" television spot launched in 1987,* showing a black-hooded Grim Reaper mowing down victims lined up like pins in a bowling alley. The shock and controversy of the ad ensured that the topic was widely discussed, and for this reason, the public health department in Australia credits it with speeding the addition of a difficult topic to the public agenda. Besides scaring people senseless, the problem with fear appeals and with calls for urgent action is that they lose their credibility with overuse. This is particularly true if both are implemented at the same time.

- Humor is another form of appeal that generally requires more skill than might be suspected because people vary so widely in what they find funny. In addition, what the public finds funny changes very quickly.

One effort that uses humor effectively to reach its youthful target audience is The Legacy Foundation's truth® campaign. truth® dissects the tobacco industry, appeals to youth through brutal honesty, buzz tactics, and heavy irony. As of this writing, their Internet site features an interactive video, "Do you have what it takes to be a tobacco company executive?"† **Box 12–2** describes the truth® campaign.

*http://www.avert.org/aids-photo-gallery.php?photo_id=552&gallery_id=9

†http://www.thetruth.com/

Box 12–2 Evolution of the truth® Campaign

By: Patricia McLaughlin, Assistant Vice President of Communications, LEGACY, Washington, DC. December 11, 2009

Where There's Smoke, There's (Creative) Fire: Evolution of the truth® Youth Smoking Prevention Campaign

How do you fight an act of rebellion like smoking? Use more rebellion. And research. And social science. And the latest online tools. And an integrated approach to marketing and communications . . .

OVERVIEW

Launched in February 2000, **truth®** is the largest national youth smoking prevention campaign and the only national campaign not directed by the tobacco industry. Legacy[SM], a national public health foundation in Washington, DC, devoted to tobacco use prevention and cessation, funds and directs the **truth®** campaign. The campaign exposes the tactics of the tobacco industry and the truth about addiction, as well as the health effects and social consequences of smoking—allowing teens to make informed choices about tobacco use by giving them the facts about the industry and its products. The campaign, marking its tenth year in 2010, is designed to engage teens by exposing Big Tobacco's marketing and manufacturing practices, as well as highlighting the toll of tobacco in relevant and innovative ways.

People know that smoking is bad for them—and teenagers are no different in knowing the ill effects of tobacco use. Yet, more than 400,000 Americans continue to die each year from tobacco-related diseases—including cancers, heart disease, emphysema and stroke. Each day, about 3,900 youth try smoking for the first time. For many, it becomes an addiction that can lead to a life of disease and, potentially, tobacco-related death.

Teenage years are a time of transition into adulthood and a quest for control. For some teens, tobacco fulfills the innate adolescent need for control. Pop culture does not help—teens regularly see images of smoking on-screen that can glamorize a deadly addiction. Research has shown that smoking in youth-rated movies influences 200,000 children and adolescents to take up smoking each year.[a] Furthermore, the tobacco industry owns some of the most powerful and recognizable brands in the world. From Joe Camel to the Marlboro Man, the industry for years has understood how to market rebellion as control and how to sell an image that is cool and appealing to teenagers.

truth® is an alternative way to meet the need to rebel—by empowering teens to rebel by *not smoking,* instead of smoking. By providing facts and information about tobacco products and the tobacco industry, the campaign gives teens tools that enable them to take control and make informed decisions about tobacco use. The campaign provides honest facts and information about tobacco products and industry marketing practices. truth® never preaches and never talks down to teenagers. Instead, it presents potentially life-saving information in a creative, attention-getting fashion, through the media teens consume and the communications tactics they employ every day in their personal relationships—all wrapped in a brand that is connected, and relevant.

TARGET AUDIENCE AND STRATEGY OF THE TRUTH® CAMPAIGN

Nearly 80 percent of smokers begin using tobacco before the age of 18; the primary focus of the truth® campaign is youth aged 12 to 17 years. The objective of truth® is to change social norms and reduce youth smoking. Recent data has shown that historic declines in youth smoking have stalled, making truth®'s life-saving messages more important than ever.

truth® directly counters messages from the tobacco industry brands. According to the Federal Trade Commission, the tobacco industry spends about $34 million each day on domestic marketing—more than truth® spends in a year! truth® can never match that spending, so instead it stays ahead by religiously tracking teens' tastes and media usage, and being more "cutting edge."

The truth® campaign uses research with teen audiences, marketing and social science research, and evidence from the most successful branding campaigns to inform its strategies. In its ten years, truth® has utilized many different forms of media and has evolved in its tactics to ensure it is reaching the teen audience most effectively. Campaign elements have included:

- television, radio and print advertising
- a Web site
- cinema advertising
- social networking sites, video sharing sites, and interactive elements
- events
- branded entertainment integrations
- partnerships with like-minded brands
- grassroots outreach through a summer tour

All marketing efforts are focused directly to teens that are most likely to smoke and need the information most. truth® ads—many of which have become iconic with the teen audience—are in-your-face and hard-hitting because teens respond to up-front and powerful messages that display courage and honesty in a forceful way. Teens are involved in testing truth® advertising concepts and provide suggestions and feedback through the truth® Web site.

For wider communications efforts around truth® and the issue of teen smoking, Legacy reaches out to key stakeholders like the media, policymakers, and academics to further publicize the campaign and reiterate the importance of keeping youth smoking high on the public health agenda.

ADVERTISING—AND MORE

truth® has been known for its edgy television ads since the campaign first took to the air. Early campaigns, such as the *infect truth®* campaign of 2001, educated teens on the facts about cigarette design and engineering. Since then, Legacy has developed more than a dozen unique television campaigns that have creatively explored the issue of tobacco. The 2005 campaign *Fair Enough* used a situational comedy set-up, featuring a cast and theme music, to reveal some of the absurdity of tobacco marketing ideas. Later campaigns like truth® *documentary* used a documentary filmmaking style to capture real people's reactions to the marketing tactics of the tobacco industry, with a correspondent and roving camera crew asking questions and recording people's real answers. In 2008, the *Sunny Side of* truth® campaign used singing and dancing numbers, animation and a comedic, ironic approach to highlight the "sunny side" of tobacco use.

---

[a]Glantz SA. Smoking in movies: A major problem and a real solution. *Lancet.* 2003;362(9380):281–285. Erratum published on January 17, 2004.

continues

Other iconic, consistently recognizable ads with the teen audiences have included a singing cowboy with a hole in his throat, and a gritty, street-style ad showing 1200 body bags being laid out at a tobacco industry headquarters, to represent the daily toll of tobacco-related deaths in the U.S.

The **truth**® campaign is everywhere in youth media—on television networks popular with teens like MTV, BET, G4, Teen Nick, fuel, VH1 and **fuse**. **truth**® can not only be seen on the small screen but the big screen as well. **truth**® campaigns have aired before films in the nation's largest theater chains including AMC Entertainment, Inc., Cinemark USA, Inc., Regal Entertainment Group, and Loews. The successful 'Singing Cowboy,' ad was featured on more than 17,606 screens in all 50 states in an effort to counter the effects of smoking depictions in movies.

Media partnerships with such media companies as **fuse**, G4, SiTV, BET and MTV allow us to further extend **truth**® by integrating the campaign's messages into existing programming—on channels and in media where teens are watching. "Branded entertainment" integrations have included several productions with MTV, as well as a partnership with the cable channel **fuse**, the nation's only viewer-driven music network.

- For MTV, **truth**® and MTV created a tongue-in-cheek spin-off of its popular reality show competition, "The Island"—a "Survivor" for the teen segment. For "The Island" spinoff—called "The Blaze"—**truth**® and MTV produced video vignettes that pitted fictional contestants against one another in challenges that mirrored those on "The Island." The challenges illustrated the marketing tactics of the tobacco industry and the dangers of tobacco use. Using satire and dark humor, Legacy showed the serious nature of the tobacco issue, by having most of the contestants wind up injured, maimed or even eaten by "sea monsters."
- For **fuse**, **fuse** produced a six-part documentary-style look at the Vans Warped Tour called "Warped: Inside & Out." **truth**® traveled with Vans as part of the campaign's summer grassroots tour. Each show featured **truth**® brand presence via the iconic orange-colored "**truth**® truck", as well as a look at activities at the **truth**® zone and interviews with **truth**® crew members.

The reach of the **truth**® campaign is also being extended through a partnership with the Centers for Disease Control and Prevention. A three-year, $3.6 million match allowed us to increase the advertising buy in rural and smaller communities that have traditionally had less exposure to the **truth**® campaign—but where smoking rates tend to be higher. Legacy is also giving grant money to some local organizations around the country, to get more teens involved in tobacco-focused educational projects. Having the financial and creative support of such well-known, credible organizations like CDC and MTV, just to name a couple—helps extend the reach of the message as well as the credibility of the campaign and helps **truth**® in its efforts to secure other partners and sources of funding.

truth® ON THE ROAD

For ten summers iconic orange **truth**® "trucks" have criss-crossed the country, making stops at popular summer musical and sporting events where teens naturally gather. During the summer of 2009 alone, the tour made stops in more than 50 cities and 27 states, touring with:

- the VANS Warped Tour—an annual summer rock festival.
- the AST Dew Tour—an action sports tour featuring the top action sports athletes in the world in skateboarding, BMX and freestyle motocross.
- Rock the Bells!—a hip hop festival, as well as some smaller festivals and events.

At each stop, a team of **truth**® crew members—young people in their early 20s who teenagers can look up to and admire—engage with teens on a peer-to-peer level. This form of grassroots marketing is never preachy, and crew members never talk down to teens. Rather, what is called the **truth**® zone—the area just around our **truth**® truck, is what can be thought of as a non-stop party! When teens visit the **truth**® truck, they can dance and listen to popular music tracks that the **truth**® DJs are spinning, get DJ lessons from the DJs, play games with the **truth**® crew members, join in on an impromptu rap session or show off their other talents on the dance floor.

Teens also can receive free **truth**® "gear"—fashion-forward giveaways like t-shirts and hats, or wallets and shoulder bags; trendy items that teens want to wear and share. But no matter how cool the gear, each piece contains a tobacco-related fact or further information on **truth**®; another way **truth**® messages are seeded in a cool and subtle way to reach teens.

Teens from across the country can also follow the **truth**® tour at the truth.com Web site, where they can get biographies of the crew members, read crew member blogs and see photos from the road. Through all of these efforts—the gear, the Web site, and the actual crew interactions—tobacco facts and information are discussed in a low-key way designed to get teens thinking about the tobacco issue, but not feel like they're being lectured to or hit over the head with anti-smoking messages.

During the course of the summer, **truth**® crew members are also interviewed by local media across the country, appearing on radio shows, morning television news programs, and in both traditional newspaper and online news sites.

The tour remains one of the best ways to bring the **truth**® campaign to life—allowing teens who watch the ads, go to the Web site, or share information through social networking sites, to really see, hear and interact with the campaign firsthand.

USE OF SOCIAL MEDIA

truth® always seeks to evolve. Teens of today are not the same as the teens of ten years ago, especially when it comes to how they receive and share information. Ten years ago, teens were watching more TV, reading more magazines and newspapers, and of course using the Internet. Today's teens are using the Internet even more—but they are also sending text messages, sharing

truth® crew members travel across the country each summer, reaching thousands of teens with important information about tobacco.

Source: Joshua Cogan Photography. truth® Crew Members, 2009 Tour.

information about themselves on Facebook and other social networking profiles, swapping photos and videos, and blogging about their lives and their opinions.

While teens still respond to traditional advertising, like TV spots found on MTV, **fuse**, and other cable channels, **truth**® realized early on that digital media could be a powerful tool in reaching teenagers and having them share information themselves. Social media and new technologies play an important role in how today's teens live, play and work. Around 97 percent of teens have electronics such as computers, cell phones, game consoles, and handheld gaming devices. In addition, 75 percent of college students and 65 percent of teens have social networking profiles.

The Web site thetruth.com is the first stop online for all things **truth**®. The site, highly interactive and in a language, style and design relevant to teens, allows teens to engage with **truth**® on their own terms.

Starting in late 2006, **truth**® launched a series of social networking homepages on such popular sites as MySpace, Hi5, Xanga, Bebo, and Piczo. The campaign is on Facebook as well—including a presence in the "Causes" section where teens can support the campaign. Social networking sites have been an ideal way for the campaign to further spread **truth**® messages quickly and cheaply. On both the truth.com Web site and social networking homepages, teens can share information, learn facts about tobacco, play games, download screensavers and desktop themes, play with do-it-yourself print tools, and participate in online discussions and polls. Many of the online components are designed to be shared, so they can spread virally through the teen community.

The Useful Cigarette

For the interactive feature The Useful Cigarette, graphics and sound effects illuminate facts about the ingredients found in cigarettes—the same ingredients that are found in familiar products such as nail polish remover, floor wipes, dynamite and rat poison. Users can click on the moving cigarette and learn how cigarettes share common ingredients with these products.

Social media efforts have also expanded to other sites. A YouTube channel plays **truth**® television advertisements and related video, including video from the annual summer **truth**® tour. Via a Twitter feed, **truth**® crew members send tweets from the road, sharing more about the **truth**® experience in real time for followers of the campaign, as well as information on tour developments and locations. Crew members also post photos from the road to the photo-sharing site Flickr™. For outreach to stakeholders and media, **truth**® and Legacy also employ separate Twitter™, YouTube™, and Flickr™ accounts, to keep information on **truth**® and the youth smoking issue flowing to media and stakeholders. Communications efforts have also included distributing e-cards and social media-friendly news releases to media and stakeholders, and submitting consumer-generated content like photographs to online publications and newspapers.

With the tobacco industry spending more than $34 million a day marketing its products, social media has been a cost-efficient—and effective—way to spread the word about **truth**®—but all the while staying true to the brand's focus on self-empowerment. The sharing aspect of online communications and social networking sites is a way to quickly and cheaply extend **truth**® messages beyond the initial consumer, to whole other networks of teens that can receive the information from friends and then share even further.

TRUTH® WORKS

A growing body of research has proven the efficacy of the **truth**® campaign in changing teens' attitudes and behaviors toward tobacco use.

Two research papers published in 2009 found that **truth**® remains highly effective as well as cost-efficient in its mission to prevent the youth of America from beginning to smoke. Two of the papers were published online in the April 2009 issue of the *American Journal of Preventive Medicine* (AJPM).

The first paper found that **truth**® was directly responsible for keeping 450,000 teens from starting to smoke during its first four years. The second study found that the campaign not only paid for itself in its first two years, but also saved between $1.9 and $5.4 billion in medical care costs to society.

In addition, in May 2007, the Institutes of Medicine presented a landmark report to Congress recommending that America implement strategies to effectively reduce and prevent smoking, and combine those efforts with a changed regulatory and policy landscape to fight the nation's number-one cause of preventable death: tobacco-related disease. The report specifically mentions the **truth**® campaign, and "concludes that a national, youth-oriented media campaign should be a permanent component of the nation's strategy to reduce tobacco."

The campaign has won more than 350 awards for advertising and public relations efficacy and has also been lauded by leading Federal and state public health officials, the U.S. Centers for Disease Control and Prevention, the U.S. Department of Health and Human Services, and former President George Bush.

Legacy and the **truth®** campaign have achieved this with only a fraction of the budget that the tobacco industry has spent on marketing its products. Currently, the foundation faces a serious budgetary drop-off that may jeopardize its ability to develop and sustain its effective mass media campaigns.

COMMUNICATIONS APPROACH

To maximize the campaign's reach, Legacy staff who work on the **truth®** campaign try to employ an integrated approach to marketing and communications. With every campaign execution, the team strives to ensure all marketing and communications elements are working in synch. While raising awareness about the campaign and its effective work, all efforts seek to reiterate the importance of smoking as a vital public health issue and the need for the **truth®** campaign to continue.

Having that clear objective for success starts with having a proven-effective campaign. To better inform learning, **truth®** regularly conducts pre-and post-research on campaign executions, as well as more targeted focus groups assessing teens' attitudes, behavior and lifestyles—helping to shape marketing and communications' strategies and tactics. Qualitative focus groups also allow campaign brand managers and communicators to garner further awareness about teen interests, trends, and awareness of **truth®** and the tobacco issue.

Communications audits help determine opportunities and challenges, and identify new tactics. Media outreach focuses on trade, national and local reporters, as well as separate messaging to youth media. While referencing specific campaign initiatives, messaging also reinforces how the campaign continues to evolve as a robust, effective way to reach teens with important messages, while maximizing assets in the face of declining funds.

truth® publicity efforts extend to a number of areas: new campaigns or advertising; new research; partnerships; grants, and summer and autumn tours. Beyond reporter outreach, information related to the campaign is also routinely posted on the Legacy Web site (legacyforhealth.org), and referenced in the monthly Legacy e-newsletter.

truth® seeks to further the campaign's awareness with other key audiences by conducting speaking opportunities on the campaign at universities, with public health and tobacco control groups, and to marketing and communication professionals. The campaign has also been cited in more than a dozen academic textbooks.

In all communications endeavors, the marketing and communications teams work closely to share information, and involve each other in early stage planning. Both also encourage collaboration and strategic thinking with and among agency partners, to help drive the campaign forward.

OVERVIEW OF LEGACY

Legacy provides funding and strategic direction for the **truth®** campaign. The campaign is produced in collaboration with agency partners Arnold Worldwide (advertising and creative production), and PHD (media buying).

Legacy^{SM} is dedicated to building a world where young people reject tobacco and anyone can quit. Located in Washington, D.C., the national public health organization helps Americans live longer, healthier lives. Legacy develops programs that address the health effects of tobacco use, especially among vulnerable populations disproportionately affected by the toll of tobacco, through grants, technical assistance and training, partnerships, youth activism, and counter-marketing and grassroots marketing campaigns. Besides **truth®**, the foundation's programs also include **EX®**, an innovative public health program designed to speak to smokers in their own language and change the way they approach quitting; and research initiatives exploring the causes, consequences and approaches to reducing tobacco use. The American Legacy Foundation was created as a result of the November 1998 Master Settlement Agreement (MSA) reached between attorneys general from 46 states, five U.S. territories and the tobacco industry. Visit www.legacyforhealth.org.

Source: P. McLaughlin, A.V.P. Communications, Legacy Foundation, Washington, DC.

- The last element in the category of tone and appeal has to do with production values. As mentioned earlier, quality shows. It is better to make one high quality piece, (and run it more), or choose a less expensive medium (e.g. radio versus television) than skimp overall on shoddy production values. (However, when we discuss budgets, there are economies of scale that must be kept in mind). **Table 12–1** features a checklist developed by the Health Communication Unit at the University of Toronto for assessing message quality.

With these thoughts guiding your overall program, let's take a look at the first piece of your final strategic plan, the creative brief.

PREPARING A CREATIVE BRIEF

We could have introduced the **creative brief**, as well as the development and pretesting of concepts and messages, in a previous chapter because these are still informed by theory. But, it is important to realize that these decisions cannot be made independent of your choice for a communication chan-

TABLE 12–1 Health Communication Message Review Tool from THCU, Canada

	Excellent	Very Good	Fair	Fail
1. The message will get and maintain the attention of the audience.				
2. The strongest points are given at the beginning of the message.				
3. The message is clear (i.e., it should be easy for the audience to point out the actions you are asking them to take, the incentives or reasons for taking those actions, and the evidence for the incentives and any background information or definitions).				
4. The action you are asking the audience to take is reasonably easy.				
5. The message uses incentives effectively (more than one type of incentive is used, the audience cares about the incentives presented, and the audience thinks the incentives are serious and likely).				
6. Good evidence for threats and benefits is provided.				
7. The messenger is seen as a credible source of information.				
8. Messages are believable.				
9. The message uses an appropriate tone for the audience (e.g., funny, cheery, serious, dramatic).				
10. The message uses an appeal that is appropriate for the audience (e.g., rational or emotional). If fear appeals are used, the audience is provided with an easy solution.				
11. The message will not harm or be offensive to people who see it. This includes avoiding 'victim blaming.'				
12. Identity is displayed throughout.				

Source: THCU, Center for Health Promotion, University of Toronto.

nel, activity, or medium. If you plan to work with healthcare providers and give them materials and training to communicate more effectively with patients, your creative brief and your entire strategy will be different than if you plan to use social media or a radio serial drama, for example. We have tried to give you a good grasp of your media channel options and how these options affect the actual message in preparation for the following discussion of the brief itself.

The term *creative brief* comes from the advertising business, where a short document was prepared by the advertising agency account manager, in consultation with the client, to brief the creative team of copywriters and artists, etc. Sometimes the term is generalized out to mean the entire communication strategy,* but we are sticking to the original meaning of a succinct document that articulates the essence of the strategy for creative interpretation. Clear thinking produces a clear creative brief and the opposite is also true. The

basic form of the creative brief used in public health communication and social marketing has evolved little since it was first introduced in the 1970s. Some agencies and organizations use different elements but the following outline reflects the general consensus.

Elements of a Creative Brief

1. *Overview of project.* This is a short summary of the overall goals of the project and its importance to the organization(s) involved.
2. *Target audience segment.* This should be one unique segment described as vividly as possible. It might include: demographic description, behavioral readiness "stage," literacy level, lifestyle information, and role in the overall communication strategy (primary audience, secondary audience, etc.).
3. *Objectives.* What specific behavior or behavioral antecedent do you want the target audiences to perform as a result of this communication? This is often

---

*This is how it is handled in the NCI "Pink Book."

phrased as what you want them to think, feel, or do, and it may be referred to as "a call to action."

4. *Obstacles.* What structural barriers, beliefs, cultural practices, social pressure, or misinformation are barriers to your audience taking this step? Is there an audience that must be approached first in order to free your intended audience to act as desired?

5. *Benefit/key promise.* What is the single most important reward (from the audience's point of view) that will result from doing the desired behavior? Is there a secondary reward? Which is more immediate and which will take longer to achieve? From the audience perspective, "what's in it for me?"

6. *Support statements/reasons.* This statement explains why the target audience should believe the promise of the key benefit. This may be scientific data, emotional data, or data drawn from the experience of others who the target audience admires or can relate to. Support statements should also provide solutions to the obstacles raised earlier.

7. *Tone.* What feeling or personality should your message or medium have? The tone set by the communication materials will influence how the target audience feels after interacting with the communications.

Examples of tones include authoritative, family-oriented, funny, loving, modern, preachy, rural, scary, sad, and so on.

8. *Distribution opportunities.* What venues, seasons, or events increase the likelihood of reaching your audience? In what other ways might this material be used? Do you need different versions to reach audiences in different settings?

9. *Creative considerations.* What else should the writers and designers keep in mind during development? What is the intended medium and channel for this product? Will a certain style of presentation resonate more with the selected target audiences: conversational, testimonial, informational, emotional, or instructional? Will the material need to be prepared in more than one language? Will known spokespersons be involved, e.g., political figures or entertainers? Are there special words or phrases to use or avoid?

10. *Other elements.* Some agencies include approval routing, timelines, and just about anything else that is needed to reach management consensus before beginning creative development.

Box 12–3 shows a completed creative brief for the folic acid campaign.

Box 12–3 Creative Briefs: Folic Acid First Campaign

Target Audience 1—Pregnancy Contemplators: Women of childbearing age, 18 to 35 years old, who were planning to get pregnant in the next year. Some of these women took a multivitamin, others did not.

Secondary audiences: The health/support systems for these women: friends, mothers, health professionals, etc. Two campaigns were implemented here, one for a general audience and one for a Hispanic audience.

Objective(s)
Convince women that they must start taking a multivitamin with folic acid (or a folic supplement) before they get pregnant.

Obstacles
- *Regarding folic acid:* Only 16% of women knew that folic acid prevented birth defects, and very few (9%) understood that it must be taken before conception to be effective.
- *Regarding multivitamin (and folic acid) supplements:* Some women did not feel that they needed a multivitamin supplement. They perceived themselves as young, healthy and not in need of any "supplementing". Most realized the need for prenatal vitamins during pregnancy but not the need for folic acid before conception. This group thought that their regular diet contained everything needed for good health.
- *Additional concerns:* Objection to taking pills, in general; fear of weight gain; inability to remember to take vitamins; fear of excessive cost.

Key Promise
If you take a multivitamin with folic acid every day before you get pregnant, you will reduce the risk of your baby being born with birth defects.

continues

Support Statements/Reasons

- Up to 75% of birth defects of the spine and head (neural tube defects) can be prevented by taking an adequate amount of folic acid before becoming pregnant.
- Folic acid is essential for the body to make cells, the very first stage of a baby's development.
- Folic acid should be taken daily for at least one month prior to conception.
- Vitamin supplements are the easiest way to get the required amount of folic acid.
- Multivitamins cost as little as 3 cents/day; folic acid supplements as little as 1 cent/day.
- Folic acid is an essential B vitamin.

Tone

It was necessary that the communication convey a sense of good health, warmth, and energy because that is how this audience saw itself. in addition, a sense of importance and urgency was needed to motivate these women to overcome their own obstacles to behavioral change

Media

Television, radio, and print.

Creative Considerations

Spots were produced in English and Spanish in order to recognize and reach diverse populations.

Target Audience 2—Pregnancy Noncontemplators: Women of childbearing age, 18 to 24 years old, who could become pregnant. These were women who were, or could be, sexually active and able to conceive. They were not planning a pregnancy in the near future and were unlikely to be taking a vitamin supplement with folic acid. However, because this group accounted for a significant percentage of pregnancies, most of which were unplanned, there was still a need for these women to take a folic acid supplement.

Objective(s)

To raise awareness among young women that taking a multivitamin or folic acid supplement is necessary, regardless of whether they are planning to become pregnant or not.

Obstacles

- *Regarding pregnancy/birth defect messages:* If a pregnancy was not planned, there was an assumption that a pregnancy would not occur. Concern over birth defects, therefore, was not a priority.
- *Regarding multivitamin/folic acid supplements:* There was the belief that a multivitamin supplement was not necessary, reinforced by the self-image of a young healthy person who needs no special supplements. Key nutrients were thought to be received through diet and that only "old people" took supplements.
- *Additional concerns:* Fear of weight gain, aversion to large pills, disruption of daily routine, cost.
- *Regarding folic acid:* Lack of knowledge of existence of folic acid, when to take it, and relevance in lifestyle.

Key Promise

If I take folic acid every day, I will look and feel better, as well as reduce the risk of my baby being born with birth defects.

Support Statements/Reasons

- Folic acid is necessary for healthy cells and most women do not get enough of it.
- If taken in sufficient amounts, folic acid can eliminate up to 75% of the most commonly disabling birth defects if taken before pregnancy and through the first month of pregnancy.
- Folic acid is an essential B vitamin.

Tone

This campaign was geared toward a younger audience and addressed them on their level, hip, youthful and energetic. A tone that conveyed a sense of good health and vibrancy was chosen because that was how this audience perceived themselves.

Media

Television, radio, and print PSAs.

Creative Considerations

Spots had to recognize a diverse population.

Source: CDCynergy Micronutrients Edition, Folic Case Study.

Use Feedback from Early Pretesting

Once again, creative briefs organize your own ideas before moving to the concept, message, and materials production phases of communication planning. When working with a creative team, either in-house (e.g., your friend the artist or yourself for a "no budget" effort, or, the media/marketing department of a public health agency or voluntary organization) or with a hired agency, it is essential to keep the artists "on message," and "on strategy." It is extremely easy to let a great creative idea steal the show. But, this is where the creative brief helps you to ensure quality.

Audiences and **gatekeepers**,* the persons who have some control over dissemination or interpretation of messages at the community or larger social level, need to be invited to **pretest** concepts before moving onto final messages and to see messages and draft materials before final production. As we will discuss later, sometimes the entire package has to be seen *in situ*, in the exact setting where it will be aired or used, in order to judge its appropriateness and effectiveness.

Even when using a participatory entertainment education strategy, where stories emerge from live role-play, the narrative can be captured in a comic strip or "story board" or presented as a scripted skit to target audience members *not* involved in the concept's creation. All material intended for mass intervention should be tested with the intended recipients and with the gatekeepers prior to distribution. No excuses.

In addition to gatekeepers, it is often important to consider who else might be sensitive to the ideas being put forward by a health communication campaign. When we think about how many things we try to "prevent" in public health, we have to be mindful of the people who already suffer from these conditions. It might be HIV. It might be a preventable birth defect or a chronic disease. Health communicators must consider how these people, or their loved ones, will feel if their condition is portrayed as something to avoid at all costs. So pretesting with persons who represent this audience of affected individuals is also advised.

A quote we are fond of in social marketing is "fail early, fail small." Some of what you think are your best ideas do not work with the intended audience, outrage the gatekeepers, or offend current sufferers. Having data from the audience pretesting is an important strategy for overcoming gatekeeper resistance to a message or media concept. (Although, sometimes you have to compromise in order to keep a communication channel open for future opportunities.) It is much better, and cheaper, to find this out with a small group of people at the concept, message, or even materials testing stage than after a multimedia campaign has been released to the public.

FROM THE CREATIVE BRIEF TO CONCEPTS

One of the most fascinating exchanges in health communication takes place when project managers meet with a creative team to discuss what is needed for the communication materials. Working through the creative brief, the managers will describe the project's overall purpose and provide all the information they have available about the intended audience. Next, they will relay the objectives of this specific communication campaign or material.

Before strategic communication became more widespread, project managers focused on a couple of key ideas that they framed as **messages**.† The message was actually the final intended behavior sought of the target audiences. It might be "Wash your hands after going to the bathroom" or "Don't send your children to school when they are sick." In the world of strategic communication, we now know that these are not the actual words that will be used to communicate this idea to the target audience, although they might be represented on some level. Instead, this idea—together with all the other information gathered about the audience—will generate a **concept**. The concept will be a creative interpretation of the information provided by the project managers about the objectives, the obstacles, the key benefits, the support statements, the tone, and the intended media channels—as well as anything else included in the creative brief.

Concepts are *gestalt*‡ interpretations—they try to grab the main idea and give it a personality. From social marketing, we have learned that the core of the concept is the most compelling benefit, and this is surrounded by the supporting information. The concept has to appeal to both the head and the heart and communicate how this idea fits into the lives of the target audience. Does it make their life easier? Is it fun? Will it seem to be a popular thing to do?§

Box 12–4 shows the first set of concepts developed in response to the folic acid creative brief.

The folic acid example demonstrates some general ideas that need to be tested during the concept testing phase. Overall, we want to identify what words and images help the target

---

*Persons who are influential in the community, particularly concerning information meant for people whom they care about, are gatekeepers. These might be health professionals, local government or religious officials, or other community leaders.

†UNICEF's Facts for Life, discussed in Chapter 15, uses this form of message in order to simplify the communication process for a global audience of health promotion managers.
‡From the German, with a meaning essentially that the whole is greater than the sum of the parts.
§To paraphrase Bill Smith.

Box 12–4 Concepts Tested for Original CDC/March of Dimes Folic Acid Campaign

Nine concepts were developed: Four were specifically designed to appeal to women hoping to become pregnant in the next year; four were for women who were not yet planning a pregnancy; and one to test its appeal to both groups.

CDC used focus groups to test the concepts. A total of 79 women participated in nine groups. The focus groups were used to determine if women could identify the main idea of each concept and to determine if the concepts motivated the target audience to increase their folic acid consumption. Five focus groups included women of different racial and ethnic backgrounds, and the remaining four groups were exclusively Hispanic women.

CONCEPTS DEVELOPED FOR PREGNANCY CONTEMPLATORS

1. "The Fetus" depicts a fetus, with the text, "Even before you realize you're pregnant, her little body is growing a spine. Begin taking folic acid when you stop taking birth control." The concept was developed in response to exploratory focus group research that indicated women were unfamiliar with the importance of folic acid *before* conception.
2. "Brussels Sprouts" displays a picture of many Brussels sprouts with the text, "To protect your unborn child from birth defects, you would need to eat this many Brussels sprouts every day. Or, take one of these. Folic Acid. It needs to start when birth control stops." The main idea of this concept was to show women how hard it was to consume enough folic acid from naturally occurring dietary folate, because women had previously stated their well-balanced diets provided them with enough folic acid.
3. "Fooling Around" depicts a man and a woman laughing with each other, while the text printed above them states, "And you thought all you needed to do was 'fool around.'" At the bottom of the concept, the text states, "Folic Acid. The pill to take when you're planning." This concept was designed to inform women that folic acid must be taken before conception.
4. "Pill Pack" depicts a pack of birth control pills at the top, and a bottle of folic acid supplements below. The text accompanying the pictures states, "When you stop taking these (picture of birth control pack), start taking these (picture of the folic acid bottle). Folic acid. The other pill." This concept's main idea was that when a woman is ready and able to become pregnant, she needs to start taking folic acid.
5. "Sanitary Napkin" featured a sanitary napkin with the text, "You may not be planning a pregnancy, but your body's been preparing for many years" written on top. Underneath the sanitary napkin, additional text stated, "Folic acid today. So your body's ready when you are." This concept was supposed to convey the idea that as soon as the body is capable of becoming pregnant, folic acid is needed.

IMPORTANT FINDINGS FROM THE CONCEPT TESTING WITH WOMEN PLANNING TO BECOME PREGNANT

1. "The Fetus" was well received as attention-getting and informative. Several women associated the image of a fetus with anti-abortion campaigns. Additionally, the image of a fetus conflicted with the idea that folic acid should be taken before conception. The image should suggest, and reinforce, the importance of taking folic acid before pregnancy, an important focus in this campaign.
2. "Brussels Sprouts" was problematic because some Hispanic women did not recognize the vegetable as something they would eat.
3. "Fooling Around" confused women because it seemed to imply that folic acid was an alternative to birth control or improved fertility.
4. "Pill Pack" was also confusing to women because it implied that folic acid was an alternative to the birth control pill. That was not the intended message.
5. "Sanitary Napkin" shocked participants, but they clearly understood the message. A different image to display the same message was suggested. It involved showing a young girl through the different stages of maturity.

CONCEPTS DEVELOPED FOR WOMEN NOT THINKING ABOUT PREGNANCY

1. "Folic Female" (version 1) was designed to convey the benefits of folic acid in promoting good health in general. An African American woman was shown sitting in a grassy meadow with the text at the top, "Folic Acid. It brings out the best in you." At the bottom of the picture, additional text asked the reader, "Are you a folic female?"

2. "Folic Female" (version 2) showed a smiling woman who was white, but could be Hispanic or any other Caucasian ethnic group with dark hair. The words "The Folic Female" were printed at the top of the concept and the text, "Folic Acid. It brings out the best in you," was printed at the bottom of the picture. These two concepts were developed in response to a large number of women in the focus groups reporting that they would be motivated to take a multivitamin with folic acid daily if it made them feel their best.

3. "Penny" featured a penny as the main visual. The headline stated, "Bring out your inner beauty for a penny a day," and the tag lines said, "Folic acid. The beauty supplement we can all afford." This concept was designed to address the concern that taking a multivitamin every day can be costly.

4. "Life happens" focused on the benefits of folic acid in preventing birth defects in future or unplanned pregnancies. The concept showed a teenager/young adult looking surprised with the caption, "Life. It's what happens to you when you're making other plans. Folic Acid. It's what prevents birth defects in babies." This concept intended to convey the main idea that girls/women need to be prepared for an unplanned pregnancy.

5. "Sanitary Napkin" was the same concept as tested for the pregnancy contemplators.

IMPORTANT FINDINGS FROM CONCEPT TESTING WITH WOMEN NOT CONTEMPLATING A PREGNANCY

1. "Folic Female" concepts conveyed the message that folic acid promoted good health and beauty, but women did not like the phrase "folic female" when seen without additional text. The question, "Are you a folic female?" was well received however, because it was not standing alone.

2. "Penny" did not convince women that folic acid was an inexpensive beauty supplement.

3. "Life Happens" clearly illustrated that women should be prepared because an unplanned pregnancy could happen, but the women did not believe that they would have an unplanned pregnancy.

4. "Sanitary Napkin" was hard for women to see (the graphic of the sanitary pad) but communicated the message most clearly. Women not planning a pregnancy both understood the message and felt it was directed to them.

TEST OF CONCEPTS WITH INDIVIDUALS AFFECTED BY SPINA BIFIDA BIRTHS

To guard against offending persons who had children with spina bifida, the primary birth defect resulting from folic acid insufficiency, the concepts were also tested with a group of mothers willing to view the materials and make comments.

1. "Sanitary Napkin." While most participants felt that the concept was powerful, some were concerned that the explicit image (the sanitary napkin) used in the example would be offensive and unappealing. It was suggested that showing someone purchasing sanitary napkins would be a gentler way of depicting the same message.

2. "Penny." Focus group members were not offended or alienated by a message focusing on beauty instead of birth defects. They felt the CDC should do whatever it took to convince people to consume folic acid.

OTHER IMPORTANT FINDINGS FROM CONCEPT TESTING WITH THIS GROUP

1. Campaign messages needed to emphasize the purpose of preventing birth defects, not saying the *people* born with birth defects could have been avoided.

2. Messages needed to avoid making parents of children with spina bifida feel guilty. Materials had to make it clear that in addition to folic acid, genetics and other factors also play a role in neural tube defects (NTDs).

3. Depictions of individuals with spina bifida (e.g., in a wheelchair or on crutches) were acceptable, as long as the individual was not portrayed as pathetic. It was also recommended that a range of severity levels be depicted.

4. Materials should make it clear that while folic acid greatly reduced the risk of having a baby with neural tube defects, it did not eliminate the risk all together. Furthermore, materials should not specify a date when the association between folic acid and NTDs was known.

5. The campaign should include scientific evidence supporting folic acid and birth defects research. Emphasis should be placed on the idea that folic acid is needed one month prior to conception in order to reduce the risk of having a baby with an NTD.

6. It was important to test campaign materials with adolescents affected by spina bifida, because they may have been particularly sensitive to images and messages.

continues

Findings from these groups were particularly revelatory for the Division of Birth Defects at CDC. In focus groups, most women said that they would want to see what the birth defect looked like,[a] and that women in general needed to see the extent of the defects to know their seriousness. At the same time, CDC was sensitive to how mothers of children with neural tube defects might feel about having their children portrayed as "what you are trying to avoid." Hence, a key challenge of the campaign was finding the balance between presenting difficult scientific information and the sensitivities of the already affected population. A decision was made to limit the more graphic images of neural tube defects to materials that would be used by physicians or other medical personal to counsel women contemplating a pregnancy.

[a]In fact, neural tube defects can be among the most frightening birth defects with some children not surviving birth, or living only a moment or two, because they lack a fully formed brain and/or head. In others, there is an opening in the back that must be surgically repaired, but this is almost always survivable in the United States.

Source: CDCynergy Micronutrients Edition, Folic Case Study.

audience understand and want to act on the issue. If a series of concepts is presented, then we try to find out:

- Which have the most appeal?
- Which prompt a reaction to think, feel, or do (the intended response)?
- Which are easy to understand?
- Which are memorable?
- Which are credible?
- Which are inoffensive?
- Which are culturally appropriate?

We will elaborate more on these factors when we discuss pretesting messages and materials. Another important goal of concept testing is to learn *what other* ideas the target audience might have; whom they see as credible spokespersons; and what media channels they feel are most appropriate for the message.

Most often concepts are tested in focus group settings; individual interviews and theater testing are alternatives. In the later, audiences view slides on a screen while the moderator speaks to them. Their collective reactions are gathered using an anonymous response system, clickers,* to tally up how many people select a particular answer to a question. At this stage, whichever testing method you select, you are exploring general concepts and themes. In the next step you will move on to messages and materials.

Box 12–5 shows the methodology and questions used in pretesting the concepts for the CDC's original folic acid campaign.

FROM CONCEPTS TO MESSAGES AND MATERIALS

Having tested your concepts, you will now build on that foundation to create bundles of words, images, and/or sounds that carry your idea to the hearts and minds of your intended recipient. The channels and activities that will use your material determine the format for production, not vice versa. You can create great audio for radio spots and video material for the Internet but you will never succeed in putting video on the radio. Similarly, materials designed for healthcare providers to counsel patients are likely to be too complex for consumers at pharmacy counters or in grocery stores.

More often than not, the actual words chosen for a message will come from your exploratory concept testing, when participants describe a problem or solution in their own words. If you are using the entertainment education approach, then messages emerge from role-plays dialogues or from finished dramatic treatment. These words are then embedded in a narrative fully articulated with characters and context. Viral or buzz marketing techniques count heavily on the intelligence and often ironic worldview of the intended (usually youthful) audience and can sometimes succeed with an "anti-message" that communicates the opposite of the actual words.

Finally, you will need many different formats of your materials, conveying different parts of your message matched to the audience and the channel. For example, you can use a "badge" on an Internet site that links to a complete Web page and a hotline phone number on that same Web page, as well as a billboard. You might get lucky and get your materials produced for free by the Advertising Council and aired as one of their top PSAs (public service announcements on radio or TV). Even better you might have the budget to pay for television, radio,

---

*Popularized by television programs such as *Who Wants to Be a Millionaire?*

Box 12–5 Methodological Overview of Concept Testing for Folic Acid Campaign[a]

CONCEPT TESTING FOR FOLIC ACID

Concepts are designed to be preliminary ideas rather than actual campaign materials. In this case, a series of 9 concepts were used to stimulate participants' thinking about what words and pictures would help them and women like them learn about folic acid and neural tube defects (NTDs), and motivate them to take folic acid daily. Concepts are not meant to stand alone, and the concepts created for this campaign might be used, for example, on the cover of a brochure, or as part of other materials that would contain additional information about folic acid and NTDs.

DESCRIPTION OF FOCUS GROUP PARTICIPANTS

The focus groups conducted for this concept-testing study included the following subgroups of women at risk:

- Women from various races/ethnicities, with specific emphasis on African American and Hispanic women (both English speaking and Spanish-speaking);
- Women between the ages of 18 and 35 years; and
- Women in lower to middle income brackets (less than $50,000 annual household income, with emphasis given to women with annual household incomes less than $30,000).

METHOD

Welcome and Introductions

The welcome and introductions section was the same for each focus group. The female moderator put the participants at ease, introduced the topic area for the discussion, and explained how focus groups work. The moderator used the opening minutes of the group to:

- Thank participants for attending and to introduce herself;
- Identify the purpose of the discussion and emphasize that the planned campaign is a public health campaign sponsored by CDC and not by a company trying to sell something;
- Stress that comments are kept confidential (names do not appear in any report) and there are no right or wrong answers;
- Explain the presence and purpose of recording devices and observers seated behind the one-way mirror.

Framing the Interview

The moderator started each discussion by displaying a foam core-mounted statement which gave participants some background information about the topic for discussion. For women planning a pregnancy, the moderator displayed the following scientific statement.

> Folic acid is a vitamin that can prevent birth defects.
> Most women don't get enough of this vitamin.
> CDC wants to talk with you about what might help convince you to take more folic acid.

This statement was chosen for women planning a pregnancy because women who matched this profile in exploratory research said they would be motivated to take more folic acid if it would help prevent birth defects.

The statement was kept on display throughout the discussion so that participants could refer to it while viewing the potential campaign concepts. This was important so that the women could provide their opinions about whether or not they felt the concepts conveyed the information presented in the scientific statement.

For women not planning on becoming pregnant, the moderator showed a different statement that exploratory research suggested might motivate women with this profile to take folic acid.

continues

---

[a]Abstracted from research report prepared by Westat for the Birth Defects and Pediatric Genetics Branch (BDPG), Division of Birth Defects, Child Development, Disability and Health at the Centers for Disease Control and Prevention (CDC), 1998. Available in its entirety on CDCynergy, Webversion, www.cdc.gov

Folic acid is a vitamin that everyone needs for good health.

Your body is producing new cells all the time and folic acid is important for this development.

Three of the concepts tested for this group were developed around motivators of feeling and looking your best, not always eating right, and preventing long-term illnesses. This statement was also displayed throughout the group discussion so that participants could refer to it when discussing if the concepts conveyed the information presented in the statement. Next, this group was also exposed to the idea of preventing birth defects through folic acid, and shown the concepts created for women planning a pregnancy.

Showing and Discussing the Concept Boards

After showing each group the initial statements, the moderator proceeded by obtaining reactions to each concept one by one. Each concept was printed in color and mounted on a large (20 by 30 inches) foam core board. Before actually viewing the concepts, participants were told that the concepts may be used to develop materials for communicating the statement they had just seen, but at this point, were preliminary ideas, not finished words or artwork. For each of the concepts, participants were asked the following questions.

- What is the main idea of the concept;
- What were your thoughts and opinions on the words and images used in each concept;
- Was there any personal relevance and motivational effect for the concept;
- Suggestions for changing the concept.

The moderator changed the order of the concepts, as well as the questions, in each group to guard against bias that may occur due to order effects.

Concept Ranking

After discussing the concepts collectively, participants were asked to rank order the concepts individually and anonymously. Each concept had a small label with a letter on it (A through E) which corresponded to the five letters listed on the sheet of paper. Participants were asked to write a #1 next to the concept letter that would most motivate them to take folic acid, a #2 next to the second most motivational concept, and so forth. Participants were also told that if none of the concepts motivated them, they should leave the sheet blank.

Wrap Up Discussion of Logo and Channels

After a group discussion of their rankings, the moderator asked about whether it would be beneficial to display a logo on the materials, such as for the CDC, the National Task Force on Folic Acid, a charitable organization, or a pharmaceutical company. The group also suggested potential channels for disseminating the information.

Conclusions

The moderator thanked the women for their time and gave them information about obtaining their incentive money following the group. After all sessions, a subject matter expert from the CDC or a local public health expert was available to answer any questions that participants had about folic acid or birth defects, and to hand out pamphlets on folic acid.

Analysis

At the time these groups were conducted, the research agency used group transcripts and notes taken during the groups to analyze themes and compare findings within and across groups. No computer aided qualitative coding system was used, although it would be recommended now.

Source: CDCynergy Micronutrients Edition, Folic Case Study.

and print production and purchase targeted air time and space. Using your best public relations strategies, you convince magazine editors to run stories on your topic. You provide sample copy and images, get the news media to cover your events on the air and get an advocacy group to run a Facebook campaign for you. The sky is the limit. The important point is that you need more than one channel—and, therefore, more than one cre-ative interpretation of the message—and you will need to test each of these as whole units.

The preliminary chapters in this textbook (Chapters 3 through 7) discuss the considerations that need to go into crafting messages that are simple, clear, and meaningful for different groups of people. The later chapters (Chapters 8 through 12) add the dimension of persuasion. You need to keep it all in mind. There really is no perfect approach, and all the do's and don'ts lists in the world will not substitute for:

- Doing your homework (the formative research and strategic planning).
- Briefing a top creative team thoroughly.
- Making sure they have access to a first-hand experience of the target audience for inspiration (e.g., focus group audio tapes or transcripts).
- Pretesting their work until you achieve the results you need.
- Allowing a bit of magic to intrude.

PRETESTING YOUR MATERIALS

Messages and creative rough production are pretested together. We are looking for many of the same results as we were in concept testing, but now we need to know if we were successful in using a *gestalt* concept to produce a specific, focused, effective message. Important factors to pretest are attractiveness, understandability and believability. Does the presentation engage the audience? Do they feel they would act in the intended manner after getting this information?

For decades, the most widespread form of pretesting materials has been the focus group or individual interview setting. Here are two common scenarios:

1. You are walking in a shopping mall and a nice person with a clipboard approaches and asks if you can spare 15 to 20 minutes. You have been selected because, unbeknownst to you, you fit a particular profile. If you say yes, you are taken to an area you didn't know existed in just about every large shopping mall in the country, the research suite. You enter a cubicle with your facilitator, and he or she shows you materials or products and usually asks you to fill in a questionnaire yourself or to complete a brief interview with the moderator. You might be given a coupon for the product, if you liked it, or some other small compensation, and you are on your way.

2. You are invited to attend a special event to test out a "pilot for a new television show." This takes place in an office suite, or perhaps a small screening room. There are anywhere from 50 to 100 people present. After the preliminary introductions, you are given a brief survey to complete that, surprisingly (because it had nothing to do with a television show), asks you to select products from different categories that you might like to have if you could have them for free to take home after the screening—that is, you are given the option of personalizing your gift for participation.

Next, you see several short segments for what seems to be a new TV show, and in-between there are commercial advertisements. Usually there are several bookending each segment. At the end of the showing, you are given another brief survey to complete that asked you questions—maybe one or two about the TV show, but, again, about the products, many of which are advertised, but some of which are not.

You realize that you can't recall if the "coffee being drunk" was actually part of the pilot television show or an advertisement. You can't actually remember if you saw a spot for a laundry detergent or orange juice, and gee, your memory isn't as good as you thought. And, you thought the show itself was pretty banal. Finally, you are again asked to check off the products you would like to have in a shopping bag to take home. One lucky participant is selected to win their shopping bag, and the rest of you go home with some small prize and the thanks of the research company. A variation of this scene would be a higher technology setting, where you would get to use an audience response system, or clickers, to respond to the interviewers' questions.

Both of these setups are used extensively in commercial marketing to pretest advertising and other marketing factors prior to a launch. This is usually a form of pretesting. In this process, participants examine the material and give their reactions out loud. The primary benefits of this form of testing are that it is relatively easy and inexpensive. You can gather the information and make corrections in your materials quickly. (The primary drawback is that participants may try to please the researcher and will say they like a message or that it will stimulate them to action, when in fact they don't and it doesn't.) After reviewing this basic, most widely used form of pretesting, we will go on to discuss high-tech and low-tech methods, from cognitive neuroimaging to role-playing.

Questions for Pretesting

Box 12–6 features some sample questions to use when pretesting a short piece such as a television or radio spot or a print piece. You'll notice that there is some redundancy in how we ask these questions. We also ask respondents to comment on how others would feel about the pieces being tested. These are deliberate attempts to get people to speak honestly. Respondents in pretests often do not want to offend the researcher and will try to say things that they believe are the "right answers," or pleasing. By asking them what others might say, there is a better chance that they might provide some negative feedback. Remember, *there is no perfect draft material*. If you come back with "No changes necessary," there was something wrong with your pretest.

Box 12–6 Questions for Pretesting in Focus Groups or Individual Interviews

1. Comprehension. Does the target audience fully understand and interpret the materials in the way you intend? Some questions that assess comprehension include:

   a. In your opinion, what is the message of this (television spot, radio spot, print piece)?
   b. Are there any words that you would change to make it easier for others to understand? Which are they?
   c. Please explain this message to your neighbor in your own words (have the respondents do so).
   d. (Indicate a particular image). Can you tell me what this is and why it might be in this picture?

2. Attractiveness. Taste obviously varies a great deal and is related to cultural factors as well as the changing times. While you are testing a rough cut of material, you should strive to make this as close as possible to the finished piece. If it is a radio spot, have someone with a good voice do the recording. If it is a story-board for a video, or a "home video" version of the script, still strive to be as professional as possible to prevent the low production value from distracting the audience. For print, you can probably produce a near-finished piece with today's simple graphics programs. Some questions that assess attractiveness include:

   a. What do you like the most about this piece?
   b. What do you dislike?
   c. How would you change this piece?
   d. What do you think others in this community would say about this piece?

3. Acceptance. This factor has more to do with norms, attitudes, and beliefs of the target audience. Can they believe the information? Is it congruent with the community's norm? Does it require a major change of opinion to act on the information? Some questions that assess acceptance include:

   a. Is there anything about this piece that you find objectionable?
   b. How about others in this community, what would they say?
   c. Do you know any people like this, or have you seen a situation like this?
   d. (Indicate a particular aspect of the piece). Is this believable to you?
   e. Can you think of anyone else, such as a religious leader or important community leader, who we should show this to before distributing it widely?

4. Involvement. The target audience should be able to recognize themselves in the materials. Based on the elaboration likelihood model, if the target audience is already concerned about the issue, then it might not be necessary to match up the imagery with their stylistic preferences. But, if you need to first focus their attention on the fact that this information is meant for them, then featuring spokespersons and images that the target audience would like to see, is important. Some questions that assess involvement include:

   a. (If using non-celebrities). Whom does this piece represent? Are these people like yourselves?
   b. (If using celebrities). Who is this? What do you feel having (Name) speak to you about _____?
   c. Do you feel that this piece is speaking to you? Why or why not?
   d. If this isn't meant for you, who do you think it is speaking to?

5. Inducement to action. All materials need a "call for action." Because we have tried to identify a behavior, attitude, or change that we think is feasible for the target audience to embrace, now is the last chance to test whether this piece will prompt them to make it. Even if we are just trying to raise awareness of a problem, we want to prompt the audience to seek more information, or tell others about what they have learned. Some questions that assess call to action include:

   a. What does this piece ask you to do?
   b. How do you feel about doing this?
   c. Would you need to do something else before you could do this?
   d. How would you explain this to a friend?
   e. How would they respond to this piece?

Source: Modified from AED Toolbox, Question 18:19–21. http://www.globalhealthcommunication.org/tool_docs/29/a_tool_box_for_building_health _communication_capacity_-_question_18.pdf.

Results

You might be surprised how much ideas change when going from concepts to media materials. **Figure 12–1** shows the two different combinations developed for the first folic acid campaign.

This is a wrap-up of the most commonly used form of pretesting in public health. Now we'll discuss a few other approaches that employ different forms of technology in pretesting.

High-Tech Pretesting

Websites: Usability Testing

There is a lot of jargon in website development. Some of it corresponds closely to what we call by other names in health communication, and the rest is unique to the information technology (IT) sector. Usability refers to how well an intended "user" (e.g., of a website, software program, or game) can learn and use the product to achieve his or her goals, as well as his or her satisfaction with the process. The central concept in usability testing is called "user-centered design," which is similar to what we've been calling a focus on the intended audience, consumer, or patient. **Table 12–2** provides explanations of what is measured in usability testing.

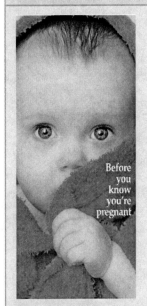

FIGURE 12–1 First Set of Materials Developed for Folic Campaign

Source: CDCynergy Micronutrients Edition, Folic Case Study.

TABLE 12–2 What Does Usability Measure?

Usability measures the quality of a user's experience with the product or system. It is a combination of factors including:

- **Ease of learning.** How fast can a user who has never seen the user interface before learn it sufficiently well to accomplish basic tasks?
- **Efficiency of use.** Once an experienced user has learned to use the system, how fast can he or she accomplish tasks?
- **Memorability.** If a user has used the system before, can he or she remember enough to use it effectively the next time or does the user have to start over again learning everything?
- **Error frequency and severity.** How often do users make errors while using the system, how serious are these errors, and how do users recover from these errors?
- **Subjective satisfaction.** How much does the user *like* using the system?

Source: http://www.usability.gov/basics/ucd/index.html.

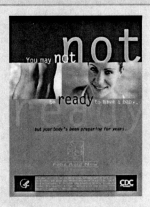

Cognitive Research

Can we really see what is going on inside a person's head? **Cognitive research** refers to a number of techniques derived from psychology that help us understand how we process information. These techniques have been applied to communication and marketing research for decades. Some involve no more than asking people questions about the questions we intend to ask other people. The federal government refers broadly to the area as the cognitive aspects of survey methodology (CASM), for which there is a large literature. Newer techniques involve use of validated questions with **Likert scales** (**Box 12–7**), which can then be subjected to statistical modeling.

Box 12–7 Likert Scales

Developed by Rensis Likert, this is the "typical" 5- (or more) point scale that asks a respondent to choose a response ranging from strongly disagree to strongly agree, strongly approve to strongly disapprove, or any other condition that can be measured in this manner. While this form of question is very popular, the points on the scale are not evenly spaced. The difference between "neutral" and "agree" might feel farther apart than "agree" and "strongly agree." Such scaled data can be ranked (they are ordinal) but not truly measured, as would be the case for body temperature, calories, and other empirical phenomena.

Finally, there are procedures to collect physiological measures, such as galvanic skin response (lie detector test), heart rate, pupil dilation, eye tracking, and even electroencephalographic (EEG) and functional magnetic resonance imaging (fMRI) data from participants asked to examine stimuli ranging from text, to images, to videos. These latter techniques are used extensively by the private sector but less so by public health organizations due to the costs involved in testing.

Next we examine how each of these techniques is used in pretesting.

Cognitive Interviewing

According to the Center for Aging at the University of California in San Francisco:

> "**Cognitive interviews** can be used to revise or develop new items so that they are appropriate to respondents' cultural context and lifestyle . . . cognitive interview methods reflect a theoretical model of the survey response process that involves four stages: comprehension or interpretation, information retrieval, judgment formation, and response editing. In other words, the respondent must first understand the question,

then recall information, then decide upon its relevance, and finally formulate an answer in the format provided by the interviewer."[10]

The National Center for Health Statistics (NCHS) of the CDC established a cognitive testing laboratory in 1985, where it reviewed and tested survey items for its own use and for collaborating agencies. NCHS championed the use of two primary techniques in cognitive testing: think-aloud interviewing and verbal probing techniques. The following sections describe these techniques.

Think-Aloud Interviewing

In the think-aloud interviewing method, the research subject is asked to literally "think out loud." Then the interviewer reads a question to the subject and records the subject's description of mental process uses to arrive at the answer. The interviewer limits probes to general encouragement ("please tell me what you're thinking") when the subject pauses. **Box 12–8** contains an example of how a research participant reflects on what appears to be the straightforward question, "How often have you spoken to a doctor in the past 12 months?" After trying this question and alternative wording out with several respondents, the researchers would arrive at a better way to gather the information.

Box 12–8 Think-Aloud Example

Question: How many times have you talked to a doctor in the last 12 months?

SUBJECT: *I guess that depends on what you mean when you say "talked." I talk to my neighbor, who is a doctor, but you probably don't mean that. I go to my doctor about once a year, for a general check-up, so I would count that one. I've also probably been to some type of specialist a couple of more times in the past year—once to get a bad knee diagnosed, and I also saw an ENT about a chronic coughing thing, which I'm pretty sure was in the past year, although I wouldn't swear to it. I've also talked to doctors several times when I brought my kids in to the pediatrician—I might assume that you don't want that included, although I really can't be sure. Also, I saw a chiropractor, but I don't know if you'd consider that to be a doctor in the sense you mean. So, what I'm saying, overall, is that I guess I'm not sure what number to give you, mostly because I don't know what you want.*

By listening to how the respondent tries to answer this question, the interviewer might conclude that this question needs to be revised due to following:

- The subject has trouble remembering whether a specific event falls within the 12-month time period. This may be too long a period for accurate recall.
- The subject does not know (a) whether the question refers only to doctor contacts that pertain to his/her health and (b) the type of physician or other provider that is to be counted.
- The subject is not certain as to what level of health professional counts as a "doctor."

Source: Based on: "Cognitive Interviewing and Questionnaire Design: A Training Manual," by Gordon Willis (Working Paper #7, National Center for Health Statistics, March 1994).

One significant problem with this seemingly easy method is that the research subjects may find it difficult to say their thoughts out loud. As a result, many researchers are moving to the more structured verbal probing approach.

Verbal Probing

In the verbal probing method, the interviewer asks the survey question and allows the subject to provide a response. Then, the interviewer asks a set of questions that elicit how the subject understood the question and arrived at the answer. **Box 12–9** provides some examples of the kinds of probes and questions.

Box 12–9 Examples of Verbal Probing

Comprehension

"What does the term 'outpatient' mean to you?"

"Can you repeat the question I just asked in your own words?"

Confidence Judgment

"How *sure are you* that your health insurance covers this treatment?"

Recall probe

"You say you went to the doctor 5 times in the past year. *How do you remember* that number?"

Specific Probe

"*Why do you think* that cancer is the most serious health problem?"

General Probes (Similar to think-aloud probes)

"How did you arrive at that answer?"

"Was that easy or hard to answer?"

"I noticed that you hesitated—tell me what you were thinking."

Source: Based on: "Cognitive Interviewing and Questionnaire Design: A Training Manual," by Gordon Willis (Working Paper #7, National Center for Health Statistics, March 1994). 2005.

Physiological Effects Testing

Galvanic Skin Response

Popularized in crime shows as part of a polygraph lie detector procedure, or more recently as a biofeedback tool, the **galvanic skin response (GSR)** is a measure of the electrical current that passes along the surface of the skin. Because perspiration conducts electricity much better than dry skin, a minute increase in perspiration resulting from an emotional response (or a menopausal hot flash) can be detected as an increase in electrical conductance. GSR is painless and can be measured easily using uncomplicated devices and computer display. In addition to its contribution to criminology, GSR has been used to gauge attention to and emotional response to media. While an emotional response can be detected with GSR, remember that there is no way to know the nature of the actual underlying emotion without asking the subject.

Pupil Dilation and Eye Tracking Technology

The eyes may not be the windows of our soul but they do give away the locus and level of our interest. **Eye tracking** is a measure of where and how long we gaze at an image (moving or still) or text. We also have an innate response of the autonomic nervous system to imminent danger or arousal that causes our pupils to dilate. Together with our blink rate (which also speeds up when we are aroused or experience fear), pupil dilation can be measured by photographic processes embedded in a computer screen. An industry leader in this area is the Danish company iMotions. They describe their technology and some of its uses in **Box 12–10**.

EEGs and fMRI

The most prevalent tool used in neuromarketing is high-density **electroencephalography (EEG)**. When groups of neurons are activated in the brain, a small electrical charge is generated, resulting in an electrical field. By placing electrodes on a person's scalp (this is painless), the resulting EEG signals can be detected and amplified for analysis. Different brain waves measure different brain processes. Ironically, EEG was initially developed by a psychiatrist to analyze behavior, but it was never widely accepted in the medical field for this use. Today the primary medical uses of EEG are for the diagnosis of epilepsy, sleep and cognitive disorders. In recent years computerized EEG analysis and mapping are being used increasingly for research and specialized applications, including neuromarketing, and now give promise of providing information about the nature, timing and localization of cognitive processes.

Functional magnetic resonance imaging (fMRI) uses a much larger and more expensive device to visualize a small regions neuronal activity associated with brain functions. This provides a high-resolution, three-dimensional image of the

Box 12–10 Examples of iMotions Eye Tracking Technology

SPOTLIGHT

Spotlight shows the distribution of attention with a transparent layer superimposed on the stimuli. Areas that have attracted more attention will be more transparent than those that have attracted less attention—the underlying image will be more visible in areas receiving highest attention. The high attention areas are classified as attention points. Spotlight measures: time spent, hit time, ratio, revisitors, revisits, residual time, and sequence of the gaze.

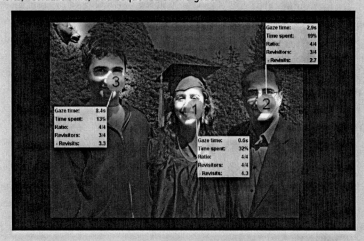

HIGHLIGHT (AOI)

Highlights (AOIs) are user-defined selections of one or many areas (areas of interest)—revealing their attention results. This is particularly useful when you need to know whether a specific area like a logo/tag line or other specific parts of a stimulus has attracted attention. Highlight measures: time spent, hit time, ratio, revisitors, revisits, residual time and sequence of the gaze.

GAZE REPLAY + FIXATION PLOT

Gaze replay shows the gaze path for an individual respondent—either based on a still or moving image stimuli—for the entire duration of the exposure time. Fixations during the gaze sequence are visualized as circles—varying in size depending on duration of a fixation. It measures: fixations points, duration of the fixation, and hit time.

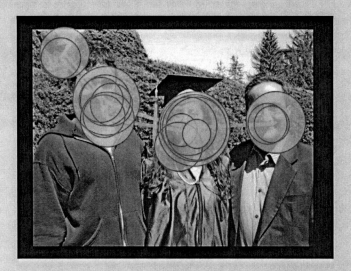

Source: "iMotions—Emotion Technology A/S 2010," http://www.imotionsglobal.com (January 2010). Analyses prepared by Jakob de Lemos, chief technology officer and co-founder. February 26, 2010.

brain's activity, including response to different products, stimuli, or situations.[11]

According to Wilson, Gaines, and Hill,

> when a person looks at a print advertisement, light activates some of the 125 million visual neural receptors, rods and cones, in each eye. . . . Using fMRI, researchers are able to image the neural activity associated with vision as well as with the cognitive and affective responses to print advertisements. . . . More than 90 private neuromarketing consulting firms currently operate in the United States. . . . The media has sensationalized many of these investigations, alleging that marketers found the "buy button in your brain" . . . and that the population is about to be "brain scammed (sic)" . . . As a result, use of neuroscience in marketing has both advocates and critics.[12]

One firm, Sands Research, has shared some of its information with us for this textbook. See **Box 12–11** for a sample run for the Super Bowl.

Testing the Final Media Package

Once we make changes based on this first round of materials testing, we move onto the real test: how the intended package performs in its "natural environment," which is a crowded media context. If we are testing a print piece intended to go in a magazine, we want to show it in a mock-up of a magazine. If we are testing a radio spot, we will play our spot along with others and some music. A television spot similarly will be sandwiched between a television show and other advertisements. Almost anyone can tell you they remember a piece of advertising if that is all they've seen. But, driving down the highway, do they really think much about the billboard, or the message they just heard on drive time radio? Do they get up and get potato chips when the spot promoting healthy eating comes on during the televised ball game?

Test Marketing

Sometimes called a **pilot test**, more thorough social marketing efforts will attempt a small-scale trial of all the elements of the strategy in a limited number of locations for a brief period of

Box 12–11 EEG Neuromarketing Example from Sands Research

EEG data is sampled continuously throughout our in-lab and mobile studies. . . . When enough sensors are used, the data can be viewed in three dimensions and plotted onto a model brain. . . . When a test subject gazes for an extended period of time at a product, activated brain areas help determine if the gaze was due to confusion or interest. In addition to the insight gained from functional brain areas, the frequency of the EEG waveforms can also provide information about attention states. A complete spectral analysis is performed on the EEG.

In hundreds of commercials with thousands of participants tested by Sands Research to date, we have seen that a good ad will always have a large spike in brain activity within the first 800 milliseconds of the ad and sustain a high plateau across the length of the commercial.

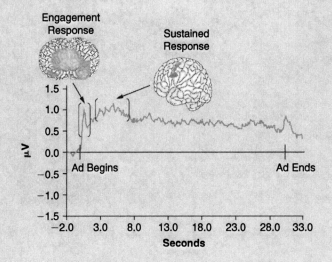

continues

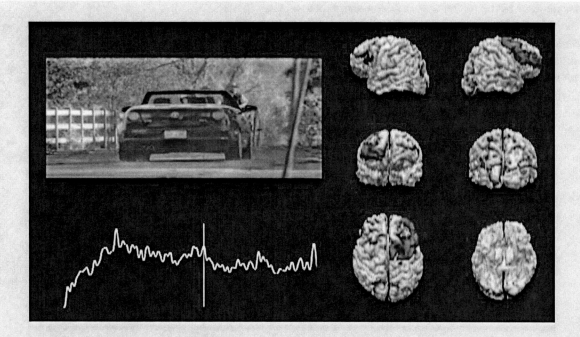

With Super Bowl advertising spots being sold for an average $2.6 to $2.7 million for 15 seconds, many companies are banking that neuromarketing pretesting will payoff.

According to developer Steven Sands, a common question in behavioral and neuromarketing research is, "What is the appropriate number of subjects needed to obtain a reliable result?" Traditional methods of market research use large numbers of respondents, and there seems to be general consensus that approximately 150–200 participants or more (depending on research objectives) are needed to obtain consistent results. With electroencephalogram methodologies (EEG) a much smaller sample size is needed to achieve a similar statistical threshold. When the number of study participants is between 30 to 40 (per target demographic grouping), there is a less than 1% chance of error, and the associated Neuro-Engagement Factor™ (NEF) score portrays an accurate and significant rating for the media stimulus in question. Sands Research utilizes the less than 1% chance of error threshold for all studies. A larger sample size could be utilized to achieve an even smaller margin of error, say .25%, although that degree of threshold does not provide us with a significant amount of "new" knowledge about the stimulus, nor is it financially efficient.

Source: Sands, S.F. White Paper: Sample Size Analysis for Brainwave Collection (EEG) Methodologies, October 2009. http://www.sandsresearch.com/.

time. Following the launch of a product in the testing phase, or an important behavior change campaign, researchers will conduct intercept interviews, or day-after recall surveys (i.e., calling people on the phone to see if they heard or saw the information) to see how the trial is going. If a tangible product is being sold, then a longer period will be used to evaluate the sales data for the product with varying degrees of promotion and other incentives (e.g., mailed coupons, media advertising, etc.). The data collected from this trial are then used to adjust the final product, its packaging, its price, its promotional campaign—or, in some cases, cancel it altogether. (Remember, "fail early, fail small.")

Pilot testing is usually used when a tangible product is close to its final form, or is being adapted to new market conditions. The technique is also used when there may be a need for a success story to conduct advocacy for the project among public or private sector partners.

CONCLUSION

Developing and testing a media strategy defines the bulk of your work as a health communication professional prior to implementing a campaign. Trends come and go in the industry. There was a time when considerable effort was devoted to formative research in order to get a message right for a particular target audience before testing occurred. Now, more time and expense is lavished on pretesting, with often outright goofy stuff presented to potential audiences to see if they like it, or not. Regardless of when audience insight is collected, the step cannot be overlooked. Methods presented in this chapter should enable you to develop a creative brief, design a message strategy, and pretest it with a sample audience. The next chapter will discuss the final planning stages of putting your entire strategy together with a budget and time line.

KEY TERMS

Cognitive interview
Cognitive research
Concept
Creative brief
Electroencephalography (EEG)
Eye tracking
Functional magnetic resonance imaging (fMRI)
Galvanic skin response (GSR)
Gatekeeper
Likert scale
Message
Message map
Pilot testing
Pretesting

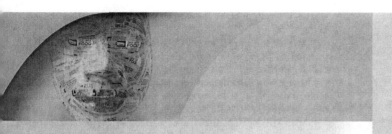

Chapter Questions

1. Why can it be difficult to be clear, accurate, and credible simultaneously?

2. Describe how tone is used in a creative brief. What do you think is the most effective tone for a children's health message?

3. What is the difference between a *concept* and a *message*?

4. What do you think is the most important part of pretesting materials?

5. What are two techniques used in cognitive interviewing?

6. What are some items that are crucial to test with users of websites?

7. How are marketers using fMRI, pupil tracking, and EEGs to measure audience response to media?

8. When would you want to implement a total pilot test of your communication strategy?

REFERENCES

1. Adapted from National Cancer Institute, Washington DC. *Making Health Communication Programs Work*. NIH Publication No. 04-5145, 2004;65–71. Available at: www.cancer.gov

2. The Health Communication Unit, University of Toronto. Health Communication Message Review Criteria. Available at: http://www.mdfile storage.com/thcu/pubs/579818192.pdf.

3. Wray R, Rivers J, Whitworth A, Jupka K, Clements B. Public perceptions about trust in emergency risk communication: Qualitative research findings. *I J Mass Emergencies and Disasters* March 2006;24,1:45–75.

4. Jones J. *Bad Blood: The Tuskegee Syphilis Experiment*, expanded edition. New York: Free Press; 1993.

5. Freimuth V S, Quinn SC, Thomas S B, Cole G, Zook E, Duncan T. African Americans' views on research and the Tuskegee Syphilis Study. *Soc Sci Med*. 2001; 2:797–808.

6. Wendler D, Kington R, Madans J, Van Wye G, Christ-Schmidt H, Pratt LA, Brawley OW, Gross CP, Emanuel E. Are racial and ethnic minorities less willing to participate in health research? *PLoS Med*. 2006 Feb;3(2):e19. Epub 2005 Dec 6.

7. Mebane F, Temin S, Parvanta C. Communicating anthrax in 2001: A comparison of CDC information and print media accounts. *J Health Commun*. 2003;8(S1):50–82.

8. The Health Communication Unit, University of Toronto. Health Communication Message Review Criteria. Available at: http://www.mdfile storage.com/thcu/pubs/579818192.pdf.

9. Witte K, Allen M. A meta-analysis of fear appeals: Implications for effective public health campaigns. *Health Educ Behav*. Oct 2000;27:591–615.

10. http://dgim.ucsf.edu/cadc/cores/measurement/Cognitive Interviews .pdf.

11. Harner RN, Personal communication, January 22, 2010.

12. Wilson R, Gaines J, Hill R.. Neuromarketing and consumer free will. *J Consumer Affairs*. 2008;42(3):389–410.

CHAPTER 13

Developing the Implementation Plan: A Summary of Section III

Claudia Parvanta

INTRODUCTION

Now that you have all the elements of your media strategy, you are ready to develop the key planning tools to manage your intervention. These are a logic model; a SWOTE analysis (the SWOT [strengths, weaknesses, opportunities, threats] model plus an "E" for ethical assessment); and an operational plan that includes your timeline, budget, and assignment of responsibilities. In theory, the logic model is developed before beginning formative research. In practice, few professionals, let alone students, can clearly define program "inputs" and "outputs" without a more complete grasp of their program.

Similarly, you wouldn't create a budget *after* you decide to run television spots during prime time; you need to know the budget before making media choices and planning dissemination. But, again, researching media options will ease the creation of a sample budget.

In public health "reality," this strategic forecasting—together with identifying stakeholders, program implementation collaborators, and potential audience gatekeepers—is all done as early as possible. We have presented them later in the sequence to make it easier to understand what is involved. Try these management tools on a small scale, in your own setting, for your own program. Using these tools with a school or community project will help you acquire the competencies to use them professionally.

PREPARING A LOGIC MODEL

Logic model gurus (e.g., Goodstadt[1] and Knowlton and Phillips[2]) have written extensively about this program management tool. The W. K. Kellogg Foundation, which funds many public health activities, has produced a *Logic Model Development Guide* in which they define a logic model as, "a picture of how your organization does its work—the theory and assumptions underlying the program."[3] Their **logic model** (there are other kinds) describes a sequence of components (boxes) that define your planned work and intended results:

- Planned work:
  - Resources/inputs.
  - Activities.
- Intended results:
  - Outputs.
  - Outcomes.
  - Impact.

You were previously exposed to some of this logic model in Chapter 2, when we talked about using the ecological model and the precede–proceed planning framework to identify a problem, contributing factors, and environmental level for creating change. The change you seek goes into the box labeled Impact. Then, in Chapter 10 you used intervention mapping and the Behave model to develop theory-based communication strategies for helping specific groups of people adopt healthier behaviors. This goes into the Outcomes box. If we just stopped with Impact and Outcome, we would have what is often called a *theory* logic model.

For an *action* logic model (Activities, Outputs), you bundle your actual media products, the channels and modes of delivery into the box called Activities. This is closely linked to another box labeled Outputs, which reflects the receipt of these activities by various users. (These can be training of health coaches or medical personnel, delivery of flyers to home mailboxes, or use of a website by consumers. Outputs are the measurement of product uptake in terms of numbers of users and how often they used the products.)

Finally you must state what you need in terms of people and resources to accomplish the activities that deliver the outputs and put them in the Resources/Inputs box. Now you have completed the program logic model by working backward from your intended impact through the intermediary boxes to the first box of resources/inputs. **Figure 13–1** shows the basic logic model as it would be implemented, now moving forward from resources to impact, just the reverse of the model development sequence described earlier.

It is a good idea to develop a logic model as a group exercise. Your ideas can first be written on cards and stuck on the wall under basic headings. Then you can move them around as you develop your ideas more completely. Once the model is completed, it should be able to fit on one printed page.* (It can be a big page.) Your colleagues, stakeholders, and partners will use this as the "big picture" of your program.

Let's add some details to these boxes.

Resources/Inputs

Inputs and Resources range from tangible items such as money, paid staff or volunteer hours, facilities, and equipment to more intangible items such as expertise, data, or the involvement of collaborators at the local, state, national or global level. Each may play a part in contributing resources to the program.

Activities

This is a description of what the program will do. A health communication program often includes the following activities:

- Mass media such as paid advertising, public service announcements, entertainment education events (plays, television program scripts, radio soap operas), blogs, YouTube videos, Facebook pages, or student classroom materials.

---

*Some say this is the only rule for logic models.

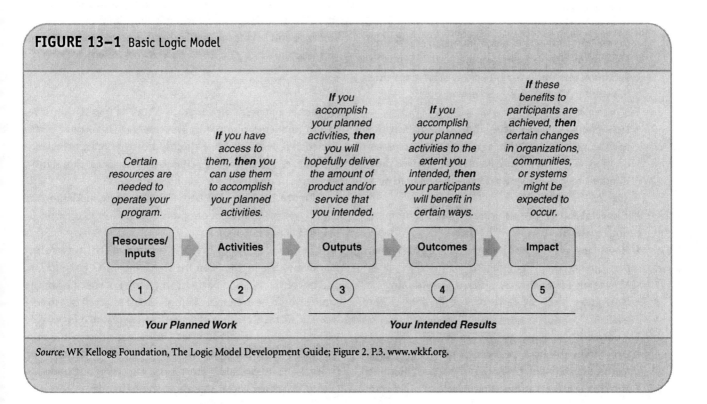

FIGURE 13–1 Basic Logic Model

Source: WK Kellogg Foundation, The Logic Model Development Guide; Figure 2. P.3. www.wkkf.org.

- Patient decision aids such as computer animations, decision software, pencil and paper flipbooks, kits, or worksheets.
- Training workshops for healthcare providers, teachers, coaches, or clergy to use media effectively.
- Outreach and education activities such as health fairs, speaking engagements, trade shows, or grocery store or drugstore promotional activities.

Numbers are associated with activities in terms of what is anticipated and budgeted. For example, conduct 10 teacher training workshops or distribute 10,000 patient decision aids.

Outputs

This measures whether the activities were delivered as planned. For example:

- For mass media:
  - If you planned to deliver 10,000 student workbooks, how many students actually received workbooks?
  - If you bought radio and television air time, when and where were your spots aired? What was the measured audience? (The television and radio stations, as well as independent media auditors, measure this).
  - If you ran a website, how many "page views," downloads or forms were completed? How long did people interact with specific pages on the site? Can you measure the exposure?
  - If you contributed to a soap opera or prime time drama television script, when and where was it aired?
  - How many people have become your "friends" on Facebook for your program's page? How many times has your YouTube video been downloaded?
- For patients:
  - How many health facilities, practices, or individual healthcare providers have agreed to use the patient decision aids? How many patients have received them?
  - If online, how many patients have downloaded or requested the materials?
- For intermediaries (people using the health communications materials to work with others):
  - How many workshops were implemented? How many participants completed pre- and posttests?
  - How many materials were ordered post-training?
  - How many feedback cards or website entries were posted?
- For outreach:
  - How many public appearances, speaking engagements, or health fairs? Where and when? Who came?
  - How many grocery stores, pharmacies, or other commercial establishments ran events with the program's materials and speakers?
  - How many trade or industry shows? Where and when? Who came and participated; who requested more information or a follow-up?

As you will see in Chapter 14 on evaluation, assessing whether your outputs were generated according to plan is an extensive part of process evaluation.

Outcomes

Outcomes are normally divided into immediate, intermediate, and long-term ranges.

Immediate outcomes for mass media might include:

- Next-day recall of message.
- Awareness of issue.
- Change in attitude or motivation to try something.

These responses would be assessed through survey research. Interactive media allow recipients to respond to website invitations, purchase, donate, or post information immediately.

Intermediate outcomes generally include changes in individual behaviors, in stages; enactment of policies; or uptake of technology or strategies by organizations. Long-term outcomes could include permanent changes in health behavior, statutes and laws, or environmental quality. Long-term outcomes may be identical to impact, although the former refers more to individuals (long-term outcome: an individual quits smoking and his life is extended) and the latter to population (impact: the death rate from tobacco goes down).

Impact

Impact is generally measured in terms of population-level health or socioeconomic improvements. This would be reflected in reductions in age-specific mortality rates, prevalence of disease, and disease-specific mortality rates. Population measures of quality of life would improve.

Figure 13–2 shows a fairly complex logic model for the CDC's optimal nutrition program, a follow-on to their original folic acid campaign.

The model shows that the optimal nutrition project planned to use inputs from the CDC, the CDC Foundation, and its contractors and partners (these are not specified or the model would be even more complicated!) to reach out to college-age women. A range of activities were planned to provide various levels of media support—some provided by the program and its partners and some created by the participating college. The immediate- (short-) and mid-term outcomes included increased knowledge about multivitamin use, positive

FIGURE 13–2 Draft Logic Model for the Optimal Nutrition Initiative Pilot Program

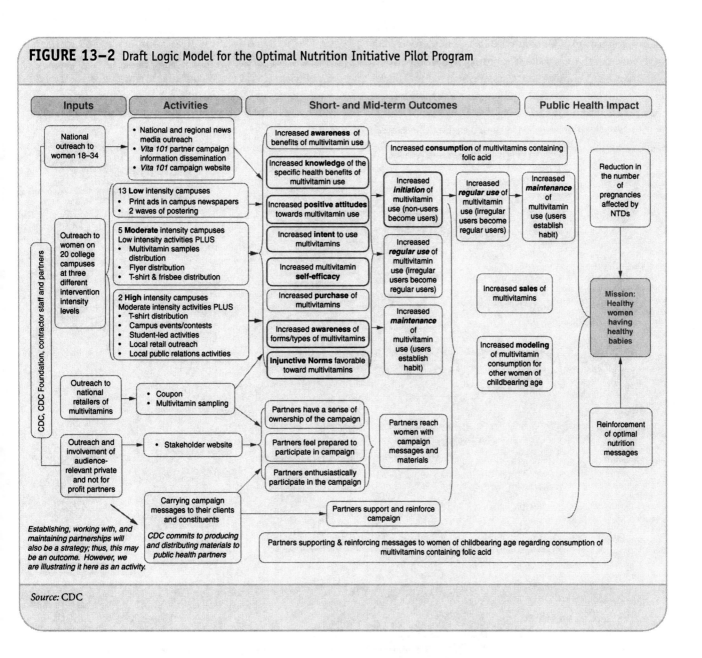

Source: CDC

attitudes toward vitamin use, and increased purchasing of multivitamins. This would lead to stages of adoption of multivitamin use as a daily habit. If and when these women became pregnant, the public health impact would be reduction in the number of pregnancies affected by neural tube defects.

Unfortunately, the optimal nutrition project was never fully implemented due to insufficient funds and a scientific disagreement concerning promotion of multivitamins—and not just folic acid alone. Thus we have an internal "weakness" in the program, in addition to the external "threat." Threats and weaknesses, together with strengths and opportunities, are discussed next.

SWOTE ANALYSIS

By now you should have a very clear idea of what you plan to do and how it's supposed to work. There is still time to modify your plans if you lack a critical resource, or if the timing is not right for your initiative. A **SWOT analysis** is the standard business tool for assessment of strengths, weaknesses, opportunities, and threats. We have added an "E" to SWOT for ethical assessment, which we describe herein. It is easy to confuse the categories, and we have seen many SWOT models that clearly do so. Strengths and weaknesses refer to conditions that are within your control, or at least inherent to you or your organization's ability to implement the program. Opportunities and threats are outside of your control. You may plan for or around them, but they will happen on their own. Ethical considerations may reside inside your organization, but it is important to assess whether intentionally, or inadvertently, your program could harm someone, limit someone's rights, or promise something that cannot be delivered.

As with the logic model discussed earlier, this exercise is best conducted with those you see as partners or stakehold-

ers in the health communication intervention. These colleagues will enable to you to assess your total assets and have a 360-degree picture of opportunities and threats. Again, you can work with cards and stick them up on the wall under the big headings, moving them around as you refine your thinking.

Box 13–1 shows a SWOTE for the folic acid program.

Box 13–1 SWOTE for Original Folic Acid Program

STRENGTHS

Issue or Product
- Birth defects, in particular, neural tube defects, were a tragic event that any political administration would support eradicating, if possible.
- There were strong scientific data to support the efficacy of folic acid to prevent neural tube defects.
- Folic acid was readily available as an inexpensive, small (easy-to-swallow) vitamin supplement; as a multivitamin; or as a component of fortified cereals and other commonly consumed foods.
- Multivitamin consumption is a fairly straightforward and simple behavior that is easy to discuss in a communication campaign.

Organizational
- The CDC Division of Birth Defects, as well as the Center housing the Division of Environmental Health, included numerous scientists, physicians, and program managers who were committed to the issue.
- Evaluation data from state and international campaigns to promote folic acid consumption were available to program planners. These indicated the need to focus on women's beliefs about the benefits and barriers of consuming enough folic acid through vitamins and/or food.
- The CDC had the capacity and financial resources to do the audience research necessary to discover motivations for folic acid consumption.
- CDC funding was available to translate research findings into draft and final health messages (i.e., prototype communication products).

WEAKNESSES

Issue or Product
- The message that all women should consume folic acid daily *if capable of becoming pregnant* posed many challenges in terms of attracting the attention of the target audience and convincing them to change behavior.
- Taking a vitamin supplement daily was considered an additional expense, or time burden, by many women.
- Many foods that contained some folate, such as orange juice or leafy greens, were thought to be adequate dietary sources for folic acid. They did *not* provide the requisite 400 μg/day unless consumed in gallons or pounds.
- At the outset (1996 or so), fortified foods, such as bread, contained too little folic acid to provide the correct dose if a normal serving were consumed. For example, a woman would have to eat 3 *loaves* of packaged white bread to receive 400 μg of folic acid per day.

Organizational
- Federal funding was limited for this program, despite congressional concern over the issue.
- Federal authorities, such as the USDA, FDA, and CDC, could not agree on the correct level of fortification in order to protect all women and prevent any potential harm. (Because folic acid is a water-soluble vitamin, the body excretes excess amounts, and it poses no problems of overdose. However, a high level of folic acid intake can prevent a clinical diagnosis of vitamin B12 deficiency. African American women, in particular, were less susceptible to NTDs and more susceptible to B12 deficiency, which is linked to macrocytic anemia.)

continues

- Changing policy is a slow process that relies on finding champions in high places.
- The CDC and all other federal agencies or organizations that receive federal funding are prohibited from lobbying Congress. Seeking more federal resources for the program, especially funding, was difficult and required extremely sensitive partners who did not have these limitations.

OPPORTUNITIES

Issue or Product
- The private sector quickly got the message and began fortifying foods or putting labels on foods that highlighted folic acid levels.
- Healthcare providers were already educating their patients about better health and pregnancy outcomes. Folic acid supplements and information were relatively inexpensive and easy to provide.
- Taking vitamins had become "trendy" as part of a fitness-, sports-, appearance-, or health-related lifestyle.

Organizational
- There were several long-established and highly reputable organizations involved in the fight against birth defects such as the National Organization of the March of Dimes, the Spina Bifida Association of America, and the American Pediatric Association. They were very willing to contribute to the campaign by providing research, data, access to target populations, and mechanisms for distribution and dissemination. They also were able to discuss the issue with their congressional representatives in their home states as well as provide and sponsor congressional briefings on the issue.
- Campaign partners agreed to disseminate messages and materials through their own channels and at their own cost.

THREATS

Issue or Product
- A seemingly "apple pie" issue such as preventing birth defects is caught up in two politically sensitive areas:
  - Unplanned, and often, premarital sexual activity.
  - Elective termination of pregnancies that are diagnosed with neural tube defects.

It was imperative that the collaborating partners, The National Council for Folic Acid, found ways to discuss the issues without suggesting that either of these activities were recommended.

- Obstetricians had been advising patients to begin taking folic acid when they confirmed pregnancy. Changing this message around was more difficult than promoting a new behavior.

Organizational
- National health communication campaigns dependent on partnerships are difficult to navigate. Implementation is completely dependent upon partners.
- Healthcare providers have less time during their patient visits to discuss many important health issues, including folic acid.

ETHICS

- A national campaign with a message saying that folic acid can help prevent serious birth defects had the potential for causing concern in several groups of women:
  - Women who had babies born with spina bifida and anencephaly. These women might feel guilty learning there was something that might have prevented this.
  - Women who were currently pregnant and hadn't taken folic acid prior to conception. They might be worried about their pregnancy.
- While fetuses with severe NTD often demise in utero, some are born in a condition that is not viable for more than a few hours or days. While physicians may advise parents to terminate such a pregnancy prior to delivery, the CDC was silent on this issue. The goal of the campaign was to prevent neural tube defects, not to prevent the birth of the babies who have those defects.
- Many children who have spina bifida receive sufficient surgery and therapy that they can overcome their disabilities and live fulfilling lives. Again, the campaign did not want to suggest that these children weren't wanted or loved.

Strengths

There are two ways to consider strengths (and weaknesses).

- *Strengths as the attributes within the organization.* These include personnel capabilities, experiences, material resources, organizational commitment, time allotted, and budget.
- *Strengths as the attributes of the intervention/communication campaign.* These include the positioning of a product or service, its cost, its attractiveness or reputation, etc. If you have a great product or service to work with (e.g., a free pizza night on a college campus), that is a program strength. If you have an unpopular idea to sell (e.g., an increase in tuition), this can be a weakness.

Weaknesses

As with strengths, there are two ways to consider weaknesses:

- *Gaps within the organization.* These include a lack of knowledge, skills, experience, or material resources. Weaknesses may also be less tangible, such as a lack of leader commitment to the intervention, a non-existent or poor reputation in the community, or within a government or other bureaucracy. And, of course, insufficient funding, or a rushed timeline are also program weaknesses.
- *Weaknesses of the actual intervention.* These may include delayed or limited availability (such as seasonal flu vaccine in some years), costs to produce (if more than the market price to sell), or distribution hurdles, or it may be that the service is unattractive to consumers in some way (e.g., think about having to promote a stool blood test or colonoscopy for colon cancer screening).

Opportunities

Opportunities are positive factors related to happenings at the time and in the place you have planned for your intervention. Partners and stakeholders may provide critical insights into opportunities (as well as threats, discussed next), which you may not know exist. Examples of opportunities include:

- *A favorable political climate.* (This often works more as a threat. For example, funding for international family planning programs nearly always diminishes during Republican administrations and builds back up under Democratic ones). At the state and local levels, the governor or congressional leaders can play an important role in supporting or thwarting health promotion activities within the state or congressional district.
- *Funding.* Some health promotion programs have benefited from federal stimulus funding. NIH research funding opportunities have cyclical deadlines as well as limited duration. Private foundations also issue time-limited calls for proposals. Funding opportunities are something of a two-edged sword. Coalitions that come together solely in response to the availability of funding often have a hard time maintaining their collaboration. For example, there have been several opportunities for academic and community partnerships to develop chronic disease prevention initiatives. Where the academic institution and community-based organizations have tried to develop initiatives already, they are more successful at both obtaining new funding—and in implementing their programs—than when the partnership is formed to "get the money."

- *Technology development and innovation.* In the health communication area, there have been enormous changes in even the past few years in terms of what is possible, as well as reductions in cost, to reach many people with more information.

- *Seasonal, entertainment, and style trends.* There are always trends (e.g., in food, clothing, skin tone) that may support (or again, threaten) an intervention. You wouldn't want to sell sunscreen, and warn about skin cancer, in winter—unless you were placing your spots on the travel channel and targeting vacationers to sunny climes.

- *Big events that draw a lot of attention.* Many, many health promotion programs (as well as commercial advertisers) have tried to link their efforts to the Olympics, for example. While the Olympics, or other major sporting events (e.g., the World Cup, for global interventions; the Super Bowl or World Series for the United States) draw huge audiences, the problem with these events is that they are focused on making the athletes and the sport the SOCO (remember Chapter 4?). Whatever time they do not manage to fill in is taken up by the major commercial sponsors. It is not a good idea to try to run a 15-second spot, which will cost a small fortune, in this big venue. What does work well is to try to develop a local angle, such as an athlete or Olympic competitor, from the community or state. This person can become a spokesperson and do much more for the health communication program before or after the event itself.

- *Celebrity endorsements.* There is a somewhat ghoulish reaction by those in health promotion when celebrities announce that they, or a loved one, have a health problem. If this person is well known, and can be seen as a positive role model, efforts are made to attract the celebrity as a spokesperson. Some well-known examples include Cindy Crawford (whose younger brother died of leukemia), Nicole Kidman, Patrick Dempsey (whose mothers died of breast cancer), and, of course,

Lance Armstrong (who suffered from testicular cancer himself). In the early days of the disease, Earvin Magic Johnson transformed the national dialogue around HIV and AIDS with his disclosure of his positive status. Because so many celebrities seem to seek meaning beyond their media careers, there are services that help match them up with agencies or issues for which they feel an affinity. So, while the celebrity has endured a personal tragedy, there is an "opportunity" to engage that person in your health issue; many celebrities find it helps them to deal with their loss in a constructive manner.

Threats

Threats are factors that could potentially delay or prevent achieving your program objectives, again, outside your immediate control. In some ways, everything listed above, if turned around, can be a threat. For example:

- *Political instability.* International work is frequently threatened by clashing political parties, including uprisings, strikes, and localized conflicts. War, while occurring in fewer places, has to be listed as the biggest threat, not only to the work of public health practitioners, but obviously, the entire planet.
- *Environmental catastrophe.* Powerful weather (e.g., hurricanes, floods) that occurs seasonally or randomly earthquakes, as well as agricultural conditions (such as droughts) all jeopardize international health communication efforts. Explosions in mines (or oil rigs) not only focus local or national attention for months, but also require use of resources planned for public health. They are thus tragedies on several levels.
- *Activity linked to risky funding, or dependent on personalities.* In the United States, organizations, academic institutions, or even small groups can all suffer externally created losses in funding or other resources. Also, the actions of one individual may threaten the reputation of an entire organization or institution. Having mentioned the opportunities posed by celebrities, too often, they are risky business. Whatever it is that keeps them in the tabloids far too often makes it difficult to rely on them for health promotion campaigns. If you are extremely careful to match your celebrity to your target audience, and they are willing to accommodate you, then their risk-taking behavior—and negative consequences—might send the right message. (Magic Johnson admitted to unprotected sexual encounters outside of his marriage as the cause of his HIV. Musicians or actors who were long-time "stoners" have regretted the drugs they did in their youth, but this seems to be less convincing to young people.)

Ethical Dimensions

Ethical dimensions in public health are derived from conflicts of philosophical and moral (i.e., cultural) principles and values. Four stand out:

- *Utilitarianism.* Defined as the "the greatest good for the greatest number of people," **utilitarianism** is central to public health, and much of public policy, in the United States. Utilitarianism requires forecasting results and presents the possibility that the "ends justify the means." An example of a highly utilitarian public health policy is quarantine and travel restrictions for infectious outbreaks. In this case, the rights of a few are restricted to protect the health of the many.
- *Deontological principles.* Much of public health is also based on **deontological** (or duty-based) **principles**. These require following rules and principles with the notion, "Stick to honorable principles, and the outcomes will take care of themselves." Many in public health believe you cannot achieve a just outcome (or end) through unjust means. A public health program that requires participants to demonstrate economic or nutritional need is an example of a deontological system as it uses rules— and not privilege (or bribery)—to distribute resources.
- *The Golden Rule.* This is probably the first ethical principle that anyone learns. In the Judeo-Christian tradition it first appears in Leviticus roughly as, "love thy neighbor as thyself," and eventually was popularized as: "Do unto others as you would have them do unto you." (Or even a client-centered, platinum rule, "Do unto others as *they* would have you do unto them.") Virtually every religion and society includes the concept of putting yourself in another's place before doing something, for good or for bad. Most public health organizations, but particularly those run by charitable organizations, put "caring" for individuals and their rights and feelings at the top of their core values.
- *Other rights and privileges.* From the Declaration of Independence, we remember: "We hold these truths to be self-evident, that all men are created equal, that they are endowed by their Creator with certain unalienable Rights, that among these are Life, Liberty and the pursuit of Happiness." Just how far an individual's right to liberty in the pursuit of happiness may go is often described, in common speech, as far as the end of someone else's nose. (Or, an application of utilitarianism to life, liberty and pursuit of happiness.)

Any student of Philosophy 101 can come up with situations where it would be impossible to apply all four of these principles simultaneously. For example, those who suggest that street drugs should be legalized might say that, "In a free country, people should be allowed to harm themselves, as long as they do not hurt anyone else in the process." This is a complicated argument that might get into comparing the damage to society from crime associated with drug dealing versus individual harm from drug ingestion. But what about the healthcare issues associated with drugs—should society bear these costs, or not? Where do harm-reduction strategies—such as a needle exchange to offset the additional risks of HIV and hepatitis infection—fall on your moral compass?

Compared with these difficult ethical dilemmas, the ones associated with health communication might seem relatively straightforward. Some have been discussed under audience research and pretesting, such as, "The communications will not stigmatize any groups" (e.g., children with birth defect, or persons with HIV), or "We will refrain from using messages that present people who engage in certain behavior in a negative way."* There is no absolute way to resolve these dilemmas, be-

*What ethical principle(s) underlie these decisions?

cause different communities, and different cultures, would apply their own values and principles. And, as mentioned previously, different political parties in the United States are associated with allowing or disallowing government-sponsored mass media pertaining to, for example, risks of tobacco, risks associated with private ownership of firearms, and use of condoms for prevention of sexually transmitted disease and birth control. And, of course, these values and associated moral codes will vary widely in international settings.

The choice of *informing* versus *persuading* may pose an ethical dilemma in some circumstances. You might think, "If I feel strongly that this harms you, or this may help you, shouldn't I use everything at my disposal to try to convince you of this?" And, the very acts of selecting a population as the focus (or target) of a health communication campaign, as well as prioritizing an issue, means that some people and some issues are left out. **Box 13–2** features a list of ethical issues identified by CDC in CDCynergy as most relevant to conducting your SWOTE for a health communications program. It is based on the framework developed by Guttman and Salmon.[4]

Box 13–2 Ethical Considerations in Public Health Communication

BIOETHICS
Bioethics is the branch of ethics, philosophy, and social commentary that discusses the life sciences and their potential impact on our society. A set of principles or guidelines that are based on bioethics can articulate and assess ethical and moral dilemmas. These ethical guidelines may include the following:

- The obligation to avoid doing harm through the actions of trying to help.
- The obligation to do good by doing one's utmost to better the health of the intended populations.
- Respect for the freedom of every person and community to make their own decisions according to what they think would be best for them.
- Ensuring adherence to justice, equity, and fairness in the distribution of resources, and providing for those who are particularly vulnerable or who have special needs.
- Maximizing the greatest utility from the health promotion efforts, especially when resources are limited and are publicly funded, and considering the good of the public as a whole.

Ethical Considerations through the Stages of Program Design and Implementation
Each facet of the intervention needs to be examined to determine whether it meets these precepts. The questions provided in the following sections can help facilitate the application of the precepts to each stage or facet of the intervention and the identification of ethical issues.

Goal-Setting Stage
- Who decides what the goals of the intervention should be?
- Who is targeted by the intervention, and who is excluded?
  - Why was the targeted population chosen?
  - Were populations with the greatest needs targeted or those who were more likely to adopt the recommendations?

continues

- Are representatives of the intervention's target population involved in goal setting?
- How will consent be obtained from the intervention's targeted populations? Are issues that are more relevant to mainstream populations given higher priority?

Designing and Implementation
- Collaboration:
  - Could collaboration with community or other voluntary organizations, with the idea of advancing participation and empowerment, actually serve to exploit these organizations by using their limited resources?
  - Are particular organizations made to feel forced to participate in the intervention's activities?
- Use of persuasive strategies and message design:
  - What kinds of persuasive appeals are used, and to what extent may they be considered to be manipulative?
  - Are the messages persuasive enough?
  - Do they unduly exploit cultural themes or symbols?
- Messages on responsibility:
  - Do messages imply that if people get an adverse medical condition, it is their fault since they did not do enough to prevent it? In other words, these kinds of messages can be viewed as potentially harmful because they may literally blame people and make them feel guilty when various circumstances prevent them from adopting the recommended practices.
  - Do the messages make it appear that one person is responsible for preventing others from taking health risks (e.g., spouse, friend, employee). That is, how much is one person responsible for others?
- Messages that may stigmatize or make people overly anxious:
  - Do messages that try to get people to avoid unwanted health conditions (e.g., AIDS, stroke, smoking) portray those who have the conditions in a negative light?
  - Does the intervention raise the level of anxiety, fear, or guilt among target populations?
- Messages that may make people feel deprived:
  - Does the intervention tell people to avoid doing certain things that give them pleasure, but not provide them with affordable and rewarding alternatives?
  - Does the campaign tell people to avoid cultural practices that are of particular significance to them?
- Messages that make promises that cannot be fulfilled:
  - Does the intervention make promises for good health when it urges people to adopt particular practices, although the promises may not be fulfilled?
  - Does the intervention contribute to increased demands on the healthcare system, which may not be able to meet the demands?
- Messages that turn health into an ultimate value:
  - Do the messages stress that health is an important value that should be vigorously pursued, and does the intervention make it sound as if those who do not pursue good health are less virtuous or have vices?
  - Does the intervention contribute to making health an ideal or a super value that people need to pursue resolutely?
- Messages that may distract:
  - Does the intervention focus on specific health topics, thus possibly serving to distract people from thinking about and pursuing activities related to other important issues?
  - Does the intervention focus on individual behavior changes, and, by so doing, distract people from thinking about the importance of social factors that influence health? That is, are downstream behaviors being blamed before upstream problems for population health?
- Control of people in work organizations:
  - Do interventions that take place in work organizations, although they may be efficient, present opportunities for employers to control the private lives of their employees?

Evaluation Stage
- Who decides the evaluation criteria and the success of the intervention?
- Are the targeted populations and the intervention practitioners involved in the assessment process?

Source: Modified from *CDCynergy*, http://www.cdc.gov/dhdsp/cdcynergy_training/Content/phase2/phase2step5content.htm. *CDCynergy*, developed by the Division of Health Communication of CDC is in the public domain.

FINAL STRATEGY ANALYSIS

Now you have a logic model and a SWOTE analysis. What do you do with them? You think about the SWOTE in terms of *when* and *how* it might affect the process described in the logical framework.

Strengths and Weaknesses

These are most likely to affect the program's "inputs."

- Is the program based on the organizational strengths and those of the intervention?
  - If not, how can these strengths featured more prominently in the intervention?
  - How can the program *fix* each weakness?
- Do the strengths and weaknesses of the partners balance each other out? This can be a critical question when deciding on partner arrangements.
- Is the proposed program too far away from the core business of the organization? (If the mission of the university is to educate students, may you conduct a health communication campaign in the community?)
- Do you need to rethink the program before too much is invested?

Opportunities and Threats

These tend to affect achievement of outputs as planned, or outcomes.

- How can the program *exploit* each opportunity?
  - What must be changed in order to exploit an opportunity?
  - What does it maximize: achievement of outputs or outcomes?
  - Do you need to build additional alliances to take advantage of an opportunity?
- How can the program *defend* against each threat?
  - How realistic are the threats, and how great a risk do they pose?
  - At what point do you need to account for the threats: between inputs and outputs or between outputs and outcomes?
  - Do you need to make additional alliances to defend against these threats?

Ethics

How can the program/organization be fair and conduct the intervention in the most ethical manner possible?

- What are the bases of these decisions?
- Again, what needs to be changed, if anything, in order to prioritize human rights, gender equity, or other ethical issues over short-term programmatic gains?

- Do you need to add partners in order to accomplish these changes?

As mentioned earlier, this analysis is best done with your partners and stakeholders. Define the S, W, O, T, and E factors and rank-order them. Normally, you need to devote most of your attention to the top five items in each of the lists. The others should not be ignored, but they will probably not need to be addressed as you plan the launch of your intervention. Comparing the strengths and opportunities for your program against the weaknesses and threats, you will make a "go/no-go" decision. Perhaps the program needs to be postponed to allow for an opportunity, to wait out a threat, or to gather a stronger alliance and attract more resources. Or, you need to move the deadline up, for some of the same reasons. These strategic decisions are part of your final plan.

PRODUCTION AND DISSEMINATION FACTORS

Having considered the timing and organizational strengths and weaknesses, now you need to do your final thinking about the quality of the communications. These are also strengths and weaknesses that can support or undermine your efforts. Thinking back to Chapter 10, we introduced a set of criteria that contribute to making health communication strategic. The list in Chapter 10 emphasized the use of scientific theory and evidence for effectiveness in message strategy development. The following is a list of criteria that apply more broadly to production and dissemination.[5]

1. **Presentability.** There is a trend in viral or buzz marketing to make media appear "home-made." But even these approaches rely on professionals to produce this somewhat shaggy, messy appearance.* How many people toss the black-and-white, photocopied brochure in the trash as they exit a health clinic? In terms of producing something that people will pay more attention to, and possibly keep, quality saves money. And, another cliché, anything worth doing—such as mass media, entertainment education, or counseling—is worth doing well. This does not necessarily mean that it has to be expensive, but that the time invested to get it right will pay off. One way to limit costs is to focus on specific audiences over a time schedule. Strategic communication does not try to be all things to all people. The surest route to reaching multiple audiences with higher-quality media is to work with partners and share the expenses.

---

*A quote that I love, attributed to Dolly Parton, expresses this concept, "You have no idea how much it costs to look this cheap."

2. **Expandability.** Almost anything will work in a small enough community with loving care lavished on every detail. The real challenge, as we've learned through RE-AIM (discussed in Chapter 14), is bringing this to a scale where there can be a genuine public health impact. In general, mass media are used to expand the scope of an intervention. This is actually the least expensive way to reach a lot of people. However, the communication is one-directional. Now, through the Internet, there are multiple, inexpensive ways of scaling up communications that allow for an exchange of views. Traditionally, the most costly intervention to bring to scale is trained counselors working with clients on behavior change. Ironically, this intervention looks to be the least expensive to do in a pilot. There are ways of bringing interpersonal communication to scale, again, by working with partners or widely spread networks of practitioners (e.g., pharmacists). But, quality control of the intervention and our ability to tie results to inputs becomes more attenuated.

3. **Sustainability.** How many public health programs have resourced a health communication campaign for six months, evaluated at one year, and been disappointed by the amount of change? As a gentle reminder, there is always advertising for Coke and Pepsi. A strategic health communication program matches partner organizations to intended audiences and spreads the costs of a campaign broadly. This enables an intervention to have a broader reach and be something that each organization can afford. It is not pointless to do something really spectacular once, or on an annual basis. But, unless it is worked into a longer-term schedule of public relations, partner counseling, or other ways of carrying the message beyond this time and place, it is not strategic.

4. **Cost-effectiveness.** Public health interventions tend to have very limited budgets, certainly compared to competing commercial campaigns for products such as tobacco, soft drinks, and fast foods. So little money is spent on sustaining health communication interventions that it is almost pointless to assess their cost-effectiveness. For those with adequate budgets, newer evaluation methods go beyond "costs per impression" (an older mass media term for number of times an advertisement is run on TV, radio, or print copy) to costs per person reached. And, if a communication strategy can be linked to health outcomes—for example, an anti-smoking campaign examined over many years against deaths due to tobacco—then costs per deaths averted can be used. Whether the metric has a short or long time scale, strategic communication uses resources creatively and to best advantage based on audience research and process evaluation.

Now you have a clear sense of what will make your health communication program more likely to succeed. How do you look at your stakeholders as true partners in the intervention? You do this by defining roles, specifying who will pay for what, and deciding how to share the credit.

DEFINING PARTNER ROLES

Thinking back to many years of international work, it went without saying that any major health communication intervention was going to be overseen by the country's health ministry. However, ministries were often organized to have subnational offices, which also had management responsibilities, assets, and liabilities distributed around the country. Furthermore, many health ministries place the financial and human resources provided by UNICEF, USAID, and other bi-lateral donors,* as well as the many nongovernmental organizations,† in different regions of the country to spread out the technical assistance and material resources available to them. Partner roles came about as a result; when planning a health communication program with a national scope, there were many partners with whom to work, who could each play a role in the project. These partners were eager to participate as the collaboration brought superior resources into their local area and they looked good—to their constituencies: the people in an area who would benefit, political administrators, and international donors—while making a relatively small investment of their own resources.

The tricky part was working each stakeholder's objectives into a unified plan so that the collective communication intervention supported individual programmatic needs. This level of negotiation could take many months (or even years) to accomplish, but it often determined whether a program would succeed or fail. The best possible programs included several key organizations that underwrote the initial stages of an intervention, while transferring responsibilities, training, and material assets down to smaller entities to continue the project on their own. This built a level of sustainability into what otherwise might have been a relatively short burst of mass media, or other communications, followed with little follow up.

*International aid programs managed by France, Germany, Sweden, and Canada were prevalent in west Africa at the time. Other countries predominate in development aid elsewhere.
†From the United States, Save the Children, CARE, Africare, and World Vision were highly visible in west Africa. Other NGOs led efforts elsewhere.

Working in the United States is not that different, except that even a very few organizations working together can often come up with sufficient resources to mount an impressive intervention. For example, the key partners for the folic acid program were the CDC and the March of Dimes, who then recruited additional organizations into the National Council for Folic Acid. Allowing organizations to contribute based on their strengths is the most strategic way to plan an intervention. In the case of the folic program, CDC contributed most of the audience research, as well as the epidemiological data tracking. The March of Dimes provided advocacy. The costs to produce the mass media spots were shared, but air time was all donated from media outlets per the rules pertaining to public service announcements. None was paid for at the time. Print materials were initially covered by the National Council for Folic Acid, and eventually, became available for partner distribution for the cost of production. CDC and the Council covered the costs of developing a partner resource guide to mount community and other small-scale interventions and, later, a media resource guide.[6] These tools, together with the website, have allowed the folic program to extend well beyond the resources available to the CDC alone, by empowering any organization concerned about the issue with facts as well as outstanding communication assets.

In planning your program, **Table 13–1** provides a model partner asset worksheet to help you think about what different partners can contribute to implementing a large- or small-scale communication intervention.

BUDGET

There are popular guidebooks available today that tell you how to do health communication and social marketing "on a shoestring." But, if you want a good result (and there is no reason to do a campaign that is not of good quality), you will need to trade off time for money—and you must create a budget. There is no reason that a dedicated group of students, for example, could not mount an effective health communication campaign using Internet-based media, live events, with potential coverage by local broadcast and print media for "nothing more" than the time and effort they devote to the campaign. Out-of-pocket expenses—such as professional talent, video and sound production, printing services, and paid placement—are what drive up costs.

Another major cost in health communication is personnel salaries for anyone with expertise that you cannot acquire for "free." For example, the salary of counselors or educators is what makes the interpersonal approach relatively expensive. The costs of various approaches and media were shown in Chapter 12.

Your budget should cover all the costs or expenses of the intervention activities. The next sections discuss categories that are normally reflected in health communication budgets.

Direct Costs

Direct costs are the part of the budget that contribute directly to a program's outputs. This line item is made up of personnel costs and out-of-pocket costs (those associated with products and services not obtained through a salaried employee).

- *Personnel costs.* These include the salaries and benefits, or portions thereof, for the people who will work on the project. Full-time employees who will work part-time on the project should be included at the appropriate percentage of time. For example, if a research assistant will spend 20 hours per week on the project for its first year, he or she should be budgeted for 50% of the total salary and 50% of the fringe benefits. (Fringe benefits include Social Security taxes, health insurance, dental insurance, and other benefits that your agency provides.) Most organizations have a calculated fringe benefit rate that can be used when developing a budget. It is often in the range of 25% to 30% of the salary.
- *Out-of-pocket/nonpersonnel costs.* These are expenses connected to program outputs that are provided by vendors. Such costs may include production services, travel, equipment, office supplies, postage, telephone expenses, etc. Some donors allow you to break out facility rental, maintenance, and insurance in your nonpersonnel costs. Others expect them to be covered by your overhead.

Indirect Costs

Also called "overhead," **indirect costs** are what it costs your agency to exist, but they are not tied directly to creating the program's outputs. Examples usually include office space, environmental management (heat, air conditioning, water, custodial services, etc.), and depreciation on equipment. Indirect costs are usually calculated as a percentage of direct costs. Institutions that have worked with the U.S. government, including many universities, have an approved overhead rate. You might be shocked to learn that it can run as high as 60% or more of the direct costs. Therefore, if you are developing a grant proposal budget, for example, and you know that the total amount of the award is fixed, you must be mindful of your indirect rate to know how much money you actually have to work with. Some donors will only pay a small percentage of indirect costs. Others, such as the National Institutes of Health, provide indirect costs on top of direct costs for research projects.

TABLE 13–1 Partner Assets Worksheet

Organization: Partnering Role(s):		Task/Objective
Assets	% Time or Yes ☑	
PEOPLE		
Leadership		
Expert staff		
Administrative support		
Students/volunteers		
EXPERTISE		
Research		
Regulatory		
Product		
Packaging		
Shipping		
Marketing		
Communication		
Meeting facilitation		
Training		
Others		
RELATIONSHIPS		
Our primary target audience		
Our secondary audience		
Donors		
Policymakers		
Community leaders/groups		
Media		
Suppliers		
Others		
RESOURCES		
Information/data (capture)		
Public health		
Environmental		
Regulatory		
Marketing		
Public opinion		
Local knowledge		
Other		
INFORMATION (DISSEMINATION)		
Electronic listserves/blogs		
Print/online publications		
Paid advertising		
News outreach (PR)		
Word of mouth		
Viral		

TABLE 13–1 Partner Assets Worksheet—continued

Organization: Partnering Role(s): Assets	% Time or Yes ☑	Task/Objective
TANGIBLES/PRODUCTS		
Food/beverage		
Ingredients		
Medicines		
IT		
Equipment		
Energy		
Transportation		
Advertising time		
Advertising creative		
Other		
ACCOMMODATIONS		
Meeting rooms (20–49)		
Meeting rooms (> 50)		
Project office		
Individual office		
High profile events		
Media setup		
Storage		

Source: Based on Box 2, Resource Map from GAIN/International Business Leaders Forum, *Partnering Toolbook,* http://tpi.iblf.org/publications/Toolbooks/partneringtoolbookdownload.jsp

In-Kind Contributions

In the nonprofit world in which public health often operates, organizations frequently consider their time, their space, use of equipment, and other in-house resources as **in-kind contributions** to a project budget. These will be used to produce program outputs but are not factored into the direct or indirect costs of the budget. Some donors will expect to see a match made of their investment through direct financial, in-kind resources or additional donations.

Total Budget

The **total budget** is the sum of direct and indirect costs, including in-kind contributions and additional donations. If the project will run for more than one year, an annual budget needs to be prepared as well as a budget for the total time period. Sometimes you will need to separate out and track funding streams into your budget. For example, if a charitable organization wants to know how you spent its contribution, you want to be able to tell them with some precision (e.g., not just, "for 30% of the project"). In addition to a spreadsheet, you often need to provide a budget narrative that describes each expenditure and its purpose. **Box 13–3** provides a sample budget and narrative for a community-based intervention.

TIMELINE

There are many software programs that enable you to develop Gantt charts or other visual tools to assign time and people to accomplish the steps in your project. **Figure 13–3** shows a sample timeline for a college communication project to promote folic acid on campus.

Most larger-scale communication programs take one year to plan and produce, including conducting formative research, developing and testing materials, and readying everything for dissemination. The actual implementation depends on the strategy being used, but a campaign of less than a few months, except in an emergency situation, is not advised. It really takes time to capture the public's attention. Following the Transtheoretical model, we know that most people would then need some time to progress through their own readiness stages before trying or adopting a behavior. Thus, you want to plan and

Box 13–3 Budget Sample and Narrative

Kididdel Hopper Community Health Center
"Kididdel Hopping Kids Project"
BUDGET NARRATIVE
January 1–December 30, 2009

SUMMARY

The total amount budgeted for the January 1 to December 30, 2009 period is $109,062, which includes an indirect cost rate of 25%, or $21,812 and direct costs of $87,250.

A. PERSONNEL

The total budget for salary expenses is $59,000. All salaries are based upon a 12-month project period.

Project Director—This position is filled by the Director of Health Promotion at a 0.2 FTE level of effort. The Director of Health Promotion position is currently filled by Sarah Parvanta, MPH. The allocated budget for this salary expense is $13,000; based upon a $65,000 annual salary and a 20% level of effort. This position is supervised by KHCHCs CEO, Dr. Claudia Kididdelhopper. The Director of Health Promotion supervises the Registered Dietitian, Youth Activity Specialist, and the Fitness Coordinator for the Center and this project.

Registered Dietitian—KHCHC's Registered Dietitian will provide individualized goal setting, nutrition education, diet planning, and weight monitoring for participants. The dietitian position is currently held by Maxine Threelegs. The allocated budget for this salary expense is $9,000; based upon a $60,000 annual salary and a 15% level of effort.

Fitness Coordinator—The Fitness Coordinator has the responsibility of providing physical activity and additional recreational programs for the participants. The position will also maintain the project website, which includes an interactive database for participants to track their fitness challenge goals and accomplishments. The Fitness Coordinator position is currently held by David Nelson, MPA, AT. The allocated budget for this salary expense is $25,000, based upon a $50,000 annual salary and a 50% level of effort.

Youth Activity Specialist—The Youth Activity Specialist has the responsibility of coordinating and leading the daily afterschool and monthly weekend programs. This position is currently held by Lola Catt, BA. The allocated budget for this salary expense is $6,400, based upon a $32,000 annual salary and a 20% level of effort.

Graduate Student Assistants—Two graduate students from the Exercise Physiology and Wellness Program at the University of the Sciences will provide formative and evaluation research assistance, as well as general assistance, to the project. Each student will provide approximately 10 hours a week for 14 weeks a semester, for a total of 560 hours provided to the project. Students are TBN (to be named).

B. FRINGE BENEFITS

A total amount of $18,290 is budgeted to pay for fringe benefits for the project director, dietitian, fitness coordinator, and youth activity specialist for the specified employment periods. (Student workers do not receive fringe benefits.) Fringe benefits include FICA, unemployment insurance, workers' compensation, and health and disability insurance. Full-time employees (must work at least 32 hours a week) receive KHCHC's standard health, dental, life and disability insurance benefit package. Fringe benefits for current employees on staff are calculated at 31.1% of gross salary.

C. TRAVEL

The total budget for travel is $2,400.

Local travel—Local travel expenses include the costs of using public transportation (SEPTA is currently $1.75 per trip) as well as private automobiles to conduct project activities. Local travel will include sending project staff out to community centers, churches, and other after-school programs within our catchment area for special events. It also supports travel to attend off-site meetings, training, and regional conference sessions.

Private automobile mileage will be reimbursed at the federally approved rate of $0.45/mile, by means of a mileage log.

The local travel budget for staff is budgeted at $1,200 for the 12-month project period.

Out-of-state travel—A travel budget of $600 is included for air and ground travel for 2 project staff to attend a professional conference related to youth obesity prevention.

Per diem and lodging—The total budget for per diem and lodging is $600. This is the estimated cost for per diem and lodging for 2 project staff to attend a professional conference related to youth obesity prevention.

D. OUT OF POCKET
The total budget for out of pocket expenses is $7,560.

The largest portion of this will be spent on Activity and Educational supplies. This includes staff curriculum materials, participant materials, parent materials, as well as outreach to promote the activity in the community. We have budgeted for the cost of two new laser printers with a year's worth of ink, as we intend to produce most of the materials in-house. We anticipate using very limited services of a graphic designer to provide a coherent look to our materials. We also intend to develop audiovisual materials to be used on-site as well as sent home with children. For this, we intend using a recording device (such as an iPod Nano), and transferring videos onto flash drives or DVDs. Finally, we will purchase sports equipment, games, light refreshments, and incentive items ($5.00 or less) for the after-school and weekend programs. We have set aside $1,000 for all office supplies, postage, and telephone services related to the project.

Kiddidelhopper "Kiddidel Hopping Kids" Project Budget Spreadsheet

Object	% TIME	Year 1
A. PERSONNEL		
Project Director	0.20	$13,000.00
Registered Dietitian	0.15	$9,000.00
Fitness Coordinator	0.50	$25,000.00
Youth Activity Specialist	0.20	$6,400.00
Graduate Student Assistants		
2 (10 hours/week) × 28 weeks × $10/hour	100.00	$5,600.00
Total Salaries		$59,000.00
B. FRINGE BENEFITS		$18,290.00
C. TRAVEL		
Local		$1,200.00
Out of state		$600.00
Per diem and lodging		$600.00
Total Travel		$2,400.00
D. OUT OF POCKET		
Activity/Educational Supplies		
Laser Printers 2 @ $250		$500.00
Paper		$2,000.00
Ink cartridges		$1,500.00
Recording software		$200.00
Recording devices		$300.00
DVDs		$200.00
Sporting equipment		$500.00
Incentives and Refreshments		$1,000.00
Other office supplies		$400.00
Postage		$240.00
Telephone service contract		$360.00
Professional services: Graphics		$360.00
Total		$7,560.00
		$0.00
E. TOTAL DIRECTS		$87,250.00
F. INDIRECT		
Negotiated rate = 0.25		$21,812.50
TOTAL BUDGET		$109,062.50

FIGURE 13–3 One Semester Time Line for College Folic Acid Communication Class Project[a]

Activity	Lead	Week 1	2	3	4	5	6	7	8[b]	9	10	11	12	13	14	15	16[c]
Familiarize team with project.	Faculty	X															
Background reading on CDC campaign, Spina bifida, Qualitative methods.	Faculty		X														
Learn formative research methods.	Faculty			X													
Learn formative research methods.	Faculty				X												
Develop & test topic guides for men's and women's focus groups.	Students				X	X											
Secure posters and materials from CDC[d] or other community or national organizations. Make arrangements with dorms, clubs, other organizations to conduct interviews.	Students w. Faculty support					X	X										
Conduct focus groups. Write up results.	Students						X	X	X								
Compare results of men's and women's groups. Develop message strategies using 'winners' from CDC materials.	Students									X							
Prepare materials for pre-testing in Central Location Interview. Make arrangements with cafeteria, gym, etc. to recruit students for interviews.	Students w. Faculty support										X	X					
Analyze results. Select final materials, produce and disseminate.	Students												X	X			
Conduct 'Next Day recall' or other short term KAP type assessment on campus.	Students														X		
Final presentation to Class on lessons learned.	Students															X	X

[a] If a class spans two semesters, more time can be devoted to pre-testing concepts and messages. Implementation can run for a month, and then a more thorough evaluation can be conducted using tools in Chapter 14. If working in an off campus community setting, anticipate needing two semesters to complete the work in order to bring partners on-board and allow for usual glitches.
[b] Many schools have a mid-semester break. Students may be using this time to complete written reports from focus groups.
[c] Many schools have final exams in week 16. This is left open for final presentations if schedule is slowed down.
[d] This can be done for any health topic. This project uses materials available from the CDC website, or developed, but not released, by the Optimal Nutrition Program. We have experience doing this project on folic acid, including print materials and test results, that will be posted on the book's website for easy adoption.

budget for several months, with up to one year of exposure, before conducting any preliminary evaluation. In Chapter 14, we discuss evaluation.

SUMMARY IMPLEMENTATION PLAN

The summary implementation plan is likely the one that will guide your program and be shown to potential collaborators or donors. For this reason, you do not want to go into all of the details included in previous sections of the book.

Your plan should include these key points:

- Background and justification, including your SWOTE analyses.
- Intended audiences.
- Communication objectives by audience.
- Messages.
- Settings and channels for conveying your messages.
- Activities (including media, materials, and other methods).
- Available partners and resources.
- Tasks and timeline (including persons responsible for each task, dates for completion of each task, resources required to deliver each task, and points at which progress will be checked).
- Budget.

You can add more, if you want. Realize that you will have more detailed planning documents for working with your media productions partners (if any), the news media (if involved), and program implementers.

Many projects need to train their partners in conducting intervention components—or at least prepare them for the launch of a mass media campaign so that they may coordinate local activities. The folic acid program prepared an outstanding guide of this nature, which has been recently reprinted; it is available at the CDC website.[7]

Box 13–4 shows a communication plan summary for a school-based physical activity campaign.

CONCLUSION

Implementation is the distillation of what you want to happen, who you plan to reach, and how you are going to proceed. Implementation is limited by how much support you have, what you can afford, external barriers, the distraction of competing influences, and imposed time limits. Implementation is

---

Box 13–4 Communication Plan Summary

BACKGROUND AND JUSTIFICATION

Heart disease is the leading cause of death among Americans. Inactivity and inadequate diet combined are the second leading cause of preventable deaths after tobacco-related deaths. (CDC's Guidelines for School and Community Health Programs, CV_physical_activity_among_young.pdf). Prevalence of overweight is at an all-time high among teens (CDC MMWR, 1997, http://www.cdc.gov/mmwr/mmwr_wk.html). Overweight in adolescence is associated with overweight in adults as well as with related chronic disease morbidity and mortality. During adolescence, physical activity decreases with age (CDC MMWR, 1997, http://www.cdc.gov/mmwr/mmwr_wk.html). Adolescents of minority groups are more likely to consume less fruits and vegetables and more high-fat foods than white teens. Minority adolescents also have higher prevalence of obesity and are more sedentary than white teens.

AUDIENCES

The target audience for this intervention (a peer advocacy training program and a communications campaign) is multiethnic teens from low-income families attending high school in five different school districts within the state. From among this target audience, certain teens were identified through key informant interviews as being "early adopters" of new behaviors, as categorized by the Diffusions of Innovations Model. Secondary audiences for the program messages include school staff and administrators, parents, and local policy makers.

COMMUNICATION GOALS AND OBJECTIVES

Communication goals were to:

- Increase healthy eating and physical activity.
- Increase advocacy activities for additional healthy food and physical activity options (i.e., to advocate for policy and environmental changes that promote healthy eating and physical activity options in the school and larger community).

OBJECTIVES

At the end of the two-year intervention (years three and four of the program), students whose high schools received the full intervention of the peer advocacy program and the communications campaign will show:

- A 40% increase in knowledge of the definition of healthy eating, its benefits, and healthy eating choices.
- A 25% increase in consumption of healthy foods, such as fruits and vegetables, low-fat products, and juices.
- A 50% increase in knowledge of the definition of physical activity, its benefits, and physical activity choices.

Disclaimer: The collaborators for the Cardiovascular Health CDCynergy adopted an existing health intervention and fictionalized it to conform to the steps of CDCynergy 2001. The Heart Healthy Program described in this case example is based loosely on the Food on the Run Program operated by California Project LEAN. The Heart Healthy Program is a fictional high school–based intervention promoting healthy eating and physical activity to multiethnic, low-income students within ten schools throughout the state. In an effort to ensure the utility and feasibility of the program examples…the information in these examples was tested with a health scientist, a cardiovascular epidemiologist, a cardiologist, two state cardiovascular health program coordinators, and additional public health professionals. This example originally appeared in CDCynergy Cardiovascular Health Edition.

continues

- A 20% increase in physical activity.
- That 70% of the teens will engage in at least one activity coordinated by the peer advocates in their schools (e.g., taste tests, cooking demonstrations, checking out workout equipment, dances) during each year of the program intervention.
- A 10% increase among full-intervention sites in the number of environmental or policy changes promoting healthy eating or physical activity.

Objectives also were established for those schools receiving the partial intervention consisting solely of the communications campaign materials (e.g., audio and video public service announcements [PSAs], posters, and countertop displays). The main goal of this intervention component was to increase knowledge among high school students of healthy eating and physical activity behaviors and choices. Therefore, behavioral change among students in schools receiving the communications campaign alone was not expected to be as great as it was among students whose schools received both the peer advocacy program and the communications campaign. Environmental and policy changes were not evaluated for the partial-intervention sites because they were not built into the goals of the communication campaign or into the messages of the campaign materials. At the end of the two-years of the intervention, students at the partial-intervention sites will show:

- A 20% increase in knowledge of the definition of healthy eating, its benefits, and healthy eating choices.
- A 10% increase in the consumption of healthy foods, such as fruits and vegetables, low-fat products, and juices.
- A 25% increase in knowledge of the definition of physical activity, its benefits, and physical activity choices.
- A 5% increase in physical activity.

CONCEPT AND MESSAGES

The concept of the program was "Simple Solutions" to eating healthy and being physically active. Program messages tied into this concept and promoted short-term benefits of these behaviors, such as increased energy, and feeling and looking better about oneself. The program also promoted the concept that the school environment affects the health behaviors of its students. Policy changes need to occur that make it easier for students to eat healthy and be physically active at school.

SETTINGS AND CHANNELS

The program was implemented in 20 high schools from five school districts throughout the state, chosen for their comparability on the demographic makeup of their student populations. Messages were communicated at individual, small-group, and organizational (school-wide) channels. The peer advocacy-training program was conducted among small groups and promoted activities among all three channels.

ACTIVITIES

Since the program's inception, participating high schools were aware that they would receive free materials from the media marketing specialist as described . . . as part of the program's intervention components. . . . Heart Healthy staff and stakeholders at the district and school levels had decided that the materials should be produced in time to be distributed at the beginning of the school year for year one of the program intervention. This gave all schools the full school year to implement the program components, which provided the foundation for the evaluation plan. Intervention materials included (1) the counter display and tip sheet, poster and public service announcement (PSA) for all 20 schools receiving only the communications campaign (partial intervention) and (2) the lesson plans and resource kit to support the peer advocacy training program for the ten schools receiving both the peer advocacy and communications campaign interventions (the full intervention).

Peer educators conducted a variety of activities on school campuses, such as:

- Taste tests and promotion campaigns of healthy foods available on campuses.
- Activities to promote physical activity among their peers, such as after-school dance lessons and sports equipment checkout tables at lunch.
- Health-related facts about nutrition and physical activity that ran in school newspapers and on school Web sites.
- School-wide surveys about what schools could do to offer healthier foods and foster increased physical activity on their campuses.
- School suggestion boxes soliciting students for their ideas, with positive suggestions promoted to the student body and school administrators.

- Letters and speeches to school boards and parents groups about desired policy changes.
- Letters to the editor and interviews with school and local media about desired policy changes.

The communications campaign components were used differently by each school. In general, closed-circuit television was used to play the video PSA, school public announcement (PA) systems and radio stations played the audio PSA, and the posters and countertop displays were put up in locations throughout each school to attract students' attention to the campaign messages. Locations for these materials included cafeterias, snack bars, concession stands, food stores, the school gymnasium, school clinics, and taste-testing tables. Posters and counter displays also were given to community locations such as teen centers, Boys and Girls Clubs, shopping mall food courts, health fairs, and to teen clinics and physicians' offices.

BUDGET (TO BE DEVELOPED)

Each year during the five-year grant period, Heart Healthy received $700,000 in funding. Major expenditures for that money included personnel, supplies, meetings and travel, formative research, materials development, and data analysis and reporting. In years one and two of the program period, more money was allocated toward research and materials development, while in years three through five of the program, the costs for meetings, personnel, and data analysis and reporting were greater.

Source: CDC, CDCynergy Web. Cardiovascular Health Edition.

---

the tip of the iceberg, supported completely by below-the-surface planning. Implementation is an extended moment of truth—the time when your planning and expectations are embodied into action. How do you know if you did well? Just turn the page: evaluation is the next step.

KEY TERMS

Bioethics
Deontological principles
Direct costs
Indirect costs
In-kind contributions
Logic model
Sustainability
SWOTE analysis
Total budget
Utilitarianism

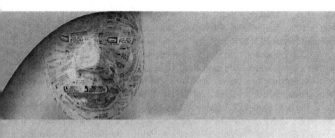

Chapter Questions

1 Describe two ways to use a logic model.

2. Which ethical principle do you think is paramount in public health?

3. What are the differences between outputs and outcomes in a logic model?

4. Why would you ever want something to have a home-made appearance?

5. What are the key elements in a budget?

REFERENCES

1. Goodstadt M. The use of logic models in health promotion practice. February 2005. Available at: http://www.course-readings-and-resources.best practices-healthpromotion.com/attachments/File/Goodstadt %20other%20 resources/Goodstadt_Introduction_to_logic_models_paper.pdf.

2. Knowlton LW, Phillips CC. *The Logic Model Guidebook: Better Strategies for Great Results*. Thousand Oaks, CA: Sage Publications; 2009.

3. W.K. Kellogg Foundation Logic Model Development Guide; 2001. Available at: http://www.wkkf.org/knowledge-center/Resources-Page.aspx?x= 42&y=6&q =logic.

4. Guttman N, Salmon CT. Guilt, fear, stigma and knowledge gaps: Ethical issues in public health communication interventions. *Bioethics.* 2004;18(6): 1467–8519 (online).

5. O'Sullivan GA, Yonkler JA, Morgan W, Merritt AP. *A Field Guide to Designing a Health Communication Strategy*. Baltimore, MD: Johns Hopkins Bloomberg School of Public Health/Center for Communication Programs; March 2003. Available at: http://www.jhuccp.org/pubs/fg/02/index.shtml. Accessed January 12, 2010.

6. The Prevention and Health Communication Team, National Center on Birth Defects and Developmental Disabilities, CDC. Media Campaign Implementation Kit. Available at: http://www.cdc.gov/ncbddd/folicacid/ documents/MediaCampaignKit.pdf.

7. Burke B, Daniel KL, Latimer A, Mersereau P, Moran K, Mulinare J, Prue C. et al. *CDC: Preventing Neural Tube Birth Defects: A Prevention Model and Resource Guide for Campaign Partners to Help in Developing a Prevention Campaign*. Available at: http://www.cdc.gov/ncbddd/orders/pdfs/09.202063-A .Nash.Neural%20Tube%20BD%20Guide%20FINAL508.pdf.

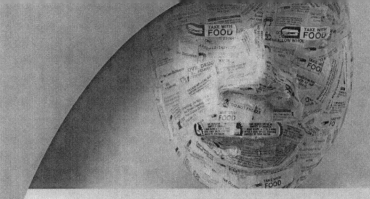

CHAPTER 14

Evaluating a Health Communication Program

May Grabbe Kennedy

INTRODUCTION

"Efficiency is concerned with doing things right. Effectiveness is doing the right things."

Peter F. Drucker, 1973[1]

Program evaluation is too often a required, dreaded procedure that renders an up-or-down verdict about the worthiness of a program. Evaluations are less stressful and much more useful when they are aimed at program improvement. Even when program improvement is the goal, evaluating health communication programs is a balancing act. An evaluator's main task is to test for a connection between program **exposure** and desired program outcomes. That sounds straightforward enough, but several important evaluation considerations involve trade-offs. See **Table 14–1** for some competing evaluation considerations.

The very use of the term "program evaluation" can be problematic. Some experts and institutions in public health draw a distinction between program evaluation and research.

Others view program evaluation as applied research. **Table 14–2** highlights some of the differences.

There is a lot of overlap in methods between rigorously conducted program evaluation and community-based intervention research. Strive for the greatest rigor possible in each set of circumstances, and be flexible about terminology.

This chapter is intended to give you an initial overview of the health communication program evaluation process, to share some lessons learned by experienced evaluators, and to point you to more in-depth resources on the topic. The chapter is aimed directly at fledgling program evaluators, but it should also be useful to staff members of programs being evaluated and to consumers of evaluation findings. It can take years of technical training and experience to become an expert health communication program evaluator. Very large, high-profile programs often hire a senior external consultant to evaluate the program or to guide internal program evaluation staff. It's a rare skill, and highly sought after.

THREE CENTRAL EVALUATION QUESTIONS

Although the process of evaluating health communication programs can be very technical, it boils down to answering three questions:

1. *Design:* Are you doing the right things?
2. *Implementation:* Are you doing them right?
3. *Outcome:* Are you doing enough of them make a difference?

TABLE 14-1 Competing Evaluation Interests

To achieve this . . .	You might have to sacrifice this, and vice versa.
The outcomes interest program decision-makers and other stakeholders.	Findings can be compared to those of other studies of programs that address the same health issue.
Measures of outcomes are credible to program stakeholders.	Comparability of findings, again.
Program insiders have detailed knowledge about the program.	Information about program performance is objective.
Reliable measures of knowledge, attitudes and other psychological determinants of health behavior often have multiple items.	Audience members have limited tolerance for lengthy questionnaires.
Getting a study design refined and approved takes time.	Evaluation results are available in time to inform key program decisions.
Health communication programs and campaigns can have several components and multiple audiences.	Evaluation resources are finite.

TABLE 14-2 Differences Between Program Evaluation and Research

Program Evaluation	Research
Intended to inform program decision makers.	Intended to produce generalizable knowledge.
Uses theory to test programs.	Sometimes just tests theory.
Emphasizes usefulness of findings.	Emphasizes study design rigor.
Sometimes exempt from Institutional Review Board (IRB) review for ethical treatment of human subjects.	Always subject to at least expedited IRB review when data are collected from program participants.
Usually allocates a larger share of available resources to the program.	Usually allocates a larger share of available resources to the study.
The program is more likely to continue after the study.	The program is less likely to continue after the study.

Doing the Right Things?

You can say that a program is doing the right things if three conditions have been met:

- First, the program intervention is either evidence based in its entirety or is made up of elements that have demonstrated their effectiveness in previous studies. If such a role has not been established in previous research, an evaluator should point this out to program planners and recommend adopting a science-based objective.

- The second design condition is that the program achieves its objectives. Before an evaluation study begins, the evaluator and program decision makers should review the logic model for the program to identify inputs, outputs, and outcomes. Key variables to measure achievement of program objectives can be discussed. As discussed later in this chapter, the measures can be qualitative, quantitative, or (preferably) both.

- The third design condition is that program procedures are acceptable to a local community. For example, an

AIDS prevention campaign that explicitly targets young gay men might not raise an eyebrow in gay bars in a major city but it could violate norms in a small town. State and local health departments organize committees to perform community standards reviews of HIV/AIDS prevention communication programs. Check with local health officials to see if this practice has been extended to your health topic of interest. If not, share program plans and draft creative copy with community representatives and confirm the acceptability of your campaign messages and materials *before* the program incurs production costs.

If sound quantitative data collected under rigorously controlled conditions show that a program worked, it has demonstrated its **efficacy**. Most of the programs in evidence-based resources (**Box 14–1**) were able to meet this standard because they were funded adequately to provide tight design and implementation.

If the same interventions *still* work when transferred to more real-world conditions, the program is referred to as **effective**. The HIV prevention interventions that have been added to a list of programs on CDC's *PRS-REP(lication)-DEBI* project (described later in this chapter) are examples of effective programs.

Unfortunately, the results of most health communication program evaluations are never published. Networking with staff from programs that are similar to yours can help you mine lessons from the gray literature for evaluation.

Doing the Right Things Right?

The implementation question isn't answered just once. Periodic data collection is necessary to verify that program activities are still faithful to the original program plan. This is called **fidelity monitoring**. When drift from the plan is detected, the reasons for the drift can be identified, and corrective action can be taken as appropriate.

Whether the program was designed by its staff or adopted from an evidence-based protocol, fidelity monitoring is an essential part of ongoing quality control (see Chapter 13). Evaluators and program staff should work together to find ways to build fidelity into the structure of a health communication program. After that, checking to make sure the program is doing the right things right should become part of standard operating procedure on an ongoing basis. See **Box 14–2** for ideas for building fidelity into a program.

Fidelity data perform a key function in outcome evaluation, too. Negative outcome evaluation results (i.e., a lack of statistically significant association between program exposure and desired outcomes) could mean that a program was based on a bad plan. On the other hand, negative outcomes could mean that the program was not implemented as conceived. Monitoring procedural fidelity during the study period will enable you to find out which of these explanations is true in a given set of circumstances.

If a program is media based, you may be able to get all the fidelity data you need from written reports of when and when ads were aired or published. However, if you are using interpersonal channels to get your messages across, you should observe the program in action from time to time.[2] One way to do this is to drop by program sites unannounced with a checklist of the activities that are supposed to be performed in a standard fashion. If you decide to regulate fidelity this way, remember to explain the reason for drop-by checks to program delivery staff *in advance.*

Box 14–1 Lists of Evidence-Based Programs, Including Health Communication Campaign

- The Guide to Community Preventive Services (http://www.thecommunityguide.org/index.html)
- The Cochran Collaboration systematic reviews of health care (http://www.cochrane.org)
- The Campbell Collaboration systematic reviews of social and educational programs (http://www.campbellcollaboration.org)
- SAMSHA's National Registry of Evidence-based Programs and Practices (http://nrepp.samhsa.gov)

Box 14–2 Building Fidelity in a Program

- Automate procedures where possible.
- Require clearance of successive generations of creative ideas for a campaign to depend, in part, on consistency with the original creative brief.
- Offer both initial and repeated "booster" staff trainings.
- Solicit staff concerns about program elements so they can be addressed in a uniform fashion that doesn't undercut the key elements of the program.

Doing Enough of the Right Things to Make a Difference?

The last central evaluation question has two levels. At a basic level, doing enough of the right things is an issue of statistical power. That is, are there data from enough exposed and unexposed audience members to detect a between-group, program-related difference of a realistic size? Many evaluators consult with a biostatistician to set a study participation target that ensures adequate statistical power to detect program effects.

A study by the CDC AIDS Community Demonstration Projects Research Group[3] shows the importance of the statistical power consideration. The intervention was a major undertaking. Over a three-year period, street outreach workers delivered a theory-based intervention individually to tens of thousands of members of high-risk groups in five cities. The goal of the project was to achieve community-level increases in (1) the use of bleach for disinfecting injection drug use equipment and (2) condoms.

Although 13,500 street intercept interviews were conducted with drug users, only four of the cities were able to contribute bleach use data to the study. The intervention was shown to have a significant community-level effect on condom use, but it was too underpowered for bleach use to detect an effect at the community level for that outcome.

Speaking more generally, the "enough right things to make a difference" question is about a program's actual impact on a disease or health problem. When impact is understood to mean disease rates, precise answers to this question are rare. They require complex mathematical modeling that goes well beyond the scope of most program evaluations. (See **Box 14–3** for program impact modeling challenges.)

Moreover, "making a difference" is, to some degree, in the eye of the beholder. Think about **5-A-Day**, the national campaign that sought to decrease rates of heart disease, diabetes, and some cancers by promoting consumption of at least five daily servings of fresh fruits and vegetables. This nutritional practice has a complicated web of barriers and facilitators, so it may not surprise you to learn that the national evaluation of the 5-A-Day campaign had mixed results. The public did become more aware of the recommendation to eat fruits and vegetables and more convinced of its importance. However, there was no overall increase in the consumption of fruits and vegetables during the campaign period.[4] There are varied opinions about whether the program really made a difference in health behavior.

Decision makers may have unrealistically high expectations about the ability of an individual program to generate evidence of impact on the prevalence of a health problem. Similarly, they may expect a credible estimate of a program's cost-effectiveness, despite the lack of the specialized economic expertise such an estimate would require (e.g., see the cost analysis of the National truth® Anti-Tobacco campaign by Holtgrave and colleagues[5]).

Don't try to go beyond the available data. Explain to stakeholders that collecting good data on the expenditures, reach, and outcomes of the program you are studying will serve two purposes. Having good basic data will make it possible to improve the program now and to contribute later to more sophisticated impact and cost studies, while the lack of it will not.

CAPTURING THE BASICS: PROGRAM EXPOSURE AND OUTCOMES

Program Exposure

It may be fairly easy to count the number of products your program distributed or service contacts it had, but measuring message exposure is more complicated. It is easy to overestimate, possibly by a large margin, the number of times audience members actually received and processed the messages you were trying to convey. Measuring both what was sent and what the audience members were aware of receiving is ideal, but it isn't always practical.

The accuracy of product distribution as a measure of message exposure depends partly on the information channel employed. Physicians who deliver messages in face-to-face exchanges with individual patients can use the "teach-back" method to verify that the messages were heard and understood[6] (see Chapter 15). By contrast, website hit counts can contain an unknown number of repeat visitors, the number of brochures distributed is not the same as the number read, and

---

Box 14–3 Program Impact Modeling Challenges

- Population level health behavior change is usually brought about by a variety of programs and other influences.
- Disease trends are affected by a host of factors beyond just individual health behaviors.
- Behavior change brought about by a mass communication intervention can be clear and widespread, but short-lived.
- Permanent behavior change can take years to be reflected in disease statistics.

the number of bus riders is not the same as the number who paid attention to posters on the bus. Measures such as website hits and bus ridership are most useful as *upper* boundaries for ranges of exposure estimates.

In media-based health communication programs, a common exposure estimate is the number of **media impressions**. This is the extent of readership or viewership or listenership claimed by a specific media outlet (e.g., radio station, website). Impressions are only *opportunities* for message exposure. In weighing the value of impressions data, bear in mind that other measures of exposure such as surveys of viewership, which do measure actual exposure, are also subject to bias and can be extremely expensive.

Data on media impressions are usually available from the media outlet that broadcast or published the messages. Sometimes the data must be purchased from another vendor that specializes in tracking (see Chapters 11 and 12). New ways to think about and track impressions will be required as health communication programs incorporate interactive media channels such as online social networking sites. See **Box 14–4** for estimates of exposure reach.

If there is a lot of room for error in an exposure estimate based on a distribution measure, it is best to supplement the estimate with self-reported exposure information from at least some target audience members. As audiences gain the ability to control broadcast timing, frequency, and content (e.g., by taping broadcasts or accessing them on websites, viewing all or parts of them more than once, and fast-forwarding through portions),[7] the whole notion of exposure will become more complex and the need for self-reported exposure data will become greater.

Be aware that gathering self-report data through traditional means is becoming more difficult. In the age of caller ID and cell phones, phone surveys are yielding lower response rates and less reliable information. Fortunately, new survey methods (e.g., large, nationally representative panels of people who agree to participate in periodic web surveys for a couple of years) are improving.

Program Outcomes

As mentioned in earlier chapters, outcomes of health communication programs can include short-term effects and longer-term effects. Among the former are increases in knowledge, attitudes, and other psychosocial factors that foster health-related behavior change such as behavioral intentions. Behavior change itself can be a longer-term effect.

Both short-term and longer-term outcomes should be measured in an evaluation. The behavioral outcomes have real public health significance, but measures of psychosocial determinants (antecedents) of behavior help show that you understand how change is being brought about. In addition, as we saw in the 5-A-Day campaign evaluation example, measuring behavioral determinants also increases your odds of capturing program effects.

Hybrid measures that incorporate both determinants and behavioral outcomes are often used in evaluations of health communication programs.[3] They can be thought of as measures of behavioral readiness (e.g., the "stages of change" Transtheoretical Model or levels of McGuire's hierarchy). **Box 14–5** lists some advantages of measuring behavioral readiness stages in an evaluation.

A website maintained by NCI is a good source for measures of behavioral readiness.* You will also find tested scales of

---

*http://dccps.cancer.gov/brp/constructs.

Box 14–4 Estimates of Exposure Reach

- The number of radio ads purchased by a campaign to promote calls to a smoking cessation counseling telephone line, multiplied by Arbitron ratings for the stations that aired the ads at the time slots of the broadcasts.
- The number of physicians trained to distribute "information prescriptions," multiplied by the average caseload of a physician in the study during the study period.
- The number of times a report from Google Analytics lists www.twitter.com as a referral site to an emergency preparedness website.

Box 14–5 Advantages of Measures of Behavioral Readiness

- They acknowledge that behavior change doesn't happen all at once.
- They are sensitive to the stage in the behavior change process that an individual is at when program exposure occurs.
- They give a program credit for spurring movement along the path to the ultimately desired behavior.
- They are fairly easy to describe and measure.

other psychosocial constructs and single-item behavioral measures that are frequently used in health communication campaign evaluations on the site.

Selecting good measures of your key evaluation variables is extremely important, but even if your measures are state of the art, your evaluation is likely to run into difficulty if the goals of the health communication program were not clearly specified in a logic model during the planning phase of the project. Translating clear goals into measurable or SMART(ER) objectives gets an evaluation off on the right foot. SMARTER objectives are Specific, Measurable, Achievable, Realistic, and Time-bound as well as Extending/challenging, and Reviewed. By *extending*, we are suggesting that you try to go beyond what might be a small, but statistically significant improvement in an outcome, and reach for something that will really make a public health impact. For example, improving children's nutrition in a developing country from −3 standard deviations below a reference norm to −2 standard deviations is statistically significant—and important. But, it still means these children are malnourished. (This is discussed later in the section on RE-AIM.) Sharing your

objectives and logic model with stakeholders for their input and critique ahead of time is what is meant by *reviewed*.

EVALUATION FRAMEWORKS

Before you put the final touches on your evaluation scheme and submit it for approval by program stakeholders, step back and consider the program and your plan for evaluating it in the larger scheme of things. A standard, formal conceptual framework can help you put program activities into a broader perspective. Spending some time viewing your program through a big-picture lens may prompt you to add to or revise your evaluation plan.

Some frameworks focus on evaluation itself, and others treat evaluation as one aspect of a program in a larger community context. Four examples are outlined next.

The CDC Evaluation Framework

The CDC framework begins with engaging stakeholders in the process of choosing evaluation outcomes and outcome measures. See **Figure 14–1**.[8]

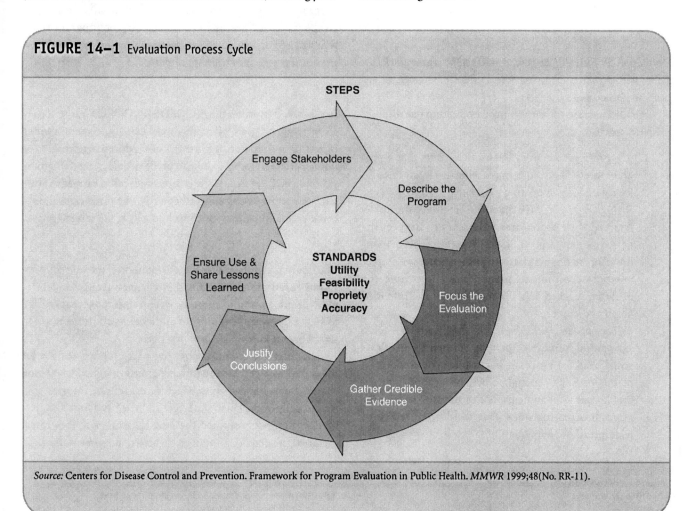

FIGURE 14–1 Evaluation Process Cycle

Source: Centers for Disease Control and Prevention. Framework for Program Evaluation in Public Health. *MMWR* 1999;48(No. RR-11).

A good evaluation provides an accurate understanding of the design, implementation, and effects of a program, but if the concerns of stakeholders are not addressed, evaluation findings will not be used to improve the program. That is why evaluations should be user focused,[9] and why most of the website links, evaluation handbooks, and other resources available on CDC's evaluation working group website* emphasize stakeholder collaboration.

Another key feature of the CDC framework is that it is a circle—a form with no endpoint—signifying that evaluation is an ongoing process. Of course, evaluating a program on an ongoing basis does not necessarily mean that you conduct the same type of study repeatedly. A better use of resources may be conducting a series of studies, each of which adds a different kind of information about how, or how well, the program is working. For example, in an initial study you might assess the effects of adding an online tutorial to a health education program that was previously limited to face-to-face instruction. If the tutorial improved program outcomes, you might conduct a subsequent study of the relative effectiveness of different versions of the online material.

The RE-AIM Framework†

Developed by Russell Glasgow, the **RE-AIM framework**, together with how to use it to improve a program's outcomes, appears in **Table 14–3**.

We can describe the three central evaluation questions in RE-AIM terms:

1. *Right things:* Can an evaluator determine that a program model is effective in *reaching* its targets and objectives, based on existing *evidence?*
2. *Right things right:* Were the core elements of the model retained if its procedures were *adapted* to meet the needs of a new target audience? Was the program monitored on an ongoing basis to ensure that it was implemented according to plan? Were the people the program reached actually members of the intended target audience?
3. *Enough of the right things:* Did the program reach a substantial number of people, enough to justify its costs? Was the program *maintained* (or could it be maintained) long enough to help bring about a measurable change in audience health status? Are the program procedures ones that lend themselves to widespread implementation?

Some suggestions for calculating variables that reflect RE-AIM concerns are listed on the website. It is not generally expected that one evaluation would encompass the entire RE-AIM framework, because it describes a process that normally spans many years of a project's lifecycle. Instead, a family of studies can address all of the relevant issues over time, and keeping the framework in mind from the beginning will help you craft a series of studies that is comprehensive from the RE-AIM perspective.

One example of bringing the full RE-AIM framework to bear systematically in an ongoing line of evaluation research and program development is CDC's *PRS-REP-DEBI* program.‡ Sponsored by the agency's Division of HIV/AIDS Prevention, the process begins with identifying an intervention that has scientifically credible evidence of efficacy. To facilitate adaptation of the program to local needs, core elements of the intervention (those that cannot be eliminated or changed without violating the integrity of the model) are identified by the original investigator. Then the intervention is replicated by someone other than the scientist who developed the model program. If it still works after "transplantation," a package of all the materials necessary to implement the program is assembled and disseminated nationwide through designated HIV prevention program training centers.

The PRECEDE–PROCEED Framework

As Chapter 2 explains, the **PRECEDE–PROCEED** framework is a systematic program planning model that guides communities in setting public health priorities and addressing them. Preliminary data collected to inform problem analysis and program planning in the *precede* phase is sometimes called formative evaluation, a topic discussed in Chapter 9. The three central outcome evaluation questions come into play at the *proceed* phase.

The Inform/Persuade Paradigm

The final conceptual model we will mention is the **inform/persuade paradigm**. As explained in Chapter 1, this model divides health communication programs into those that set out to deliver new information to audiences and those that attempt to put knowledge into practice.

Because the intended objective of a program should be measured well and thoroughly, programs designed to inform should assess the degree to which new, accurate information was actually imparted to the target audience and how long audience members retained the new information. Programs designed to persuade should be evaluated in terms of message

*http://www.cdc.gov/eval.
†http://www.re-aim.org.

‡http://www.cdc.gov/hiv/topics/prev_prog/rep/index.htm.

TABLE 14–3 RE-AIM Questions to Ask and Ways to Enhance Program Impact

RE-AIM Dimension	Questions to Ask of Potential Programs	Possible Ways to Enhance Dissemination
Reach (Individual Level)	What percent of the target population comes into contact?	Formative evaluation with potential users and with decliners
	Does program reach those most in need?	Small scale recruitment studies to test methods
	Will participants reflect the targeted population?	Identify and reduce barriers
		Use multiple channels of recruitment
Effectiveness (Individual Level)	Does program achieve key targeted outcomes?	Incorporate more tailoring to individual
	Does it produce unintended adverse consequences?	Reinforce via repetition, multiple modalities, social support and systems change
	How will impact on quality of life (QOL) be assessed?	Use stepped care approach
		Evaluate adverse outcomes and QOL for program revision and cost-to-benefit analysis
Adoption (Setting/Organizational Level)	What percent of target settings and organizations will use?	Conduct formative evaluation with adoptees and settings that decline
	Will organizations having underserved or high-risk populations use it?	Recruit settings that have most contact with target audience
	Does program help the organization address its primary mission?	Provide different cost options and customization of intervention
		Develop recruitment materials outlining program benefits and required resources
Implementation (Setting/Organizational Level)	How many staff within a setting will try this?	Provide delivery staff with training and technical assistance
	Can different levels of staff implement the program successfully?	Provide clear intervention protocols
	Are different components delivered as intended?	Consider automating all or part of the program
		Monitor and provide staff feedback and recognition for implementation
Maintenance [Individual (I) and Setting (S) Levels]	Does the program produce lasting effects at individual level?	Reduce level of resources required
	Can organizations sustain the program over time?	Incorporate "natural environmental" and community supports
	Are those persons and settings that show maintenance those most in need?	Conduct follow-up assessments and interviews to characterize success at both levels
		Incorporate incentives and policy supports

Source: RE-AIM. http://www.re-aim.org/2003/t_3b.htm

credibility and attitude change at a minimum. When persuasive communication is part of a multipronged strategy to change behavior by altering its actual and/or perceived costs and benefits, the entire effort should be evaluated in terms of behavior change, perceived costs and benefits, and other major theoretical predictors such as intentions.[10]

DISTINGUISHING AMONG AND COMBINING TYPES OF DATA

Evaluation data can be *qualitative* (i.e., based on rich, in-depth data from a few people or about a few cases), *quantitative* (i.e., numeric responses to a limited number of questions from a larger group of people), or both. Program evaluations that rely wholly on qualitative data are often called case studies. Qualitative data can also play an important secondary role when a study is mainly quantitative; quotes, insights and themes make numeric findings more interpretable.

CDC's Prevention Marketing Initiative (PMI) Demonstration Project illustrates a type of value added by qualitative data to a quantitative study. This coalition-based social marketing intervention was designed to reduce sexual risk of HIV among adolescents. As part of its evaluation, an anonymous random-digit-dial telephone survey was conducted in 15 Zip codes in Sacramento, California. The survey data showed that teens who were exposed to PMI were 26% more likely to have used a condom at last sex with their main partners than teens who had not been exposed. Teen condom use increased more than twice as much in Sacramento than in the rest of the country that year, but another program or event in Sacramento could have brought about the observed increase. That possibility was considered unlikely on the basis of data from key informant interviews.[11]

QUANTITATIVE STUDY DESIGNS AND METHODS

Several research study designs have been used to evaluate the outcomes of health communication interventions. You can find more complete information on study designs and the threats to the validity of conclusions to which each design is subject in books such as *Evaluating Health Promotion Programs*[12] and *Quasi-Experimentation*.[13]

Experiments

In the simplest version of a true experiment (or **randomized controlled trial, RCT**), each participant is randomly assigned to either a treatment or a control condition. Those in the treatment condition are exposed to some stimulus, and then outcomes are measured in both groups. The RCT design provides the soundest logical basis for drawing the conclusion that a specific intervention caused certain effects.

An RCT can be a feasible evaluation design for a health communication program if control of message exposure is a real possibility. The ability to avoid cross-condition exposure "contamination" is rare in communitywide programs, but not unusual if messages are being sent to audiences electronically, delivered by physicians directly to patients, or conveyed by health education instructors to classes.

A study of message tailoring strategies conducted by Matthew Kreuter and his colleagues offers an example of using an RCT in evaluating a health communication intervention.[14] They randomly assigned more than 1,000 African American women to a usual care control condition or to one of three groups that received a series of magazines along with usual care. The magazines contained messages about mammography and another health issue. The messages were demographically tailored, culturally tailored, or tailored both ways. Mammography increased when the messages were tailored both ways, but neither demographic tailoring nor cultural tailoring alone had significant effects. Because of the RCT design, you can have confidence in the conclusion that, for women in that sample of that population at that point in time, the dual tailoring really caused the increase in mammography uptake.

It is nearly impossible to use an RCT to evaluate a mass communication program. Experiments that have a comparison group but no truly randomized control condition (quasi-experiments) are not feasible when communication campaigns cover extremely large areas. There is no truly adequate comparison area for the United States as a whole, for example. See **Box 14–6** for a list of challenges to conducting RCTs with a mass media intervention.

Box 14–6 Challenges to RCTs for Full-Coverage Programs with Media

- Lack of initially comparable control areas for national or other very large programs.
- Prohibitive cost and analysis challenges (e.g., group clustering) of randomizing at the community level of analysis.
- Difficulty of limiting exposure in a given community to just one specific target audience.
- Community resistance to no-treatment control status when an intervention has face validity and the health issue is urgent.
- Unpredictable activities in the control community that parallel intervention activities.

Correlational Studies

When broadcast channels are used to deliver messages to large target audiences, evaluators often use surveys to collect information on (1) program exposure as it occurred in the real world, (2) the outcome of interest, and (3) other variables that could affect the relationship between exposure and outcomes (e.g., demographics). Correlations or odds ratios are then calculated to assess the association between exposure and outcomes; regression and other multivariate methods are often used to control statistically for as many potentially confounding factors as possible. This kind of study is referred to as "observational" because the evaluator lacks control over program exposure and is relegated to observing associations that may or may not be a function of program effects.

Correlational studies can include one or more waves of data collection. Multiwave studies can be longitudinal (i.e., follow and re-interview a "cohort" of respondents over time) or cross-sectional (i.e., interview different respondents in each survey wave). Often, the data collection occurs immediately before, immediately after, and several months after exposure to the program, but sometimes there are many points of data collection.

The results of quasi-experiments are considered more interpretable than the results of one-group correlational studies. Nonetheless, to save money and preserve the anonymity of respondents, single-wave, cross-sectional, post-program designs are often employed. Outcomes among exposed respondents are compared with those of unexposed respondents.

There are serious threats to the validity of causal conclusions drawn from single-wave, cross-sectional studies. These threats are listed in another volume in this series[15] and in books on study design.[12,13] Evaluators relying on correlational data must attempt to rule out rival causal explanations of changes for which program sponsors would like to take credit (or avoid blame). **Box 14–7** lists some ways to counter threats to validity.

Interrupted Time-Series

When multiple observations of the same population are made over a fairly long period of time, including the period before a program began, you can compare observations made before and after the "interruption" constituted by the program. If a change occurred in the average value of the variables or their slope when the program was introduced, you can infer that the program was responsible for the change. The inference is strengthened if an analogous set of observations made at the same times in a comparison community show no discontinuity in values. According to Cook and Campbell,[13] the advantage of the interrupted time-series design over other observational measures is that it allows you to see if a trend in the outcome you are trying to affect was already in place before your intervention began. If there was a preprogram trend, adjustments for it can be made in the data analysis.

You can collect your own data for a time-series study, use data that are routinely collected for program management purposes and archived, or use what is sometimes called *indicator* data. These data come from surveillance activities that track a health problem or behavior using a set of standard methods at regular intervals. Surveillance is usually funded by a government agency. One example is the Behavioral Risk Factor Surveillance System, a state-based survey funded and analyzed by the CDC.* Another surveillance survey called HINTS† was developed by the National Cancer Institute specifically to inform health communication efforts.

Indicator data reflect the cumulative effects of all programs and influences on an outcome. Sometimes you can arrange to have a questionnaire item (or a new response alternative for an existing item) added to a standard survey to tap

---

*http://www.cdc.gov/BRFSS/.
†http://hints.cancer.gov.

Box 14–7 Ways to Counter Threats to Validity of Nonexperimental Study Conclusions

- Collect data from a comparison community to show that positive outcomes in the program community were not just a function of historical or "secular" trends that would have unfolded with or without the program.
- Include measures of exposure dosage in surveys; outcomes that increase with exposure dosage help legitimize causal inferences.
- Time survey waves to be able to show that outcomes rise and fall in synchrony with campaign waves.
- Consider using statistical techniques to control for an exposure bias called "self-selection." If a survey contains enough information about respondents, "propensity scoring" can help to rule out the possibility that people were more likely to notice a health message if they were already primed to change a relevant behavior.[16]

exposure to your program. In any event, if your campaign did enough of the right things to make a difference and there is a coincidental spike in indicator data, you can use other sources to try to make the case that your program contributed to the change in the surveillance data pattern.

Direct Observations

Some evaluation studies depend on direct observation of behavior. The subjects being observed may or may not be aware of the observation. A hypothetical evaluation of a campaign to prevent smokeless tobacco use among Little League baseball players provides a vivid example of unannounced or unobtrusive observations.

Imagine that you are evaluating a program based in two very similar and adjacent small towns. It is a smokeless or "spit" tobacco prevention intervention delivered through coaches to at-risk Little League baseball players. You toss a coin to determine which town gets the messages during the study and explain to stakeholders in the other town that the program will be replicated there if the evaluation shows it works. Before and after the campaign, you send first-year graduate students out to make postgame counts of spit tobacco wads in the dugouts and on the ground of Little League ball parks in both towns.

This is an example of an unobtrusive observation. Its advantage over self-report measures such as surveys and interviews is that it avoids "social desirability" bias—answers tainted by what subjects think you want to hear. A disadvantage of unobtrusive observation is that you may not have access to all settings in which the behavior could be performed.

Sampling

Regardless of the study design you use, you are unlikely to collect evaluation data from every member of a target population. Instead, the population is sampled. **Sampling** involves the selection of a small group of individuals chosen to have the same overall characteristics as the population from which they were taken. Samples of phone numbers or addresses are typically purchased from commercial vendors that specialize in this service. Once the sample is drawn, other vendors can be hired to administer the survey to sample members via mailed questionnaires, telephone interviews, or newer electronic means. **Table 14–4** displays some types and characteristics of different samples.

CONCLUSION

Evaluation of health communication programs follows some conventions and includes some "tricks of the trade." The following recommendations are based on guidance from national experts in health communication evaluation who were convened by the CDC.[10]

TABLE 14–4 Types and Characteristics of Different Samples

Random samples	Yield results that can be generalized to an entire target population
Convenience samples*	Can be adequate to inform program decisions
Snowball samples†	Appropriate when communication exposure and/or outcomes have an inherent network dynamic

*e.g., passers-by in a mall
†e.g., friends of friends and relations

- *Cognitive test your interview or questionnaire.* Words and questions may not mean the same thing to you as they do to the target audience. Find this out by asking a small sample of audience members to think out loud as they read a questionnaire and translate the questions into their own words.

- *Evaluate effects of exposure to the campaign overall, not through specific channels.* Health communication interventions work best when they convey new information and send the information out through multiple channels.[17] But memories of the number of times a person has been exposed to a message through a specific traditional channel are notoriously unreliable. This may prove to be equally true of new channels (e.g., social networking media such as YouTube, or Internet 2.0 media such as wikis).

- *Make and measure program signal intensity.* One of the major reasons health communication programs fail is that the messaging signal generated is too small or infrequent to cut through the noise of the other messages that bombard us. Did your program expose enough members of the target audience enough times to register? Quantifying program outputs is critically important in understanding a program's effects.

- *Determine when it's time to refresh a campaign.* Nothing works forever. Examine data from periodic tracking "pulse-checks" (e.g., media ratings, low-cost surveys of convenience samples) to detect a fall-off in campaign response.

- *Measure both recognition and recall.* It is easier to recognize something you have been exposed to than to supply it—to "fill in the blank" instead of make a choice from a list of options—but recognition is more subject to "false-positive" responses.

- *Add "ringer" exposure items* (e.g., questions about exposure to an ad that wasn't really broadcast) to estimate the percentage of false exposure reporting. That enables you to correct for false reporting in your final numbers and adds credibility to your evaluation.
- *Use multiple measures of key outcomes.* Asking the most important questions several ways does not add a great deal of length to the questionnaire and makes it more likely that you will capture any effect your program caused.
- *Track both intended and unintended campaign effects.* This is both an ethical and a political consideration. For example, parents are not going to support sustaining a program that increased condom use among teens unless there is good evidence that it didn't increase teen sexual activity.
- *Be aware of low-cost qualitative and quantitative data collection strategies.*[18]
- *Stay abreast of the increasingly prominent role informatics* (as described in Chapter 3) *can play in evaluation.* **Box 14–8** lists several.

KEY TERMS

5-A-Day campaign
Correlational studies
Effectiveness
Efficacy
Exposure
Fidelity monitoring
Inform/persuade paradigm
Media impressions
PRECEDE–PROCEED model
Randomized controlled trial (RCT)
RE-AIM framework
Sampling

Box 14–8 Examples of Informatics in Evaluation

- Employ terminology consistent with Controlled Medical Vocabularies to make your results more comparable and accessible to those of other studies.
- Use electronic medical records to track exposures and outcomes in interventions that use healthcare providers as channels.
- Assess features of online clinical decision support systems.
- Measure the effects on physical activity levels of handheld, GPS-equipped devices that prompt users to take the stairs instead of an elevator when they enter a multistory building.

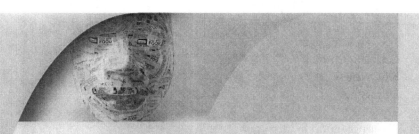

Chapter Questions

1. What is the basic purpose of a health communication program evaluation?

2. What are the central research questions a health communication program evaluation asks?

3. At what points and how should stakeholders be involved?

4. Which major study designs are used to evaluate health communication programs?

5. What does the RE-AIM framework bring to the program design and evaluation approach?

REFERENCES

1. Drucker PF. *Management: Tasks, Responsibilities, Practices*. New York: Harper & Row; 1973: 45.

2. Evans SW, Weist MD. Implementing empirically supported treatments in the schools: What are we asking? *Clin Child Fam Psychol Rev*, 2004;7(4): 263–237.

3. CDC AIDS Community Demonstration Projects Research Group. Community-level HIV intervention in 5 cities: Final outcome data from the CDC AIDS Community Demonstration Projects. *AJPH*, March 1999;(89)3: 299–301.

4. Stables G, Subar AF, Patterson BH, et al. Changes in fruit and vegetable consumption and awareness among U.S. adults: Results of the 1991 and 1997 5-A-Day for better health program surveys. *J Am Diet Assoc*. 2002;102:809–817.

5. Holtgrave DR, Wunderink KA, Vallone DN, Healton CG. Cost-utility analysis of the national truth campaign to prevent youth smoking. *AM J Prev Med*. May 2009;36(5):385–388.

6. Osbourne H. In other words . . . confirming understanding with the teach-back technique. American Medical Foundation. Available at: http://www.healthliteracy.com/article.asp?PageID=6714, accessed June 15, 2009.

7. Heeter C. Interactivity in the context of designed experiences. *J Interactive Advert*, 2000;1(1), Available at: http://www.jiad.org/article2, ISN 1525-2019, accessed June 15, 2009.

8. Centers for Disease Control and Prevention. Framework for Program Evaluation in Public Health. *MMWR* 1999;48(No. RR-11).

9. Patton MQ. *Utilization-Focused Evaluation: The New Century Text* (3rd ed.). Thousand Oaks, CA: Sage; 1997.

10. The Communication Evaluation Expert Panel, Abbatangelo J, Cole G, Kennedy MG. Guidance for evaluating mass communication health initiatives: Summary of an expert panel discussion sponsored by CDC. *Eval Health Prof*. 2007;30(3):229–253.

11. Kennedy MG, Mizuno Y, Seals BF, Myllyluoma J, Weeks-Norton K. Increasing condom use among adolescents with coalition-based social marketing, *AIDS*. 2000;14(12),1809–1818.

12. Valente TW. *Evaluating Health Communication Programs*. New York: Oxford; 2002.

13. Cook TD, Campbell DT. *Quasi-Experimentation: Design & Analysis Issues for Field Settings*. Boston: Houghton Mifflin; 1979.

14. Kreuter MW, Sugg-Skinner C, Holt CL, Clark EM, Haire-Joshu D, Fu Q, Booker AC, Steger-May K, Bucholtz D. Cultural tailoring for mammography and fruit and vegetable intake among low-income African-American women in urban public health centers. *Prev Med*. July 2005;41(1):53–62.

15. Edberg M. *Essentials of Health Behavior: Social and Behavioral Theory in Public Health*. Sudbury, MA: Jones & Bartlett; 2007.

16. Yanovitsky I, Zannuto E, Hornik R. Estimating causal effects of public health education campaigns using propensity score methodology. *Eval Program Plann*. 2005;28:209–220.

17. Snyder LB, Hamilton, MA, Mitchell EW, Kiwanuka-Tondo J, Fleming-Milici F, Proctor D. A meta-analysis of the effect of mediated health communication campaigns on behavior change in the United States. *J Health Commun*. 2004;9(6 Suppl 1):74–96.

18. Fitzpatrick JL, Sanders JR, Worthen BR. *Program Evaluation: Alternative Approaches and Practical Guidelines* (3rd ed.). Boston: Allyn & Bacon; 2003.

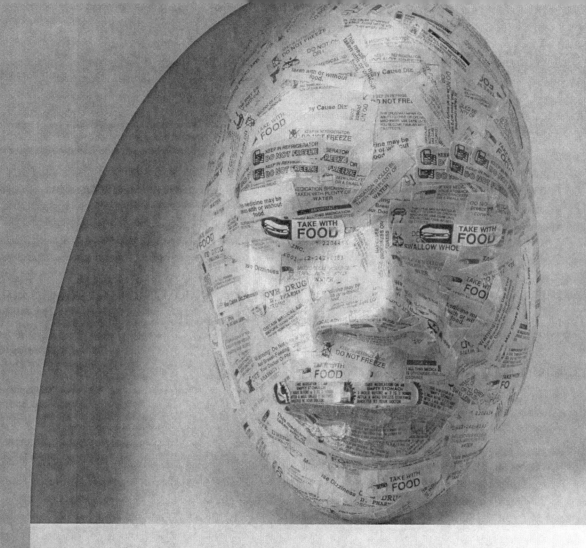

SECTION IV

Special Contexts

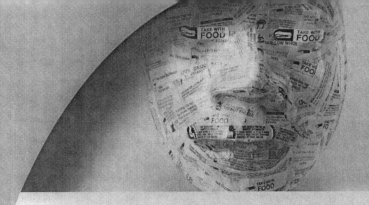

CHAPTER 15

Patient–Provider Communication

Richard N. Harner

LEARNING OBJECTIVES

By the end of this chapter, the reader will be able to:

- Describe the relationship between healthcare patients and providers in terms of multiple goals, barriers, and levels of communication.
- Identify key tools the healthcare provider may use to communicate effectively with the patient.
- Practice empathetic and effective listening and speaking with a model patient.

INTRODUCTION

This chapter focuses on **patient–provider communication (PPC),** the face-to-face communication between a healthcare provider and his or her client. Fifty years ago, this would have been mostly about the doctor–patient relationship.[1–5] Since then, the nature of doctor–patient communication has changed. New technologies and new demands on time have reduced the amount of energy that physicians deliver to the patient encounter. In parallel, and in part as a consequence, new health professions have arisen; nurses have become nurse practitioners, assistants have become physician assistants, and emergency medical technologists have become independent practitioners. When we add on an increasing interest in improving public health, through interventions at the level of pharmacy, government, and others, we find that the spectrum of healthcare providers who are communicating with individual patients is greatly broadened.[6,7]

Physicians, other clinicians, and healthcare workers in general all must communicate effectively with individual patients (clients?—see **Box 15–1**) in order to diagnose, treat, care for, and assist those in need. We develop a conceptual framework for

Box 15–1 Client or Patient?

What distinguishes a patient from a client? Wing wrote that, "the question of patient autonomy versus medical paternalism is occasionally raised as a possible reason to justify the use of 'client,'" but concluded that people sought out the protection and care of a physician, and did not want to think of themselves as clients or "consumers" of medical services.

Source: Wing PC. Patient or client? If in doubt, ask. *Can Med Assoc J* 1997;157287–157289.

PPC, emphasize the multifaceted, bidirectional nature of the process, and outline the steps toward more effective interaction.

CONCEPTUAL FRAMEWORK FOR EFFECTIVE PATIENT–PROVIDER COMMUNICATION

As we begin, keep in mind four dichotomies that help frame the interaction between patients and healthcare providers. These dichotomies, along with goals, barriers, levels, modes, tools, and externals, to be discussed later, form the conceptual framework for effective PPC (**Figure 15–1**).

Dichotomies

- *Health/disease:* Are we approaching our interaction from a predominately health-oriented or a predominately disease-oriented perspective—the annual physical examination or an evaluation of recent weight loss and abdominal pain?

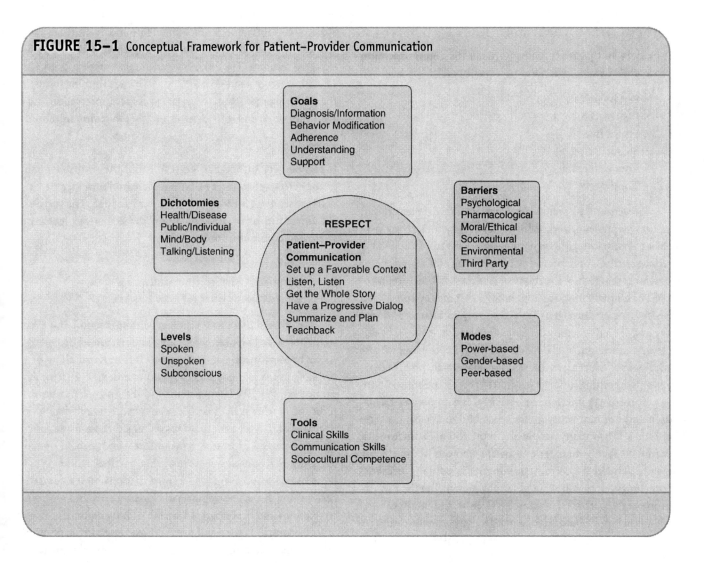

FIGURE 15–1 Conceptual Framework for Patient–Provider Communication

Goals
Diagnosis/Information
Behavior Modification
Adherence
Understanding
Support

Dichotomies
Health/Disease
Public/Individual
Mind/Body
Talking/Listening

RESPECT

Patient–Provider Communication
Set up a Favorable Context
Listen, Listen
Get the Whole Story
Have a Progressive Dialog
Summarize and Plan
Teachback

Barriers
Psychological
Pharmacological
Moral/Ethical
Sociocultural
Environmental
Third Party

Levels
Spoken
Unspoken
Subconscious

Modes
Power-based
Gender-based
Peer-based

Tools
Clinical Skills
Communication Skills
Sociocultural Competence

- *Public/private:* Is our intervention at the public level or predominately at the individual/private level? In this chapter we focus on the individual level.
- *Mind/body:* While mind cannot easily be separated from body, it is helpful to consider them separately to ensure that both views are considered fully, even though the initiating event may seem wholly physical or mental.
- *Talking/listening:* We cannot overemphasize the essential bi-directional nature of effective PPC. We want to talk, but we must also listen. As we will see later, most often listening should form the larger part of the intervention to achieve the goals of patient-centered communication.

Goals

We may also view a patient–provider encounter as in an exercise in goal-setting. What do patients and providers want? Consider the following goals, all or most of which are relevant to every provider–patient encounter:

- Diagnosis/information.
- Behavior modification.
- Adherence to treatment.
- Understanding.
- Support.

When the patient comes to a physician for diagnosis and treatment of headaches, a different set of priorities are involved than when a provider approaches a client in an attempt to change behavior for obesity control. The problems of adherence to treatment programs are very particular and have major implications for public as well as individual health.

Finally, the goals of promoting patient understanding and support need to be emphasized. At least equal importance should be given to these "soft" goals in their own right as well as to enhance the achievement of "hard" goals of direct patient care. We will discuss goal-setting and sharing later in detail.

Barriers

Providers and patients alike approach the communication process with a set of barriers:

- Psychological.
- Pharmacological.
- Ethical/moral.
- Sociocultural.
- Environmental.
- Third party.

Barriers at the psychological level include disinterest, fear, anxiety, depression, and reality distortion by underlying psychosis. Pharmacologic intervention such as overmedication may reduce alertness and interaction. Overriding ethical and moral standards may reduce the ability of clinicians to take certain actions or for patients to respond in ways that may be considered healthy. Sociocultural barriers accompany sociocultural diversity and include issues with language, gender, income, health literacy, education, intellect, and ethnicity. Environmental distractions are relevant; excessive noise, inadequate time, and inappropriate settings or dress may interfere with communication.

Third-party interference with PPC is common with children and not rare with adults. It is useful to ask yourself the question, "How many people are in the room?" Sometimes a dominant family member or a friend who can be affected or even offended by certain statements is actually present. Sometimes the person is not physically present, but their words drone in the patient's (or clinician's!) head and interfere with what otherwise would have been effective communication

There are many barriers to successful PPC, but all is not lost!

GETTING STARTED

If two natural communicators were to meet with a shared healthcare goal, their interaction might be simple, brief, and effective. For the rest of us, we need to keep in mind the multiple levels in which communication takes place and the multiple goals that may be present within the minds of both the sender and receiver in the communicative process.

When entering into a healthcare encounter, both provider and patient must be prepared to shift between providing information and giving feedback in a flexible and progressive fashion.[8–16] The provider may juggle goals and approaches to achieve the overall communication goal.

Much has been written about interpersonal communication. While communication in relation to health shares some features—such as effective give and take, agenda setting, and the like—the context of the health encounter often sets a difficult tone. Often, emotional issues are overriding, bringing relief, de-spair, or euphoria into an encounter. Life and death issues may charge seemingly harmless words with great intensity and unexpected meaning. The following paragraphs make explicit some of the features of successful PPC.[17–22] Threads running through the following discussion will relate to respect, motivation, momentum, story, and soft-focus approaches to communication.

Levels

It can be very difficult to keep in mind the multiple goals brought to an encounter by both patient and provider, particularly when time is short and emotions run high. The successful communicator will engage on three distinct levels of goal/need communication:

- Spoken (what is said).
- Unspoken (what is left unsaid).
- Subconscious (what is below awareness).

We all tend to focus on spoken communication. But even well-chosen, well-spoken words are best interpreted in context. As we become more aware of context our understanding of a patient's needs and goals can expand to a degree "that words cannot express." We begin listening to the unspoken communication, to what is *not* said. The patient who faces a diagnosis of cancer and never asks about his or her short-term and long-term prospects is expressing a major fear—and perhaps signaling a desire to not know more at that particular time. What remains unspoken also provides information about a patient's background, fears, upbringing, political concerns, and religious convictions and beyond. It is a wealth of information.

Subconscious goals and needs are expressed in the posture, movements, and expressions that make up our body language. In addition to body language, dress, punctuality, and the choice of accompanying persons provide information about unconscious needs and goals. The mythical perfect communicator knows and uses all of this information. For the rest of us, it helps to begin by consciously searching for communication opportunities at all levels until the search becomes implicit in our own communication behavior.

Modes

There are three modes of PPC in common use:

- Power based.
- Gender based.
- Peer based.

Authoritarian, power-based doctor–patient interaction has a long history. We now know that physicians are not infallible and that diagnoses, treatments, opinions, and technical skills can vary widely. Still, according to surveys of public opinion, the respect given to physicians and other healthcare providers infuses their direct communication with the power to produce change beyond that of any other healthcare channel.

A second factor in PPC relates to gender roles.[23–25] Gender differences and similarities influence the encounter at spoken, unspoken, and unconscious levels, offering opportunities and risks for the participants. Historically, a paternalistic role for physicians has been assumed and expected by patients seeking care for their illness. When the provider is a woman, a maternalistic relationship may result. Patients do assign roles that empower providers, but these roles also complicate PPC and the patient–provider relationship. Hall and colleagues have shown that gender-based communication is a factor in patient satisfaction and adherence to treatment programs.[19–22] Women as providers are often more effective in this regard and women now account for more than half of medical school applicants and a third of practicing physicians.

A viewing of the recent television program *Private Practice* (2007–2010, American Broadcasting Co.) gives a current example of peer-based PPC. Ties and white shirts are avoided, long white coats as well. Doctors become friends and advisors, and the less formal peer–peer communication is used to effect change.

Shorn of the power and respect inherent in the classic doctor–patient model, the provider must earn respect and empowerment through effective communication and actions. This can take a while.

Power-based, gender-based, and peer-based communications all have the power to enhance communication and have associated risks.[26] Their use depends on the background and spirit of the communicators, patient and provider alike. The best approach is a flexible one, in which the provider chooses or changes modes to best fit the needs of the patient and the skills of the provider.

Tools

Each provider can bring to bear a variety of tools to deal with the many barriers to effective communication just described. These can be grouped under three headings:

- Clinical skills.
- Communication skills.
- Sociocultural competence.

In the classical doctor–patient relationship, the physician brings a broad spectrum of knowledge and clinical skills to bear on the patient's problems and provides answers and therapeutic plans and addresses questions of concern on behalf of the patient. Relevant clinical skills remain the cornerstone of patient care.

In recent decades, faced with increasing demands on their professional time and startling expansion of the medical knowledge base, generalists and specialists alike are finding their medical knowledge increasingly incomplete.[27–30] At the same time, patients have become more knowledgeable about their own diseases, diagnosis, and treatment—especially through widespread availability of information on the Internet. As the knowledge differential between patient and provider diminishes, the provider–patient interaction is altered. To put it another way, because information can now be easily obtained from a variety of sources, the provider has become less a source of information and more of an advisor, an organizer, a facilitator. This means that any provider, whether medically trained or not, will need to have full array of communication skills in addition to clinical competence in his/her chosen area.

The third element in the tool set for PPC is that of **sociocultural competence,** the ability to understand and relate to behavioral patterns that are determined in part by membership in racial, ethnic and social groups. This term is used here in preference to the more widely used "cultural competence" to emphasize the major role of social factors (age, income, gender, living circumstance, etc.) in successful PPC.[31] (Cultural competence should have the same meaning but too often is limited to racial and ethnic issues by common usage.)

It is the rare healthcare encounter that does not have a significant element of social and cultural determination of ultimate outcome. This requires, especially on the part of the provider:

- Awareness and acceptance of the need for social and cultural competence.
- Language and social skills that allow cultural barriers to be franchised.
- Cross-cultural training and/or experience whenever possible.

Numerous sociocultural factors affect communication, including, community, customs, morals, ethics, income, language, style, and body language. For example, norms for body language, eye contact, and choice of interpersonal distance for communication are culturally determined.[32–35] To be unaware of the potential for a mismatch in such cultural norms risks being misunderstood or even giving offense with a simple gesture or movement.

Externals

While externals in the encounter environment are usually less important than the interpersonal considerations described earlier, location, time of day, environmental factors such as noise, distraction, furnishings, dress, lighting, and more can facilitate or impair communication. Emergency care in the middle of a busy street is a setting in which PPC is vital but difficult. In a controlled setting such as a doctor's office, PPC can be facilitated by supportive personnel and environments for reception, waiting, examining, and consultation.

To this point we have outlined dichotomies, goals, barriers, levels, modes, tools, and externals that relate to PPC. While it may seem detailed, the purpose is to underline the multiple factors that contribute to effective PPC. As we learn how to apply this framework, the details will be replaced by implicit PPC skills.

PATIENT–PROVIDER ENCOUNTER

Each of the following is an important consideration in the patient–provider encounter:

- Respect.
- Preparation.
- Listen first.
- The "story."
- Progressive dialogue.
- Review and summation.

We will use a new patient visit to a doctor's office to illuminate the process. The "doctor" may be another type of clinician such as a nurse practitioner or a physician assistant. The patient is a stranger, unknown to the doctor.

Respect

As Purtilo and Haddad (2007) state, "Respect is the thread that weaves together discussions regarding professional and patient encounter in the healthcare environment." Throughout the health encounter, the need and search for respect on the part of provider and patient alike are never absent. Respect sets the tone of PPC before the first word is spoken and then allows one to listen, think, move, speak, disagree, cajole, encourage, plan, share, and more—respectfully. Respect for values, customs, language, education, economic, age, and gender diversity are essential to the application of sociocultural competence to PPC. R-E-S-P-E-C-T, Respect. To get it you've got to give it. It is the essence of effective PPC.

Preparation in Environment, Body, and Mind

If the patient feels valued from the moment of entry into the encounter environment, that feeling will enhance the subsequent face-to-face communication. If the wait is long, the staff abrupt, or the waiting area less than serene, the effect on PPC may be negative. Even the face-to-face communication process begins before any words are spoken.[36] Do you place a big desk between you and your patient, or talk across the corner of a small table, or sit on the floor with a child?

Nonverbal cues such as dress, demeanor, grooming, and touch are extremely important. The first impressions of doctor and patient alike will influence the rest of the discussion in a more powerful way than might ordinarily be appreciated.[37]

The prime factor in selection of dress should be meeting the patient's needs. In support of earlier and (still continuing)

patients' need to place the doctor at a higher level, long white coats, white shirts, ties, and the like are required. Open shirts and casual attire help to establish a peer-based PPC. An active patient-oriented choice on the part of the provider is required for best PPC. When it comes to grooming and cleanliness, there is no choice. Bad grooming and lack of cleanliness are always negative.

When possible and appropriate, some type of tactile contact can be useful in setting the tone for a verbal communication (**Box 15–2**). First, the doctor must quickly establish the limits of any touch that is to be extended to the patient, based on a sociocultural awareness and nonverbal cues

In Western cultures, an offered handshake is often worth a try, even with children. If nonverbal cues of fear or distance are perceived or suspected, the touch communication will have to wait or be avoided altogether.

Listening

From the physician's standpoint, listening is the next step.[38] In order to listen, the patient must be talking; for the patient to be talking, the patient has to be motivated. Both doctor and patient will need to listen carefully to what the other person is saying in order to find out what communication channels will be open. The best approach is to establish some simple communication at the level of, "How are things," or "How is your day going?" Sometimes, a physician can initiate patient verbalization by simply waiting or making a welcoming gesture that

Box 15–2 Touch and More

A patient reports, "We have been building our relationship for more than 15 years. I've had a lot of medical problems: a broken hip, a blood clot, bypass surgery, shingles. When my doctor comes into the room he always breaks the ice by greeting me and giving me a light touch. He asks how I am doing and is interested in who I am as a person. He'll take my hand and say, "We're going to take care of this." He has given me his home number because he knows I won't abuse it. He shares things with me about his interests and his life. I don't feel like a number or a co-pay. I get more than just a prescription and a bill. He treats me as he would treat his own mother.

I have a lot of faith in my doctor. Why can't all doctors have that level of compassion for their patients? Don't they learn that in medical school?"

Source: American Academy of Family Physicians. http://www.aafp.org/afp/20080515/closeups.html

seems to say, "What can you tell me?" Much is to be gained by not forcing a particular direction or focus on the conversation. Sometimes a nonmedical question is needed to break the ice, as in **Box 15–3**.

It is often useful to say to a patient, "What was going on *before* all of this started?" to focus on the possibly related events leading up to the onset of symptoms.

Story

Once a health encounter is initiated, and one has obtained some sense of the levels (spoken, unspoken, unconscious) on which the patient is communicating, the next step is to obtain the story. The value of the narrative in health communication has been the subject of considerable interest.[39,40] Indeed, the illumination of narrative is what we seek. How did it all start? What was the context? What happened next? Then what? After that? Now? Feelings? Fears? However, the narrative in actual practice is usually disjointed, delayed, confused, and difficult to obtain. Typically, the patient cannot tell you the story of his or her problem in one pass with any of the clarity that you would like. So, you have to work with various bits and pieces through the entire encounter, which may be an hour or so, letting the details drift in before a coherent narrative can be formulated.

Box 15–3 "How 'Bout Them Phillies!"

Consider, at an appropriate point, taking a moment with your patient. Make yourself ask an unscripted question: "Where did you grow up?" Or: "What made you move to Boston?" Even: "Did you watch last night's Red Sox game?" You don't have to come up with a deep or important question, just one that lets you make a human connection. Some people won't be interested in making that connection. They'll just want you to look at the lump. That's Okay. In that case, look at the lump. Do your job. You will find, however, that many respond because they are polite, or friendly, or perhaps in need of human contact. When this happens, try seeing if you can keep the conversation going for more than two sentences.

If the patient comes in and asks, "I want you to take a look at this bump," you may well do so, but add, "How are things going otherwise?" This focuses on the patient's needs but also allows for useful information to arrive from sources yet unknown.

Source: Gawande A. *Better.* New York: Metropolitan Books, Henry Holt and Company, 2007, p. 151.

It may be difficult for a patient to stay in focus. Patients arrive with a bewildering array of symptoms and complaints, supplemented with a list of doctor's visits and medications. While all of these things are important, it is sometimes (that is to say, almost always) useful to focus on the narrative or story of the illness, if indeed diagnosis is one of the goals of the encounter.

A useful approach, developed in the 1950s by Carl Rodgers,[41] involves the use of nondirective statements whenever possible, rather than asking questions. How does one get information if no questions are asked? One way to get the patient talking is through a simple statement such as, "Tell me about it," or "Tell me more." Then as the patient begins to talk, brief, affirmative, repetitive, or conjunctive statements ("OK . . .," "you felt weak . . .," "and . . .") can be used to maintain the flow. When a patient says something dramatic, a silent response may allow the patient to develop the drama in terms that he or she understands better than you.

The patient's idea of narrative may be less useful than desired. For example, the patient may see the story of his or her illness as a series of doctor's visits, tests, test results, and treatments prescribed. From a medical standpoint—and a socialcultural standpoint—we look for something else; we look for what is going on within the patient more than what has been done to the patient. It is often useful to say to the patient, "It would help to hear more about you and your symptoms than about your previous medical opinions and treatments." This is often a difficult point to get across but an important one if the underlying story of the disease and the person is to be developed coherently.

With a focus on the patient symptoms and feelings (rather than diagnoses and treatments), the details of the patient's personal life are presented along with disease symptoms and provide a broader understanding of the illness (the individual's response to disease) to be diagnosed and treated. This is **patient-centered health communication.**[42–45]

During this time and during subsequent encounters, emphasis should be placed on patient verbalization. Quantitative studies of doctor–patient communication indicate that some doctors are talking 70% while patients are speaking 30% of the time or less. Patients ordinarily view these interactions as unrewarding.[46–48] It is first goal of the provider to encourage patient verbalization before turning to a list of need-to-know questions.

This next step may be called the "interrogative step," at which point one begins to ask specific details about symptoms, treatments, circumstances, medications, and responses and beyond. At the same time, the patient's background needs to be filled in; we need to know about their local and extended family. We need to know about their work circumstance, which may be directly related to the disorder for which the patient is seeking help.

Physicians are taught that the **past medical history (PMH)** and the review of symptoms (ROS) are crucial features of the medical history. However, specific questions about

PMH and ROS need to be delayed until the most of the story has been told to avoid biasing or even obliterating the crucial story of the patient and the illness.

Toward the end of a successful health encounter, the patient and physician are beginning to develop a mutual understanding of the story of the illness and can start to formulate plans for the next step in health care. But before that step can be taken, the provider will widen his or her scope to look for important information that may have been left out or inappropriately included. It is at this point where the symptom checklist that is often given in the waiting room may be usefully reviewed, but not before.

Expert communicators will develop a sense of timing and patience in obtaining information from a patient about his or her disease or life. Often, specific or sensitive questions about medical history and symptoms can be usefully delayed, even until the time of physical examination. In any case, simple questions are often of more value than complex questions, leading questions, or questions containing medical jargon.

Physical Examination

If this is a medical visit for a new patient, then a physical examination needs to take place. However, the history taking and the story telling does not stop, but is rather is stimulated by the examination itself. As one examines the eyes, ears, nose, throat, chest, abdomen, legs, and beyond, regional questions or comments can elicit information relevant to the "story."

To prevent the examination from interfering with interpersonal communication and actually enhance it, it is important to begin an examination with nonthreatening behavior. The inexperienced doctor who immediately takes out an ophthalmoscope and shines its bright light directly in the eye of the patient knows that it is important to look at someone's eyes but is not aware of the fear that can be induced from having such a bright and sharp object an inch from one's eye.

Perhaps the best way to begin a physical examination is to take patients' hands and gently raise both arms to a forward extended position and ask that the position be maintained. This allows an initial touch, which can be comforting and reassuring, and also allows the physician to gauge any weakness or instability or inability to follow directions on the part of the patient. This tactile contact can be used as part of the overall PPC as well as the in the systematic physical examination.

Progressive Dialogue

During a doctor–patient visit, a progressive dialogue develops that is second in importance only to the story itself. As information is shared, symptoms, causes, and needs are clarified. A mutual momentum and motivation are established, leading to goals that are shared rather than imposed. An effective progressive dialogue makes the process of later planning, encouragement, or persuasion much easier.

Review and Summation

All the work (and fun!) of PPC culminates in the explicit summation of what has been learned, what is to be done, and how to go about it. Sometimes, it helps to say just that, "Let's sum up where we are and what we need to do." The summation process is facilitated by keeping key steps in mind:

- Inform.
- Teach-back.
- Support.
- Comfort.

The provider provides information, opinions, and plans based on everything learned in the encounter, choosing words that are *informed* by what has been learned during the encounter about the language, sociocultural background, and goals of the patient. Then the patient is asked to say what he or she understands to have been said. This is the crucial **teach-back** (see Chapter 7, Box 7–2). These steps are iterated as necessary to enhance mutual understanding at best, or at worst to lead to the recognition that communication is incomplete.

In either case, the provider gives *support* for the patient and the patient's point of view, and avoids recrimination for any failures to communication or understanding. In every case, the patient must leave with the feeling that "The doctor understands me." When the provider has gained some understanding and when this is associated with unfeigned empathy, a patient begins to feel comforted. Patient *comfort* is always a goal in itself but is also an aid in producing behavior change, adherence to treatment program, or acceptance of unachievable goals for the individual patient.

SPECIAL CASES

Language Barriers

Of all the sociocultural barriers to PPC, language is the most obvious. Language barriers can be due to a patient's age, disease, emotional factors, education, or simply not speaking the language of the provider. It is the responsibility of the provider to find the best means of communication, using patience, words, gestures, and/or an interpreter.[49,50] A few shared words of a common language can enhance trust and respect and perhaps even communication.

The use of an interpreter deserves special mention because additional elements of uncertainty are added by the translation. Is the interpreter translating exactly? Can the words even be translated? Is the interpreter adding a personal bias to the translation? Most often, a family member serves as an *ad hoc* interpreter. Lack of training and family biases can obscure or alter the patient's needs and symptoms as well as the provider's intentions and opinions. In the case of recent immigrants, their children often end up as interpreters. This may prevent a patient from expressing feelings or problems that they consider inappropriate for their child's ears.

The best interpreters translate accurately without adding or removing words or phrases (see **Box 15–4**). Only if they know the culture as well as the language they are translating are supplementary comments on the cultural significance of words or body language appropriate.

Patient and provider alike should be alert for signs of inappropriate translation. If several sentences of speech are translated by, "She says No," then you can be sure that you have missed the flavor of that negative response and know to be alert for other mismatches.

Informed Consent

An extensive literature has developed concerning **informed consent**—obtaining the permission, or consent, of a patient or guardian before performing a medical procedure or service. How much information for informed consent is enough? How much information is too much? Often, the answer to these questions can be found in the early and progressive understanding of the patient's needs and goals. Then tailoring of information to the patient's understanding, attention, and language can be most successful. In fact, consent forms are not tailored but prepared ahead of time in order to obtain institutional approval. Such consent forms are often too long, covering all the

---

Box 15–4 Using an Interpreter

Medical interpretation is a two-way process. The interpreter must understand not only the culture and language of the patient but also that of the provider. This is why experts agree that asking family members to interpret should be avoided. "What if the relative does not know medical terminology and the doctor says appendicitis?" says Dharma E. Cortés, PhD, who trains medical interpreters at Cambridge College. "You don't know how the family member is translating that to the patient. If a child is interpreting for a parent, the child may be experiencing an undue emotional burden as he learns more about his parent's health in the process of translating the conversation between his parent and the doctor. Also, a parent may not disclose information relevant to his/her medical condition because he/she may not want his/her child to know about it."

Source: Dharma E Cortés, personal communication, January 22, 2010.

---

possible medical and legal aspects. While these documents are necessary to protect the patient (and the physician), they require unhurried explanation to avoid serious misunderstanding or non-acceptance on the part of the patient.

If progressive dialogue is important in all patient–provider encounters, it is of paramount in obtaining informed consent. In this situation as in perhaps in no other, the presence of a third party, a patient advocate in the room, can be of value. Obtaining informed consent requires a high level of both clinical and communication skills to be successful. This is not a task to be delegated to the unaccompanied student, trainee, or intern. The provider must be willing to evaluate the consent form paragraph by paragraph, providing excellent explanation where necessary and an explanation of options at all times. This is always easier if the provider is known to the patient and has already established a working level of mutual communication.

The Dying Patient

The counseling of a dying patient causes concern to arise at the individual, family, social, cultural, religious, and political levels. Witness the intense political debate in Congress in 2009 when a new health program was to contain provisions for financial support for counseling of the dying patient. The dispute is based on the potential for conflicting goals of the dying patient and those of other "interested" parties. How much should the government say about how we choose to die? How much influence should the doctor or family have on the patient's exit?

While it is easy to support the supremacy of the patient's own wishes, it is also impossible to ignore the societal pressures that bear on such decision. No one prescription can be given to navigate this potentially treacherous path.[51–57] Perhaps the most useful path would be a return to the PPC encounter process. The patient's story remains central. The patient's needs and goals at spoken, unspoken, and unconscious levels are clarified. Third-party interests are addressed. Mutual understanding is sought. Then final decisions are made, based on the patient's interests, within the constraints of local, legal, and sociocultural limits.

PROSPECTS

As discussed earlier, recent decades have seen a progressive increase in the role of nonphysician healthcare providers in PPC. Part of this results from a reduction of PPC by physicians because of diminishing time and increasing technical needs of the medical diagnostic and therapeutic process. It is not just the external constraints. Physicians in the past had little specific training in communication. They learned by observing their elders: some were good communicators and some were not. The past social climate allowed physicians to be less than good communicators if their medical skills were exemplary.

Things have changed. We have expectations for our physicians at all levels now, and expectations that cannot really be met. Doctors still do not have enough time to see patients. The amount of information that a doctor is required to know is beyond the capacity of most physicians and specialists unless their focus is in a very narrow field. This means that even specialist physicians are becoming more and more like general practitioners. This is, in part, because of the sobering impossibility of a complete knowledge of medical science for generalist and specialists alike. In this setting, the importance of communication and cultural skills looms larger and larger.[28]

As a by-product, other clinicians, especially nurse practitioners and physician assistants, are playing an increased role and gaining parity with physicians in promoting good health and health communication. The burdens and opportunities of interpersonal healthcare communication will be increasingly shared among health profession from a variety of backgrounds. All are joined by the idea of developing of mutual two-way PPC that facilitates diagnosis, treatment, and long-term health care for individuals and the communities at large.

A concept that combines several aspects of health information and health communication into a potentially viable working model is that of the **patient-centered medical home (PCMH)** as described in **Box 15–5.** Whole-person, patient-centered PPC is essential to the concept.

Box 15–5 Patient-Centered Medical Home

The PCMH is a patient-centered healthcare setting that facilitates partnerships among individual patients and their personal physicians, and, when appropriate, the patient's family.

PRINCIPLES

Personal physician: Each patient has an ongoing relationship with a personal physician trained to provide first contact, and continuous and comprehensive care.

Physician-directed medical practice: The personal physician leads a team of individuals at the practice level who collectively take responsibility for the ongoing care of patients.

Whole-person orientation: The personal physician is responsible for providing for all the patient's healthcare needs or taking responsibility for appropriately arranging care with other qualified professionals. This includes care for all stages of life: acute care, chronic care, preventive services, and end-of-life care.

Care is coordinated and/or integrated across all elements of the complex healthcare system (e.g., subspecialty care, hospitals, home health agencies, nursing homes) and the patient's community (e.g., family, public and private community-based services). Care is facilitated by registries, information technology, health information exchange, and other means to ensure that patients get the indicated care when and where they need and want it in a culturally and linguistically appropriate manner.

Quality and safety are hallmarks of the medical home:

- Practices advocate for their patients to support the attainment of optimal, patient-centered outcomes that are defined by a care planning process driven by a compassionate, robust partnership among physicians, patients, and the patient's family.
- Evidence-based medicine and clinical decision-support tools guide decision making.
- Physicians in the practice accept accountability for continuous quality improvement through voluntary engagement in performance measurement and improvement.
- Patients actively participate in decision-making, and feedback is sought to ensure patients' expectations are being met.
- Information technology is utilized appropriately to support optimal patient care, performance measurement, patient education, and enhanced communication.
- Practices go through a voluntary recognition process by an appropriate nongovernmental entity to demonstrate that they have the capabilities to provide patient-centered services consistent with the medical home model.
- Patients and families participate in quality improvement activities at the practice level.

Enhanced access to care is available through systems such as open scheduling, expanded hours, and new options for communication among patients, their personal physician, and practice staff.

Payment appropriately recognizes the added value provided to patients who have a patient-centered medical home.

Source: Patient-Centered Primary Care Collaborative. http://pcpcc.net/content/joint-principles-patient-centered-medical-home

Opportunities and challenges occur on the patient side as well. Given the rise in complexity of health care and healthcare communication, patients need to be active participants in PPC, not just passive receivers. The PPC process needs all the help it can get! As an example, The Ask Me 3™ program encourages active self-advocacy for patients (**Box 15–6**).

Many patients are now informed health seekers whose search of the Internet offers a panoply of options. The burden of too much information is real. One may read about a disease one week and as a result develop the symptoms the next. We are suggestible as a species. The need for restraint and judgment before jumping to medical conclusions is greatly needed. Restraint can be developed, but judgment can only be realized by a broad clinical training in symptom analysis and the spec-

trum of underlying disease. Still, for all its problematic features, the Internet does provide a remarkable source of medical information that reduces the chance that important aspects of health and disease will go unconsidered. PPC partners with mediated (media-based) health communication to provide overall motivation toward the improved future health of the community.

The rapid influx of non-English-speaking groups into the United States provides a good example for a need of cross-cultural training at all levels of healthcare interaction. Patients and providers who misunderstand even the simplest of words and bring disparate cultural background to PPC represent a challenge not easily met. The first step toward meeting this challenge is to recognize and address cultural differences before jumping to conclusions about understanding, diagnosis, or intervention.

CONCLUSION

This chapter develops a conceptual framework for patient–provider communication (PPC); emphasizes the multifaceted, bidirectional nature of PPC; and outlines the steps toward more effective PPC. The most important concepts to take away are (1) the PPC framework, (2) the respect for the PPC process and its participants, (3) the need to care and learn how the patient communicates, (4) the value of listening and silence in communication, (5) the power of story to inform, (6) the humility to put the patient first, and (7) the satisfaction of making it all work. If you are motivated by these ideas, then you already have within your grasp the opportunity to dramatically improve health and the healthcare experience, one life at a time.

KEY TERMS

Informed consent
Past medical history (PMH)
Patient-centered health communication
Patient-centered medical home (PCMH)
Patient–provider communication (PPC)
Sociocultural competence
Teach-back

Box 15–6 Ask Me 3™

Ask Me 3 is a patient education program designed to promote communication between healthcare providers and patients in order to improve health outcomes. The program encourages patients to understand the answers to three questions:

1. What is my main problem?
2. What do I need to do?
3. Why is it important for me to do this?

Patients should be encouraged to ask their providers (doctors, nurses, pharmacists, therapists) these three simple but essential questions in every healthcare interaction. Likewise, providers should always encourage their patients to understand the answers to these three questions.

Studies show that people who understand health instructions make fewer mistakes when they take their medicine or prepare for a medical procedure. They may also get well sooner or be able to better manage a chronic health condition.

Source: Partnership for Clear Health Communication at the National Patient Safety Foundation. http://www.npsf.org/askme3/

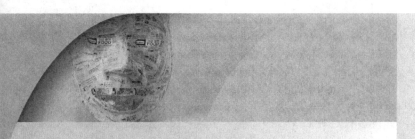

Chapter Questions

1. What are the three main levels of patient–provider communication interaction?

2. Name three ways of facilitating verbal communication with the patient.

3. How would the approach to patient–provider communication described in this chapter apply to a health communication trainee delivering door-to-door surveys on obesity in the inner city?

4. Could the suggestions to providers for improved communication given in the chapter also be used by patients? If so, how?

ADDITIONAL RESOURCES

Here is a list of references and resources that address the extensive literature relating to PPC. The specifics of application to different settings are interesting and rewarding to appreciate.

- Doctor–patient communication has a real impact on health. *Science Daily.* April 10, 2007. http://www.science daily.com/releases/2007/04/070409144754.htm
- Doctor–patient communication: When things go wrong. *Medical College of Wisconsin HealthLink.* http://health link.mcw.edu/article/1031002495.html
- Hicks R. Doctor–patient communication. *BBC Health.* February 2007. http://www.bbc.co.uk/health/talking_to_ your_doctor/gp_communication.shtml
- Houghton A, Allen J. Understanding personality type: Doctor–patient communication. *BMJ Career Focus.* 2005; 330:36-37. http://careerfocus.bmj.com/cgi/content/full/ 330/7484/36
- Ong LM, de Haes JC, Hoos AM, Lammes FB. Doctor–patient communication: A review of the literature. *Soc Sci Med.* 1995;40(7):903–918.
- Teutsch C. Patient–doctor communication. *Med Clin North Am.* 2003;87(5):1115–1145.
- University of Pittsburgh Institute for Doctor-Patient Communication. http://www.dgim.pitt.edu/idpc
- Mutha S, Allen C, Welch M. *Toward Culturally Competent Care: A Toolbox for Teaching Communication Strategies.* San Francisco: Center for the Health Professions, University of California, San Francisco; 2002. 186 pages.

REFERENCES

1. Fritz PA, Kent State University. Television Center. *Doctor, Patient Communications.* 1981.
2. Charney E. Patient–doctor communication. Implications for the clinician. *Pediatr Clin North Am.* 1972;19(2):263–279.
3. Ziegler JL. *Ethical Dilemmas in the doctor–Patient Relationship.* Lexington, VA: Washington and Lee University; 1976.
4. Hasler J, Pendleton D. *Doctor–Patient Communication.* London; New York: Academic Press; 1983.
5. Reiser DE, Rosen DH. *The Doctor–Patient Relationship.* Baltimore: University Park Press; 1984.
6. Purtilo, R. and Haddad. A. *Health Professional and Patient Interaction,* 7th ed. St. Louis: Saunders Elsevier; 2007.
7. O'Toole G. *Communication: Core Interpersonal Skills for Health Professionals.* Philadelphia: Churchill Livingstone; 2009.
8. Adler RB, Rosenfeld LB, Proctor RF II. *Interplay: The Process of Interpersonal Communication.* New York: Oxford University Press; 2009.
9. Beebe SA, Beebe SJ, Redmond MyCommunicationLab MV. *Interpersonal Communication: Relating to Others,* 6th ed. Boston: Allyn & Bacon, Series; 2010.
10. DeVito JA. *Interpersonal Messages: Communication and Relationship,* 2nd ed. Boston: Allyn & Bacon, MyCommunicationKit Series; 2010.
11. Baxter LA, Braithwaite DO (Eds.). *Engaging theories in interpersonal communication.* Thousand Oaks, CA: Sage; 2008.

12. Monaghan L, Goodman J. *A Cultural Approach to Interpersonal Communication: Essential Readings.* Malden, MA:Wiley-Blackwell; 2007.
13. Lustig MW, Koester J. *Intercultural Competence: Interpersonal Communication Across Cultures,* 6th ed. Sudbury, MA: Allyn & Bacon; 2009.
14. Knapp ML, Daly JC. *Interpersonal Communication.* Thousand Oaks, CA: Sage, Sage Benchmarks in Communication; 2010.
15. Trenholm S, Jensen A. *Interpersonal Communication.* New York: Oxford University Press; 2007.
16. Verderber KS, Verderber RF, Berryman-Fink C. Inter-Act: *Interpersonal Communication Concepts, Skills, and Contexts.* New York: Oxford University Press; 2006.
17. Kalbfleisch PJ, Cody MJ. *Gender, Power, and Communication in Human Relationships.* Hillsdale, NJ: Erlbaum; 1995.
18. Blanch DC, Hall JA, Roter DL, Frankel RM. Medical student gender and issues of confidence. *Patient Educ Couns.* 2008;72(3):374–381.
19. Hall JA, Irish JT, Roter DL, Ehrlich CM, Miller LH. Satisfaction, gender, and communication in medical visits. *Med Care.* 1994;32(12):1216–1231.
20. Hall JA, Irish JT, Roter DL, Ehrlich CM, Miller LH. Gender in medical encounters: An analysis of physician and patient communication in a primary care setting. *Health Psychol.* 1994;13(5):384–392.
21. Hall JA, Roter DL. Do patients talk differently to male and female physicians? A meta-analytic review. *Patient Educ Couns.* 2002;48(3):217–224.
22. Hall JA, Roter DL, Katz NR. Meta-analysis of correlates of provider behavior in medical encounters. *Med Care.* 1988;26(7):657–675.
23. Roter D, Lipkin M,Jr, Korsgaard A. Sex differences in patients' and physicians' communication during primary care medical visits. *Med Care.* 1991;29(11):1083–1093.
24. Roter DL, Hall JA. Physician gender and patient-centered communication: A critical review of empirical research. *Ann. Rev Public Health.* 2004; 25:497–519.
25. Roter DL, Hall JA. How physician gender shapes the communication and evaluation of medical care. *Mayo Clin Proc.* 2001;76(7):673–676.
26. Power GR, Asymmetry and Decision-Making in Medical Encounters. In: R. Gwyn *Communicating Health and Illness.* London: Sage Publications; 2002.
27. Lloyd M, Bor R. *Communication Skills for Medicine,* 3rd ed. Edinburgh; New York: Churchill Livingstone/Elsevier; 2009.
28. Patak L, Wilson-Stronks A, Costello J, et al. Improving patient-provider communication: A call to action. *J Nurs Adm.* 2009;39(9):372–376.
29. Wright KB, Sparks L, O'Hair D. *Health Communication in the 21st Century.* Malden, MA: Blackwell Publications; 2008.
30. Bergmo TS, Kummervold PE, Gammon D, Dahl LB. Electronic patient-provider communication: Will it offset office visits and telephone consultations in primary care? *Int J Med Inform.* 2005;74(9):705–710.
31. Wissow L. Assessing socio-economic differences in patient-provider communication. *Patient Educ Couns.* 2005;56(2):137–138.
32. Ngo-Metzger Q, Telfair J, Sorkin DH, et al. *Cultural Competency and Quality of Care.* The Commonwealth Fund; vol 39, October, 2006.
33. Stewart J, Zediker KE, Witteborn S. *Together: Communicating Interpersonally: A Social Construction Approach.* New York: Oxford University Press; 2004.
34. Nápoles-Springer A, Pérez-Stable EJ. The role of culture and language in determining best practices. *J Gen Intern Med.* 2001;16(7):493–495.
35. Spencer-Oatey H. *Culturally Speaking: Managing Rapport through Talk Across Cultures.* London; New York: Continuum; 2000.
36. Philippot P, Feldman RS, Coats EJ. *Nonverbal Behavior in Clinical Settings.* New York: Oxford University Press; 2003.
37. Amer A, Fischer H. "Don't call me 'mom'": How parents want to be greeted by their pediatrician. *Clin Pediatr (Phila).* 2009;48(7):720–722.
38. Hart V. *Patient–Provider Communications: Caring to Listen.* Sudbury, MA: Jones and Bartlett; 2010.
39. Gwyn R. *Narrative and the Voicing of Illness.* Thousand Oaks, CA: Sage Publications; 2002:139.

40. Hinyard LJ, Kreuter MW. Using narrative communication as a tool for health behavior change: A conceptual, theoretical, and empirical overview. *Health Educ Behav.* 2007;34(5):777–792.

41. Rogers CR. *Client-Centered Counselling.* Boston: Houghton-Mifflin; 1951.

42. Wilson EV. *Patient-Centered e-Health.* Hershey PA: Medical Information Science Reference; 2009.

43. Chapman BP, Duberstein PR, Epstein R, Fiscella K, Kravitz RL. Patient centered communication during primary care visits for depressive symptoms: What is the role of physician personality? *Med Care.* 2008;46(8):806–812.

44. Keselman A, Logan R, Smith CA, Leroy G, Zeng-Treitler Q. Developing informatics tools and strategies for consumer-centered health communication. *J Am Med Inform Assoc.* 2008;15(4):473–483.

45. Stewart A. *Patient-Centered Medicine—Transforming the Clinical Method,* 7th ed. Thousand Oaks, CA: Sage Publications; 1995.

46. Ellington L, Roter D, Dudley WN, et al. Communication analysis of BRCA1 genetic counseling. *J Genet Couns.* 2005;14(5):377–386.

47. Roter D, Larson S. The roter interaction analysis system (RIAS): Utility and flexibility for analysis of medical interactions. *Patient Educ Couns.* 2002; 46(4):243–251.

48. Roter DL, Hall JA. Studies of doctor-patient interaction. *Ann Rev Public Health.* 1989;10:163–180.

49. Aranguri C, Davidson B, Ramirez R. Patterns of communication through interpreters: A detailed sociolinguistic analysis. *J Gen Intern Med.* 2006;21(6):623–629.

50. Hudelson P. Improving patient-provider communication: Insights from interpreters. *Fam Pract.* 2005;22(3):311–316.

51. Hunt LM, de Voogd KB. Are good intentions good enough? Informed consent without trained interpreters. *J Gen Intern Med.* 2007;22(5):598–605.

52. Mayer GG, Villaire M. *Health Literacy in Primary Care: A Clinician's Guide.* New York: Springer Publications; 2007.

53. Curtis JR, Patrick DL, Caldwell E, Greenlee H, Collier AC. The quality of patient–doctor communication about end-of-life care: A study of patients with advanced AIDS and their primary care clinicians. *AIDS.* 1999;13(9): 1123–1131.

54. Mack JW, Hilden JM, Watterson J, et al. Parent and physician perspectives on quality of care at the end of life in children with cancer. *J Clin Oncol.* 2005;23(36):9155–9161.

55. Yedidia MJ. Transforming doctor–patient relationships to promote patient-centered care: Lessons from palliative care. *J Pain Symptom Manage.* 2007;33(1):40–57.

56. Formiga F, Chivite D, Ortega C, Casas S, Ramon JM, Pujol R. End-of-life preferences in elderly patients admitted for heart failure. *QJM.* 2004;97(12): 803–808.

57. Barnard D, Quill T, Hafferty FW, et al. Preparing the ground: Contributions of the preclinical years to medical education for care near the end of life. Working group on the pre-clinical years of the national consensus conference on medical education for care near the end of life. *Acad Med.* 1999;74(5):499–505.

Risk and Emergency Risk Communication: A Primer

David W. Cragin and Claudia Parvanta

LEARNING OBJECTIVES

By the end of this chapter, the reader will be able to:

- Define the difference between risk and emergency risk communication and know the challenges of both.
- Define risk assessment terms used by the Environmental Protection Agency.
- Use Hill's criteria to evaluate causality.
- Describe processes to undertake before, during, and after a public health emergency.
- Apply key theories to crafting emergency risk messages.
- Use tools for organizing a communication response:
  - An emergency communication plan.
  - Message maps.
  - Q&A techniques.
- Understand factors that affect how the public responds during an emergency.
- Follow basic guidance for presenting emergency risk communication to the public.

INTRODUCTION

Those of us working in the Office of Communication at the CDC were as shocked as the rest of the world on September 11, 2001. The campus was evacuated, and I (CFP) remember sitting in my car, stuck in the parking lot for about an hour, wondering if Atlanta was to be a target. What I didn't know that day, and of course, none of us did, was that we were about to become the "*Emergency* Health Communication Office" for the next four years or so. It was barely a month later when my boss, Vicki Freimuth, who held the senior communication position at the CDC, received a phone call telling her that a man working at American Media Inc. in Florida had been di-

agnosed with a *probable* case of anthrax disease. I was sitting in her office at the time and didn't understand the significance of that information. But we were about to learn much more than we ever wanted to know about anthrax—and about emergency risk communication on a national and international scale.

The CDC's communication experience with anthrax has been published.[1] It transformed the agency in terms of what and how the CDC communicated with many different audiences, not the least of which, the public. By 2003, the CDC also had communicated about severe acute respiratory syndrome (SARS) and received the following vote of approval from an independent CDC critic:

> Director Julie Gerberding of the U.S. Centers for Disease Control and Prevention is a master at not over-reassuring us, at helping us hold onto good news while worrying about bad news, at acknowledging uncertainty. Her frequent SARS "telebriefings" for journalists have been the most consistently good SARS risk communication we've seen.[2]

The CDC had to change quickly from an agency that rarely spoke directly to the public, (preferring instead to work through state and local intermediaries) to one frequently on the nightly news. Its whole view of preparing materials for the public also changed from epidemiologists resisting having to "dumb it down," to understanding their roles as "subject matter experts (SMEs)" teamed up with communication and health literacy professionals. The "docs" also learned that when conducting investigations, people considered them to be "healthcare providers," and they upgraded their interpersonal communication skills accordingly (see Chapter 15).

In between anthrax and SARS, the CDC spent considerable time managing a "first responder/healthcare provider" smallpox vaccination program, which required an enormous investment in communication to various audiences. Shortly after, the CDC began its preparations for pandemic flu, as well as preparing strategies and materials for terrorist-induced or naturally caused public health emergencies. These prevention efforts were mirrored around the country through grants made to state, local, territorial, and tribal health departments[*] and preparedness centers (academic partners).[†] As of this writing, the ability of communication officers working in health departments to mount a coordinated response for most emergencies should be excellent.[‡]

In 2001, the scientists and program managers working in the CDC's sister agency, the Agency for Toxic Substances and Disease Registry (ATSDR), as well as those in several divisions of the National Center for Environmental Health of the CDC, had much more experience in speaking to an often angry, and always worried, public. Their work in investigating environmental hazards (e.g., explaining the complexity of risks associated with building over the site of an old thermometer factory or living "down wind" from a nuclear reactor) provided a valuable blueprint from which the CDC built its communication response. Some of the experts who had long advised the private sector in environmental crisis communication, such as Peter Sandman, quoted earlier, and Vince Covello,[§] became the CDC's new gurus for what became known as **emergency risk communication (ERC).** It is not possible to disentangle the contributions of these experts, or their colleagues, such as Baruch Fischoff[ǁ] at Carnegie Mellon, or Paul Slovic[¶] at the University of Oregon, from what became the CDC's approach to emergency risk communication.

Following the same learning progression, we will discuss normal risk communication first, followed by emergency risk communication (ERC). Both provide information to people so that they may protect themselves. Risk communication (RC) can be done quietly by a toxicologist, a healthcare provider, or with an online program; ERC adds crisis proportions and speed to the challenge.

A BASIC RISK FRAMEWORK[#]

Most health risk discussions concern **causality,** "Does A (thing) cause B (disease)," or **risk,** "If you are exposed to A, what is your likelihood of suffering disease B." The Environmental Protection Agency (EPA) has developed a framework for distinguishing between hazard and risk, and exposure and toxicity, as shown in **Box 16–1.**

The distinctions in Box 16–1 are important. Toxicity is innate to the substance, whereas hazard, risk, and exposure are situation specific. For example, lead is toxic, but brief exposure to a block of lead is not hazardous and presents a very low health risk. On the other hand, prolonged exposure to very fine, absorbable particles of lead is very hazardous and presents a high risk of poisoning. A small amount of ethanol dissolved in water presents no fire hazard, whereas pure ethanol is highly flammable.

Many in risk assessment use the criteria developed by Hill, discussed in Chapter 4. Hill developed these while trying to demonstrate the causal association between tobacco and a specific disease.[3] Hill himself said, "None of my nine viewpoints can bring indisputable evidence for or against the cause-and-effect hypothesis and none can be required *sine qua non.*" With that disclaimer, the more of these criteria that are satisfied in a particular event, the stronger the likelihood of causation. (Refer back to Table 4–2.)

[#]Most of this section prepared by David Cragin.

Box 16–1 EPA Framework for Risk

Useful definitions:

Hazard—*Qualitative* likelihood of an adverse event occurring under a specific set of conditions. Generally, hazard = danger.

Risk—*Quantitative* likelihood of an adverse event occurring under a specific set of conditions. Risk is a function of probability.

Exposure—Contact with a chemical or physical agent by a person or animal.

Toxicity—the intrinsic ability of a substance to cause adverse health effects.

Source: *U.S. Environmental Protection Agency's Risk Assessment Guidance for Superfund (RAGS).* Washington, DC: Environmental Protection Agency; 1989.

---

[*]http://emergency.cdc.gov/cotper/coopagreement/10/FinalPHEP_BP10_Guidance_508%20Version.pdf.
[†]http://emergency.cdc.gov/cotper/cphp/centers.asp.
[‡]As measured against these performance measures, http://emergency.cdc.gov/cotper/coopagreement/09/pdf/performance_measures_guidance_bp9.pdf.
[§]http://www.centerforriskcommunication.com/staff.htm.
[ǁ]http://sds.hss.cmu.edu/src/faculty/fischhoff.php.
[¶]http://www.decisionresearch.org/people/slovic/.

Now you should have a vocabulary to describe risk, hazards, toxicity, and exposure, as well as likelihood of causality, to other scientists. Later we will present arguments as to why, in some cases, logic and clarity may not trump other techniques when communicating risk to the public. But first it is important to understand the logic underlying a risk assessment and how it is presented.

PRESENTING RISK

It is not always that easy to calculate, much less present, a risk accurately and clearly. **Figure 16–1** shows the procedure used to calculate the risk of dying from various chronic diseases based on smoking status, with **Table 16–1** presenting the results. You will note there are different tables for men and women.

The correct way to interpret Table 16–1 is to say something like, "People who share these traits, and are in other ways similar, collectively carry this risk. Out of 1,000, *N* are predicted to die from this disease in this age group over a 10-year period." That's a pretty complicated statement, and people want to know what "their" risk is. Of course, their individual risk is unknown. But, the typical way of interpreting this table is to say a 50-year-old man has about a 1% chance of dying from heart disease if he never smoked and a 3% chance of dying from heart disease if he currently does. When all the diseases in the table are combined, the 50-year-old male smoker

has a 13% chance of dying compared to the 5% chance carried by the man who never smoked. While 13 compared to 5 is nearly a three-fold increase in risk, some people would shrug this off. Ironically, they might be the same people who would consider a 10% to 15% chance of surviving a complicated operation to be "good," and 5% "not so good." Perception of risk is partially shaped by the positive or negative frame, survival versus death, as mentioned in previous chapters. But, it also has to do with our information processing abilities and the psychology of risk.

How the Public Deals with Risk

As discussed in Chapter 7, the vast majority of people in the United States have never studied statistics, epidemiology, toxicology, nor any of the other scientific disciplines that relate to risk assessment. And, we know that far too many of us have difficulty with a train schedule or with interpreting a food label, let alone a "confidence interval." While a scientist may consider "less than a tenth of one part per million" of a toxic substance in drinking water to be absolutely safe; much of the public will hear this as "millions of parts" of something dangerous contaminating the water. Others hold the mistaken belief that, "If you can't say zero, then it's not safe." So, part of the challenge in risk communication is translating fairly complex statistical concepts into pictures and language that can be broadly understood.

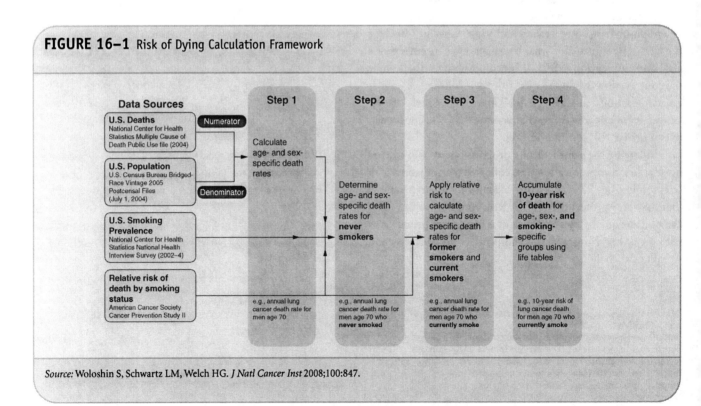

FIGURE 16–1 Risk of Dying Calculation Framework

Source: Woloshin S, Schwartz LM, Welch HG. *J Natl Cancer Inst* 2008;100:847.

TABLE 16–1 Risk of Dying, Multiple Causes, M/W, Smokers and Never Smoked

Risk Chart for Men (Current and Never Smokers)*

Find the line closest to your age and smoking status. The numbers tell you how many of 1,000 men will die in the next 10 years from . . .

		Vascular Disease		Cancer			Infection			Lung Disease	Accidents	All Causes Combined
Age	**Smoking Status**	**Heart Disease**	**Stroke**	**Lung**	**Colon**	**Prostate**	**Pneumonia**	**Flu**	**AIDS**	**COPD**		
35	Never smoker	1	1						2		5	15
	Smoker	**7**	**1**	**1**		**Less than 1 death**			2		5	**42**
40	Never smoker	3	1	1	1				2		6	24
	Smoker	**14**	**2**	**4**	**1**				**2**	**1**	**6**	**62**
45	Never smoker	6	1	1	1				2		6	35
	Smoker	**21**	**3**	**8**	**1**		**1**		**2**	**1**	**6**	**91**
50	Never smoker	11	1	1	2	1	1		1		5	49
	Smoker	**29**	**5**	**18**	**2**	**1**	**1**		**1**	**3**	**5**	**128**
55	Never smoker	19	3	1	3	2	1		1	1	5	71
	Smoker	**41**	**7**	**34**	**3**	**1**	**2**		**1**	**7**	**4**	**178**
60	Never smoker	32	5	2	5	3	2		1	1	5	115
	Smoker	**56**	**11**	**59**	**5**	**3**	**3**		**1**	**16**	**4**	**256**
65	Never smoker	52	9	4	8	6	3			3	6	176
	Smoker	**74**	**16**	**89**	**7**	**6**	**5**			**26**	**5**	**365**
70	Never smoker	87	18	6	10	12	6			5	7	291
	Smoker	**100**	**26**	**113**	**9**	**10**	**9**			**45**	**6**	**511**
75	Never smoker	137	32	8	13	19	11			6	11	449
	Smoker	**140**	**39**	**109**	**11**	**15**	**16**			**60**	**9**	**667**

*A never smoker has smoked fewer than 100 cigarettes in his life and a current smoker has smoked at least 100 cigarettes or more in his life and smokes (any amount) now. The numbers in each row do not add up the chance of dying from all causes combined because there are many other causes of death besides the ones listed here.

TABLE 16–1 Risk of Dying, Multiple Causes, M/W, Smokers and Never Smoked—continued

Risk Chart for Women (Current and Never Smokers)*

Find the line closest to your age and smoking status. The numbers tell you how many of 1,000 women will die in the next 10 years from . . .

Age	Smoking Status	Vascular Disease		Cancer					Infection			Lung Disease	Accidents	All Causes Combined
		Heart Disease	Stroke	Lung Cancer	Breast Cancer	Colon Cancer	Ovarian Cancer	Cervical Cancer	Pneumonia	Flu	AIDS	COPD		
35	Never smoker	1			1						1		2	14
	Smoker	1	1	1	1						1		2	14
40	Never smoker	1			2	1					1		2	19
	Smoker	4	2	4	2						1	1	2	27
45	Never smoker	2	1	1	3	1	1				1		2	25
	Smoker	9	3	7	3	1	1				1	2	2	45
50	Never smoker	4	1	1	4	1	1						2	37
	Smoker	13	5	14	4	1	1					4	2	69
55	Never smoker	8	2	2	6	2	2	1	1			1	2	55
	Smoker	20	6	26	5	2	2	1	1			9	2	110
60	Never smoker	14	4	3	7	3	3	1	1			2	2	84
	Smoker	31	8	41	6	3	3	1	2			18	2	167
65	Never smoker	25	7	5	8	5	4	1	2			3	3	131
	Smoker	45	15	55	7	5	3	1	4			31	3	241
70	Never smoker	46	14	7	9	7	4	1	4			5	4	207
	Smoker	56	25	61	8	6	4	1	7			44	4	335
75	Never smoker	89	30	7	11	10	5	1	8			6	7	335
	Smoker	99	34	58	10	9	4		14			61	7	463

Less than 1 death (for cells in the upper region)

*A never smoker has smoked fewer than 100 cigarettes in her life and a current smoker has smoked at least 100 cigarettes or more in her life and smokes (any amount) now. The numbers in each row do not add up the chance of dying from all causes combined because there are many other causes of death besides the ones listed here.

Source: Woloshin S, Schwartz LM, Welch HG. *J Natl Cancer Inst* 2008;100:849–850.

We have discussed health literacy and numeracy issues adequately in Chapter 7 and in Appendix 7A. You should apply this guidance in all of your risk and emergency risk communication work. For example, you could turn the numbers in Table 16–1 into an icon array or pie chart to help explain the risk to people who had difficulty with computation.

But simplifying language and visual aids are not enough. The psychology of risk provides an added set of rules that apply to both normal risk and emergency risk communication.

The Psychology of Risk Perception

Researchers have been studying **risk perceptions** for decades. As a result, we have a long list of characteristics that are associated with how the public will perceive different kinds of hazards. There are some factors that seem obvious in how they affect a person's perception of risk, such as immediate danger to oneself or one's family. But other factors are not that obvious. See **Table 16–2**.[4]

In a recent review, Fischoff discusses studies using multidimensional scaling techniques to identify factors that position various hazards in people's minds. The most important seem to be "unknown" and "dread," which, Fischoff says, "capture the cognitive and emotional bases of people's concern, respectively. . . .When a third factor (dimension) emerges, it appears to reflect the scope of the threat, labeled *catastrophic potential*."[5] These factors represent the biggest three for risk. Bioterrorism can rank at the very top of all three of these scales.

While these factors clearly influence how the public will generally react to a risk assessment, there is one factor that modifies their perception above all others: their level of trust in the information source. You are often presenting information to people who do not trust you because you work for "the government." Or, sometimes they do trust you for the same reason. Institutional or organizational trust is critical to engaging the public in a frank discussion of the risks associated with a particular hazard. From surveys run during the anthrax attacks, the CDC learned that it, the EPA, and most local health departments stood in good stead with the public, as did personal physicians and clergy. Elected officials (with Rudolph Giuliani post–9/11 as the outstanding exception) and industry spokespersons are generally not seen as credible sources for risk assessments.[6]

PRESENTING A RISK ASSESSMENT
Report Content

Risk assessments in the health field have primarily examined environmental or toxicological risk—that is, the risks of drugs, industrial chemicals, pollutants, food additives, and the like. We will walk through the sections of a typical report from a risk assessment.[7]

If you are assessing a nonenvironmental exposure, then some concepts such as "dose–response" may not be relevant.

1. *Introduction:* Provide an overview of the risk question to give the reader context for the risk assessment. If there are two schools of thought on the issue, discuss them both up-front.
2. *Hazard identification (and possibly benefit identification):* This step identifies the agents(s) of concern (drugs, pesticides, pollutants, etc.) or other factors related to a risk. Hazard identification is the *primary filtering step* in the report. Every risk issue has many facets. Delving into unrelated or unimportant issues will detract from the focus of the report. The hazard identification step identifies only those hazards that are relevant for the risk assessment you are conducting. Hazard identification is a judgment process. (Remember: hazard assessment is a *qualitative process*; risk assessment is a *quantitative process*.)

    For example, if you are examining the potential cardiac benefits of oral aspirin, it does not matter that powdered aspirin can be an eye irritant. In contrast, if you are examining the hazards to workers who manufacture aspirin, the eye irritation potential of aspirin is relevant while the potential for stomach irritation is much less so. Similarly, although the needle used in smallpox vaccination is a "hazard," the hazard it presents is miniscule compared to the risks of smallpox or the vaccination itself. Use the hazard identification step to eliminate insignificant hazards from further consideration.

    A basic concept in risk assessment is that if you protect people from the adverse effect that occurs at the lowest dose, you will protect them from effects that occur at higher doses. Another aspect of hazard identification is determining the most important health effect in the time frame of interest. Are you assessing acute, subchronic, or chronic health effects (or all three)? What health endpoint is relevant for each? For salt exposure to a population, chronic health effects are likely of interest. In contrast, acute effects might be of concern if you are addressing health effects for workers in salt processing plant. Cigarettes generally present subchronic and more importantly chronic risk. In contrast, most street drugs present acute and subchronic risks. Although infectious diseases often do not fit neatly into any single category, most present an acute or subchronic hazard. Similarly, the benefit identifica-

TABLE 16–2 Sources of Public Concern

Term	Explanation	Example
Benefit unclear	People are more concerned about hazardous activities that are perceived to have unclear benefits than about hazardous activities that are perceived to have clear benefits.	Taking drug with possible side effects for prophylaxis versus drugs to cure illness. (In U.S., polio vaccination versus measles vaccination.)
Causation (Also called *attributability*)	People are more concerned about risks that are perceived to be due to human actions than about risks that are perceived to be natural in origin.	Industry accidents, terrorism versus hurricanes, earthquakes.
Catastrophic potential	Fatalities and injuries that are grouped in time and space cause more concern than fatalities and injuries that are scattered or random in time and space.	Airplane crashes versus automobile accidents.
Children involved	Activities that are perceived as putting children specifically at risk cause more concern than activities not generally so perceived.	Kidnapping, online child endangerment versus adult disappearance, online exploitation of adults.
Controllability (*voluntariness* of exposure is similar term)	Risks that are perceived to be not under individuals' personal control engender more concern than risks that are perceived to be under their personal control.	Traveling as a passenger in an airplane or automobile versus driving an automobile. Smoking cigarettes versus secondhand smoke. Exposure to unlabeled food additives versus sunbathing.
Dread	The public is more concerned about risks that evoke a response of fear, terror, or anxiety than about risks that are more common and likely, but not especially dreaded.	Exposure to potential carcinogens from toxic waste dumps, nuclear radiation, or a terrorist attack versus car crashes, household accidents, and flu.
Equity	People are more concerned about activities that are characterized by a perceived inequitable distribution of risks and benefits than about those characterized by a perceived equitable distribution of risks and benefits.	Distribution of antibiotics during anthrax attack: Cipro (first) to Senate, amoxicillin (later) to postal workers.
Familiarity	People are more concerned about risks that are unfamiliar than about risks that are familiar.	Genetically modified food versus chlorine bleach.
Future generations	People are more concerned about activities that pose risks to future generations than about risks that are not perceived to pose risks to future generations.	Genetic effects due to exposure to radiation versus binge drinking. Smoking during pregnancy versus smoking as a single adult.
Identifiable victims	People are more concerned about risks to identifiable victims than about risks to statistical victims.	Astronauts, coal miners versus thousands of vehicle fatalities. Individual soldiers versus U.S. forces in Iraq and Afghanistan.
Media attention	People are more concerned about risks that receive a lot of media attention versus those that receive little.	Airline crashes versus worksite accidents. Violent crimes versus domestic violence.
Understanding/uncertainty	Activities characterized by poorly understood exposure mechanisms or processes cause more concern than those that are seemingly well understood.	Nuclear radiation versus solar UVA and UVB radiation. Genetically modified food versus cross-breeding.

Source: Modified from: McCallum D. Risk communication: A tool for behavior change. In: Becker, TE, David, SL, Saucy, G. *Reviewing the Behavioral Science Knowledge Base on Technology Transfer.* National Institute on Drug Abuse (NIDA) Research Monograph 155; 1995, Figure 1, pp. 70–71.
Copyright: Public Domain, NIH. Downloaded from: http://www.nida.nih.gov/pdf/monographs/155.pdf, January 13, 2010.

tion seeks to determine the primary benefits that may occur from a particular action. What are the health, financial, or other benefits relevant to the action that will be taken? Many risk assessments do not include a benefit analysis, so include this only if it is relevant to your risk question.

3. *Exposure assessment:* In this section, identify the human receptors likely to be exposed to chemicals of concern. For assessing chemical risks, you need to identify the receptors that are likely most sensitive to the effect you are assessing—that is, are the young or the old, pregnant women, or others most sensitive to the adverse effect (or outcome) you are assessing? For example, Reye's syndrome associated with aspirin is relevant for infants and not relevant for adults. If you are assessing risk of inducing Reye's syndrome (a severe systemic disorder related to aspirin administration in children), you would identify children as the receptors and discount the need to assess adult risks. This aspect of the discussion of adult versus infant sensitivity to aspirin may also be relevant for the introduction and the hazard identification. In contrast, if you are examining the risks associated with aspirin administration for prevention of stroke and myocardial infarction, infants would not be a relevant receptor.

4. *Dose–response assessment:* This is a description of the relationship between the magnitude of exposure (dose) and the risk (probability) of occurrence of adverse health effects (response) associated with the chemical(s) of concern.

5. *Risk characterization:* In this step, the results of the exposure assessment are integrated with the dose–response assessment to provide quantitative estimates of risk. This is often a very short section. It should have little or no commentary and should be presented in an objective format.

6. *Conclusions:* Include a summary of the findings of the preceding assessment.

7. *Uncertainty analysis:* This section discusses uncertainties associated with the calculated exposures and potential health risks. Any aspects of the assessment that may have biased the results should be discussed here. For example, which elements of the risk assessment might have under- or overestimated potential risks? Which factors are less certain or may have a bias?

8. *Risk management:* This is a discussion of the potential actions that could be taken to mitigate risks identified in the report. Technically, this discussion is not part of a risk assessment, but it is often included.

The Written Document

Because the risk assessment is often both lengthy and detailed the written report should begin with an executive summary. This is a much shorter, stand-alone document that conveys the basic methodologies and findings addressed in the risk assessment. Many people will only read the executive summary. The summary should include:

- Why the risk assessment was done.
- How it was done (in general terms).
- Major conclusions.

You do not need to reference other parts of the report or provide detailed information on methodology or data. Try to keep it to one page. While it comes first in a written report, most people prepare this last. The written document will also include full citations for references cited in the report. A reference section is preferable to citations within text because it is easier to read.

Oral Presentation

Presenting a risk assessment to a community requires good preparation, practice, and thick skin. The classic town meeting is held in an auditorium with large numbers of seats. Speakers present to the audience from a podium or stage. Usually, a series of specialists will present what they know about the different facets of the investigation. Sounds good but when asked how he runs an effective town meeting, the head of community affairs at one chemical company replied, "You don't. Town meetings don't work." Why not?

In the town meeting format, a few vocal individuals can completely dominate the discussion. Often these are very angry individuals. Even if the majority of the audience supports the organization that is running the meeting, many will be unwilling to speak up against an extremely upset individual. In addition, a town meeting format presumes that everyone in the audience will arrive on time to hear all of the presentation and that the audience listens to every part. It also presumes that every audience member will be willing to speak up and voice his or her questions of concern.

A more effective alternative is a poster session, similar to what we use at scientific meetings. The room is set up with posters around the periphery with an expert manning each one. This allows the audience members to meet the experts on a one-on-one basis and greatly facilitates questions and answers. An individual too shy to ask what they perceive to be a "stupid" question in an open auditorium is much more likely to speak on an individual basis, particularly if the expert has made the effort to promote dialog. In addition, poster sessions give the experts a chance to solicit the opinions and feelings of large numbers of participants. The participants get a chance to see the experts as people. For more on poster sessions, see **Box 16–2.** Depending on the situation, a hybrid town-meeting/poster session may be appropriate. For example, it might facilitate discussions for the experts to give very concise up-front talks and then direct the audience to talk with them at each of their posters.

When You Can't Be There in Person

First of all, all efforts should be made to meet with the concerned community in person. But, there might be a time when the best expert needs to be elsewhere and, therefore, cannot personally attend a meeting. There are few alternatives. Online discussion platforms are available (e.g., the YouTube and Facebook interventions during the recent presidential debates) but have not yet been tried for risk assessment. They may be inappropriate in many cases, given the reputation of social media for triviality and the need to be seen as giving serious consideration to a serious subject. However, using a monitored discussion blog is a way to respond to a large number of questions from the public in an open and accountable manner that could be used in conjunction with more direct means. During anthrax, when not offering a televised briefing with live journalist questions, the CDC used a monitored conference call system. Everyone could hear the questions and responses but callers were activated to speak by the telephone operating system and could only speak one at a time. This proved to be an equitable, civilized, and time-efficient way to interact with the media, many of whom could not attend a meeting in person. This approach could be adapted for smaller communities as well.

We will now discuss what happens when risk communication has to be done during a crisis or emergency.

EMERGENCY RISK COMMUNICATION*

ERC, also called CERC (crisis and emergency risk communication), is a term the CDC coined to describe the process of communicating about risk with various publics during a complex emergency. It has been a key element in their cooperative agreements with state, local, territorial, and tribal health departments for health emergency preparedness.[8] The CDC is careful to note that ERC/CERC is not "tactical communication," which involves communication *among responders* such as the military, police, fire, and other local emergency units.

The CDC and its partners have developed many resources to support ERC and CERC.[†] These have been used extensively

---

*Most of this section prepared by Claudia Parvanta.
[†]Part of the distinction in nomenclature is that the Division of Health Communications with Oak Ridge National Laboratories took the lead on creating the CDCynergy tool for ERC, while Barbara Reynolds, originally in the Media Relations Division, and her contractor, Prospect Associates, put together the original version of CERC. The CERC manual and associated courses are what the CDC currently supports out of the Coordinating Office for Terrorism Preparedness and Emergency Response (COTPER). http://emergency.cdc.gov/cotper/.

Box 16–2 Conducting Poster Sessions for Risk Assessments

Poster sessions cater to both visual and auditory learners. Those who would like to read to learn can do so. Those who would prefer to talk with the expert can do so. Poster sessions offer excellent opportunities for blended learning. They also give the control to the audience—that is, the individual can decide which posters to visit and which information matters most to them.

Another strength of poster sessions is that they accommodate extremely busy individuals whose schedules don't allow them to spend an entire night in a town meeting. With a poster session, a participant can arrive at any time or leave at any time and not miss key information.

Poster sessions also offer the best possible forum to engage your worst critics in discussion. These discussions can also help you identify key allies in the community. For example, you may be able to identify a professor, schoolteacher, or other highly respected member of the community who can contribute to the discussions.

Considerations to enhance the value of poster sessions:

1. Offer a handout at each poster.
2. Ensure that each expert has training in risk communication.
3. Assess the content of posters: Do they provide the appropriate level of detail? Are they too complex/too simplistic?
4. Provide a refreshment area, including some healthy snacks. Food promotes discussion and also acknowledges that people may have come directly from work to attend the sessions and skipped their meal. Hunger makes people angry.

to develop this section of the book.[9] We need to stress that this chapter *in no way* represents everything you would need to know about ERC or CERC, and we advise you to examine the references mentioned if, in fact, you are working in a health department and need to have a professional level of competency in this domain. Throughout this chapter, we use ERC to refer to the generic activity and CERC when using CDC source material. The terms mean the same thing in this chapter. Another useful resource for working with the media during a crisis has been developed by Hyer and Covello for the World Health Organization.[10]

What Distinguishes ERC from Routine Health Communication?

(Let's Not Call Them Target) Audiences

The first major difference between ERC and routine health communication is the characterization of the audience. **Figure 16–2** shows the concentric nature of audience segments associated with a disaster. As you can see, different audiences have different needs for information. We will describe the specifics—for example, what is meant by vicarious rehearsal—in more detail later.

Channels and Media Choices

An important aspect of ERC is that two-way communication is required to make it successful. As the CDC notes,

> [The public is] a key partner in preventing, preparing for, responding to, and recovering from public health emergencies. Public involvement and cooperation are required to facilitate critical response activities such as evacuation, sheltering in place, social distancing, and queuing at Points of Dispensing (POD). CERC can be effective in influencing how the public responds to these activities.[11]

As an interactive process, ERC needs to provide accurate, credible, and timely information to the many different population groups who need it to make the best decisions possible

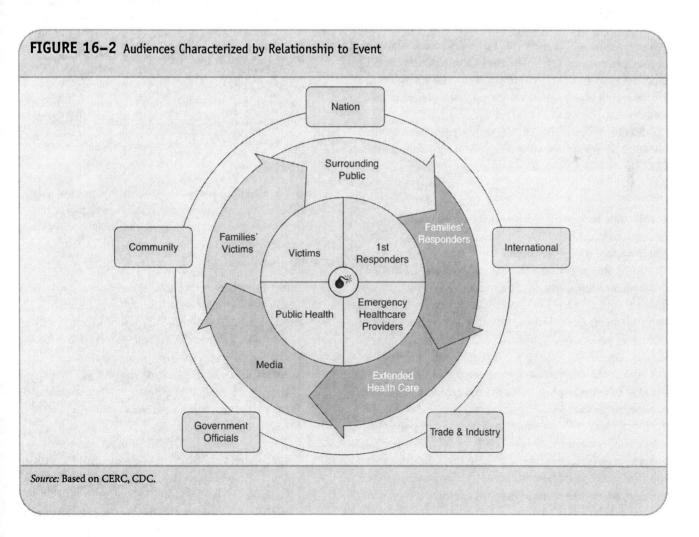

FIGURE 16–2 Audiences Characterized by Relationship to Event

Source: Based on CERC, CDC.

during emergencies. This means making important media choices and generating multiple forms of content at the right reading level, as well as specific versions for different cultural and linguistic audiences. The public needs to be able to call, go online, or ask someone in person about their concerns. These communication efforts need to be monitored to ensure that information is received, understood, and acted upon. While Figure 16–2 indicated audiences by their proximity to an event, **Table 16–3** displays audiences by potential media channels, communication products, and considerations beyond their primary information needs.

Psychological Needs during a Disaster

Each emergency creates its own psychological wake. Ideally, a health communicator should have some background in psychology in order to anticipate the psychological needs and stresses that the population is experiencing and use ERC strategies to best effect. Or, better yet, bring in a qualified psychologist used to dealing with stress-related disorders to advise you during the emergency. It is not that hard to imagine that people caught up in the throes of an emergency, such as an earthquake, hurricane, or terrorist attack, are fearful and anxious, possibly stripped of their home, access to money, or even identity. And, those are the lucky ones. Surrounding them are people who are either trying to help them, or who are observing what is going on from some distance, but still concerned.

Box 16–3[12] presents some key psychological variables that influence how people react during a crisis, according to the CDC.

The Stages of ERC

The diagram in **Figure 16–3** is issued with guidance[13] on applying for a grant from the CDC to do CERC as part of integrated emergency preparedness.

You'll note that it begins with an "incident" (something bad happens.) But emergency risk communication starts when things are quiet. In a not too optimistic way, this is referred to as the *pre-event phase*. Following that come the *event*, and an evaluation period we optimistically call (this time) *post-event*. We focus on pre-event planning in this textbook. During an actual event, you would work through the steps in Figure 16–3, trying to follow your plans to the extent possible. Of course, as in a combat setting, most plans are completely revised within the first 48 hours of any emergency. As a junior person in a public health team, you would largely be following instructions during an actual emergency. During the post-event phase, you can gather and learn a lot about what went right and wrong in order to make modifications in materials and plans for the next time.

Pre-Event Planning

If you are not actively dealing with an emergency, you are in a pre-event phase, even if you are still mopping up (in post-event) from the last one. This is because you will feed everything you learned from the last emergency into what you prepare for the next.

While it might seem somewhat daunting, the CDC's Emergency Communication Checklist, shown in **Table 16–4,** summarizes everything you need to have ready to manage a communication response during a public health emergency.

If you look carefully, you will see that the rest of the checklist is just the details in response to item 1.1, "Does your organization have an emergency response/crisis communication operational plan . . . ?" And, unless they have worked through most of this checklist, then the answer is no.

Your objective during the pre-event phase is to imagine the unimaginable—the various disasters that could occur. These are listed under Checklist item "II. Messages and Audiences in the Checklist." You also need to work out your logistical, partnership, resource, and personnel arrangements and commit these to printed (yes, old-fashioned paper) as well as online plans. You'll want to create and preposition (post electronically, distribute to partners, print out, make camera ready, record videos, etc.) content you would need in the first 48 hours of a disaster.

If you were to start from scratch, here are some of the tools you could use to develop your operational plan for ERC. (Refer to Table 16–4.)

Who's in Charge?

Much of the plan deals with coordination of plans, spokespersons, and public information officers, at all emergency response agencies, public health departments, and government offices that would be involved in an emergency. This requires meetings and development of:

- Lists that are turned into listservs, phone-trees, blast faxes, and any other form that can be used instantly to connect with one and other. This should include after-hours (cell phone) contacts for all PIOs (public information officers) as well as supervisory officials.
- Memoranda of understanding that designate lines of authority, subject matter experts, spokespersons, clearance procedures, training and resource availabilities, etc.
- What is needed to get the job done?
  - *Training.* While you have the time, train everyone in ERC principles. In particular, work with SMEs and officials on being a community or media spokesperson.
  - *Resources.* Have you identified space, facilities management (i.e., heat and light), equipment, and people

TABLE 16–3 Audiences by Channels and Products

	AUDIENCES			
	Unaffected Public (General)	**Affected Communities**	**Public Health Professionals**	**Clinical Care/First Responders**	**Civic Leaders: Local, State, National**

C O N C E R N S	Vicarious rehearsal readiness	Personal and family safety Pet safety Property protection Interruption of normal activities Stigmatization	Personal safety Resources to accomplish response and recovery Treatment recommendations Media talking points	Personal safety Resources to accomplish response and recovery Treatment recommendations Media talking points	Quality of response and recovery Informing constituents Statutes and laws Opportunities for expressing concern Impact on trade, industry Media talking points
C H A N N E L S	Agency website News media Public inquiry phone hotline TV/radio PSAs (optional)	On-site responders[1] State/local websites Local news Phone hotline (dedicated or general) TV/radio PSAs	Agency listserve Agency website Conference calls PHIN* Health alerts (HAN)[†] Webcasts EpiX[2] MMWR[3] Preparedness center sites (by state) As appropriate, clinical networks	Agency listservs Agency website Webcasts Conference calls Phone hotline Medical Association host sites PHIN Health alerts (HAN) Webcasts EpiX MMWR	Telebriefings Agency listserve Dedicated agency subsite HAN News media

Communication Products Typically Requiring Clearance during Emergency					
P R O D U C T S	Responses to media questions (Q&As) Scripts for public information line PSA scripts, storyboards Fact sheets Backgrounders Website content	Spokesperson talking points (If not lead SME) Risk communication materials Informed consent documents Patient education sheets	Health alerts Fact sheets Information sheets for channel specific distribution	Triage guidelines Post-exposure Prophylaxis Diagnosis, treatment Short-term follow-up patient care Long-term follow-up	Talking points Website content

Other Communication Considerations					
I S S U E S	Literacy level Language Disability requirements	Fear/outrage Spokespersons Media options Literacy level Language Disability requirements	PHIN, EpiX access Local area networks Level of BT communication preparedness	Computer/Internet access Needs for patient materials (literacy, language)	Federal, state policy Localized data

[1]Direct communication to on-site responders and clinical care team handled by Emergency Response Command and Subject Matter Experts (SMEs) according to role.

[2]EpiX has separate emergency clearance procedures—included as channel in table for audience.

[3]MMWR has separate emergency clearance procedures—included as channel in table and articulates tightly with others as source of cleared materials.

*PHIN http://www.cdc.gov/PHIN/

[†]HAN http://www2a.cdc.gov/HAN/Index.asp

Box 16–3 Psychological Reactions during a Crisis

It is important for the communicator to understand that in crisis, people often manifest the following psychological reactions:

- Vicarious rehearsal.
- Denial.
- Stigmatization.
- Fear and avoidance.
- Withdrawal, hopelessness, and helplessness.

Vicarious Rehearsal

Interestingly, experience has shown that people farther away (by distance or relationship) from the threat may exercise less reasonable reactions than those who are facing the crisis more directly. The communication age allows some people to vicariously participate in a crisis without risk and "try on" the courses of action presented to them. These "armchair" victims have the luxury of time to choose a course of action and may become hypercritical about the value of a recommendation. In some cases, they reject the proposed course of action, choose another, or insist that they are also actually at risk and need the recommended remedy, such as a vaccination or a visit to an emergency room. In its most troublesome form, these "worried well" will heavily tax the recovery and response.

Denial

Members of the community will experience denial. Some people:

- Avoid getting the warnings or action recommendations.
- Become agitated or confused by the warning.
- Believe the threat is not real.
- Believe the threat does not apply to them.

An individual experiencing denial may not take recommended steps to ensure his or her safety until the absolute last moment, sometimes when it is too late. This maladaptive crisis response is often associated with the sudden, deep feeling that the universe is no longer a rational and orderly system.

Stigmatization

In some instances, victims may be stigmatized by their communities and refused services or public access. A *stigma,* is a negative characterization of an individual or group because of disease, behavior, or background (e.g., tuberculosis, people with piercings, ethnicity) that leads to fear, avoidance, even violence on the part of others. Stigmatization will hamper community recovery and affect evacuation and relocation efforts. In a disease outbreak, a community is more likely to separate from those perceived to be infected.

Fear and Avoidance

Fear in the affected population is an important consideration in the response to a crisis. The fear of the unknown or the fear of uncertainty may be the most debilitating of the psychological responses to disaster. With fear at the core, an individual may act in extreme, and sometimes irrational, ways to avoid the perceived or real threat.

Withdrawal, Hopelessness, and Helplessness

Some people can accept that the threat is real, but the threat looms so large that they feel that the situation is hopeless. They feel helpless to protect themselves and so, instead, they withdraw.

For more on the range of emotional reactions that a crisis can provoke, and ways to deal with these various emotions, see Dr. Peter Sandman, *Beyond Panic Prevention: Addressing Emotion in Emergency Communication,* http://www.orau.gov/cdcynergy/erc/Content/activeinformation/resources/BeyondPanicPrevention.pdf.

Source: CDCynergy Emergency Risk Communication. Phase 1, Essential Principles: Psychology. Available at www.orau.gov/cdcynergy.

FIGURE 16–3 Crisis and Emergency Risk Communication (CERC) with the Public "Process Map"

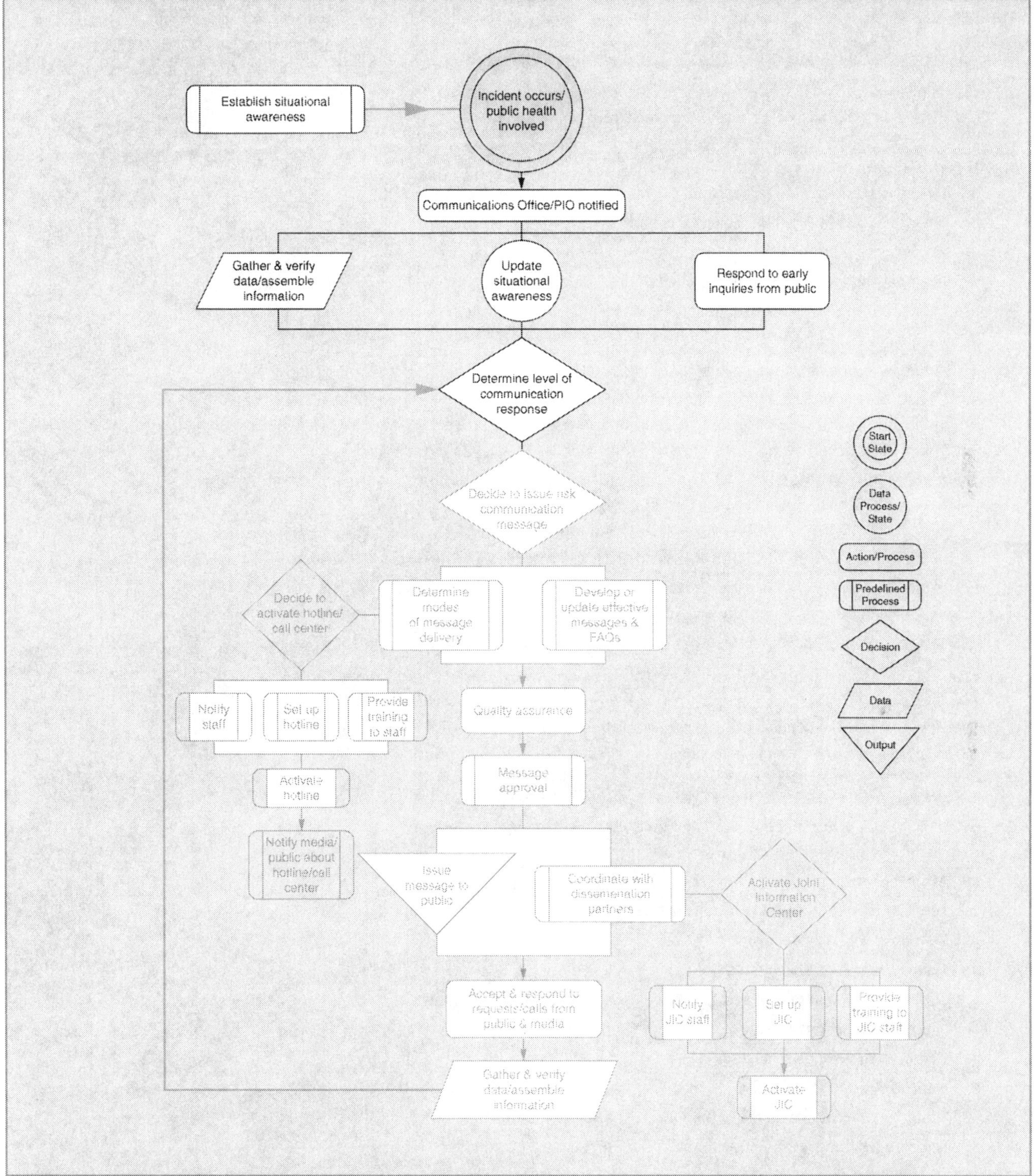

Source: CDC, Public Health Emergency Preparedness Cooperative Agreement. Budget Period 9 (BP9) Performance Measures Guidance, November 2008; p. 42.

TABLE 16–4 Emergency Risk Communication Checklist

Use this comprehensive checklist to help assess your organization's preparedness for responding to an emergency.		
I. Planning, Research, Training, and Evaluation	Yes	No
1.1 Does your organization have an emergency response/crisis communication operational plan for public information and media, partner, and stakeholder relations?		
If yes, does the plan have the following elements:	**Yes**	**No**
a. Designated line and staff responsibilities for the public information team?		
b. Information verification and clearance/approval procedures?		
c. Agreements on information release authorities (who releases what/when/how)?		
d. Regional and local media contact list (including after-hours news desks)?		
e. Procedures to coordinate with the public health organization response teams?		
f. Designated spokespersons for public health issues in an emergency?		
g. Public health organization emergency response team after-hours contact numbers?		
h. Contact numbers for emergency information partners (e.g., governor's public affairs officer, local FBI public information special agent in charge, local or regional department of agriculture or veterinarian public information officers, Red Cross and other nongovernment organizations)?		
i. Agreements/procedures to join the Joint Information Center (JIC) of the emergency operations center (if activated)?		
j. Procedures to secure needed resources (space, equipment, people) to operate the public information operation during a public health emergency 24 hours a day/7 days a week, if needed?		
k. Identified vehicles of information dissemination during a crisis to public, stakeholders, partners (e.g., e-mail list servs, broadcast fax, door-to-door leaflets, press releases)?		
	Yes	**No**
1.2 Have you coordinated your planning with the community or state emergency operation center?		
1.3 Have you coordinated your planning with other response organizations or competitors?		
1.4 Have designated spokespersons received media training and risk communication training?		
1.5 Do the spokespersons understand emergency crisis/risk communication principles to build trust and credibility?		
II. Message and Audiences	Yes	No
2.1 Are any of the following types of incidents (disasters) likely to require intense public information, media, and partner communication responses by your organization:		
a. Airborne infectious disease outbreak (e.g., pandemic influenza)?		
b. Foodborne infectious disease outbreak (e.g., listeria)?		
c. Waterborne (Cryptosporidiosis)?		
d. Vector borne (West Nile virus)?		
e. Outbreak with potential to spread outside your region or to your region?		
f. Unknown infectious agent?		
g. Chemical or toxic material disaster?		
h. Natural disasters?		
i. Unknown infectious agent (international) with potential to spread to the United States?		
j. Known infectious agent (international) with potential to spread to the United States?		

continues

TABLE 16–4 Emergency Risk Communication Checklist—continued

		Yes	No
k.	Large-scale environmental crises?		
l.	Radiological event?		
m.	Terrorist event		
	m.1 Biological (suspected or declared)?		
	m.2 Chemical?		
	m.3 Radiological?		
	m.4 Mass explosion?		
n.	Site-specific emergencies		
	n.1 Laboratory incident with laboratory worker?		
	n.2 Laboratory incident/release of material in community?		
	n.3 Death of employee/contractor/visitor while on campus/premises?		
	n.4 Hostage event with/by employee/contractor on campus/premises?		
	n.5 Bomb threat?		
	n.6 Explosion/fire—destruction of property?		
	n.7 Violent death of an employee/contractor or visitor on campus/premises?		
		Yes	No
2.2	Have you **identified special populations** (e.g., elderly, first language other than English, tribal communities, border populations)? List any specific sub-populations that need to be targeted with specific messages during a public health emergency related to your organization (e.g., tribal nations, persons with chronic respiratory illness, unvaccinated seniors).		
2.3	Have you **identified your organization's partners who should receive direct information and updates** (not solely through the media) from your organization during a public health emergency?		
2.4	Have you **identified all stakeholder organizations** or populations (groups or organizations that your organization believes have an active interest in monitoring activities—to whom you are most directly accountable, other than official chain of command) who should receive direct communication during a public health–related emergency?		
2.5	Have you **planned ways to reach people according to their reactions** to the incident (fight or flight)? Are messages, messengers, and methods of delivery sensitive to all types of audiences in your area of responsibility?		
2.6	Are there **mechanisms/resources in place to create messages** for the media and public under severe time constraints, including methods to clear these messages within the emergency response operations of your organization (include cross clearance)?		
2.7	Have you identified how you will perform **media evaluation, content analysis, and public information call analysis in real time** during an emergency to ensure adequate audience feedback?		
		Yes	No
2.8	Have you developed **topic-specific pre-crisis materials** for identified public health emergency issues, or identified sources of these materials if needed:		
a.	Topic fact sheet (e.g., description of the disease, public health threat, treatment, etc.)?		
b.	Public questions/answers (Q/As)?		
c.	Partner questions/answers?		
d.	Resource fact for media/public/partners to obtain additional information?		
e.	Web access and links to information on the topic?		
f.	Recommendations for affected populations?		
g.	Background beta video (B-roll) for media use on the topic?		

TABLE 16–4 Emergency Risk Communication Checklist—continued

	Yes	No
h. List of subject matter experts outside your organization who would be effective validators to public/media regarding your activities during a public health emergency?		
III. Messenger	**Yes**	**No**
3.1 Have you identified public health spokespersons for media and public appearances during an emergency?		
If yes, have you:		
a. Identified persons by position to act as spokespersons for multiple audiences (e.g., media spokesperson, community meeting speaker, etc.) and formats about public health issues during an emergency?		
b. Ensured that the spokespersons understand their communication roles and responsibilities and will incorporate them into their expected duties during the crisis?		
IV. Methods of Delivery (Information Dissemination) and Resources	**Yes**	**No**
4.1 Does your organization have **go kits** for public information officers who may have to abandon their normal place of operation during a public health emergency or join a JIC?		
If yes, does the kit include:	**Yes**	**No**
a. A computer(s) capable of linking to the Internet/e-mail?		
b. A CD–ROM or disks containing the elements of the crisis communication plan (including media, public health, and organization contact lists, partner contact lists; information materials, etc.)?		
c. A cell phone or satellite phone, pager, wireless e-mail, etc.?		
d. A funding mechanism (credit card, etc.) that can be used to purchase operational resources as needed?		
e. Manuals and background information necessary to provide needed information to the public and media?		
f. Care and comfort items for the public information operations staff?		
4.2 Have you identified the mechanisms that are or should be in place to ensure **multiple channels of communication to multiple audiences** during a public health emergency?		
If yes, do they include:	**Yes**	**No**
a. Media channels (print, TV, radio, Web)?		
b. Websites?		
c. Phone banks?		
d. Town hall meetings?		
e. Listserv e-mail?		
f. Broadcast fax?		
g. Letters by mail?		
h. Subscription newsletters?		
i. Submissions to partner newsletters?		
j. Regular or special partner conference calls?		
k. Door-to-door canvassing?		
4.3 Are **contracts/agreements** in place to post information to broadcast fax or e-mail systems?		
4.4 Have **locations for press conferences** been designated and resourced?		
V. Personnel	**Yes**	**No**
5.1 Have you identified employees, contractors, fellows, interns currently working for you or available to you in an emergency who have skills in the following areas:		
a. Public affairs specialist?		
b. Health communication specialist?		
c. Communication officer?		

continues

TABLE 16–4 Emergency Risk Communication Checklist—continued

		Yes	No
d.	Health education specialist?		
e.	Training specialist?		
f.	Writer/editor?		
g.	Technical writer/editor?		
h.	Audio/visual specialist?		
i.	Internet/Web design specialist?		
j.	Others who contribute to public/provider information?		
5.2	Have you identified who will provide the following expertise or execute these activities during a public health emergency (including backup):		
Command and control:		**Yes**	**No**
a.	Directs the work related to the release of information to the media, public, and partners?		
b.	Activates the plan, based on careful assessment of the situation and the expected demands for information media, partners, and the public?		
c.	Coordinates with horizontal communication partners, as outlined in the plan, to ensure that messages are consistent and within the scope of the organization's responsibility?		
d.	Provides updates to organization's director, Emergency Operations Center (EOC) command and higher headquarters, as determined in the plan?		
e.	Advises the director and chain of command regarding information to be released, based on the organization's role in the response?		
f.	Ensures that risk communication principles are employed in all contact with media, public, and partner information release efforts?		
g.	Advises incident-specific policy, science, and situation?		
h.	Reviews and approves materials for release to media, public, and partners?		
i.	Obtains required clearance of materials for release to media on policy or sensitive topic-related information not previously cleared?		
j.	Determines the operational hours/days, and reassesses throughout the emergency response?		
k.	Ensures resources are available (human, technical, and mechanical supplies)?		
Media:		**Yes**	**No**
a.	Assesses media needs and organizes mechanisms to fulfill media needs during the crisis (e.g., daily briefings in person, versus a Website update)?		
b.	Triages the response to media requests and inquiries?		
c.	Ensures that media inquiries are addressed as appropriate?		
d.	Supports spokespersons?		
e.	Develops and maintains media contact lists and call logs?		
f.	Produces and distributes media advisories and press releases?		
g.	Produces and distributes materials (e.g., fact sheets, B-roll)?		
h.	Oversees media monitoring systems and reports (e.g., analyzing environment and trends to determine needed messages; determining what misinformation needs to be corrected; identifying concerns, interests, and needs arising from the crisis and the response)?		
i.	Ensures that risk communication principles to build trust and credibility are incorporated into all public messages delivered through the media?		
j.	Acts as member of the JIC of the field site team for media relations?		
k.	Serves as liaison from the organization to the JIC and back?		

TABLE 16–4 Emergency Risk Communication Checklist—continued

Direct public information:	Yes	No
a. Manages the mechanisms to respond to public requests for information directly from the organization by telephone, in writing, or by e-mail?		
b. Oversees public information monitoring systems and reports (e.g., analyzing environment and trends to determine needed messages; determining what misinformation needs to be corrected; identifying concerns, interests, and needs arising from the crisis and the response)?		
c. Activates or participates in the telephone information line?		
d. Activates or participates in the public e-mail response system?		
e. Activates or participates in the public correspondence response system?		
f. Organizes and manages emergency response Web sites and Web pages?		
g. Establishes and maintains links to other emergency response Websites?		
Partner/stakeholder information:	Yes	No
a. Establishes communication protocols based on prearranged agreements with identified partners and stakeholders?		
b. Arranges regular partner briefings and updates?		
c. Solicits feedback and responds to partner information requests and inquiries?		
d. Oversees partner/stakeholder monitoring systems and reports (e.g., analyzing environment and trends to determine needed messages; determining what misinformation needs to be corrected; identifying concerns, interests, and needs arising from the crisis and the response)?		
e. Helps organize and facilitate official meetings to provide information and receive input from partners or stakeholders?		
f. Develops and maintains lists and call logs of legislators and special interest groups?		
g. Responds to legislator/special interest groups requests and inquiries?		
Content and material for public health emergencies:	Yes	No
a. Develops and establishes mechanisms to rapidly receive information from the EOC regarding the public health emergency?		
b. Translates EOC situation reports and meeting notes into information appropriate for public and partner needs?		
c. Works with subject matter experts to create situation-specific fact sheets, Q/As, and updates?		
d. Compiles information on possible public health emergency topics for release when needed?		
e. Tests messages and materials for cultural and language requirements of special populations?		
f. Receives input from other communication team members regarding content and message needs?		
g. Uses analysis from media, public and partner monitoring systems, and reports (e.g., environmental and trend analysis to determine needed messages; what misinformation need to be corrected; and identify concerns, interests, and needs arising from the crisis and the response) to identify additional content requirements and materials development?		
h. Lists contracts/cooperative agreements/consultants currently available to support emergency public/private information dissemination?		
VI. Suggestions to Consider about Resources	Yes	No
Do you have space:		
a. To operate your communication teams outside the EOC? (You need a place to bring media on site, separate from the EOC.)		
b. To quickly train spokespersons?		

continues

TABLE 16–4 Emergency Risk Communication Checklist—continued

		Yes	No
c.	For team meetings?		
d.	For equipment, exclusive for your use? (You cannot stand in line for the copier when media deadlines loom.)		
Have you considered the following contracts and memoranda of agreement:		**Yes**	**No**
a.	A contract with a media newswire?		
b.	A contract with a radio newswire?		
c.	A contract for writers or public relations personnel who can augment your staff?		
d.	A contract for administrative support?		
e.	A phone system/contractor to supply a phone menu that directs type of caller and level of information desired, including:		
	e.1 General information about the threat?		
	e.2 Tip line, listing particular actions people can take to protect themselves?		
	e.3 Reassurance/counseling?		
	e.4 Referral information for healthcare/medical facility workers?		
	e.5 Referral information for epidemiologists or others to report cases?		
	e.6 Lab/treatment protocols?		
	e.7 Managers looking for policy statements for employees?		
Do you have the following recommended equipment:		**Yes**	**No**
a.	Fax machine (with a number that's preprogrammed for broadcast fax releases to media and partners)?		
b.	Website capability 24/7? (You should attempt to have new information posted within 2 hours; some say within 10 minutes.)		
c.	Computers (on local area networks [LANs] with e-mail listservs designated for partners and media)?		
d.	Laptop computers?		
e.	Printers for every computer?		
f.	Copier (and backup)?		
g.	Tables? (You will need a large number of tables.)		
h.	Cell phones/pagers/personal digital devices and e-mail readers?		
i.	Visible calendars, flow charts, bulletin boards, easels?		
j.	Designated personal message board?		
k.	Small refrigerator?		
l.	Paper?		
m.	Color copier?		
n.	A/V equipment?		
o.	Portable microphones?		
p.	Podium?		
q.	TVs with cable hookup?		
r.	Video recording and playing capability?		
s.	CD–ROMs or flash drives?		
t.	Paper shredder?		

TABLE 16–4 Emergency Risk Communication Checklist—continued

Do you have the following recommended supplies:	Yes	No
a. Copier toner?		
b. Printer ink?		
c. Paper?		
d. Pens?		
e. Markers?		
f. Highlighters?		
g. Erasable markers?		
h. Shipping and postal supplies?		
i. Sticky note pads?		
j. Tape?		
k. Notebooks?		
l. Poster board?		
m. Standard press kit folders?		
n. Organized B-roll in media ready format (keep VHS copies around for meetings)?		
o. Formatted computer disks?		
p. Color-coded items (folders, inks, etc.)?		
q. Baskets (to contain items you're not ready to throw away)?		
r. Organizers to support your clearance and release system?		
s. Expandable folders (alphabetized or days of the month)?		
t. Staplers?		
u. Paper punch?		
v. Three-ring binders?		
w. Organization's press kit or its logo on a sticker?		
x. Colored copier paper (for door-to-door flyers)?		
y. Paper clips (all sizes)?		

Source: CDC Emergency Risk Communication *CDCynergy*

who can operate an office, possibly 24/7, if needed? What if it needs to be far away from your present location? You might need to set up contracts with vendors (including local universities) for language translation, printing, photocopying, door-to-door dissemination, media monitoring, survey research, and other services on an as-needed basis.

Message and Audience

The list in section 2.1 of the ERC Checklist is scary and thorough. About the only thing you might be able to cross off the list are emergencies dealing with laboratories, if you do not support one. But that's about all you can rule out ahead of time. A good use of this list is to prioritize your preparations. How can you say that a terrorist event with a chemical agent is less important to prepare for than an airborne infectious disease outbreak? If it is a terrorist event, it is likely that the FBI and the CDC will take charge and you will basically follow their lead and use their materials. Many of the disasters on the list are actually "routine" emergencies for public health departments, and most choose to focus on these first, if using their own resources. (If they have received money for terrorism preparation, it goes to support that.) You might also need to tailor your notification, operations, and other lists by type of incident. Waterborne chemical agents require a different network, including the local water management officials, than an explosion at a fuel refinery.

ERC Checklist sections 2.2, 2.3, and 2.4 deal with finding and reaching specific populations. Many government offices, local Chambers of Commerce, or other organizations maintain websites that contain many community details. Many local organizations have formed networks of "block captains," people who will go door-to-door in the case of an emergency and tell their neighbors what do to. It will be very helpful to know the organizations that established and maintain this structure and to find a way to shoot materials to them.

In addition, the CDC has an interactive database, "Snap Shots of State Population Data, Version 1.5" or SNAPS[14] on the emergency sub-site at www.CDC.gov. According to the webpage,

> SNAPS provides a "snap shot" of key variables for consideration in guiding and tailoring health education and communication efforts to ensure diverse audiences receive critical public health messages that are accessible, understandable, and timely.

Box 16–4 shows a typical set of data generated by SNAPS.

The material in Box 16–4 is derived from the U.S. Census, and will be updated every 10 years. Census data provide a rough estimate of the community needs in terms of overall population size, broken down by reported sex, race, religious affiliations, disabilities, language needs, and educational levels. Data on heating fuel, vehicle ownership, and phones are more relevant to other emergency planners, but the SNAPS database can be queried for more specific data on economic indicators and a few other variables. This is a good starting point to know what religious organizations and community groups need to be involved in order to plan appropriate meeting sites, as well as to help identify partners to train. A full list of all broadcast media is also generated (the list in the example is truncated for space). Together with information on businesses, schools, and any other potential stakeholder organizations, you would develop plans and lists, as you did in Section I, to have a rapid communication network ready in case of an emergency. And you would use these or more customized data to plan your materials in the ERC Checklist section 2.8.

Topic-Specific Pre-Crisis Materials ERC Checklist section 2.8 lists a number of pre-crisis materials that you can prepare and have ready to go in the event of an emergency. It was mentioned earlier that you want to have both electronic and printed-out copies of your materials. Print versions are needed in case your power is cut off, or the Internet has been sabotaged, and you need to produce photocopies the old-fashioned way. Paper in a file folder is really great for this. So are DVDs, flash drives, and other more permanent records of materials. You cannot count on having access to the Internet (or electricity, unfortunately) in an emergency!*

The good news is that the CDC, and other organizations, have been working with increased intensity on materials preparation since September 11, 2001. There is now a good repository of fact sheets, Q&As (question-and-answer sets), clinical guidelines, and other information that you could use within the first 48 hours of a response. The CDC has focused on this time period because things might initially feel chaotic. After this you will need to update the materials with what you have learned about the specific incident. To get out of the starting gate, however, there are templates and topic-specific materials ready to go.

Through a cooperative agreement with several schools of public health, the CDC was able to develop sets of materials for specific populations across the United States,† including American Indians, African Americans, Hispanics, and persons with lower literacy abilities in English. There are also multiple language translations (e.g. Spanish, Russian, Vietnamese, French, etc.) for many materials. According to your community's needs, you would download these, print them out, and store them on flash drives so you have them ready to go, wherever you might have to set up shop.

Boxes 16–5 and **16–6** present a few sample materials from this site and CDCynergy ERC.

Message Maps Particularly for planning oral presentations, some people find it very useful to prepare **message maps.** The CDC learned about message mapping for health emergencies from Vincent Covello.[15] You use a message map to organize complex information into units and to help a speaker to focus on key points. They also are designed to automatically provide sound bites for the media. Messages are presented in three short sentences that convey three key messages in 27 words. (These limits were developed based on research that front-page media and broadcast stories usually carried three key messages in less than nine seconds for broadcast media or 27 words for print.) While this approach predates Twitter, such compact emergency messages could be "tweeted."

Message maps should be written at a sixth-grade reading level. Each primary message has three supporting messages that can be used when and where appropriate to provide

---

*You might want to consider having an old-fashioned typewriter and mimeograph machine around, if you can find them.
†http://emergency.cdc.gov/firsthours/intro.asp.

Box 16–4 Typical SNAPS Output for Communication Planning

Generated by entering Montgomery County, PA, into SNAPS system at: http://www.bt.cdc.gov/snaps/.

State Health Department:

- Pennsylvania Department of Health: P.O. Box 90, Harrisburg

Population:

- Total population: 750,097
- Males: 361,969; Females: 388,128

Ethnicity:

    White: 640,575
    Black/African American: 54,686
    Hispanic: 15,463
    Native American/Eskimo: 894
    Asian: 29,381
    Hawaiian / Pacific Islander: 252
    Other: 811
    Two or more: 8,035

Top Five Languages Spoken at Home:

1. English only (635,060)
2. Spanish (14,170)
3. Korean (7,940)
4. Italian (7,025)
5. German (4,545)

Top Five Religions by Adherents:

1. Catholic Church (263,375)
2. Jewish Estimate (59,550)
3. Evangelical Lutheran Church in America (43,735)
4. Presbyterian Church (U.S.A.) (16,964)
5. United Methodist Church, The (16,214)

Heating Fuel:

    Total reported: 286,098
    Utility gas: 138,395
    Bottled or LP gas: 4,215
    Electricity: 57,269
    Fuel oil, kerosene: 83,353
    Coal or coke: 544
    Wood: 998
    Solar energy: 14
    Other fuel: 938
    No fuel used: 372

Vehicles Available:

- Total reported: 541,869
- One or more vehicle: 509,351
- No vehicle: 32,518

Education Attainment:

- No school: 2,234
- No high school: 13,415
- Some high school: 43,658
- Some college: 85,342
- Associate's degree: 30,596
- College degree: 118,910
- Master's degree: 49,634
- Professional degree: 21,324
- Doctoral degree: 9,919

Household Phones:

- Households reporting: 286,098
- Owners with phone: 209,808
- Owners without phone: 429
- Renters with phone: 74,723
- Renters without phone: 1,138

10 Closest Counties:

1. Philadelphia County, Pennsylvania
2. Delaware County, Pennsylvania
3. Bucks County, Pennsylvania
4. Chester County, Pennsylvania
5. Camden County, New Jersey
6. Gloucester County, New Jersey
7. Lehigh County, Pennsylvania
8. Northampton County, Pennsylvania
9. Salem County, New Jersey
10. New Castle County, Delaware

Zip Codes in County:

18041, 18054, 18070, 18073, 18074, 18076, 18084, 18915, 18918, 18924, 18936, 18957, 18958, 18964, 18969, 18971, 18979, 19001, 19002, 19003, 19004, 19006, 19009, 19012, 19025, 19027, 19031, 19034, 19035, 19038, 19040, 19041, 19044, 19046, 19066, 19072, 19075, 19090, 19095, 19096, 19401, 19403, 19404, 19405, 19406, 19407, 19408, 19409, 19415, 19420, 19422, 19423, 19424, 19426, 19428, 19429, 19430, 19435, 19436, 19437, 19438, 19440, 19441, 19443, 19444, 19446, 19450, 19451, 19452, 19453, 19454, 19455, 19456, 19462, 19464, 19468, 19472, 19473, 19474, 19477, 19478, 19483, 19484, 19485, 19486, 19490, 19492, 19505, 19525

Licensed Broadcast Media Outlets:

- WDBD (TV) Bala Cynwyd, PA
- WTLH (TV) Bala Cynwyd, PA
- WPXT (692 TV) Bala Cynwyd, PA
- WQMY (704 TV) Bala Cynwyd, PA
- WOLF-TV (722 TV) Bala Cynwyd, PA
- WDSI-TV (752 TV) Bala Cynwyd, PA, and about 40 more radio stations

Source: Author generated at http://www.bt.cdc.gov/snaps/

Box 16–5 Message Examples for Emergency Communication

MESSAGE TEMPLATE FOR THE FIRST MINUTES FOR ALL EMERGENCIES

The following suggested template could be used in the first minutes after a suspected terrorism incident when little is known.

1. Please pay close attention. This is an urgent health message from [your public health agency].
2. Officials [emergency, public health, etc.] believe there has been a serious incident [describe incident including time and location] in _____ area.
3. At this time, we do not know the cause or other details about the incident.
4. Local officials are investigating and will work with state and federal officials to provide updated information as soon as possible.
5. Stay informed and follow the instructions of health officials so you can protect yourself, your family, and your community against this public health threat.
6. [Give specific information about when and how the next update will be given.]

When more information is known, additional messages could be added about what is happening, the specific terrorist agent, the actions people should take to protect themselves and others, and where to go for more information. Because these messages were developed to be effective for a variety of scenarios, they will need to be adapted to the specific event.

MESSAGE DEVELOPMENT WORKSHEET

Step 1: Determine audience, message purpose, and delivery method by checking each that applies.

Audience
- Relationship to event
- Demographics (age, language, education, culture)
- Level of outrage (based on risk principles)

Purpose of Message
- Give facts/update
- Rally to action
- Clarify event status
- Address rumors
- Satisfy media requests

Method of Delivery
- Print media release
- Web release
- Through spokesperson (TV or in-person appearance)
- Radio
- Other (e.g., recorded phone message)

Step 2: Construct message using six basic emergency message components

1. Expression of empathy:

2. Clarifying facts/call for action:

Who:

What:

Where:

When:

Why:

How:

3. What we don't know:

4. Process to get answers:

5. Statement of commitment:

6. Referrals:

Step 3: Check your message for the following:

Does your message use . . .	Yes	No
Positive action steps?		
An honest/open tone?		
Risk communication principles?		
Simple words, short sentences?		
Does your message avoid . . .		
Jargon?		
Judgmental phrases?		
Humor?		
Extreme speculation?		

**GENERAL CHEMICAL AGENT EXTENDED MESSAGE
HEALTH AND SAFETY INFORMATION FOR THE FIRST HOURS**

Grade Level: 8.2

Points:
1. What is happening?
2. What to do if you are near the release of the chemical—either in the immediate area or the surrounding area.
3. What to do if you have symptoms or think you have had contact with a chemical.
4. Can the illness caused by a chemical agent be spread from person to person?
5. What are the symptoms of contact with various chemical agents?
6. What to do if you are in a car that is in the immediate area of the release.
7. What to do if you are concerned about *xxx* [add name] chemical agent.
8. What is being done and how to get more information.

continues

NOTE TO USERS: Initial health and safety information is almost identical for all chemical agents, with the exception of symptoms. These messages are general for all categories of chemical agents. Specific symptoms are listed by category of agent. It will be necessary to carefully review and revise the messages during an actual event once the agent is confirmed.

What is happening?

- This is an urgent health message from the U.S. Department of Health and Human Services (HHS). Please pay careful attention to this message to protect your health and that of others.
- Public officials suspect that a chemical agent has been released in the *xxx area* or *xxx building*.[add information]
- *xxx number* [add information] of cases have been reported, with symptoms of [chemical agent]. These symptoms include: [list of symptoms].

NOTE TO USER: Give description of agent (e.g., colorless gas, odorless, or mild smell of garlic or almond), depending upon the agent.

- If the chemical was released in your building, follow emergency personnel's instructions. You should leave the building as quickly as possible.
- How people were exposed to this chemical or the full extent of the problem is unclear.
- Local, state, and federal officials, including HHS, FBI, and Homeland Security, are working together to find out more about this situation. Updates will be made as soon as officials know more.
- If you are near the *xxx area* [add information], protect yourself and your family by staying home or where you are and wait for further instructions.
- If you are not close to the *xxx area* [add information], stay where you are and avoid unnecessary travel until further instructions.
- We have challenges ahead, and we are working to find out more about this situation. By staying informed and following instructions from health officials, you can protect yourself, your family, and the community against this public health threat.
- For more information on chemical agents, go to the HHS Web site at www.hhs.gov, the Centers for Disease Control and Prevention's Chemical Emergencies Web site at http://www.bt.cdc.gov/chemical/, or call the CDC Hotline at 1-800-CDC-INFO for the latest updates.
- This message contains additional information that can help protect your health and the health of others.

What to do if you are near the release of the chemical—either in the immediate area or the surrounding area.

- If you are outdoors, emergency personnel may ask you to leave the area or find shelter nearby. If you are told to go indoors or you are already inside a shelter, follow these instructions:
- *Go to the highest level of the building*. Find a room with as few windows and doors as possible.
- *Reduce air flow from outside to inside*. Close vents, air conditioning, fireplace dampers, and anything else that exposes the room to outside air.
- *Seal the room*. Use plastic and duct tape to close all openings, including windows, doors, vents, and electrical outlets. Even if you cannot seal all openings, follow the other instructions.
- *Eat only sealed, stored food and water*. Do not eat or drink anything that may have been exposed to the chemical.
- *Turn to the radio, television, or Internet news for updated health and safety announcements*. Announcements will be made about when it is safe to go outside.

What to do if you have symptoms or think you have had contact with a chemical.

- Do not touch other people to prevent getting the chemical on them.
- Remove your outer layer of clothing.
- Do *not* remove clothes over your head. If necessary, cut clothes off.
- If possible, put clothes inside a bag and seal it. Put this sealed bag into another bag and seal again.
- Wash your hair and body thoroughly with soap and water right away.
- If eyes are burning or irritated, rinse with water for 10–15 minutes. Do not use soap in your eyes.
- After you have followed these instructions, call your doctor or local public health department right away at *xxx-xxx-xxxx* [add information]. They will tell you how and where to get more help.

Can the illness caused by a chemical agent be spread from person to person?

- The *illness* caused by a chemical agent *cannot* spread from person to person. It is *not* a contagious disease that can be spread by coughing or sneezing.
- People can spread the *chemical* if it is on their skin, clothing, or hair. People can also spread the *chemical* if it is in their body fluids, such as vomit. If someone else comes into contact with the chemical in these ways, they may become ill.
- Once exposed people take off their clothes and shower, most of the chemical will be removed and is much less likely to be spread by these people.

What are the symptoms of contact with various chemical agents?
Symptoms of contact with a blister agent:

- Contact with this type of chemical causes blistering on the skin and in the nose, mouth, and throat.
- After contact with a blister agent, symptoms may occur immediately or may take up to 24 hours to appear.
- First symptoms may include red, itchy, or painful skin, followed by blisters.
- Later symptoms may include pain or swelling in the eyes and lungs, tears in the eyes, and trouble breathing.

Symptoms of contact with a blood agent:

- Contact with this type of chemical deprives the blood and organs of oxygen.
- After contact with a blood agent, symptoms may occur immediately or may take up to 24 hours to appear.
- In general, symptoms may include rapid breathing, nausea, convulsions, and loss of consciousness.

Symptoms of contact with a nerve agent:

- Contact with this type of chemical can damage the nervous system and affect movement and breathing.
- After contact with a nerve agent, symptoms may appear immediately or up to 18 hours later.
- Symptoms include seizures, drooling, eye irritations, sweating or twitching, blurred vision, and muscle weakness.

Symptoms of contact with a choking agent:

- This type of chemical attacks the respiratory system and causes difficulty breathing.
- After contact with a choking agent, symptoms may occur immediately or may take 24 to 48 hours to appear.
- In general, symptoms may include coughing; burning in the eyes, nose, or throat; blurred vision; upset stomach; fluid in the lungs; and difficulty breathing.

NOTE TO USERS: Officials might offer particular instructions for reducing exposure if people are in their cars. Following is a message for staying in the car and pulling over.

If you are in your car in xxx [add information] area, you can help prevent being exposed to the chemical by following these steps:

1. Pull over to the side of the road in a manner that will not block or interfere with the movement of emergency vehicles.
2. Temporarily turn off the engine and shut down any vents that draw outside air, including those of the air conditioner. Running the engine and driving pull outside air into the car and could expose you to additional chemicals.
3. To minimize the amount of chemical you inhale, cover your mouth and nose with a cloth, such as a scarf or a handkerchief.
4. Listen for further instructions from emergency personnel on the scene or listen for news on the radio.

What to do if you are concerned about xxx [add information] chemical agent.

- It is natural to be concerned or afraid at a time like this. Staying informed and following instructions from public health officials will help you stay as safe and healthy as possible.
- Many chemical agents are commonly used in industry and household products. In this situation, [chemical agent] may have been released deliberately. We are not sure at this time if this is the case.
- If you near the *xxx area* [add information], protect yourself and your loved ones by staying home or where you are and wait for further instructions from officials.
- If you are not close to the *xxx* [add information] area, stay where you are and avoid unnecessary travel until further notice.
- Stay informed by turning to the radio, television, or Internet news for updated health and safety announcements.

continues

What is being done and how to get more information.

- Federal, state, and local health officials are working together to find and treat people who have symptoms or who may have had contact with *xxx* [add information] chemical agent. They are also taking actions to prevent others from being exposed.
- Officials will share information and give more instructions as the situation develops and they learn more.
- Go to [insert local media information here] to hear the latest information from local officials.
- For more information on botulism, visit the HHS Web site at http:www.hhs.gov, the Centers for Disease Control and Prevention's Chemical Emergencies Web site at http://www.bt.cdc.gov/chemical/, or call the CDC Hotline at 1-800-CDC-INFO for the latest information.

GENERAL CHEMICAL AGENT SHORT MESSAGE
HEALTH AND SAFETY INFORMATION FOR THE FIRST HOURS

Grade Level: 9.3

- This is an urgent health message from the U.S. Department of Health and Human Services.
- Public officials suspect that a chemical agent has been deliberately released in the *xxx area* or *xxx* building [add information].
- *xxx* [add information]number cases have been reported with symptoms of [chemical agent]. These symptoms include: [list of symptoms].

NOTE TO USERS: Give description of agent (e.g., colorless gas, odorless or mild smell of garlic or almond), depending upon the agent.

- If you are outdoors in the *xxx area* [add information], emergency workers will ask you to leave the area or find shelter nearby.
- If you are indoors in the *xxx area* [add information], go to the highest level of the building and close windows, doors, and fireplace dampers. Turn off heating and cooling systems and close vents so that the room is not exposed to outside air.
- If the chemical was released in your building, follow emergency personnel's instructions.
- How people were exposed to this chemical or the full extent of the problem is unclear.
- Local, state, and federal officials, including HHS, FBI, and Homeland Security, are working together to find out more about this situation. Updates will be made as soon as officials know more.
- If you are near the *xxx area* [add information], protect yourself and your family by staying home or where you are and wait for further instructions.
- We have challenges ahead, and we are working to find out more about this situation. By staying informed and following instructions from health officials, you can protect yourself, your family, and the community against this public health threat.
- Go to [insert local media information here] to hear the latest information from local officials.
- For more information on chemical agents, go to the HHS Web site at www.hhs.gov, the Centers for Disease Control and Prevention's Chemical Emergencies Web site at http://www.bt.cdc.gov/chemical/, or call the CDC Hotline at 1-800-CDC-INFO for the latest updates.

Source: CDC. http://emergency.cdc.gov/firsthours/intro.asp

context for the issue being mapped. **Box 16–7** shows one of 65 message maps developed by the U.S. Department of Health and Human Services for avian influenza and pandemic influenza.[16]

Some communication experts feel that message maps can be confining and make the speaker sound too rehearsed. They recommend that spokespersons keep a list of the key points available instead. Message maps probably work best when used to prepare materials ahead of time to ensure that the most important concepts are presented prominently, succinctly and in simple language. Having more than 10 maps for a subject will also likely lead to confusion.

COMMUNICATING DURING AN EMERGENCY

In an emergency, what you can *not* do is wait until all the information is in to craft the perfect message. CERC's motto is, "Be First. Be Right. Be Credible." And we learned that getting to the audience and establishing a trusting partnership will set the tone for how they hear and respond to what you say. Your first communications need to let the audience know:

Box 16–6 Anticipated Questions-and-Answers Worksheet

Use these worksheets to write anticipated questions about a specific event; then develop appropriate answers for the public and sound bites for the media.

Step 1: Review the following list of questions commonly asked by the media. The spokesperson should have answers to these questions prepared and change/update as necessary throughout the duration of the crisis:

Questions Commonly Asked by Media in a Crisis (Covello, 1995)

- What is your (spokesperson's) name and title?
- What effect will it have on production and employment?
- What happened? (Examples: How many people were injured or killed? How much property damage occurred?)
- What safety measures were taken?
- When did it happen?
- Who is to blame?
- Where did it happen?
- Do you accept responsibility?
- What do you do there?
- Has this ever happened before?
- Who was involved?
- What do you have to say to the victims?
- Why did it happen? What was the cause?
- Is there danger now?
- What are you going to do about it?
- Will there be inconvenience to the public?
- Was anyone hurt or killed? What are their names?
- How much will it cost the organization?
- How much damage was caused?
- When will we find out more?

Step 2: Using the following Answer Development Model, draft answers for the public and sound bites for the news media in the space provided after the model. Then go back and check your draft answers against the model. Don't forget that sound bites for the news media should be eight seconds or less and framed for television, radio, or print media.

ANSWER DEVELOPMENT MODEL

In your answer/sound bite, you should . . .	By . . .
1. Express **empathy and caring** in your first statement	<ul><li>Using a personal story</li><li>Using the pronoun "I"</li><li>Transitioning to the conclusion</li></ul>
2. State a **conclusion** (key message)	<ul><li>Limiting the number of words (5–20)</li><li>Using positive words</li><li>Setting it apart with introductory words, pauses, inflections, etc.</li></ul>
3. **Support** the conclusion	<ul><li>At least two facts</li><li>An analogy</li><li>A personal story</li><li>A credible third party</li></ul>

continues

4. **Repeat** the conclusion

5. Include **future action(s)** to be taken

- Using exactly the same words as the first time

- Listing specific next steps
- Providing more information about
  - Contacts
  - Important phone numbers

Source: CDC. http://emergency.cdc.gov/firsthours/intro.asp

- You are aware of the emergency.
- You care about the people who were harmed and their loved ones.
- You are putting a response in place.
- Here is what you know now.
- This is how you know it.
- Here is what you do not know.
- This is why you do not know it.
- Here is what you are doing to find out the rest.

You do not want to speculate about what you do not know, because the public will latch onto these numbers and expect them to be borne out. When they are not, credibility goes down. It is also critically important that experts agree on facts and speak with one voice. Inconsistent messages will increase anxiety and quickly diminish experts' credibility. Finally, and most importantly, the first words out of your mouth need to show your empathy and caring.

Box 16–7 Pre-Event Message Map for Pandemic Influenza

Stakeholder: Public and Media
Question or Concern: How is pandemic influenza different from seasonal flu?

Key Message 1:	Key Message 2:	Key Message 3:
Pandemic influenza is caused by an influenza virus that is new to people.	The timing of an influenza pandemic is difficult to predict.	An influenza pandemic is likely to be more severe than seasonal flu.
Supporting Fact 1-1: Seasonal flu is caused by viruses that are already among people.	**Supporting Fact 2-1:** Seasonal flu occurs every year, usually during winter.	**Supporting Fact 3-1:** Pandemic influenza is likely to affect more people than seasonal flu.
Supporting Fact 1-2: Pandemic influenza may begin with an existing influenza virus that has changed.	**Supporting Fact 2-2:** Pandemic influenza has happened about 30 times in recorded history.	**Supporting Fact 3-2:** Pandemic influenza could severely affect a broader set of the population, including young adults.
Supporting Fact 1-3: Fewer people would be immune to a new influenza virus.	**Supporting Fact 2-3:** An influenza pandemic could last longer than the typical flu season.	**Supporting Fact 3-3:** A severe pandemic could change daily life for a time, including limitations on travel and public gatherings.

Source: HHS Pandemic Influenza Message Maps. Available at http://www.orau.gov/hsc/picw/PrePandemicMessages/Pandemic%20Flu%20Pre-event%20Message%20Maps.pdf.

SEVEN RECOMMENDATIONS

These recommendations, selected by the CDC Office of Communication, are a subset of recommendations developed* in the wake of the anthrax crisis.

- Be careful with risk comparisons.
- Do not over-reassure.

*http://www.psandman.com/col/part1.htm.

- Use sensitive syntax.
- Acknowledge uncertainty.
- Give people things to do.
- Stop trying to allay panic.
- Acknowledge people's fears.

Box 16–8 summarizes Sandman's recommendations on these seven issues. It intersperses his words with those of the ERC CDCynergy authors.[17]

Box 16–8 Sandman's Communication Advice for Emergencies

These are selected from among 26 recommendations made by Peter Sandman to the CDC in the aftermath of the anthrax attacks. The full set of recommendations is available on his website,* and it remains the most thoughtful work you can find on the subject.

RECOMMENDATION 1: BE CAREFUL WITH RISK COMPARISONS

The true risk and perceived risk can be quite different. The source of the risk can be as troubling as the degree of risk. People do not like injustice. If they perceive that the risk has been imposed on them, that they have been unfairly singled out to experience the risk, or that a fellow human being deliberately put them in the position to be exposed to the risk, they are likely to perceive the risk with more concern or outrage. Dr. Peter Sandman cautions about risk comparisons in the following way by exploring both the true risk and the perception of that risk. He defines "hazard" as the seriousness of a risk from a *technical* perspective:

"Outrage" is the seriousness of the risk in *nontechnical* terms. Experts view risk in terms of hazard; the rest of us view it in terms of outrage. The risks we overestimate are high-outrage and low-hazard. The risks we underestimate are high-hazard and low-outrage.

When technical people try to explain that a high-outrage, low-hazard risk is not very serious, they normally compare it to a high-hazard, low-outrage risk. "This is less serious than that," the experts tell us, "so if you are comfortable with that, you ought to be comfortable with this." In hazard terms, the comparison is valid. But the audience is thinking in outrage terms, and viewed in outrage terms the comparison appears false. Although "this" is lower *hazard* than "that," it is still higher *outrage*.

Terrorism is high-outrage and (for most of us, so far) low-hazard. You cannot effectively compare it to a low-outrage, high-hazard risk, such as driving a car—which is voluntary, familiar, less dreaded, and mostly under our own control. Even naturally acquired anthrax fails to persuade as a basis for comparison. People are justifiably more angry and frightened about terrorist anthrax attacks than about other natural outbreaks, even if the number of people attacked is low.

High Hazard	High Outrage
Low Hazard	Low Outrage

A volatile risk comparison can work if it is clear that you are trying to inform the public's judgment, not coerce it. If you are trying to inform the public about a risk, the most effective thing to do would be to bracket the risk: bigger than "X," smaller than "Y." If you only report that the risk is smaller than "Y," your audience can tell that they are being coerced.

To use risks for comparison, they should be similar in the type and level of emotion they would generate. Here is a risk comparison that can work:

Research indicates that a person is 10 times more likely to be killed by brain damage from a falling coconut than to be killed by a shark. In this case, the risks are both natural in origin, fairly distributed, exotic, and outside the control of the individual. Although

continues

*http://www.psandman.com/col/part1.htm

being killed by a shark may cause greater terror or emotion, its comparison to being killed by a coconut helps the individual to see that he or she may be perceiving the risk as greater than it is. Most people have never considered their risk of dying by coconut.

Remember that all risks are not accepted equally. The following are examples:

- Voluntary versus involuntary
- Controlled personally versus controlled by others
- Familiar versus exotic
- Natural versus manmade
- Reversible versus permanent
- Statistical versus anecdotal
- Fairly versus unfairly distributed
- Affecting children versus affecting adults.

If you use risk comparisons, be sure to tell people how confident you are. Acknowledge uncertainty, especially beforehand (talking about future possible risks), but also in mid-crisis. The worst thing about risk comparison is the implication that you actually know how big the risk is, and thus can compare it to another risk. For more on Dr. Sandman's argument against over reassuring, see the section "Being alarming versus being reassuring . . . ," of his article, "Dilemmas in Emergency Communication."

RECOMMENDATION 2: DO NOT OVER-REASSURE

Expect high outrage if an emergency event is catastrophic, unknowable, dreaded, unfamiliar, in someone else's control, morally relevant, and memorable. Too much reassurance can backfire. For example, when people are in outrage, reassurance can increase their outrage because their perception is that you are either not telling them the truth or you are not taking their concerns seriously. An example of this is the CDC's experience in Puerto Rico. Instead, tell people how scary the situation is, even though the actual numbers are small, and watch them get calmer.

Even if reassurance worked, which it does not, it is important to remember that an over-reassured public is not your goal. You want people to be concerned, vigilant, and even hyper-vigilant at first. You want people to take reasonable precautions: feel the fear, misery, and other emotions that the situation justifies.

During a crisis, if you have to amend the estimate of damage or victims, it's better to have to amend down, not up. It is "less serious than we thought" is better tolerated by the public than "it is more serious than we thought."

(It is important to note that the recommendation to "not over-reassure" is considered controversial and is not universally accepted.)

RECOMMENDATION 3: SENSITIVE SYNTAX: PUT THE GOOD NEWS IN SUBORDINATE CLAUSES

The previous section does not mean that you shouldn't give people reassuring information. Of course you should! But do not emphasize it. Especially do not emphasize that it is "reassuring," or you will trigger the other side of your audience's ambivalence.

One way to avoid this is to use "sensitive syntax." Sensitive syntax means putting the good news in subordinate clauses, with the more alarming information in the main clause. Here is an example of using sensitive syntax:

Even though we have not seen a new anthrax case in X days *(subordinate clause with good news)*, it is too soon to say we are out of the woods *(main clause with cautioning news)*. The main clause is how seriously you are taking the situation or how aggressively you are responding to every false alarm.

RECOMMENDATION 4: ACKNOWLEDGE UNCERTAINTY

Acknowledging uncertainty is most effective when the communicator both shows his or her distress and acknowledges the audience's distress: "How I wish I could give you a definite answer on that . . ." "It must be awful for people to hear how tentative and qualified we have to be, because there is still so much we do not know. . . ." More information on acknowledging uncertainty can be found in Yellow Flags: The Acid Test of Transparency (http://www.psandman.com/col/yellow.htm) and in the section "Tentativeness vs confidence . . . ," of Dr. Sandman's article, "Dilemmas in Emergency Communication."

RECOMMENDATION 5: GIVE PEOPLE THINGS TO DO

Action helps with fear, outrage, panic, and even denial. If you have things to do, you can tolerate more fear.

In an emergency, some actions communicated are directed at victims, persons exposed, or persons who have the potential to be exposed. However, those who do not need to take immediate action will be engaging in "vicarious rehearsal" regarding those recommendations and may need to substitute action of their own to ensure that they do not prematurely act on recommendations not meant for them. In an emergency, simple actions will give people back a sense of control and will help to keep them motivated to stay tuned to what is happening (versus denial, where they refuse to acknowledge the possible danger to themselves and others) and prepare them to take action when directed to do so.

When giving people something to do, give them a choice of actions matched to their level of concern. Give a range of responses: a minimum response, a maximum response, and a recommended middle response. For example, when giving a choice of actions for making drinking water safe, you could give the following range of responses:

Response Type	Example
Minimum response	"Use chlorine drops."
Maximum response	"Buy bottled water."
Recommended middle response	"We recommend boiling water for two minutes."

Another way of looking at this is a three-part action prescription:

1. You must do X.
2. You should do Y.
3. You can do Z.

This type of clarity is very important in helping people cope with emergencies.

Some of the "things to do" are different types of behaviors:

- *Symbolic behaviors:* things that don't really help externally, but help people to cope (attending a community vigil).
- *Preparatory behaviors:* things to do now that will minimize your risk if bad things happen.
- *Contingent/"if then" behaviors:* things to do not now, but only if bad things happen (implementing a family disaster plan).

The section "Democracy and individual control vs. expert decision-making" of Dr. Peter Sandman's article, "Dilemmas in Emergency Communication," provides further information on these issues.

RECOMMENDATION 6: STOP TRYING TO ALLAY PANIC

Panic is much less common than we imagine. The literature on disaster communication is replete with unfulfilled expectations of panicking "publics." Actually, people nearly always behave extremely well in crisis.

The condition most conducive to panic is not bad news; it is double messages from those in authority. People are the likeliest to panic (though still not very likely) when they feel that they cannot trust what those in authority are telling them; when they feel misled or abandoned in dangerous territory. When authorities start hedging or hiding bad news in order to prevent panic, they are likely to exacerbate the risk of panic in the process.

Experience shows that in a true emergency (matter of life and death), people do respond exceptionally well. However, it also seems that the inverse is true; that the further away the public is from the real danger (in place and time), the more likely they are to allow their emotions full range. This vicarious rehearsal ("How would I feel in an emergency? What would I do? Does this advice work for me?") can be overburdening in an emergency. Therefore, the communicator must recognize the differences among audiences. The person anticipating the "bad risk" is much more likely to respond inappropriately than the person "in the heat of the battle" who is primed to act on the information and does not have quite the same amount of time to mull it over.

The section "Planning for denial and misery vs. planning for panic" of Dr. Peter Sandman's article, "Dilemmas in Emergency Communication," provides further discussion of these issues.

RECOMMENDATION 7: ACKNOWLEDGE PEOPLE'S FEARS

When people are afraid, the worst thing to do is to pretend they are not. The second worst thing to do is to tell them they should not be afraid. Both responses leave people alone with their fears.

Even when their fear is totally unjustified, people do not respond well to being ignored; nor do they respond well to criticism, mockery, or statistics. And when the fear has some basis, these approaches are still less effective. Instead, you can acknowledge people's fears even while giving them the information they need to put those fears into context. Giving people permission to be excessively alarmed about a terrorist threat, while still telling them why they need not worry, is far more likely to reassure them.

Source: Sandman, P. ERC CDCynergy

CONCLUSION

You may hope that you will never have to deal with a disease outbreak, a hurricane, a toxic chemical spill, a terrorist strike with a dirty bomb, a chemical attack, or bioterrorism. But if you work in public health, chances are you will need to one day, even if it's "just" an outbreak of meningitis at an area college or a toxic run-off from an upstream CAFO.* For timely risk communication, public health departments need to keep their all hazards preparations up-to-date, including having solid communication plans and draft materials ready to go.

---

*Concentrated animal feeding operation. Yes, we mean, yuck!

While emergencies are never routine, the practiced expert risk communication response can be. You can become expert at emergency communication, just as you can in creating health promotion campaigns to combat child obesity or prevent neural tube defects caused by a lack of folic acid.

KEY TERMS

Causality
Emergency risk communication (ERC)
Message maps
Risk
Risk assessment
Risk perception

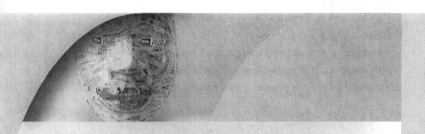

Chapter Questions

1. What is the difference between a hazard and a risk?

2. When someone asks you what the chances are from dying of a particular disease or calamity, how can you respond to their question?

3. How would you characterize "nano-particles" in make-up and the potential harm they can do to our bodies in terms of how the public appraises hazards?

4. Which of the most common concerns in risk do you worry about the most?

5. What is the difference between how we think about audiences during routine health communication and emergency risk communication?

6. What is the risk from "stigmatization" during an emergency?

7. How could you use a database like SNAPS to plan your communications?

8. Use the message template and draft an emergency message for the release of a toxic chemical on your campus.

9. Why can't you just tell everyone, "There's nothing to worry about"?

REFERENCES

1. Kennedy M (Issue Editor), *Journal of Health Communication International Perspectives.* 2003;8(Suppl. 1).

2. Sandman PM, Lanard J, *Fear Is Spreading Faster Than SARS—And So It Should!* Available at: http://www.psandman.com/col/SARS-1.htm

3. Hill AB, The environment and disease: association or causation? *Proc Roy Soc Med.* 1965;58:295–300.

4. McCallum, D. Risk communication: A tool for behavior change. In: Becker TE, David SL, Saucy G. *Reviewing the Behavioral Science Knowledge Base,* Monograph 155; 1995, Figure 1, pp. 70–71. Downloaded January 13, 2010, from http://www.nida.nih.gov/pdf/monographs/155.pdf.

5. Fischhoff B. (2009). Risk perception and communication. In Detels R, Beaglehole R, Lansang MA, Gulliford M (Eds), *Oxford Textbook of Public Health,* 5th ed. (pp. 940–952). Oxford: Oxford University Press. Reprinted in Chater NK (Ed.), *Judgement and Decision Making.* London: Sage.

6. Pollard, WE. Public perceptions of information sources concerning bioterrorism before and after anthrax attacks: an analysis of national survey data. *Journal of Health Communication International Perspectives.* 2003;8(Suppl. 1).:93–103; discussion 148–151.

7. *U.S. Environmental Protection Agency's Risk Assessment Guidance for Superfund (RAGS).* Washington, DC: Environmental Protection Agency; 1989.

8. CDC, Public Health Emergency Preparedness Cooperative Agreement. Budget Period 9 (BP9) Performance Measures Guidance, November 2008.

Accessed January 12, 2010, from: http://www.bt.cdc.gov/cotper/coopagreement/09/pdf/performance_measures_guidance_bp9.pdf.

9. http://emergency.cdc.gov/cerc/index.asp.

10. Hyer RH, Covello VT. Effective Media Communication During Public Health Emergencies. *WHO Handbook.* WHO/CDS/2005.31. Available at: http://www.who.int/csr/resources/publications/WHO%20MEDIA%20HANDBOOK.pdf.

11. McCallum. Risk communication.

12. CDCynergy Emergency Risk Communication. Phase 1, Essential Principles: Psychology. Available at: www.orau.gov/cdcynergy

13. CDC, Public Health Emergency Preparedness Cooperative Agreement. p. 42.

14. http://www.bt.cdc.gov/snaps/.

15. Covello VT. (2006) Risk communication and message mapping: A new tool for communicating effectively in public health emergencies and disasters. *J Emer Manage.* 2006;4(3):25–40.

16. HHS Pandemic Influenza Message Maps. Available at: http://www.orau.gov/hsc/picw/PrePandemicMessages/Pandemic%20Flu%20Pre-event%20Message%20Maps.pdf.

17. CDCynergy ERC Phase 1, Essential Principles: Psychology. Available at: http://www.orau.gov/cdcynergy/erc/Content/activeinformation/essential_principles/EP-psychology.htm.

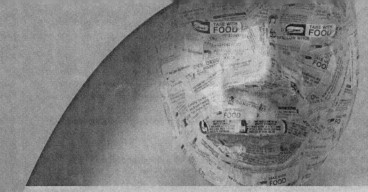

Glossary and Common Abbreviations

Many of the words used in health communication and informatics have "real-world" meanings that are somewhat different from how we use them in the field. The definitions provided here are based on *our* jargon. Unless otherwise indicated, the definitions are adapted from *CDCynergy*, the NCI "Pink Book," or other resources in the public domain such as HHS or EPA. If a definition refers to a specific organization (e.g., The Advertising Council), the definition comes from that organization's website. Definitions marked with an * come from the American Marketing Association online dictionary (http://www.marketingpower.com/_layouts/dictionary.aspx).

5-A-Day	The national campaign seeking to decrease rates of heart disease, diabetes, and some cancers by promoting consumption of at least five daily servings of fresh fruits and vegetables.
Acculturation	1. The learning of the behaviors and mores of a culture other than the one in which the individual was raised. For example, acculturation is the process by which a recent immigrant to the United States learns the American way of life. 2. The process by which people in one culture or subculture learn to understand and adapt to the norms, values, lifestyles, and behaviors of people in another culture or subculture.*
Action Theory	Guides the development of health promotion interventions by spelling out concepts that can be translated into program messages and strategies. Action Theory is different from Causal Theory in that Causal Theory helps you understand the contributing factors to a health problem, while Action Theory guides what you do about the problem. Also referred to as Change Theory or Theory of Action.
Activities	Methods used within a channel to deliver a message (e.g., the activity of holding training classes to help seniors start their own walking clubs is an example of using a community channel).
Address	A unique identifier for a computer or site online, usually a URL for a website marked with an @ for an e-mail address. Literally, it is how your computer finds a location on the information highway.*
Adopters	When we promote a new behavior, we refer to the people who take it up as "adopters." E. Rogers classified adopters into five groups according to the timing of their adoption of an innovation: (1) innovators (the first 2% to 5%); (2) early adopters (the next 10% to 15%); (3) early majority (the next 35%); (4) late majority (the next 35%); (5) laggards (the final 5% to 10%).

Advertisement

Any announcement or persuasive message placed in the mass media in paid or donated time or space by an identified individual, company, or organization.*

Advertising Council

A nonprofit organization devoted to development and placement of public service media in the United States. Its legacy includes Smokey the Bear's "Only you can prevent forest fires," the "Tearful Indian" campaign against pollution, the crash test dummies for motor safety, "A Mind Is a Terrible Thing to Waste" (for the United Negro College Fund), and more recently, "Buzzed Driving Is Drunk Driving." You may find them online at: www.adcouncil.org.

Advocacy

Any attempt to influence public opinion and attitudes that directly affect people's lives. An individual can act on his or her own to advocate for a particular cause or belief, or may be part of a highly organized network of individuals joined by a common cause.[1] Media advocacy amplifies an issue so that it is heard. Advocacy bring an issue up to a decision-making level, be it for one school, a community, or an elected official.

Affect

1. The feelings a person has toward an object such as a brand, advertisement, salesperson, etc. Affect is growing in importance in attempts to understand and predict consumer behavior. 2. The affective response itself, including emotions, specific feelings, and moods that vary in level of intensity and arousal.*

Anthropology

The study of humans, past and present. To understand the full sweep and complexity of cultures across all of human history, anthropology draws upon knowledge from the social and biological sciences as well as the humanities and physical sciences.[2] Anthropologists use "ethnographic" methods to understand the deep cultural meaning of human behavior in a specific context, be it spatial or temporal.

Appeal

A message quality that can be tailored to one's target audience(s). This term refers to the motivation within the target audience that a message strives to encourage or ignite (e.g., appeal to love of family, appeal to the desire to be accepted by peer group, fear appeal).

Arbitron ratings

Arbitron Inc. is an independent media and marketing research firm serving the media—radio, television, cable, and out-of-home—as well as advertisers and advertising agencies. They can be accessed at www.arbitron.com.
- For radio, there are two basic ratings: AQH Persons and Share.
- Average Quarter-Hour Persons (AQH Persons): The average number of persons listening to a particular station for at least 5 minutes during a 15-minute period.
- Share: The percentage of those listening to radio in the metropolitan area who are listening to a particular radio station.

[AQH persons to a station / AQH persons to all stations] $\times$ 100 = Share (%)

Ask Me 3

A patient education program designed to promote communication between healthcare providers and patients in order to improve health outcomes. The program encourages patients to understand the answers to three questions: "What is my main problem?", "What do I need to do?" and "Why is it important for me to do this?" Developed and maintained by Pfizer for the Partnership in Clear Health Communication.[3]

Association of Schools of Public Health (ASPH)[4]

The Association of Schools of Public Health represents the Council on Education for Public Health (CEPH)-accredited schools of public health located in North America. ASPH promotes the efforts of schools of public health to improve the health of every person through education, research, and policy. Based upon the belief that *"you're only as healthy as the world you live in,"* ASPH works with stakeholders to develop solutions to the most pressing health concerns and provides access to the ongoing initiatives of the schools of public health.

Attitudes

An individual's predisposition toward an object, person, or group that influences his or her response to be either positive or negative, favorable or unfavorable.

Audience

The people to whom communications are directed. (See *primary, secondary,* as well as *target audience.*)

Audience profile

A formal description of the characteristics of the people who make up a target audience. Some typical characteristics useful in describing segments include media habits (magazines, TV, newspaper, radio, and Internet), family size, residential location, education, income, lifestyle preferences, leisure activities, religious and political beliefs, level of acculturation, ethnicity, ancestral heritage, consumer purchases, and psychographics.

Audience segment(s)

A group of people who are enough alike on a set of predictors that one can develop program elements and communication activities that will likely be equally successful with all members of the segment, be it a school, a community, or an elected official.

Audience segmentation

Division of a large group of people into smaller more homogenous groupings based on shared characteristics for the purpose of communication.
• Partner-based segmentation (i.e., working through intermediary groups, which include a target audience as a constituency).
• Channel segmentation reflects personal preferences for media.
• Stage-based segmentation.
• Demographic, sociodemographic, and geographic segmentation.
• Theory-based segmentation.

Association

An observed relationship or statistical dependence between two or more events, characteristics, or variables. Association is broader than correlation and not equal to causality.

Attributes (product)

The characteristics by which products are identified and differentiated. Product attributes usually comprise features, functions, benefits, and uses. These are not equivalent to the *benefits* of the product, which are perceived by the consumer.

ATSDR

Agency for Toxic Substances and Disease Registry (part of the U.S. Department of Health and Human Services [HHS]).

Baby Boomers

Children born during the period from the end of World War II until the early 1960s (between 1943 and 1964), when the number of births increased significantly, resulting in a population surge. There was an "echo boom" beginning in 1975 of the children of the Baby Boomers (see *Millennials; Generation Y*). The group in between is referred to as *Generation X.*

Bandwidth

A measure of the amount of information (text, images, video, sound) that can be sent through a connection, usually measured in bits-per-second (bps). A full page of text is about 16,000 bits. A fast modem can move approximately 15,000 bits in one second. Full-motion full-screen video requires about 1 to 10 million bps, depending on resolution and compression.*

Banner ad   A graphical Internet advertising tool. Users click on the graphic to be taken to another website. The term "banner ad" refers to a specific size image, measuring 468 pixels wide and 60 pixels tall (i.e., 468 × 60), but it is also used as a generic description of all graphical ad formats on the Internet.*

Barriers   Hindrances to desired change. These may be factors external or internal to audience members themselves (e.g., lack of proper healthcare facilities or the belief that fate causes illness and is inescapable).

Baseline study   The collection and analysis of data regarding a target audience or situation prior to intervention. Generally, baseline data are collected in order to provide a point of comparison for an evaluation.

BEHAVE framework   A simple and widely used framework for describing an audience, a behavioral change, a motivation, and a mechanism for change developed by the Academy for Educational Development (AED).

Behavior   The overt acts or actions of individuals or groups that can be directly observed.

Behavior change theories   Theories used to explain and predict behavior. These predictors are often made up of psychosocial constructs such as attitudes, beliefs, personal characteristics, and social and environmental factors.

Behavioral lever   The crucial, rate-limiting step in a complex behavior that makes it impossible for a person to perform a desired behavior or, alternately, a facilitating step (or resource acquired) that allows the remaining steps to follow in sequence without further thought.

Belief   A term that encompasses knowledge, opinion, or faith. Also, the perceived association between two concepts. A belief is based on knowledge or meaning that refer to consumers' interpretations of important concepts. Unlike an attitude, a belief is emotionally or motivationally neutral.*

Beneficiary   The person or group of people who would benefit most directly by an intervention. Sometimes the audience and the beneficiary are the same. Sometimes others are asked to act on behalf of a third-party beneficiary, as when mothers are asked to adopt behaviors that benefit their children.

Benefit   The value provided to a customer by a product feature. It is the consumer's perceptions that define a benefit.

Best practices   A loose term that refers to interventions or strategies that have been evaluated and found to be effective in more than one trial. When sufficient evidence exists of adequate quality, these are referred to as evidence-based interventions. Best practices are not based on the highest quality evaluation data, but are recommended because of cost, ease of use, or other criteria.

Bioethics   The branch of ethics, philosophy, and social commentary that discusses the life sciences and their potential impact on our society.

Bioterrorism   The deliberate use of viruses, bacteria, or other biological agents by those wishing to cause illness or death in people, animals, or plants, thereby causing widespread fear, panic, and terror.

Blog   A hybrid form of Internet communication that combines a column, diary, and directory. The term, short for "Web log" refers to a frequently updated collection of short articles on various subjects with links to further resources.

Bounce-back cards	A preprinted, preaddressed, prepaid postcard distributed with program materials. Recipients are asked to respond to a few simple questions about the materials and then return the postcard by mail.
Branding	Like a cattleman's mark, a brand symbolizes "ownership" of a product. When a set of communication materials are branded, it usually means they carry the same format, color palette, logo, slogan, or other identifying marks to indicate where they came from. A brand has also taken on the meaning of a reputation for consumers who associate a level of quality with a particular brand. A "brand is a promise made by an organization to the consumer."[5] Many organizations have developed brands for public health programs or initiatives over the past decade.
BRFSS	Behavioral Risk Factor Surveillance System. Surveillance system managed by the Centers for Disease Control and Prevention (CDC) to assess and track health behavior, risk behavior, and health status in the population through state-based phone interviews.
Broadcast quality	The media industries' standard for material that can be aired. Technical format and content are both aspects of broadcast quality. For example, 3/4-inch video tape is broadcast quality; VHS tape is not. Publicity submissions that are not broadcast quality generally will not be used.*
B-roll	Videotaped footage that is not included in the final edited version of a video news release (VNR). B-roll is given to television stations along with the VNR to give the stations the option of putting together their own version of the story, giving more time to aspects the station feels will be of particular interest to its viewers.*
Buzz marketing	A strategy "to capture the attention of consumers and the media to the point where talking about the brand or company (or offering) becomes entertaining, fascinating and newsworthy." Source: Hughes, M. (2005). *Buzz Marketing. Get People to Talk About Your Stuff.* New York: Penguin Group, p. 2.
Case-control study	This involves collecting data, often through surveys, about past exposures among a population with some type of health issue (e.g., "cases" with a disease or condition) and comparing these data with similar data collected from a comparable control group without the disease or condition.
Causal Theory	Describes the factors that influence a behavior or situation and identifies why a problem exists. Causal theory guides the search for modifiable factors such as knowledge, attitudes, self-efficacy, social support, or lack of resources. Also referred to as problem theory, explanatory theory, or theory of the problem.
Causality	"The relating of causes to the effects they produce. . . . A cause is termed 'necessary' when it must always precede an effect. . . . A cause is termed 'sufficient' when it inevitably initiates or produces an effect. Any given cause may be necessary, sufficient, neither, or both." Source: Last, J. M. (1995). *A Dictionary of Epidemiology* (3rd ed.). New York: Oxford University Press, p. 25.
CDC	Centers for Disease Control and Prevention. The U.S. government agency dedicated to protecting health and promoting quality of life through the prevention and control of disease, injury, and disability. The CDC is an operational unit of the Department of Health and Human Services (HHS).
CDCynergy	A software tool to help program planners develop and implement health communication programs. More information at www.cdc.gov/healthmarketing/cdcynergy/.

CERC	Crisis and Emergency Risk Communication. A term the CDC coined to describe the process of communicating about risk with various publics during a complex emergency. It has been a key element in its cooperative agreements with state, local, territorial, and tribal health departments for health emergency preparedness. (See also *ERC.*)
Central-location intercept interviews	A method used for pretesting messages and materials. It involves "intercepting" potential intended audience members at a highly trafficked location (such as a shopping mall), asking them a few questions to see if they fit the intended audience's characteristics, showing them the messages or materials, and then administering a questionnaire of predominantly closed-ended questions. Because respondents form a convenience sample, the results cannot be projected rigorously to a wider population. Also called mall intercept interviews.
Channel	The conduit or route of information delivery (e.g., interpersonal, small group, organizational, community, mass media).
Cochrane Reviews[6]	Cochrane Reviews investigate the effects of interventions for prevention, treatment, and rehabilitation in a healthcare setting. They are designed to facilitate the choices that doctors, patients, policymakers and others face in health care. Most Cochrane Reviews are based on randomized controlled trials, but other types of evidence may also be taken into account, if appropriate. Reviews are published in the Cochrane Library, by the Cochrane Collaboration, which is a global network of volunteers.
Cognitive interview	A qualitative method that asks participants to comment on their own thought processes in reference to some stimuli, such as a survey. Often used in the development or pre-testing phase. Two primary techniques are the think-aloud interview and verbal probing.
Cognitive research	A number of techniques derived from psychology that help us understand how we process information. These techniques have been applied to communication and marketing research for decades.
Cohort studies	These consist of a group of individuals for whom data are either collected prospectively (going forward) or for whom historical data of some type exist (retrospective or looking backward). Data are examined for changes over time, such as in a subgroup exposed to some sort of "treatment," or stimulus (e.g., a chemical in an occupational environment), compared with an unexposed subgroup.
Communication	The use of messages to transmit meanings within and across various contexts, cultures, channels, and media.[7]
Communication theory	Explores how messages are created, transmitted, received, and assimilated. When applied to public health problems, the central question that theories of communication seek to answer is, "How do communication processes contribute to, or discourage, behavior change?"
Community	A group of persons joined together for a common purpose, be it geographical, social, or cultural or because they share and want to discuss an illness, a condition, or a hobby. Can exist in real space and time, or in virtual settings using communication channels, such as the Internet. In public health, the term usually refers to geographically local residents who participate in, and/or own and manage an intervention.
Community-Based Organizations	CBOs offer services at a community level and are usually, but not always, without a profit motive. They often serve a larger geographic area than one neighborhood.

Community Guide[8]   The *Guide to Community Preventive Services* is a free resource offering systematic reviews that answer these questions: Which program and policy interventions have been proven effective? Are there effective interventions that are right for my community? What might effective interventions cost, and what is the likely return on investment? Reviews are prepared by the Task Force on Community Preventive Services, an independent body of researchers and practitioners.

Competence/competency   Measured by observable characteristics of a skill or ability, competency is the standardized requirement for an individual to properly perform a specific task. It encompasses a combination of knowledge, skills, and behavior.

Competition   In social marketing, this refers to what the intended user is doing now, or using now, instead of the behavior or product promoted to improve their health. Sometimes this is just using brand X over brand Y. But, sometimes competition comes from outside the same category, such as drinking sugary soda in place of low-fat milk.

Comprehension   The degree to which transmitted messages are understood. Can be estimated qualitatively (e.g., low comprehension) or measured quantitatively (e.g., 30% comprehension).

Concepts   Ideas that can be communicated symbolically or artistically for discussion, sometimes referring to something broad (like germ theory) or something new (e.g., nanorobotics).

Concept testing   The process of exposing representatives of the target audience to creative interpretations of ideas on which you might base your message. This process usually requires qualitative research, such as focus groups.

Confirmation bias   A tendency to interpret messages as confirmation of what we already believe (i.e., "He only hears what he wants to hear").

Consensus (scientific)   Agreement by body of scientists about best or optimal strategy in a particular situation, often sought when definitive data are not available. May be based on a meta-analysis, independent studies, or other forms of comparative research.

Consumer   Traditionally, the ultimate user or consumer of goods, ideas, and services. The term is also used to refer to the buyer or decision-maker rather than the ultimate consumer. A mother buying cereal for a small child to eat is often called the consumer, although she is not the ultimate user.*

Consumer-Generated Media (CGM)   Websites that are created using Web 2.0 technologies (such as blogs, wikis, and social networking sites) often use their membership to generate at least a portion of the site's content. This is generally referred to as user-generated content (UGC), user-created content (UCC), or CGM.

Convenience sample   Collection of respondents in research studies that are typical of the target audience and are easily accessible. No attempt is made to collect a probability sample, and convenience samples are not statistically representative of the entire population being studied. Therefore, findings from studies using convenience samples are not generalizable.

Correlational studies   A term from psychology describing a series of studies to examine the association of variables.

Creative brief   A document that includes information that will be needed by a creative team in order to develop concepts and messages. The brief contains information about your primary target audience as well as settings, channels, and activities for reaching them. Promising message variables and thoughts on what materials will be needed are included. Secondary audiences are also profiled.

Credibility

A quality that allows a messenger to be trusted by the recipient of the message. Some components of credibility include whether the message source is trustworthy, believable, reputable, competent, and knowledgeable.

Cross-sectional studies

This involves collecting data from subjects at one time, the most typical cross-sectional study being a survey. The major drawback of this type of study design is that data are collected on potential exposures and outcomes at the same time, making it difficult to determine if exposures actually *preceded* potential outcomes of interest.

Culture

The acquired knowledge people use to interpret experience and generate behavior. (Spradley, J. (1998). Participant observation. In R. Bodgdan & S. Biklen. *Qualitative research for education: An introduction to theory and methods* (3rd ed.). Boston: Allyn and Bacon.). Culturally constructed phenomena are any experiences that we shape by our perceptions, values, attitudes, and beliefs. We take many things for granted as "natural" that are actually cultural constructions, such as definitions of sickness and health.

Delivery (assessment)

Studies the functioning of components of program implementation. Includes assessments of whether materials are being distributed to the right people and in the correct quantities, the extent to which program activities are being carried out as planned and modified if needed, and other measures of how and how well the program is working. Sometimes referred to as process evaluation.

Delphi method

A small-group research technique that seeks a consensus among experts through sequential rounds of data collection and reduction.

Demographics

Individual descriptors such as sex, age, ethnicity, income, or education that can be collected from a target audience and that can be useful for defining the target audience and understanding how to communicate more effectively with the target audience.

Deontological principles

Duty-based principles. They require honorably following rules, due to the belief that you cannot achieve a just outcome (or end) through unjust means.

Description

In journalism, refers to providing the basic facts of who, what, where, and when. Answering "why" and "how" often gets into explanation or interpretation.

Diffusion of Innovations

A theory by E. Rogers that addresses change in a group rather than an individual. This could be a classroom, an organization, or a community. The theory describes how new ideas, or innovations, are spread within the group. According to this theory, innovations spread via different communication channels within social systems over a specific period of time. Source: Rogers, EM. (1995). *Diffusion of innovations* (4th ed.). New York: Free Press. (See *adopters.*)

Direct costs

The part of the budget that contributes directly to a program's outputs. Direct costs are made up of personnel costs (salary and benefits) as well as "out-of-pocket" costs associated with products and services not obtained through a salaried employee. (See also *Indirect costs.*)

Document

Term used in literacy studies to refer to text presented in tables, forms, graphs, or other structured formats. Contrasts with "prose," which is written in sentences and paragraphs.

Doer versus non-doer analysis   The anthropological concept behind this marketing term is "positive deviance."[9] Formative research technique that involves identifying individuals performing a desirable trbehavior and finding out how and why they are doing it. These "doers" are compared to individuals not performing the behavior to see if their experiences can be promoted to the others to inspire them to also adopt the behavior.

Downstream   A term used in social or health policy to describe making a change near the end point of an ecological process, such as at the community or individual level. (See also *upstream*). Also refers to a story about a project that is completed for advocacy purposes.

Earned media   Usually mass media coverage of a story that is earned through public service methods. While no money changes hands between the sponsor and the media broadcast company, there is usually an agency that develops and places the story for a fee, or *pro bono (for the good; i.e., no charge)*.

Ecological Model   The public health principle that health and well-being are affected by *interaction* among multiple determinants including biology, behavior, and the environment. Interaction unfolds over the life course of individuals, families, and communities. An ecological *approach* to health is one in which multiple strategies are developed to impact determinants of health relevant to the desired health outcomes.

Ecologic studies   These typically involve correlating or comparing two types of population-level data. While they can be valuable for generating hypotheses (e.g., smoking prevalence tends to be higher in areas where populations have lower socioeconomic status), they can produce misleading results because data correlation does not mean causation.

Ecology   The study of the relations among living species and their physical and biotic environments, particularly adaptations to environments through the mechanisms of various systems.

EEG   See *electroencephalography*.

Effectiveness   The ability of an intervention to produce the desired beneficial effect in a real-world setting (see, in contrast, *efficacy*). Usually refers to the performance of a drug taken by patients in a nonconstrained situation.

Effects evaluation   A measure of the extent to which a program accomplished its stated goals and objectives. Also called impact, outcome, or summative evaluation.

Efficacy   The ability of an intervention to produce the desired beneficial effect in expert hands and under ideal circumstances. Usually refers to the performance of a drug under controlled metabolic trial. Sometimes used casually to mean effectiveness.

Elaboration Likelihood Model (ELM)   This suggests that if you are already engaged in an issue, you will pay more attention to new information about this issue. If you are not engaged, you need peripheral stimuli to grab your attention.

Electroencephalography (EEG)   When groups of neurons are activated in the brain, small electrical currents are generated, resulting in electrical fields. Using electrodes on the scalp, EEG signals can be detected and amplified for analysis over time. These brain waves measure different brain processes.

Enabling factors   Part of PRECEDE analysis. Enabling factors are largely structural, such as the availability of resources, time, or skills that allow someone to perform a behavior.

Entertainment education The process of purposely designing and implementing a media message to both entertain and educate; a communication strategy to bring about behavioral and social change.

EPA Environmental Protection Agency. The federal agency formed in 1970 that regulates the amount of pollutants manufacturers can emit.

ERC Emergency Risk Communication. The process of communicating about hazards and risks during an emergency. Involves three stages of planning, implementation, and follow-up evaluation. (See also *CERC*.)

Ethnography What cultural anthropologists do when they study a group of people and their life-ways. Also refers to the published study.

Evaluation Assessment of components of an intervention by comparing what was expected to what was observed. Types of evaluation discussed in text include formative, delivery/implementation, cost/benefit, exposure/reach, effects, and theory-based evaluation.

Evidence-based intervention An intervention that has been tested in several different settings and that has demonstrated both efficacy and effectiveness.

Eye-tracking technology Using a head-mounted camera and computer screens designed for this purpose, it is possible to detect and measure eye movements and gaze fixation as we look at an image (moving or still) or text. Our innate response to imminent danger, or arousal, causes our pupils to dilate and our blink rate to change. All can be measured photographically and can be used to measure reading ease as well as a subject's interest in an image, video, or text.

Executive summary An overview of a project, evaluation, or research findings generally presented at the beginning of a report that highlights such issues as activities that took place, why a study was conducted, how it was carried out, and results and recommendations.

Experimental studies These studies involve researchers "exposing" a group of subjects (e.g., people or animals) to an intervention and comparing the results to those of a statistically similar group of unexposed subjects.

Expert review Examination and critique of program plans or materials by selected people who are knowledgeable in a relevant content area.

Exposure Contact by a person or animal with a chemical or physical agent.

Exposure (media) Measures the extent to which a message was disseminated (i.e., how many members of the target audience encountered the message). However, this type of evaluation does not measure whether audience members paid attention to the message or whether they understood, believed, or were motivated by it. A part of process evaluation.

External validity One criterion by which an experiment is evaluated. Refers to the extent to which populations, settings, and observed experimental effects can be generalized.

Fear A mental state that motivates problem-solving behavior if our intuitive "fight or flight" options are available. If these options are not available, it motivates other defense mechanisms such as denial or suppression, which are antithetical to rational decision making.

Fear appeals	Messaging that attempts to elicit a response from the target audience using fear as a motivator (e.g., fear of injury, illness, loss of a loved one). Fear appeals were once very popular before we fully understood their negative consequences.
FCC	Federal Communications Commission. The federal regulatory agency responsible for supervising radio and television broadcasting, including cable and satellite television.
FDA	Food and Drug Administration. This federal agency was created by the Pure Food and Drug Act of 1906. The FDA has the power to set standards for foods and food additives, to establish tolerances for deleterious substances and pesticides in foods, and to prohibit the sale of adulterated and misbranded foods, drugs, cosmetics, and devices. All new drugs must be submitted to the FDA for approval, and applications must be supported by extensive laboratory testing indicating efficacy and safety.
Fidelity monitoring	Ensuring that program activities are still faithful to their original objectives through periodic data collection.
Focus group	A formative research technique that convenes a small group of people (usually 8 to 10) who share certain characteristics for a discussion of selected topics. It generally follows a prepared guide and is led by a trained moderator. Focus groups provide creative themes and user language. The qualitative results may be extremely useful even though they are not necessarily representative of a larger audience.
Folic acid	A B-vitamin that is essential to human health. It is required for the body to make DNA and RNA, the blueprints for development of all cells. It is especially vital to a developing embryo because rapid cell division occurs early in fetal development. Consuming folic acid before conception and through the first month of pregnancy will prevent 50% to 75% of neural tube defects from occurring.
Formative research	The information-gathering activities conducted prior to developing a health communication strategy. Includes measurement of the extent to which concepts, messages, materials, activities, and channels meet researchers' expectations with the target audience.
Fotonovela	From the Spanish *foto* = photo + *novela* = short novel. Fotonovelas are typically soap opera–like stories told through the use of photos of characters with their thoughts or conversations written in "balloons" or in captions, as in comic books. Very popular medium for role model approaches. A medium that has moved from south of the border to "El Norte" in terms of its popularity.
Framing	Words (or sometimes images) used to put a message or a data point in a desired context. For example, if your chances of winning the lottery are 1 in 1 million, a positive frame states that 1 person out of 1 million will be a big winner. A negative frame states that 999,999 people out of 1 million will lose. Different frames lead people to draw different conclusions, even when the same data are being discussed.
Framing bias	When questions or answers are phrased in a way that, while technically accurate, still misleads people to interpret information incorrectly. The use of relative versus absolute risk is often used this way. For example, if a treatment increases five-year survival from 1% to 2%, it is misleading to say that survival has been doubled. The risk of death in five years remains 98%!
Free listing	A formative research technique in which a respondent is asked to list out all the examples of a particular kind of thing that they know about. For example, you might ask for a list of "appropriate foods

for young children," "the most important qualities in a man," or "flu-like symptoms." The researcher records these items, usually onto separate index cards.

Functional Magnetic Resonance Imaging (fMRI)	Regional cerebral blood flow is directly related to regional brain activity. Functional magnetic resonance imaging measures the change in blood flow in regions of the brain by means of the increased magnetic resonance of oxygenated blood in contrast to nonoxygenated blood. This provides high-resolution, three-dimensional images of brain activity, including its response to different products, stimuli, or situations.
Gallup Poll[10]	See *polls.*
Galvanic skin response (GSR)	Commonly known as a lie-detector test, GSR is a measure of the electrical current that passes along the surface of the skin. Because perspiration conducts electricity much better than dry skin, a minute increase in perspiration resulting from an emotional response can be detected as an increase in electrical conductance. GSR is painless and can be measured easily using uncomplicated devices and computer display. In addition to its contribution to criminology, GSR has been used to gauge attention to and emotional response to media. While an emotional response can be detected with GSR, there is no way to know the nature of the actual underlying emotion without asking the subject.
Gatekeepers	Persons who have a reputation, or perceived responsibility, for upholding standards in a community. They can help support a behavior change goal if they agree with it, or prevent its adoption if they disagree. Very often, popular clergy members, business leaders, or healthcare providers may be community gatekeepers, and it is wise to seek their input when planning an intervention.
Generalizable finding	A study result from which you can make reliable inferences about a larger population of people, places, or settings similar to those included in the sample for the study (i.e., all the criteria for external validity have been satisfied).
Generation X	Children born following the Baby Boom. (See *Baby Boomers.*)
Generation Y	Children of the Baby Boomers. Also known as *Millennials.*
Gestalt (German)	A wholeness. With the added meaning that the whole is greater than the sum of the parts. The *gestalt* effect refers to the process whereby the brain takes in incomplete sensory data and, based on prior experience, completes it to form a perceived object. This is the basis for many optical illusions and some of the differences in audience perception and observer bias. (See *image.*)
Gray literature	Unpublished reports, usually prepared for government agencies. Not peer-reviewed but often accurate and authoritative. More commonly available now on program websites or through agency resources.
GRP	Gross Rating Point. One percentage point of a specified target audience. Total GRPs for a campaign can be calculated by the following formula: Reach × Average frequency. This is a measure of the advertising weight delivered by a medium or media within a given time period. A given total of gross rating points may be arrived at by adding together ratings from many different spots. GRPs may, thus, sum to more than 100% of the total target audience.*
Harris Interactive Poll	See *polls.*
Hazard	The real qualitative possibility of an adverse event occurring under a specific set of conditions. Generally, hazard = danger. (See also *toxicity* and *risk.*)

Headline	The top component of a newspaper, magazine, online article, or print advertisement that is meant to attract the reader's attention and provide a very brief summary of the information.
Health	A state of complete physical, mental, and social well-being and not merely the absence of disease or infirmity. (World Health Organization, 1948)
Health 2.0	The use of social software and its ability to promote collaboration among patients, their caregivers, medical professionals, and other stakeholders in health.
Health behavior	An action performed by an individual that can negatively or positively affect his or her health (e.g., smoking, exercising).
Health Belief Model (HBM)	This model was first developed to explain individual public health behaviors, such as participation in free tuberculosis screening programs. In the HBM, individual beliefs motivate or discourage health behaviors such as perceived susceptibility, perceived severity, perceived benefits of interventions, perceived costs of intervention, cues to activate behavior change, perceived ability to act (self-efficacy).
Health communication	The study and use of communication strategies to inform and influence individual and community decisions that enhance health. (See also *public health communication*.)
Health literacy	The ability to understand and use complex health information.
Heuristic	The simplified "rules of thumb" by which decisions are made.*
Hierarchy of Effects (HOE) Model	With a "source" sending information out to a "receiver," the lower-level effects sought by McGuire were exposure, attention, interest, and comprehension. A higher-order set of effects included acquisition of skills, changes in attitude, short-term retention of information, long-term retention, decision making, one-time performance of a behavior, reinforcement of the behavior, and maintenance of the behavior indefinitely through complex life changes.
HTML	Hyper Text Markup Language is a coding language used to make hypertext documents for use on the Web. HTML resembles old-fashioned typesetting code, where a block of text is surrounded by codes that indicate how it should appear. HTML allows text to be "linked" to another file on the Internet.*
Image	The consumer perception of a product, institution, brand, business, or person that may or may not correspond with "reality" or "actuality." For marketing purposes the "image of what is" may be more important than "what actually is."*
Impact evaluation	See *effects evaluation*. Impact is generally an assessment of health results and not behavioral change.
Impression	Term of art used in advertising to refer to a single view or display of an ad. Ad reports list total impressions per ad, which tells you the number of times your ad was served by the search engine when searchers entered your keywords (or viewed a content page containing your keywords). (*Synonym: media impressions*.)*
IMR	Infant Mortality Rate. The number of deaths of children under one year of age per one thousand live births in the same year. IMR = 1,000 × Infant deaths/Live births.[11]
In-depth interviews	A qualitative research method involving a one-on-one discussion between an interviewer and a respondent about selected topics. The structure and interviewing style are more flexible than in surveys using a questionnaire.

Indirect costs	Also called "overhead," these are expenses that it costs your agency to exist, but that are not tied directly to creating the program's outputs. Examples usually include office space, environmental management (heat, air conditioning, water, custodial services, etc.), and depreciation on equipment. Indirect costs are usually calculated as a percentage of direct costs. Institutions that perform work under government contract negotiate and set their indirect cost rate annually.
Informatics	"The effective organization, analysis, management, and use of information."[12] (See also *public health informatics.*)
Information processing theory	The mental processes by which consumers interpret information from the environment to make it meaningful and integrate that information to make decisions. A communication theory that focuses on how the mind receives, stores, retrieves, and uses information, addressing, for example, the mental processes by which consumers interpret and integrate information and use it in decision making.
Informed consent	Studies involving human subjects need to be reviewed by Institutional Review Boards (IRBs) for this purpose. This is referred to as "IRB approval." An important aspect is how you inform the participants about the study, and their ability to give consent based on this information.
Inform/persuade paradigm	A categorization of health communication programs into those that intend to provide new information to audiences, and possibly facilitate decision making, from those that promote behavior change. Put differently, communications that seek to build knowledge in contrast to those that seek to prompt action. This is a *paradigm* because either choice has its own set of principles and guidelines for success.
In-kind contributions	In the nonprofit world in which public health often operates, organizations frequently consider their time, their space, use of equipment, and other in-house resources as "in-kind" contributions to a project budget. These will be used to produce program outputs but are not factored into the direct or indirect costs of the budget. Some donors will expect to see a match made of their investment through direct financial, in-kind resources or additional donations.
Integrative Model	The most important assumption of the IM is that the best predictor of behavior is *intention* to perform the behavior. Thus, this model focuses on the antecedents, or predictors, of an individual's intention to perform (or not perform) a behavior.
Intention	A cognitive plan to perform a behavior or action ("I intend to go shopping later"), created through a choice/decision process that focuses on beliefs about the consequences of the action.*
Interpersonal channel	A communication channel that involves dissemination of messages through one-on-one communication (e.g., mentor to student, friend to friend, pharmacist or doctor to patient).
Interval scale	An equal interval scale involves assignment of values with a natural distance between them, so that a particular distance (interval) between two values in one region of the scale meaningfully represents the same distance between two values in another region of the scale (e.g., for temperature, date of birth).[11] A linear scale has equal intervals, like a ruler. A logarithmic scale does not, nor do many qualitative scales.
Involvement	The degree of personal relevance a consumer perceives a product, brand, object, or behavior to have. High-involvement products are seen as having important personal consequences or as useful for achieving important personal goals. Low-involvement products are not linked to important consequences or goals.*

JIC	Joint Information Center. Used in emergency communication. A facility established to coordinate all incident-related public information activities. It is the central point of contact for all news media at the scene of the incident. JICs gather information, verify it, and produce news products for the media and other stakeholders. Other tasks for the JIC include (1) monitoring news coverage to ensure accurate information is being disseminated and received properly, while correcting incorrect information about the emergency response that appears in the news media; (2) managing news conferences and press operations for disaster area tours; (3) providing basic facilities to assist the news media in disseminating information to the public and to credential media representatives; (4) providing all stakeholders directly or indirectly affected by the emergency with access to timely and accurate information about response, recovery, and mitigation activities and their limitations; and (5) ensuring government communication resources are managed effectively and duplication of effort by departments is minimized.[13]
JPEG	Joint Photographic Experts Group. JPEG (also JPG, pronounced "jay peg") is a graphics format, newer than GIF, which displays photographs and graphic images with many colors. It also compresses well and is easy to download.
Joke	Something that you find funny. This is a joke. (Really. This is a joke.) Humor is a form of appeal that requires more skill than might be suspected, because people vary so greatly in terms of what they find funny. What seems funny in a small group may be interpreted very differently by the audience of a large media campaign. (Think about the difference between telling someone something and sending them an e-mail!)
Key informants	Persons or organizations whose opinions can be seen as representative of a community or target audience because of their experience or expertise with the target audience.
Keyword stuffing	Generally refers to the act of adding an inordinate number of keyword terms into the HTML or tags of a Web page.*
Latent need	Something that you didn't realize you needed. A marketing concept for stimulating desire in a consumer for a product.
LEP	Limited English Proficiency. When clients or patients do not speak English well enough to understand instructions or questions. Often (incorrectly) used to refer to people, and not their abilities.
Likert-type scales	The typical five-point (or more) scale that asks a respondent to choose a response ranging from strongly disagree to strongly agree, strongly approve to strongly disapprove, or any other condition that can be measured in this manner.
Literacy	The ability to use printed and written information to function in society, to achieve one's goals, and to develop one's knowledge and potential. Refers to an individual's ability to make sense of information in any form in which it is presented. While it was once sufficient to sign your name to be considered literate, the definition has acquired a larger meaning of social competence.
Living room language	Using commonplace words and analogies to explain phenomena that are outside most persons' experience.
Logic Model	A visual design of how a problem will be solved through an intervention; the structured flow of inputs, outputs, outcomes, and goals obtained.

Macro plan	A preliminary plan that includes the analysis of the problem, the ecological setting, the affected populations, the core intervention strategy, and any additional research necessary to understand those persons affected by the problem and/or with whom you plan to communicate.
Market research	The systematic gathering, recording, and analyzing of data with respect to a particular market, where *market* refers to a specific customer group in a specific geographic area.*
Materials	Tangible products, using a medium, that contain the message to be delivered to the target audience (e.g., a brochure, a PSA tape, or a script for an oral presentation).
Maven	A Yiddish word meaning "expert." Malcolm Gladwell uses this term to describe an *opinion leader* (see definition of that term) in *The Tipping Point* (2000).
Media (*pl.* medium)	Any material or format used to convey a message. In health communication, predominantly print, electronic, audio, or visual. Sometimes used to refer to broadcast journalism.
Media advocacy	Using the mass media strategically to advance a social or policy initiative. Often involves staging events that the news media cover including protest gatherings, release of a report or survey, or other gatherings of people who seem concerned about an issue. In the political arena, it has become the predominant strategy, including purchased advertising. May also involve use of public service announcements. (See *PSA*.)
Media impressions	The extent of readership or viewership or listenership claimed by a specific media outlet (e.g., radio station, website). Impressions are only *opportunities* for message exposure.
Media kit	A package for journalists that includes items for print or broadcast that provides press releases, contact information, camera-ready copies of print materials, video and audio formats, and a backgrounder with more in-depth information.
Media literacy	"An informed, critical understanding of the mass media. It involves examining the techniques, technologies and institutions involved in media production; being able to critically analyze media messages; and recognizing the role audiences play in making meaning from those messages."[14] Improving media literacy is a health communication strategy has been used effectively with middle school students to enable them to evaluate tobacco, food, and other advertising directed toward them as consumers.
Media relations	The management of communication between an organization and its publics, primarily through the news media. In a large organization, it may be a large group that releases information to the news as well as responds to media and online questions.
Media tracking	The monitoring of radio, television, and print media over a specified period of time for a specific topic or message. Data gathered can be analyzed for content or trends in amount in coverage.
Message	The memorable, explanatory words or images that convey an idea. In health communication, the literal words or images that communicate what you want people to know, feel, or do.
Message map	A visual framework used to organize a body of information into simple, short talking points. Message maps have been predominantly used in emergency risk communication. A typical map is directed to a specific audience (e.g., the public, emergency victims) and answers one question with up to three key messages. The map provides a handy reference for a spokesperson, and multiple spokespersons

can work from the same message map to ensure the rapid dissemination of consistent and core messages. In addition, using maps minimizes the chance of a speaker saying something inappropriate or not saying something that should have been said. A printed message map allows spokespersons to check off the talking points as they are covered. This helps to prevent omissions of key facts or misstatements that could provoke misunderstandings, controversy, or outrage.[15]

Meta-analysis	A study in which a researcher analyzes a body of published results on a specific topic. Using a set of well-defined rules for selecting studies and data sources, statistical approaches are used to pool data from multiple studies on the same topic and calculate a summary measure estimating the level of association between two variables. Meta-analyses extend the value of review articles, which may offer no pooled quantitative data. They are being used increasingly as the basis for evidence-based recommendations.
Meta-message	The larger context shaping the interpretation of a message. Without getting too complicated, it is often the part of a statement that is not said, but what you are "trying to say." For example, if you make a lot of statements about the need to support the troops in Iraq and Afghanistan, you are sending a meta-message of patriotism.
Millennial generation	Sometimes referred to as Generation Y (following Generation X), or the echo Baby Boom; the children born between 1982 and 1995.
Mixed methods	A research design that combines quantitative and qualitative methods. These may be sequenced or done at the same time and compared, or "triangulated," to draw an additional conclusion.
Moderator's guide	A set of questions, probes, and discussion points used by a focus group moderator to help him or her facilitate the group. A guide can also contain reminders of which questions are most important to the research to help the moderator use discussion time effectively.
Morbidity	Rate of disease, infirmity, or disability. Often expressed as the number of cases per 1,000 individuals per year.
Mortality	Rate of death, often expressed as the number of deaths per 1,000 individuals per year.
***Morbidity and Mortality Weekly Report* (MMWR)**	Catchy title of the CDC's weekly release of epidemiological findings, special studies, or recommendations pertaining to disease and death in the United States or globally.
NAAL	National Assessment of Adult Literacy.
National Cancer Institute (NCI)	Established under the National Cancer Institute Act of 1937; the federal government's principal agency for cancer research and training. NCI oversees the National Cancer Program. Over the years, legislative amendments have maintained the NCI's authorities and responsibilities and added new information dissemination mandates, as well as a requirement to assess the incorporation of state-of-the-art cancer treatments into clinical practice. NCI is a Center within the National Institutes of Health (NIH), an operating unit of the Department of Health and Human Services (HHS).[16]
Neuromarketing	Marketing research that uses methods and data derived from neuroscience such as EEG, fMRI, galvanic skin response (GSR), and the like to predict audience response to media and messages. (See *neuroscience*.)

Neuroscience   The study of the nervous system, which includes the brain, the spinal cord, and networks of sensory nerve cells, or neurons, throughout the body. Neuroscientists use tools ranging from computers to special dyes to examine molecules, nerve cells, networks, brain systems, and behavior. From these studies, they learn how the nervous system develops and functions normally and what goes wrong in neurological disorders.[17]

News peg   The main point of a news release that justifies to the media the value of using the story. A news peg generally links the story to current events or concerns. It may be of use for a few hours to a few days, but apart from a long-term event (e.g., political campaign), the main news peg is relevant to something that just happened.

Nielsen   Nielsen describes itself as "The world's leading marketing and media information company." Nielsen measures and analyzes how people interact with digital platforms, traditional media, and in-store environments—locally as well as globally. It has long been known for estimating the size of television audiences, with "Nielsen" ratings determining which shows stay on the air or are discontinued.

Nominal scale   Classification into unordered qualitative categories (e.g., race, religion, country of birth).[11]

Numeracy   The ability to think and express oneself quantitatively. In reference to health literacy, it encompasses the knowledge and skills required to estimate quantities from food labels, use a glucometer or thermometer correctly, measure medicine doses, or any other mathematical operation necessary for nonhealth professionals to manage their own or a loved one's health care or wellness.

Objective   The desired or needed result to be achieved by a specific time. In health communication, an objective is more specific than a program goal. SMART objectives are Specific, Measurable, Actionable, Realistic, and Time-bound.

Observational study   A study in which individuals are observed in a natural setting with minimal observer interaction (e.g., observing shoppers in a grocery store to see if they are reading nutrition labels on packages).

Op-ed   An opinion letter, statement, or short essay submitted to a newspaper editor by a reader or representative of an organization. These pieces are featured opposite the editorial page, hence the name "op-ed" (opposite the editorial).

Open-ended questions   Questions worded to allow an individual to respond freely in his or her own words.

Opinion leader   Not all individuals in a group or all consumers in a society wield equal personal influence on the attitudes, opinions, and behavior of others. The most influential are termed the opinion leaders—that is, the ones to whom others turn for advice and information.*

Ordinal scale   Classification into ordered qualitative categories (e.g., Likert scale from strongly disagree to strongly agree, 1 to 5). While there is a distinct order ($3 > 2 > 1$), there is no measured distance between their possible values.[11]

Page view   A request to load a single HTML page. Often used as a measure of website traffic.

Partners   Individuals or organizations that combine their efforts for a common goal. In public health, partners can have a variety of roles (e.g., contribute data, share skills, provide various resources, or reach out to specific audiences).

Past Medical History (PMH)	This is a dated list of prior medical care, hospitalizations, treatments, and diagnoses obtained as part of the medical history typically obtained during a patient visit. Other parts of the classical medical history are the chief complaint, history of present illness, past medical history, review of systems, medications, social history and family history. While this sequence of subheadings is useful for preparing a medical report, it should not be used as an outline for obtaining the history, but rather used later in the process to supplement the narrative history.
Patient-centered (health) communication	"Communication that is respectful of and responsive to a health care user's needs, beliefs, values and preferences. Any communication that affects health care users can be patient-centered, including oral, written and nonverbal communications between individuals and practitioners, individuals and health care organizations, and between and among health care practitioners and health care organizations." Source: American Medical Association. An Ethical Force Program Consensus Report. *Improving Communication—Improving Care.* 2006. Accessed from: http://www.ama-assn.org
Patient-Centered Medical Home (PCMH)	A cooperative patient-centered healthcare setting that facilitates partnerships among healthcare facilities, individual patients, and their personal physicians, and when appropriate, the patient's family. Electronic sharing of health-related information is a key feature.
Patient–Provider Communication (PPC)	The interpersonal, often face-to-face communication between a healthcare provider and a patient.
People and Places Model of Social Change	Model developed by Maibach, Abroms, and Marosits that asks, "What about the people, and what about the places, needs to be happening in order for the people (and the places) to be healthy?" Forces that affect people at the individual, social network, community, or population level are referred to as "people fields of influence." Those that are linked inextricably to location, at a local level, or a higher administrative level (state, nation, world) are referred to as "place fields of influence." Source: Maibach EW, Abroms LC, Marosits M. Communication and marketing as tools to cultivate the public's health: a proposed "people and places" framework. *BMC Public Health* 2007;7. DOI: 10.1186/1471-2458-7-88. Available at: http://www.biomedcentral.com/1471-2458/7/88.
Performance objective	Intervention mapping term that defines exactly what you hope the recipient of an intervention will do.
Peripheral route to persuasion	A key component of the Elaboration Likelihood Model. In the peripheral route, the consumer does not focus on the central message in an ad (or other material) but on other stimuli such as attractive or well-known celebrities or popular music. The presence of these other stimuli may change the consumer's beliefs and attitudes about the information or product.*
Personal Health Record (PHR)	Contains information about your health compiled and maintained by you. This is different from the medical records that contain information about your health compiled and maintained by your healthcare providers.[18] This may be maintained in print or in an on-line form.
Personal medical record	See *Personal Health Record.*
Persuasion/persuasive	Convincing someone to do what you suggest. A critical component of behavior change communication.
Pile sorting (also called card sorting)	A rapid ethnographic (cognitive) technique for organizing cards or other visual indicators into groups of like and unlike. Used to explore categories and relationship of items according to another person's worldview.
Pilot testing	(See *test market.*)

Pink Book	Nickname for the National Cancer Institute's publication, *Making Health Communication Programs Work*, because the original print cover is bright pink.
PIO	Public Information Officer. The lead communicationperson for an organization or agency responsible for interfacing with the media and other publics.
Point-of-Purchase (POP)	The promotional materials placed at the immediate area where a consumer will select an item, or complete a purchase, that are designed to attract consumer interest or call attention to a special offer.
Policymaker	In effect, anyone who makes a decision that affects others. In this book, we refer chiefly to elected officials (e.g., city council members, state legislators, U.S. Representatives and Senators) as policymakers.
Polls	An inquiry into public opinion conducted by interviewing a random sample of people. Two well-known polling companies that provide much of the data to the government and media are Gallup[19] and Harris Interactive.
Portal	A site featuring a suite of commonly used services, serving as a starting point and frequent gateway to the Web (Web portal) or a niche topic (vertical portal).*
Positive deviance	An anthropological approach that is based on the identification of successful behaviors or practices of the most successful members of a group in an area and/or population that is largely unhealthy or unsuccessful at negotiating their environment. The successful group members deviate from the norm in a positive way. This is an excellent first step in promoting successful behavior in the group as the innovation comes from within and is already suited to the environment and culture, for the most part.
Practice strategy	In Intervention Mapping, a term meaning the way to deliver a theory-based method in an intervention. (See *theory-based method*.) An example of a practice strategy is Entertainment Education (EE) as a way to deliver role modeling, which is a method informed by Social Cognitive Theory.
Precaution Adoption Process Model (PAPM)	A stage-based model that predicts how an individual will adopt or refuse a risk reduction intervention. According to its originators (Weinstein and Sandman, 2000) the stages are (1) unaware of the issue, (2) aware of the issue, (3) deciding what to do, (4) planning to act, (5) deciding not to act, (6) acting, and (7) maintenance. It is very similar to the Transtheoretical Model, apart from having a stage of deciding not to act entirely.
PRECEDE–PROCEED Model	Developed by Green, Kreuter, and associates in the 1970s,[20] the model works backward from a desired state of health and quality of life and asks what about the environment, behavior, individual motivation, or administrative policy is necessary to create that healthy state. *Precede* stands for predisposing, reinforcing, enabling constructs in educational/ environmental diagnosis and evaluation. *Proceed* stands for policy, regulatory, and organizational constructs in educational and environmental development. Precede–proceed has nine steps: (1) social assessment, (2) epidemiological assessment, (3) behavioral and environmental assessment, (4) educational and ecological assessment, (5) administrative and policy assessment, (6) implementation, (7) process evaluation, (8) impact evaluation, and (9) outcome evaluation.
Predisposing factors	Label for the group of factors included in the educational diagnosis of *Precede*. It includes existing beliefs, attitudes, and values (e.g., cultural or ethical norms) that influence whether a person will adopt a behavior. (See also *enabling* and *reinforcing factors*.)

Pretesting   A type of formative research that involves systematically gathering target audience reactions to messages and materials before they are produced in final form.

Primary audience   When planning a communication intervention, you may decide it is most effective to share information directly with the group of people most affected by a problem, and whose behavior you hope to change. This group is defined as the primary audience. (See *audience segmentation*.)

Prospect Theory   Developed by Tversky and Kahneman, it posits that people will take risks if they think there is something to be lost, but avoid risks if they think there is something to be gained as a result of their decision (i.e., people are risk averse unless they think they will lose something by not taking the risk). Source: Kahneman, D. & Tversky, A. (1979). Prospect Theory: An Analysis of Decision under Risk. *Econometrica*, XLVII, 263–291.

PSA   Public Service Announcement (or advertising). PSAs are typically aired or published without charge by the media. Can be in print, audio, or video form.

Public domain   Any information or media that is not under copyright to any person or entity. These materials and text can be reproduced and used without obtaining permission from the producer or paying fees or royalties. Unless specifically stated otherwise, items produced by the federal government, or employees of the federal government, are in the public domain.

Public health communication   An integrated cycle of health data collection, interpretation, and communication to support public health objectives.

Public health informatics The systematic application of information and computer science and technology to public health practice, research, and learning.

Public relations   The methods and activities employed in persuading the public to understand and regard favorably a person, business, or institution.

Qualitative research   Research that collects data that appear in words rather than numbers. Useful for collecting information about feelings and impressions. Focus groups and in-depth personal interviews are common types of qualitative research.

Quality of life   A sense of well-being about a person's or society's way of life and lifestyle, often estimated by social indicators. The governing factors include income, wealth, safety, recreation facilities, education, health, aesthetics, leisure time, and the like.*

Quantitative research   Research designed to count and measure knowledge, attitudes, beliefs, and behaviors. Yields numerical data that are analyzed statistically. Surveys are a common type of quantitative research.

Random sample   A sample of respondents in which every individual in the population has an equal chance of being selected.

Randomized controlled trial (RCT)   Generally considered the most scientifically rigorous method of hypothesis testing available, subjects are randomly assigned to receive or not receive some intervention. The outcomes of interest are measured in both groups.

Readability testing   Applying a formula to written materials to predict the approximate reading grade level a person must have achieved in order to understand the material.

RE-AIM	Framework for assessing the Reach, Effectiveness, Adoption, Implementation and Maintenance of an intervention. Developed by Russell E. Glasgow.
REALM	Rapid Estimate Of Adult Literacy in Medicine. A widely used tool for estimating health literacy. (See also *TOFHLA*.)
Recall	The extent to which respondents remember seeing or hearing a message that was shown in a competitive media environment; usually centers on main idea or copy recall. (See *unaided recall*.)
Recurring costs	Costs for planning, implementing, and evaluating health communication efforts that occur at regular intervals (e.g., salaries, utility bills).
Reinforcing factors	A set of factors in the *PRECEDE* model that encourage or discourage adoption of a behavior. These include family and community approval or discouragement.
Risk	Quantitative likelihood of an adverse event occurring under a specific set of conditions. Risk is a function of probability. (See also *hazard* and *toxicity*.)
Risk assessment	Human health risk assessment is the characterization of the potential adverse health effects of human exposures to environmental hazards. Risk assessments can be either quantitative or qualitative in nature. The elements of a human health risk assessment consist of planning and scoping, acute hazards, evaluating toxicity, assessing exposures and characterizing risks. Source: Environmental Protection Agency. www.epa.gov
Risk perception	True to the proverb, "one man's meat is another man's poison," people appraise the risk of different hazards according to personal psychological recipes. The actual probability for harm is often not part of this thinking. For example, more people worry about flying in an airplane that traveling in an automobile. Risk perception is also the scientific study of how people go about characterizing different threats, and how they might respond under various circumstances.
Rothschild's behavioral management model	A behavioral management model contrasting perceived costs and benefits against education, marketing, and law as influencing behavior.
Rough	A mockup of a print advertising layout or an early version of a television storyboard prepared by art directors and copywriters to help them realize the advertising idea and discuss it with others in the advertising agency and sometimes with clients.
RSS	Rich Site Summary or Really Simple Syndication. An XML format for distributing news headlines on the Web.*
Run-of-Press (ROP)	The positioning of ads anywhere within the pages of a newspaper or magazine as the staff of the publication prepares the various pages for printing, in contrast to advertisers paying premium prices for ads that are to be placed in specific locations in a magazine or newspaper.*
Sample	"A selected subset of a population. A sample may be random, or non random and may be representative or non-representative." Source: Last, J. M. (1995). *A Dictionary of Epidemiology* (3rd ed.). New York: Oxford University Press, p. 150.
Sampling	"The process of selecting a number of subjects from all the subjects in a particular group or 'universe'. Conclusion based on sample results may be attributed only to the population sampled...."

Source: Last, J. M. (1995). *A Dictionary of Epidemiology* (3rd ed.). New York: Oxford University Press, p. 151.

SARS — Severe Acute Respiratory Syndrome is respiratory disease that is often fatal in the elderly and is caused by a coronavirus, SARS-CoV. There was a near pandemic from November 2002 to July 2003 that originated in China. No cases have been reported since 2004.

Saturation — Achievement of a message gaining wide coverage and high frequency designed to achieve maximum impact. Also used in qualitative research to describe the point in data collection when no new information is uncovered about a specific topic.

Science — A body of knowledge learned through systemic study using agreed-upon methodologies by others in the same field and that attempts to discover generalized truths about phenomena using hypotheses and deductions.[3]

Screener — An instrument containing short-answer questions used in the recruitment process for research methods such as focus groups and central location intercept interviews. Interviewees' answers to the questions determine who is eligible to participate in the research.

Search Engine Optimization (SEO) — SEO is the process of including terms in a website that will result in high placement on search engine lists. High placement translates into more hits, higher web traffic and more exposure for your message or product.

Secondary audience — A group(s) of individuals that can help reach or influence the intended audience segment and is not considered part of the problem. Secondary audience(s) should be identified through profiles created for the primary audience(s). (See *audience segmentation*.)

Secondary research — Research that involves obtaining, synthesizing, and analyzing existing data concerning the problem and/or population. See also meta-analysis.

Selective exposure — Limiting media exposure to channels that offer information and opinions with which the individual agrees.

Self-administered questionnaires — Questionnaires that are filled out by respondents. These can be distributed by mail, handed out in person, or programmed into a computer enabling respondents to enter answers electronically.

Setting — A location or environment where the target audience can be reached with a communication effort (e.g., a grocery store is a setting where audience members can be reached with educational pamphlets).

Sigma encoding — A process in which an electronic device is attached to each videotape copy of a public service announcement sent to television stations. When the PSA is aired, a signal is sent to a central location where records are kept on when, where, and how often the PSA appears.

Small-group channel — A communication channel in which messages are disseminated at the small-group level (e.g., meetings on health topics, cooking demonstrations).

SMART objectives — See *objectives*.

SNAPS — Snap Shots of State Population Data. A website hosted by the CDC that provides local-level community profile information nationwide. It can be browsed by county and state and searched by ZIP code.

Social Cognitive Theory (SCT)   Developed by Albert Bandura, this hypothesizes that individual behavior is the result of constant interaction between the external environment and internal psychosocial characteristics and perceptions. This idea has been dubbed reciprocal determinism. There are numerous constructs in SCT, including self-efficacy, that have migrated into other theories, as well.

Social marketing   "The design, implementation and control of programs aimed at increasing the acceptability of a social idea, practice [or product] in one or more groups of target adopters. The process actively involves the target population who voluntarily exchange their time and attention for help in meeting their needs as they perceive them."[21] In this text, social marketing does not refer to the use of social media or social causes to promote commercial products and services. Both of these uses are making their way into popular vernacular.

Sociocultural competence   The ability to understand and relate to behavioral patterns that are determined in part by membership in racial, ethnic and social groups. This term is used to emphasize the major role of social factors (age, income, education, living circumstance, etc.) in successful health communication. (Cultural competence should have the same meaning but often is limited to gender, ethnic, and nationality issues by common usage.)

SOCO   The Single Overriding Communication Objective worksheet asks for the message in one sentence, a few sentences, and a paragraph. Originated by the CDC Division of Media Relations for authors publishing in the MMWR. The implication of being "socked" by the message is intended.

Source credibility   The reliability of a source of scientific information assessed along two dimensions: (1) individual scientists and their respective institutions and (2) the publication or publisher of the information. The credibility of individual researchers is based on their prior research, reputation within their field among other scientists, and the institution at which they work.

Strategy   A systematic plan of action that leads to accomplishment of a goal. A strategy may encompass several activities.

Stratify   To arrange the population at large into population groups that can be targeted for an intervention. In study design, stratified random sampling is often used to increase the likelihood that a random sample will fully represent important strata (e.g., gender, age, income, health, etc.) in the population at large and improve the power of statistical analysis.

Style   A message quality that can be tailored to one's target audience(s). This is a general term that refers to such issues as presenting cartoon figures versus detailed graphs, or using flowery, embellished text versus short or pithy text.

Summative evaluation   See *effects evaluation.*

Surgeon General's Report (SGR)   The U.S. Surgeon General serves as a highly regarded health communicator by providing Americans the best scientific information available on how to improve their health and reduce the risk of illness and injury. Official publications of the Office of the Surgeon General include the SGR, Calls to Action, and other documents. Of these, SGRs tend to be thorough (and therefore lengthy) summaries of research and may provide policy direction and recommendations. They often set a course of action for the Public Health Service.

Surveillance systems   Data collection systems established at national, state, and local levels to record and monitor events or assess trends in health statistics on an ongoing basis.

Sustainability	Commonly defined as the ability to keep something going by replenishing the resources that are removed, as in environmental sustainability. In health program jargon, often refers to the ability of a local community, or even a national government, to afford the human and material resources to continue activities once donor funding is withdrawn.
SWOTE analysis	Classical SWOT analysis is a plan developed in the 1960s for assessment of a program's internal Strengths and Weaknesses, Opportunities and Threats. CDC health communicators added an "E" for ethical assessment.
Tailored health communication/ tailoring	As in sewing, tailoring refers to custom fitting a health communication material or message to one person's needs based on information about that individual. Tailoring is often based on theoretical constructs (such as readiness stage, health beliefs, and self efficacy), demographic factors, factors specific to a health behavior or condition, and personal information deemed relevant to the intervention.
Talking points	Prepared notes used by a speaker to guide his or her presentation.
Target audience	In health communication, the persons who are the intended recipients of specific messages. These people often have critical features in common, such as demographic factors, risk behaviors, or roles to play in enabling or facilitating change for others.
Targeted health communication	Communications media that use demographic, cultural, or other group references in the media or channel strategy to reach specific audiences. For example, using MTV or BET are both channel strategies to reach youth and African American audiences. Church-based outreach to promote breast cancer screening among older African American women is another targeted channel strategy. Billboards and print advertising frequently feature models of recognizable ethnicities, sex, and age to appeal to target market segments. (In the past, group targeting was also called tailoring. True individually tailored communication has only recently become feasible on a large scale through the Internet and informatics applications.)
Teach-back	Patient-centered communication techniques to check if patient or client understands information provided by health care provider. Asks patient to explain information in own words as if teaching the provider what to do.
Tertiary audience	A group that affects the behavior of an intermediate audience that in turn may affect the behavior of a primary audience. The "public at large" is often considered a tertiary audience in communications directed to patients (as primary audiences) and providers or caregivers (as secondary audiences).
Test market	A geographically limited area used to test a new or modified product, service, or promotion, usually with all strategy elements in place. Usually the last step in a "fail early, fail small" strategy before taking an intervention to scale.
Theater testing	A research method in which a large group (60 to 100, sometimes up to 300) is gathered in a theater-style setting to view and respond to audiovisual materials such as commercials or PSAs. Control audiovisual materials are also shown to lend realism and help check how memorable materials being tested are in comparison.
Theoretical constructs	Pieces of a theory that can stand alone, much like atomic elements, but are most effective when used in combination with the other elements (or constructs) of a theory (e.g., constructs are to theory as hydrogen and oxygen are to water).

Theory-informed method   An intervention mapping term that describes translation of a behavior change theory into an action. One example of a theory-informed method is using "vicarious learning" (learning from another's experience) to promote constructs from social cognitive theory. A practice strategy delivers this method in an intervention.

Theory of Reasoned Action (TRA)   The theory of reasoned action (developed by Fishbein and Ajzen) states that individual performance of a given behavior is primarily determined by a person's intention to perform that behavior. This intention is determined by two major factors: the person's attitude toward the behavior (i.e., beliefs about the outcomes of the behavior and the value of these outcomes) and the influence of the person's social environment or subjective norm (i.e., beliefs about what other people think the person should do, as well as the person's motivation to comply with the opinions of others). Sources: (1) Ajzen I., Albarracin D., & Hornik, R. (2007). *Prediction and Change of Health Behavior: The Reasoned Action Approach.* Mawah, NJ: Lawrence Erlbaum Associates. (2) Fishbein, M., & Ajzen, I. (1975). *Belief, Attitude, Intention, and Behavior: An Introduction to Theory and Research.* Reading, MA: Addison-Wesley.

TOFHLA   Test of Functional Health Literacy in Adults. A widely used tool for estimating health literacy. (See also *REALM.*)

Tone   A message quality referring to the manner of expression along chiefly emotional lines (e.g., a fatherly tone, an alarming tone, a friendly tone).

Total budget   The sum of direct and indirect costs, including in-kind contributions and additional donations.

Toxicity   The intrinsic ability of a substance to cause adverse health effects. For example, lead is a toxic substance for humans, but brief exposure to a block of lead is not hazardous and presents a very low health risk. Chronic ingestion (e.g., of paint chips) is very hazardous and can increase the risk of anemia or brain damage.

Trademarks   Distinctive symbols, pictures, or words that identify a specific product or service. Received through registration with the U.S. Patent & Trademark Office. Tier I search engines prohibit bids on trademarks as keywords if the bidder is not the legal owner, although this keyword bid practice is still allowed by Google.*

Traditional media   Any communications medium used before the advent of the internet to communicate with populations (i.e., excludes telephones and other means of accessing individuals) such as television, radio, movies, newspapers and magazines, as well as outdoor advertising staples such as billboards, bus cards, and stadium signs. New media include everything available through the internet, as well as mass use of cell phone technology. (See *media.*)

Traffic   Refers to the number of visitors a website receives. It can be determined by examination of web logs,* often by use of a proprietary program such as Google-based Adsense.

Transtheoretical Model (TTM)   According to TTM, individuals move through a specific process when deciding whether to change their behavior and when actually changing their behavior. The stages are: precontemplation, contemplation, preparation, action, and maintenance.

Trialability   This is a marketing term reflecting the extent to which a product can be tried and tested by the consumer (e.g., free samples in supermarkets, airplane toiletries, small-size products).

Twitter   "A real-time short messaging service that works over multiple networks and devices" connected to the Web at twitter.com. Source: http://www.alexa.com/siteinfo/twitter.com

UGC   User-Generated Content, (See *consumer-generated content.*)

Unaided recall   In survey research, when the respondent states a fact, name, or message without prompting from the researcher (e.g., a list is not read). Considered the strongest form of recall of a message.

URL   Uniform Resource Locator. The location of a resource on the Internet. This term is often used interchangeably with "domain" and "Web address."

Usability testing   A research step in the design and launch of a website, where users evaluate the ease of use of a website's navigation, layout, and other attributes.*

USP   1. United States Pharmacopeia. A nongovernmental, official public standards–setting authority for prescription and over-the-counter medicines and other healthcare products manufactured or sold in the United States. USP also sets widely recognized standards for food ingredients and dietary supplements. 2. Unique Selling Proposition (or point). An approach to developing the advertising message that concentrates on the uniquely differentiating characteristic of the product that is both important to the customer and a unique strength of the advertised products when compared to competing products.* An emphasis of benefits over costs.

Utilitarianism   "The principle of utility states that an action is 'right if it produces as much or more of an increase in happiness of all affected by it than any alternative action, and wrong if it does not.' Its basis is the idea that pleasure and happiness are intrinsically valuable, that pain and suffering are intrinsically not, and that anything else has value only in its causing happiness or preventing suffering. A utilitarian is someone who accepts the principle of utility—and is therefore concerned with maximising the value (utility) of the universe—which makes utilitarianism a *consequentialist* (goal-based) theory of ethics, as opposed to a *deontological* (rule-based) theory. Source: http://www.utilitarian.org/utility.html#note

Value   Commonly used to mean good value for the money. Perceived benefits outweigh costs. (See also *values,* which is different.)

Value proposition   The sum total of benefits a customer is promised to receive in return for the associated payment (or other value transfer).*

Values   Beliefs widely shared by members of a culture about what is desirable or good (e.g., thrift, free speech, or honesty) and what is undesirable or bad (e.g., arson, bigotry, deceit). If a value is accepted by the individual, it can become a major influence on his or her behavior. Values are the important, enduring ideals or beliefs that guide behavior within a culture or for a specific person. For example, health and fitness have recently become important values for Americans.

Video News Release (VNR)   A publicity device designed to look and sound like a television news story. The publicist prepares a 60- to 90-second news release on videotape, which can then be used by television stations as is or after further editing.*

Viral marketing   A marketing strategy that facilitates and encourages people to pass along a message through social networks. Nicknamed "viral" because it relies on a small number of people initially exposed to a message passing on the message to others, like a virus or disease. "Buzz marketing" is term used more often now.

Web 2.0	A term that refers to a second generation of Internet-based services. These usually include tools that let people collaborate and share information online, such as social networking sites, wikis, communication tools, and folksonomies.*
Website	A collection of one or more electronic "pages" at a single address on the Internet and used to provide information about a company, organization, cause, or individual.*
Widget	A live update on a website, webpage, or desktop. Widgets contain personalized, neatly organized content or applications selected by its user. (Also an old-school marketing term meaning the thing you are trying to sell, your product).
Wiki	A Web application that allows users to add content, as on an Internet forum, but also allows anyone to edit the content. Wiki also refers to the collaborative software used to create such a website.*
Word-of-Mouth (WOM) communication	Occurs when people share information about products or promotions through a social network. May be positive or negative. Viral or buzz marketing can be seen to either stimulate genuine WOM or create artificial WOM.
Worldview	This refers to how people perceive their level of control over their own lives and how they think power and wealth are distributed. Examples include fatalism, individualism, egalitarianism, or respect and trust for authority.
XML	eXtensible Markup Language. A data delivery language, used widely to create content on the internet for data intensive internet-based applications.
Zapping/zipping	Using a remote control to change television stations when commercials appear or to fast-forward through advertisements on video recordings. Users of PSAs have to consider this behavior as well as commercial advertisers.
Zine	A magazine that is published digitally on the Internet, rather than on paper. Some zines are mainstream; others appeal to a very small niche of readers.
Zip code	A geographical classification system developed by the U.S. government for mail distribution consisting of a 5 + 4 scheme. The first five digits, which indicate state, county, and post office, are not very useful for targeted, demographic marketing because they cover wide areas, but the ending 4 code provides a smaller, normally more economically cohesive unit.

REFERENCES

1. http://www.ebasedtreatment.org/treatment/toolbox/advocacy/advocacy-definition
2. http://www.aaanet.org/about/WhatisAnthropology.cfm
3. http://www.npsf.org/askme3/
4. http://www.asph.org/document.cfm?page=100
5. This idea is everywhere, with no clear first reference. According to Tom Asacker in his blog, "A brand is the customer's *evolving* expectation of value; value the way he or she subjectively intuits it. It is *not* your slow-to-change, inside-out declaration or 'promise.'" http://www.acleareye.com/sandbox_wisdom/2009/06/a-brand-is-a-promise.html, accessed October 26, 2009.
6. http://www.cochrane.org/index.htm

7. National Communication Association.
8. http://www.thecommunityguide.org/index.html
9. PD Health website. www.positivedeviance.org
10. http://www.gallup.com/home.aspx
11. Last JM. *Dictionary of Epidemiology,* 3rd ed. New York: Oxford University Press; 1995.
12. American Medical Informatics Association.
13. U.S. Department of Homeland Security. Crisis Communications Planning: Establishing Joint Information Centers; 2005. Retrieved from https://www.llis.dhs.gov.
14. Shepherd R. Why teach media literacy. *Teach Magazine,* Quadrant Educational Media Services, Toronto, ON, Canada, October/November 1993.
15. http://www.epa.gov/nhsrc/news/news040207.html
16. http://www.cancer.gov/aboutnci/overview/mission
17. http:///www.sfn.org
18. http://www.nlm.nih.gov/medlineplus/personalmedicalrecords.html
19. http://www.gallup.com/home.aspx
20. Green LW, Kreuter MW. *Health Promotion Planning: An Educational and Ecological Approach,* 3rd ed. New York: McGraw-Hill, 1999.
21. LeFebvre C, Flora J. *Health Education Quarterly* 1998;15:299–315.

*http://www.marketingpower.com/_layouts/Dictionary.aspx

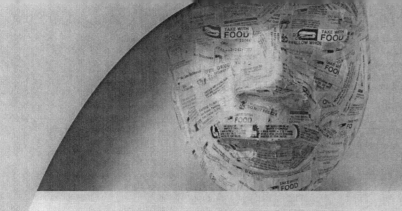

Index

Figures, tables, and boxes are indicated by *f*, *t*, and *b* following page numbers.

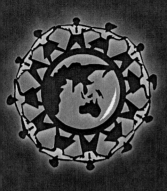

ESSENTIAL PUBLIC HEALTH

The
ESSENTIAL PUBLIC HEALTH SERIES
from Jones & Bartlett Learning

Essential Public Health is an introductory series that captures the full range of issues that affect the public's health from the impact of AIDS to the cost of health care. Edited by Richard Riegelman, the series takes the big picture "population health" perspective by introducing concepts and content that are fundamental to the study and practice of public health. The series is closely tied to the new public health core competencies, which serves as the basis for the certifying examination by the National Board of Public Health Examiners.

CURRENT AND FORTHCOMING TITLES IN THE SERIES

Public Health 101: Healthy People–
Healthy Populations
Richard Riegelman, MD, MPH, PhD

Epidemiology 101
Robert H. Friis, PhD

Global Health 101, Second Edition
Richard Skolnik, MPA

Case Studies in Global Health: Millions Saved
Ruth Levine, PhD & the What Works Working Group

Essentials of Public Health, Second Edition
Bernard J. Turnock, MD, MPH

Essential Case Studies in Public Health:
Putting Public Health into Practice
Katherine Hunting, PhD, MPH &
Brenda L. Gleason, MA, MPH

Essentials of Evidence-Based Public Health
Richard Riegelman, MD, MPH, PhD

Essentials of Infectious Disease Epidemiology
Manya Magnus, PhD, MPH

Essential Readings in Infectious Disease
Epidemiology
Manya Magnus, PhD, MPH

Essentials of Biostatistics in Public Health,
Second Edition
Lisa M. Sullivan, PhD (with Workbook: *Statistical*
Computations Using Excel)

Essentials of Public Health Biology:
A Guide for the Study of Pathophysiology
Constance Urciolo Battle, MD

Essentials of Environmental Health, Second Edition
Robert H. Friis, PhD

Essentials of Health, Culture, and Diversity
Mark Edberg, PhD

Essentials of Health Behavior:
Social and Behavioral Theory in Public Health
Mark Edberg, PhD

Essential Readings in Health Behavior:
Theory and Practice
Mark Edberg, PhD

Essentials of Health Policy and Law
Joel B. Teitelbaum, JD, LLM & Sara E. Wilensky, JD, MPP

Essential Readings in Health Policy and Law
Joel B. Teitelbaum, JD, LLM & Sara E. Wilensky, JD, MPP

Essentials of Health Economics
Diane M. Dewar, PhD

Essentials of Global Community Health
Jaime Gofin, MD, MPH & Rosa Gofin, MD, MPH

Essentials of Program Planning and Evaluation
Karen McDonnell, PhD

Essentials of Public Health Communication
Claudia Parvanta, PhD; David E. Nelson, MD, MPH;
Sarah A. Parvanta, MPH; & Richard N. Harner, MD

Essentials of Public Health Ethics
Ruth Gaare Bernheim, JD, MPH & James F. Childress, PhD

Essentials of Management and Leadership in
Public Health
Robert Burke, PhD & Leonard Friedman, PhD, MPH

Essentials of Public Health Preparedness
Rebecca Katz, PhD, MPH

ABOUT THE EDITOR:

Richard K. Riegelman, MD, MPH, PhD, is Professor of Epidemiology-Biostatistics, Medicine, and Health Policy, and Founding Dean of The George Washington University School of Public Health and Health Services in Washington, DC. He has taken a lead role in developing the Educated Citizen and Public Health initiative which has brought together arts and sciences and public health education associations to implement the Institute of Medicine of the National Academies' recommendation that "…all undergraduates should have access to education in public health." Dr. Riegelman also led the development of George Washington's undergraduate major and minor and currently teaches "Public Health 101" and "Epidemiology 101" to undergraduates.

CPSIA information can be obtained
at www.ICGtesting.com
Printed in the USA
LVOW09s0811081117
555487LV00011B/309/P